Orthopedic Traumatology

Orthopedic Traumatology

Edited by **Sharlton Pierce**

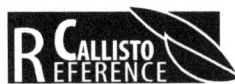

R CALLISTO
REFERENCE

New York

Published by Callisto Reference,
106 Park Avenue, Suite 200,
New York, NY 10016, USA
www.callistoreference.com

Orthopedic Traumatology
Edited by Sharlton Pierce

International Standard Book Number: 978-1-63239-650-1 (Hardback)

The publisher's policy is to use permanent paper from mills that operate a sustainable forestry policy. Furthermore, the publisher ensures that the text paper and cover boards used have met acceptable environmental accreditation standards.

Trademark Notice: Registered trademark of products or corporate names are used only for explanation and identification without intent to infringe.

Printed in the United States of America.

Contents

Preface

Orthopaedic traumatology refers to the treatment of shock or trauma suffered by a person under extreme circumstances or life threatening events. It consists of two procedures first, assessment of the patient, his mental condition, shock he is enduring, and second, assessment of the wound inflicted on him, the depth, width, shape, etc. This book will provide significant information of this field to help develop a good understanding of orthopaedic traumatology. It presents researches and studies performed by experts across the globe in this subject. This book attempts to assist those with a goal of delving into this area. It will prove to be a beneficial source of knowledge for students and researchers alike.

This book unites the global concepts and researches in an organized manner for a comprehensive understanding of the subject. It is a ripe text for all researchers, students, scientists or anyone else who is interested in acquiring a better knowledge of this dynamic field.

I extend my sincere thanks to the contributors for such eloquent research chapters. Finally, I thank my family for being a source of support and help.

Editor

Single locking compression plate fixation of extra-articular distal humeral fractures

Malhar N. Kumar · M. R. Ravishankar · Ravikiran Manur

Abstract

Background Earlier literature on fixation of distal third humeral fractures describes the use of elaborate modification of existing implants, custom-made implants and dual plating. These modifications have the disadvantages of limitations of hardware availability and cost as well as longer surgical exposure to accommodate the plates. The aim of this study was to assess the effectiveness of osteosynthesis of extra-articular diaphyseal fractures of the distal third of the humerus using a single 4.5-mm locking compression plate (LCP) with two-screw purchase in the distal fragment.

Materials and methods We performed internal fixation of distal third extra-articular humeral fractures in 22 adult patients using 2–3 lag screws neutralized with a single 4.5-mm locking compression plate with only two screws in the distal fragment. The mean follow-up period was approximately 1.6 years.

Results Fractures united in all 22 patients with minimal complications. The mean time to union of fracture was 13 weeks. The Mayo elbow score and the DASH scores were in the excellent and good category in all patients at final follow-up.

Conclusions Our study showed that it is possible to obtain excellent outcomes in distal third fractures using only a single 4.5-mm LCP with two-screw (4-cortices) purchase in the distal fragment. The disadvantages inherent in the previous methods can be avoided with the use of the present technique. This technique obviates the need for the use of customized distal humeral implants and modified implants in most patients.

Level of evidence Level IV.

M. N. Kumar (✉) · M. R. Ravishankar · R. Manur
HOSMAT Hospital, 45, McGrath Road, Bangalore 560025, India
e-mail: docmnkumar@gmail.com

Keywords Distal humerus fractures · Locking compression plate · Plate osteosynthesis of humerus · Metaphyseal fractures of humerus

Introduction

Fractures of the distal third of the humerus are challenging injuries due to their peri-articular location, small size of the distal bone fragments, and the osteopenic quality of the bone in older adults. Methods of management of distal humerus fractures include conservative management using plaster cast immobilization or functional bracing, plate osteosynthesis and intra-medullary nailing [1–4]. Stewart et al. proposed that fractures of the distal-third humerus shaft should not be treated by hanging cast because angulation is difficult to control [1]. Sarmiento et al. treated 85 extra-articular comminuted distal-third humeral fractures with a functional brace. The nonunion rate in their series was 4 % and the malunion rate was 16 % (varus angulation in the majority). A decrease in the range of motion at the elbow and shoulder was another significant problem in their series [2]. Jawa et al. compared the use of functional bracing and plate fixation for extra-articular distal-third diaphyseal fractures of the humerus. They concluded that for extra-articular distal-third diaphyseal humeral fractures, surgical treatment achieves more predictable alignment and potentially quicker return of function but risks iatrogenic nerve injury and infection and the need for reoperation [3].

It is difficult to manage extra-articular distal humerus fractures with locking intra-medullary nails. The flat cross section of the distal humerus with a narrow medullary canal makes it difficult to insert intra-medullary nails and increases liability for comminution of the distal fragment during nail insertion. The short distal fragment makes it difficult to achieve stable fixation with distal interlocking. Radial nerve injury, if present, cannot be addressed without a separate incision. Plate osteosynthesis has distinct advantages in the distal humerus, and compression plating has been established as a successful modality for the surgical treatment of humerus fractures [4].

Recommendations for improving stability of plate fixation include plate thickness of >3.5 mm (a large-fragment plate) for most adults, and at least four screw holes in both the proximal and distal fragments [5]. However, adhering to these principles becomes difficult in distal humeral shaft fractures, especially those around the metaphyseal transition zone between the shaft and the supracondylar ridges. Fixation with three or four screws in the distal fragment is difficult as longer plates tend to impinge on the olecranon fossa.

Livani et al. reported the use of percutaneous osteosynthesis in a small series of six patients with distal humerus fractures with preoperative radial nerve palsy [6]. They used a dynamic compression plate for fixation (with two screws on either side of the fracture). The purpose of our study was to assess the effectiveness of a contoured standard 4.5-mm locking compression plate (LCP), with the use of only two screws in the distal fragment, in the management of distal-third fractures of the humerus. Interfragmentary screws were used wherever possible and the plate was used as a neutralization plate. If this method is effective in achieving fracture union with minimal rates of complications, it offers the advantages of the use of a standard and easily available implant, avoiding fixation beyond the olecranon fossa and avoiding extension of the incision beyond the elbow crease.

Materials and methods

A prospective study was conducted between October 2011 and December 2012. Permission was obtained from the hospital ethics committee prior to commencing the study. Informed written consent was obtained from the patients prior to the study. The patient cohort consisted of 22 patients with distal-third diaphyseal humerus fractures. All adult patients with closed extra-articular fractures of the distal third of the humerus were included in this study. Patients with open fractures, pathological fractures, fractures with articular or intercondylar extension, floating elbow injury and children with distal humerus fractures were excluded from the study. The mean age of the patients was 32.6 years (21–58 years); almost 60 % of the patients were aged 21–30 years. 14 fractures were on the left side and 8 on the right side. The predominant mode of injury was road traffic accident (17 patients). In three patients, the fracture was the result of a fall and in two patients, the fracture was due to assault. All patients were operated on

Table I Orthopaedic Trauma Association (OTA) classification of fractures

OTA fracture subtype	No. of patients	Percentage
12A1.3	5	22.7
12A2.3	2	9.1
12B1.3	7	31.8
12B2.3	5	22.7
12B3.3	1	4.5
12C1.3	2	9.1
Total	22	100

within 48 h of injury. The fractures were classified based on the anteroposterior and lateral radiographs. The OTA classification is shown in Table 1. An LCP was chosen (even though the bone quality of our patients was good due to the younger age) to ensure reliable fixation with only two screws distally.

All patients were treated with LCP fixation with a posterior midline triceps-splitting approach. The patient was positioned in the lateral decubitus position with the elbow flexed over a well-padded radiolucent bolster. The incision stopped short of the tip of the olecranon. The triceps was split in the midline until the apex of the olecranon fossa, and no dissection was performed distally. The triceps was not reflected from the medial or lateral supracondylar ridges. The radial nerve was dissected in the region of the spiral groove, traced until the junction of the middle and distal thirds of the humerus. The fracture was stabilized using two or three 3.5-mm lag screws, and a 4.5-mm LCP was used as a neutralization plate (Figs. 1, 2, 3). Two lag screws were used in 14 patients with short oblique fracture patterns. Three lag screws were used in the remaining eight patients with a long oblique/spiral fracture pattern. The plate was contoured intra-operatively to match the dorsal surface of the humerus accurately. Bending was performed at the site of the dynamic compression hole. Following plate fixation, the radial nerve was repositioned superficial to the plate and the wound was closed in layers. A long arm slab was applied for 3 weeks following the operation for pain relief. Physiotherapy including active assisted range of motion exercises was started 1 week post-operatively. Between 1 and 3 weeks following the operation, an active and gentle passive range of motion exercises was performed twice a week under the direct supervision of the surgeon (the slab was removed and reapplied). From the fourth week onwards, patients were allowed to perform active and gentle passive exercises on their own with the aid of the physiotherapist. Lifting of light weights was permitted only after complete radiological union was seen at the fracture site.

Patients were followed up clinically and radiologically every 6 weeks until fracture union. Functional outcome

Fig. 1 a Anteroposterior and lateral views showing an oblique fracture with medial butterfly fragment. **b** Immediate post-operative radiographs showing fixation with two lag screws and pre-contoured LCP with two locking screws in the distal fragment

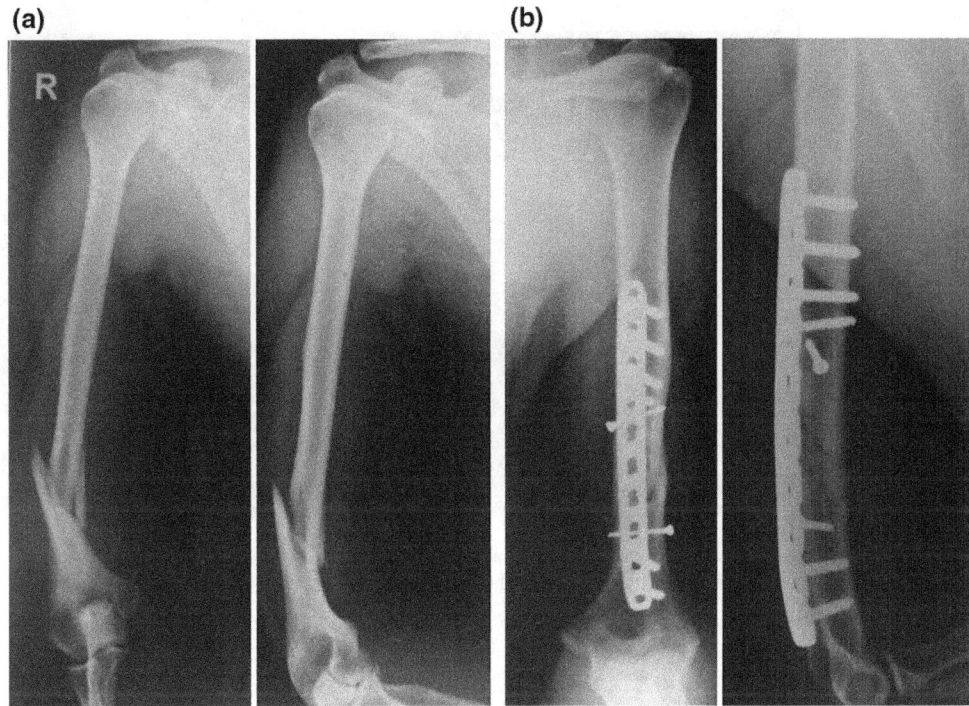

Fig. 2 a Anteroposterior and lateral views showing a transverse fracture of the distal third of the humerus. **b** Post-operative anteroposterior and lateral radiographs showing sound union at 5 months following fixation with LCP

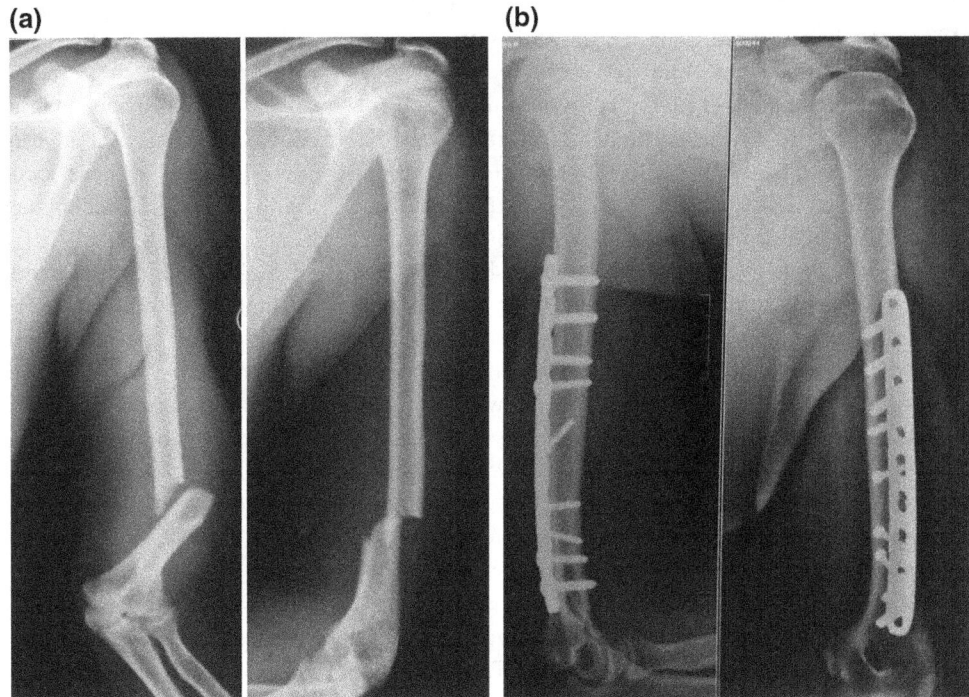

was measured by the 'Mayo Elbow Performance Index' (MEPI) and the 'Disabilities of Arm, Shoulder and Hand' (DASH) questionnaire at final follow-up. The MEPI is one of the most commonly used physician-based elbow rating systems [7]. This index consists of four parts—pain (with a maximum score of 45 points), ulnohumeral motion (20 points), stability (10 points) and the ability to perform five functional tasks (25 points). The DASH questionnaire is a standardized questionnaire which evaluates impairments and activity limitations, as well as participation restrictions for both leisure activities and work [8]. It includes questions about symptoms and disabilities of upper limb (30 items). Statistical analysis was performed using SPSS 20.0 software [version 17 Chicago, IL: SPSS, Inc.; 2008].

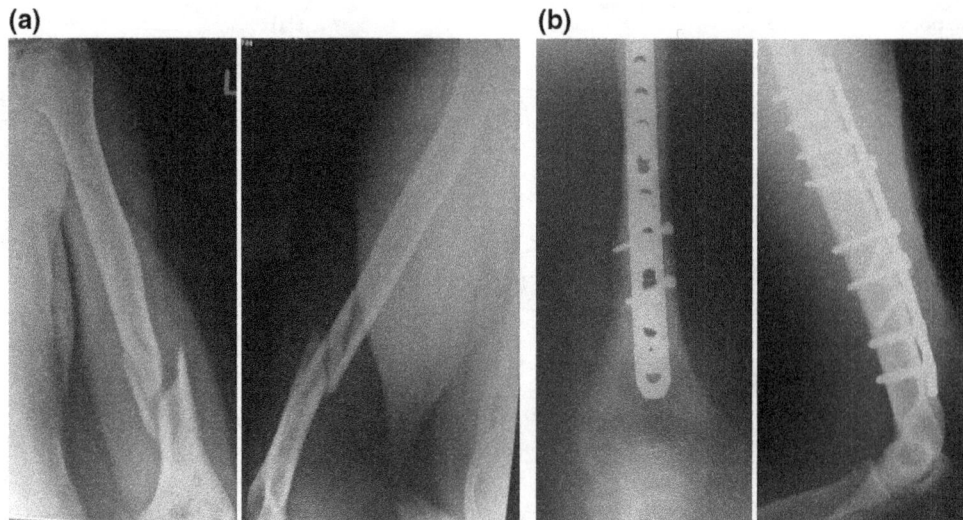

Fig. 3 a Anteroposterior and lateral views showing a distal-third fracture with medial comminution and proximal extension of the fracture line. b Post-operative anteroposterior and lateral views showing complete union at 4.5 months; only two locking screws are in the distal fragment

Results

The mean duration of surgery was 110 ± 15.3 min (90–150 min). Average blood loss was 155 ± 25.5 ml (130–240 ml), measured using the surgical swab weighing technique. The mean duration of follow-up was 15.3 ± 1.3 months (14–17 months), with a minimum follow-up period of 14 months. Radiological union was evident by an average of 13.5 ± 1.46 weeks (10–17 weeks). Complications were found in 2 of the 22 patients—one patient had signs of early myositis ossificans and another patient had a broken lag screw (the fracture had clinically and radiologically united). There were three patients with pre-operative radial nerve palsy, diagnosed in the emergency department; operative findings showed radial nerve contusion in all the three patients. There were no postoperative/iatrogenic radial nerve palsies. The three patients with pre-operative radial nerve palsy recovered within a mean period of 5 months. All patients had full range of shoulder and elbow motion, except one patient who had loss of extension of 10 degrees in the elbow.16 out of 22 patients (72.7 %) in our series had excellent scores and six (27.3 %) had good scores on the MEPI scoring system. The mean DASH score in our series was 14.3 (SD ± 8.3). The DASH score was <15 in 16 out of 22 patients (5.0–14.20) and between 15 and 30 in six patients (15.80–29.20).

Discussion

At present, there is a paucity of literature on the management of distal-third diaphyseal fractures of the humerus. The current study deals with lower metaphyseal fractures of the humerus (extra-articular distal humerus fractures) treated using a 4.5-mm LCP (contoured intra-operatively) as a neutralization plate with 3.5-mm lag screws, using the posterior triceps-splitting approach. Various modifications of plate osteosynthesis have been introduced. These include the use of a modified lateral tibial head buttress plate, custom-made 'hybrid' locking plates, double reconstruction plates and anterior plating of the distal humerus [9–11]. Each of these methods has its own disadvantages both in surgical techniques as well as in the choice of implants. Levy et al. [9] modified the Synthes® Lateral Tibial Head Buttress Plate for use at the distal humerus. An ipsilateral Lateral Tibial Head Buttress Plate was modified using a high-speed rotary diamond-cutting tool to remove the posterior hole of the proximal expanded section of the plate. The resulting sharp edges were rounded off with a diamond-cutting wheel. The plate was then bent so that the bend in the proximal section of the plate was reversed. This resulted in a 4.5-mm limited contact dynamic compression plate (LC-DCP) with a distal angular offset of approximately 22° that allowed the modified plate to be placed on the lateral column of the distal humerus. The authors reported good results in their series. The problem with this approach is the necessity for elaborate modification of an existing design or the necessity for bulk production of such a modified design.

Spitzer et al. [10] used a custom-made 'hybrid' locking plate for difficult fractures of the meta-diaphyseal humeral shaft. This was a special plate prepared for use by the author with 4.5-mm locking holes at one end and a cluster of 3.5-mm locking holes at the other end (distal).The outcome was excellent in their series; however, this approach also involves modification of existing designs and their bulk production for universal use. Zhiquan et al. [11] treated 13 distal third humeral shaft fractures with minimally invasive percutaneous osteosynthesis (MIPO). Fractures were reduced by closed means and fixed with a long narrow 4.5-mm dynamic compression plate introduced through two small incisions away from the fracture site. The plate was fixed on the anterior aspect of the humerus under fluoroscopy guidance. The radial nerve was not exposed during this procedure. They reported that the fractures united with a mean healing time of 16.2 weeks, a little longer than the reported time of 9–12 weeks in posterior open plating of the humerus. Disadvantages of this approach are that the radial nerve is not visualized directly during the exposure and, biomechanically, the posterior surface of the humerus is considered better for plate application especially of distal-third fractures. Schatzker and Tile listed four reasons for plating the distal humerus posteriorly—the posterior surface of the distal humerus provides a flat surface suitable for plating; placement of the most distal screws from a posterior approach allows direct visualization and avoids the antecubital fossa; posterior placement allows for the plate to extend distally permitting additional screw placement; and the posterior approach provides the option of double plating [12]. Livani et al. [6] obtained good results following minimally invasive percutaneous DCP fixation of distal humerus fractures in six patients with radial nerve palsy. We chose an LCP due to the presence of significant comminution in many of our patients. The open surgical approach that we used required more soft tissue stripping which made stable fixation mandatory. Since the majority of our patients had no radial palsy pre-operatively, nerve exploration and protection required an open approach.

Prasarn et al. [13] treated extra-articular fractures of the distal third of the humerus with dual plates from a single posterior midline incision (2.7- and 3.5-mm pelvic reconstruction plates). The average time to union was 11.5 weeks and the mean elbow flexion/extension arc was 4°–131°. Possible disadvantages of this approach are the necessity to reflect the triceps to accommodate plate application on the lateral column, and the need for using two plates to secure reduction. The 2.7- and 3.5-mm plates used in this series tend to be less strong than 4.5-mm compression plates.

Advantages of our technique are that fracture stabilization is achieved with a single 4.5-mm LCP without any modification of the implant except for slight contouring. The posterior approach dissection was limited up to the olecranon fossa hence avoiding triceps fibrosis/elbow stiffness as it was not necessary to expose the lateral column until the distal tip. Use of a 4.5-mm LCP obviates the need for double plating and simplifies the procedure. Contouring allows the plate to match the posterior surface

of the humerus and prevents the tip of the plate from rising above the humerus just proximal to the olecranon fossa. Secondly, it minimizes stress on the skin and soft tissues overlying the plate [14]. Bending was performed at the level of the dynamic hole in the plate as recommended by Smith et al. [15]. Since the distal fixation relies on only two screws, quality of bone is important and the technique is best avoided in elderly patients with poor bone quality and in highly comminuted fractures. Our results were excellent in terms of fracture union as well as elbow and shoulder range of motion. We had two complications, namely breakage of a lag screw in one patient and early myositis ossificans in the second patient; however, the patients were not seriously affected and the quality of the results did not suffer due to these complications. Our post-operative protocol consisted of immobilization of the elbow in a long arm slab for 3 weeks. However, the slab was removed every week and the elbow was mobilized under the direct supervision of the surgeon. This subsequently proved to be helpful in the early recovery of range of movement. There is no need for elaborate modification of existing implants and no need for the use of custom-made implants. It can be argued that use of only two screws in the distal fragment might compromise the stability of fixation. It has been shown by Hak et al. [16] that two locking screws per segment are sufficient and the addition of a third screw in the locked plate construct did not add to the mechanical stability in axial loading, bending, or torsion. It is possible to insert at least two locking screws in the distal fragment in the vast majority of distal humeral fractures.

We conclude that the use of one or two lag screws along with a single posteriorly placed 4.5-mm contoured locking compression plate having at least two locking screws in the distal fragment provides sufficient rigid fixation in distal metaphyseal fractures of the humerus. The dissection does not extend beyond the apex of the olecranon fossa. The implant stops well short of the olecranon fossa. Excellent results can be achieved in these fractures without the use of dual plating and without the need for expensive customized implants or elaborately modified implants. Careful patient selection is important for this technique and indiscriminate use of single-plate fixation should be avoided. Physiologically, young patients with good bone quality and good motivation for post-operative physiotherapy are suitable for this technique. Patients with open fractures, highly comminuted fractures, fractures with intercondylar extensions and pathological fractures are not suitable for this type of fixation.

Conflict of interest Authors have not received any funding for this study.

Ethical standards Written informed consent was obtained from the patients prior to enrolling them in the study. The study was approved by hospital ethics committee and performed in accordance with the ethical standards of the 1964 Declaration of Helsinki as revised in 2000.

References

1. Stewart MJ, Hundley JM, Tennessee M (1955) Fractures of the humerus-A comparative study in methods of treatment. J Bone Joint Surg Am 37-A(4):11
2. Sarmiento A, Horowitch A et al (1990) Functional bracing for comminuted extra-articular fractures of the distal third of the humerus. J Bone Joint Surg Br 72(2):283–287
3. Ring D, Harris M, Doornberg J, McCarty P, Jawa A (2006) Extra-articular distal-third diaphyseal fractures of the humerus. A comparison of functional bracing and plate fixation. J Bone Joint Surg Am 88-A:2343–2347
4. McKee MD (2006) Fractures of the shaft of the humerus. In: Bucholz RW, Heckman JD, Court-Brown CM (eds) Rockwood and green's fractures in adults. Lippincott Williams & Wilkins, Philadelphia, pp 1117–1159
5. Archdeacon MT, Cannada LK, Herscovici D, Anglen JO (2008) Avoiding complications in the treatment of humeral fractures. J Bone Joint Surg Am 90-A:1580–1589
6. Livani B, Belangero WD, Castro de Medeiros R (2006) Fractures of the distal third of the humerus with palsy of the radial nerve: management using minimally-invasive percutaneous plate osteosynthesis. J Bone Joint Surg Br 88(12):1625–1628
7. Morrey BF, An KN, Chao EYS (1993) Functional evaluation of the elbow. In: Morrey BF (ed) The elbow and its disorders, 2nd edn. W. B. Saunders, Philadelphia, pp 86–89
8. Atroshi I, Gummesson I, Andersson B, Dahlgren E, Johansson A (2000) The disabilities of the arm, shoulder and hand (DASH) outcome questionnaire. Acta Orthop Scand 71:613–618
9. Levy JC, Kalandiak SP, Hutson JJ, Zych G (2005) An alternative method of osteosynthesis for distal humeral shaft fractures. J Orthop Trauma 19:43–47
10. Spitzer AB, Davidovitch RI, Egol KA (2009) Use of a ''hybrid'' locking plate for complex metaphyseal fractures and non unions about the humerus. Injury 40:240–244
11. Zhiquan A, Bingfang Z, Yeming W, Chi Z, Peiyan H (2007) Minimally invasive plating osteosynthesis (MIPO) of middle and distal third humeral shaft fractures. J Orthop Trauma 21:628–633
12. Schatzker J, Tile M (1996) The rationale of operative fracture care, 2nd edn. Springer, Toronto, pp 83–94
13. Prasarn ML, Ahn J, Paul O, Morris EM, Kalandiak SP, Helfet DL, Lorich DG (2011) Dual plating for fractures of the distal third of the humeral shaft. J Orthop Trauma 25:57–63
14. Südkamp NP, Niemeyer P (2006) Principles and clinical application of the locking compression plate (LCP). Acta Chir Orthop Traumatol Cech 73:221–228
15. Smith WR, Ziran BH, Anglen JO, Stahel PF (2007) Locking plates: tips and tricks. J Bone Joint Surg Am 89A:2298–2307
16. Hak DJ, Althausen P, Hazelwood SJ (2010) Locked plate fixation of osteoporotic humeral shaft fractures: are two locking screws per segment enough? J Orthop Trauma 24:207–211

The effect of locally delivered recombinant human bone morphogenetic protein-2 with hydroxyapatite/tri-calcium phosphate on the biomechanical properties of bone in diabetes-related osteoporosis

Frank A. Liporace · Eric A. Breitbart ·
Richard S. Yoon · Erin Doyle · David N. Paglia ·
Sheldon Lin

Abstract

Background Recombinant human bone morphogenetic protein-2 (rhBMP-2) is particularly effective in improving osteogenesis in patients with diminished bone healing capabilities, such as individuals with type 1 diabetes mellitus (T1DM) who have impaired bone healing capabilities and increased risk of developing osteoporosis. This study measured the effects of rhBMP-2 treatment on osteogenesis by observing the dose-dependent effect of localized delivery of rhBMP-2 on biomechanical parameters of bone using a hydroxyapatite/tri-calcium phosphate (HA/TCP) carrier in a T1DM-related osteoporosis animal model.

Materials and methods Two different doses of rhBMP-2 (LD low dose, HD high dose) with a HA/TCP carrier were injected into the femoral intramedullary canal of rats with T1DM-related osteoporosis. Two more diabetic rat groups were injected with saline alone and with HA/TCP carrier alone. Radiographs and micro-computed tomography were utilized for qualitative assessment of bone mineral density (BMD). Biomechanical testing occurred at 4- and 8-week time points; parameters tested included torque to failure, torsional rigidity, shear stress, and shear modulus.

Results At the 4-week time point, the LD and HD groups both exhibited significantly higher BMD than controls; at the 8-week time point, the HD group exhibited significantly

higher BMD than controls. Biomechanical testing revealed dose-dependent, higher trends in all parameters tested at the 4- and 8-week time points, with minimal significant differences.

Conclusions Groups treated with rhBMP-2 demonstrated improved bone mineral density at both 4 and 8 weeks compared to control saline groups, in addition to strong trends towards improvement of intrinsic and extrinsic biomechanical properties when compared to control groups. Data revealed trends toward dose-dependent increases in peak torque, torsional rigidity, shear stress, and shear modulus 4 weeks after rhBMP-2 treatment.

Level of evidence Not applicable.

Keywords rhBMP-2 · Calcium phosphate · Hydroxyapatite · Diabetes · Fracture · Osteoporosis

Introduction

Diabetes mellitus is a devastating and life-altering disease, affecting over 20 million people in the USA [1]. Ten percent of those 20 million people suffer from type 1 diabetes (T1DM), in which a 20 % prevalence of osteoporosis with significant bone loss has been reported when compared to healthy, age-matched subjects. Multiple T1DM animal models have been used to further observe and understand T1DM-related osteoporosis. Related animal models have exhibited weakened and altered bony architecture, with potential causes secondary to lack of vascular supply, and osteocalcin receptor malfunction [2–4].

With a clear clinical need to identify targets to combat T1DM-related osteoporosis, bone morphogenetic proteins (BMPs) have become an obvious research target [5]. BMPs

F. A. Liporace (✉) · R. S. Yoon
Division of Orthopaedic Trauma, Department of Orthopaedic Surgery, NYU Hospital for Joint Diseases, 301 E 17th Street, Suite 1402, New York, NY 10003, USA
e-mail: liporace33@gmail.com

E. A. Breitbart · E. Doyle · D. N. Paglia · S. Lin
Division of Orthopaedic Trauma, Department of Orthopaedic Trauma, UMDNJ, New Jersey Medical School, Newark, NJ 07101, USA

are important in bone metabolism and exert their effects on bone through the tightly coupled processes of osteoclastogenesis and osteoblastogenesis [6–8]. The BMP family, in addition to being the largest member of the transforming growth factor (TGF)-β superfamily, is also involved in almost all processes related to skeletal development, morphogenesis, angiogenesis, and homeostasis [9–12]. Because of BMPs' essential role in bone regeneration, several delivery models have been studied, including the utilization of hydroxyapatite/tri-calcium phosphate (HA/TCP) as a primary delivery platform and scaffold [13–18]. With the frequent use of HA/TCP in the fragility fracture setting, this is an obvious delivery model and early results as an osteogenic promoter have been promising [15, 18].

Given the prevalence of T1DM-related osteoporosis and the lack of safe and effective anabolic therapies, studying a corollary between BMP-2 and its possible effect on T1DM-related osteoporosis seems like a natural progression to a potentially beneficial clinical modality [19]. This study evaluated the dose-dependent effect of local rhBMP-2 on biomechanical parameters of bone in the T1DM-related osteoporotic state by combining its possible improved efficacy with a HA/TCP delivery carrier, and using the spontaneous diabetic BB Wistar rat model.

Materials and methods

Animals, preoperative preparation, and cohort formulation

Male BB Wistar rats were used in this study; these rats develop T1DM through an autoimmune, selective destruction of the pancreatic beta cells. The BB Wistar rat currently represents a close homology of human T1DM in a laboratory animal [20]. The BB Wistar rats were obtained from a breeding colony established at the senior author's institution with breeding pairs obtained from BioBreeding (Toronto, Canada). The Institutional Animal Care and Use Committee (IACUC) approved all research protocols. The diabetes-prone BB Wistar rats develop diabetes at an incidence rate of approximately 30–45 % at 70–120 days of age. Urine from the diabetic BB Wistar rats was checked for glycosuria three times a week. Once glycosuria was detected, blood specimens obtained from tail veins were tested for blood glucose levels greater than 250 mg/dl. If the reading exceeded this value, an insulin implant (Linplant®) which provided constant insulin release for approximately 30 days was aseptically placed subcutaneously in the dorsal neck. Blood glucose levels were determined by the glucose-oxidase method (Accu-Chek Advantage, Roche Diagnostics, Indianapolis, IN, USA) obtained through the posterior dorsal tail vein. The diabetic rats were treated with insulin to maintain blood glucose levels between 300 and 450 mg/dl, representing a poorly controlled state of diabetes with glycosuria but no sign of ketonuria. All animals were evaluated for blood glucose levels in the first 24 h after insulin implantation. If the desired blood glucose level was not achieved, an additional amount of insulin implant was given to achieve the appropriate level. The blood glucose levels were evaluated three times a week for the appropriate level of blood glucose control and animals were treated accordingly. Using the model based on Verhaeghe et al. [21], animals were considered osteoporotic 12 weeks after onset of diabetes. Surgery was performed 12 weeks after onset of diabetes in all groups.

All groups except for the saline group required preparation of the HA/TCP carrier for injection. The procedure is as follows: first, 0.2 g HA/TCP (particle size <0.53 μm) was mixed with 100 μl of the appropriate rhBMP-2 dose. The mixture was allowed to stand for 15 min to allow the rhBMP-2 to bind to the HA/TCP carrier. After 15 min, 100 μl of buffer solution was added and mixed. The mixture was then drawn into a 1-ml syringe ready for injection into the femoral canal. Note that the HA/TCP control group received buffer solution twice in place of rhBMP-2. All groups received approximately 0.1 ml injections into the femur.

A surgical procedure was performed in which injections of varying doses of BMP-2, saline, and HA/TCP carrier (particle size <0.53 μm) were injected into the intramedullary (IM) canal of the femur. There were four different treatment groups:

A. diabetic w/saline
B. diabetic w/HA/TCP carrier
C. diabetic w/HA/TCP carrier + rhBMP-2 Low Dose: 0.11 mg/ml (approximate actual dose applied: 2.75 μg per femur)
D. diabetic w/HA/TCP carrier + rhBMP-2 High Dose: 0.22 mg/ml (approximate actual dose applied: 5.5 μg per femur)

Group A consisted of diabetes-related osteoporotic rats receiving an intermedullary injection of saline to determine whether the reaming of the IM canal had any effect. Group B consisted of diabetes-related osteoporotic rats receiving an IM injection of the HA/TCP carrier alone to determine whether there is a carrier-dependent effect. Groups C and D consisted of diabetes-related osteoporotic rats that received IM injections of the HA/TCP carrier with two different doses of rhBMP-2: 0.11 mg/ml for the low dose (LD) and 0.22 mg/ml for the high dose (HD). All groups received approximately 0.1 ml injection of the appropriate treatment into the IM canal of the femur.

The study cohorts consisted of 48 rats divided into four different experimental groups at both 4- and 8-week time-points, with $n = 6$ per group (Table 1). Losses included death from anesthesia given for Linplant insulin treatment, which occurred with two animals (accounting for two groups with $n = 5$). The 8-week saline group had 3 extra ($n = 8$) animals, as they were available for surgery before rhBMP-2 was obtained.

Surgical method

The surgical procedure for the rhBMP-2 treatment in the diabetes-related osteoporotic model is as follows: general anesthesia was administered by intraperitoneal injection of ketamine (60 mg/kg) and xylazine (8 mg/kg). After adequate anesthesia, each rat was shaved and prepped with Betadine® and 70 % alcohol. A 4-mm longitudinal skin incision was made over the patella. The patella was then dislocated laterally and the interchondylar notch of the distal femur was exposed. An entry hole was made with an 18-gauge needle and the IM canal was then reamed. At this time the appropriate treatment was administered by injecting either saline, HA/TCP carrier, low-dose BMP-2 and HA/TCP or high-dose BMP-2 and HA/TCP into the IM canal followed by wound closure with a 4-0 vicryl. The rats were allowed to ambulate freely post-surgery.

Postoperative evaluation

Radiographs were taken immediately after surgery to ensure that the IM canal was properly entered without damage to the femur as well as to detect the presence of material in the canal. Radiographs were taken using a Model 804 Faxitron (Field Emission Corp., McMinnville, OR, USA) and 8 × 10 Kodak Min-R 2000 mammography film (Eastman Kodak Co., Rochester, NY, USA) with an exposure time of 30 s at 55 peak kilovoltage (kVp). Subsequent radiographs were taken at 2-week intervals to observe any effect changes in the bone as well as to check for infection. The animals were killed and both right and left femurs were resected, and magnified radiographs of both anterior–posterior (AP) and lateral (L) views were taken. Radiographs were not used for quantification but

were used for qualitative observation. Micro-computed tomography (CT) imaging studies were performed on all samples in order to provide a higher quality imaging study for additional qualitative evaluation to calculate BMD.

Animals were killed at 4 and 8 weeks post-surgery. The treated femora as well as the contralateral femora were resected and stored at −20 °C in saline (0.9 % NaCl)-soaked gauze. Prior to testing, all femora were removed from the freezer and allowed to thaw to room temperature. Samples were cleaned of soft tissue and femur dimensions were measured using calipers. Proximal and distal ends of the femora were then embedded in ¾-inch (6-mm) square nuts with Wood's metal (Alfa Aesar, Ward Hill, MA, USA), leaving an approximate gauge length of 14 mm. The samples were then torsionally tested to failure using a servo hydraulics machine (MTS Systems Corp., Eden Prairie, MN, USA) with a 20 N m torque cell (Interface, Scotsdale, AZ, USA) at a rate of 2.0°/s. Maximum torque to failure and angle of failure were obtained from the torque force to angular displacement data. Standard equations modeling each femur as a hollow ellipse were used to calculate polar moment of inertia. Peak torque to failure (T_{max}), angle of failure (θ), gauge length (L), and polar moment of inertia (J) were used to calculate maximum torsional rigidity (TR), shear modulus (SM), and maximum torsional shear stress (SS). Mechanical testing values were normalized to minimize inter-animal variability. Normalized data is presented as a percentage and was calculated by dividing treated femur values by the contralateral untreated femur values.

Statistical analysis

Data was analyzed using the Sigma Stat (version 3.0) statistical analysis program. Analysis was performed using one-way ANOVA at each time point (4 and 8 weeks) for all four treatment groups. A 2-sample t test was used to compare combined LD and HD rhBMP-2 groups against combined control groups. In all cases significance was determined as a p value of less than 0.05. Power analysis was performed using the Pass power analysis software (6.0, NCSS, Kaysville, UT, USA).

Results

Inclusion of animals in this study was based upon 12 weeks duration of poorly controlled T1DM in the spontaneous diabetic BB Wistar rat, at which point the animal was considered osteoporotic. Average blood glucose levels, age at surgery, weight at surgery, weight at death, and weight change for all four treatment groups showed no statistical differences when compared within their respective time points (Table 2).

Table 1 Experimental groups

Groups	Testing time-point	
	4 weeks	8 weeks
Diabetic + saline	5 rats	8 rats
Diabetic + HA/TCP + buffer	6 rats	6 rats
Diabetic + HA/TCP + low-dose rhBMP-2	5 rats	6 rats
Diabetic + HA/TCP + high-dose rhBMP-2	6 rats	6 rats

Radiographic images were analyzed independently by two blinded reviewers, who were asked to compare the thickness of the cortices of left (untreated) and right (treated) femurs. Qualitative analysis revealed cortical thickening in the diaphysis in over 75 % of the femurs (18/23) treated with rhBMP-2 in both the LD (9/11) and HD (9/12) groups (Fig. 1) compared to the untreated femur, significantly higher than in the saline control (4/13) and HA/TCP control (5/12) groups ($p < 0.01$). To supplement these plain radiographs, microCT was performed, with similar observations noted amongst the experimental groups (Fig. 2).

In regards to bone mineral density, at the 4-week time point a significant improvement in BMD was seen in both the LD and HD rhBMP-2 groups compared to the saline control ($p = 0.007$ and $p = 0.002$, respectively). At the 8-week time point a significant improvement was maintained in the HD group only ($p = 0.03$) compared to the saline control group (Table 3).

The effect of locally delivered rhBMP-2 with a HA/TCP carrier on the biomechanical properties of osteoporotic bone was measured by torsional mechanical testing. As expected with intact femora, torsional testing to failure consistently resulted in mid-diaphyseal spiral fractures (Fig. 3). Although statistical analysis of general health parameters between treatment groups showed no significant differences, the inclusion criteria (based upon onset of T1DM) used in this study inherently created variability of age, weight, and weight change within treatment groups. Due to this variability, mechanical testing values were normalized to the contralateral limb, thus providing a more accurate assessment of the effects of rhBMP-2 treatment on biomechanical properties of the bone.

The treated femur values and normalized values for both time points showed no statistical differences between the four treatment groups in all categories except maximum torque to failure and peak shear (Tables 4, 5). While the statistical analysis lacked significance ($p > 0.05$), normalized data for both 4-week rhBMP-2-treated groups revealed strong trends toward dose-dependent improvement of peak torque, maximum torsional rigidity, maximum shear stress, and shear modulus (Table 4). Comparison of the combined rhBMP-2 groups and combined control groups demonstrated substantial differences close to statistical significance. Combined 4-week LD and HD rhBMP-2-treated groups showed 15 and 20 % increases in peak torque ($p = 0.056$) and torsional rigidity ($p = 0.072$), respectively, when compared to combined 4-week saline and HA/TCP groups (Table 6).

Normalized values from the 8-week LD rhBMP-2 group revealed a continued significant improvement in peak torque, and revealed significant improvement in peak shear (Table 5). Conversely, the normalized values for the 8-week HD rhBMP-2 group did not maintain the trend towards improved biomechanical properties seen in the 4-week HD rhBMP-2 group. The HA/TCP group, although not statistically significant, did perform better at 8 weeks than at 4 weeks in maximum torsional rigidity and exhibited comparable results to the 8-week LD rhBMP-2 group (Table 5).

Discussion

To our knowledge, this study is the first to extend research on rhBMP-2 into a non-fracture DM-related osteoporosis model with HA/TCP as a carrier. Numerous studies have investigated locally delivered rhBMP-2 in fracture, segmental defect, and ectopic bone formation models but few have studied its effects on intact bone [14, 18].

Table 2 General health at 4- and 8-week time-points	Groups	Blood glucose* (mg/dl)	Age at surgery (days)	Weight at surgery (g)	Weight at death (g)	Weight change (g)
	Saline ($n = 5$)					
	4 weeks	444 ± 40	182 ± 15	408 ± 36	404 ± 28	−4 ± 17
	8 weeks	421 ± 44	184 ± 11	369 ± 30	401 ± 30	33 ± 24
	Buffer + HA/TCP ($n = 6$)					
	4 weeks	493 ± 22	187 ± 12	398 ± 40	385 ± 45	−13 ± 43
The data represent average values ± standard deviation	8 weeks	433 ± 14	175 ± 20	394 ± 33	404 ± 35	10 ± 16
	Low-dose rhBMP-2 + HA/TCP ($n = 5$)					
* Blood glucose data represents mean data from animals in each	4 weeks	478 ± 38	174 ± 10	401 ± 15	407 ± 18	6 ± 7
treatment group resulting from	8 weeks	440 ± 37	161 ± 8	383 ± 60	383 ± 60	2 ± 17
measurements taken from blood	High-dose rhBMP-2+ HA/TCP ($n = 6$)					
drawn two or three times per	4 weeks	474 ± 44	176 ± 13	404 ± 27	387 ± 32	−16 ± 22
week from each animal from onset of T1DM up to death	8 weeks	430 ± 27	177 ± 13	425 ± 23	416 ± 11	−8 ± 18

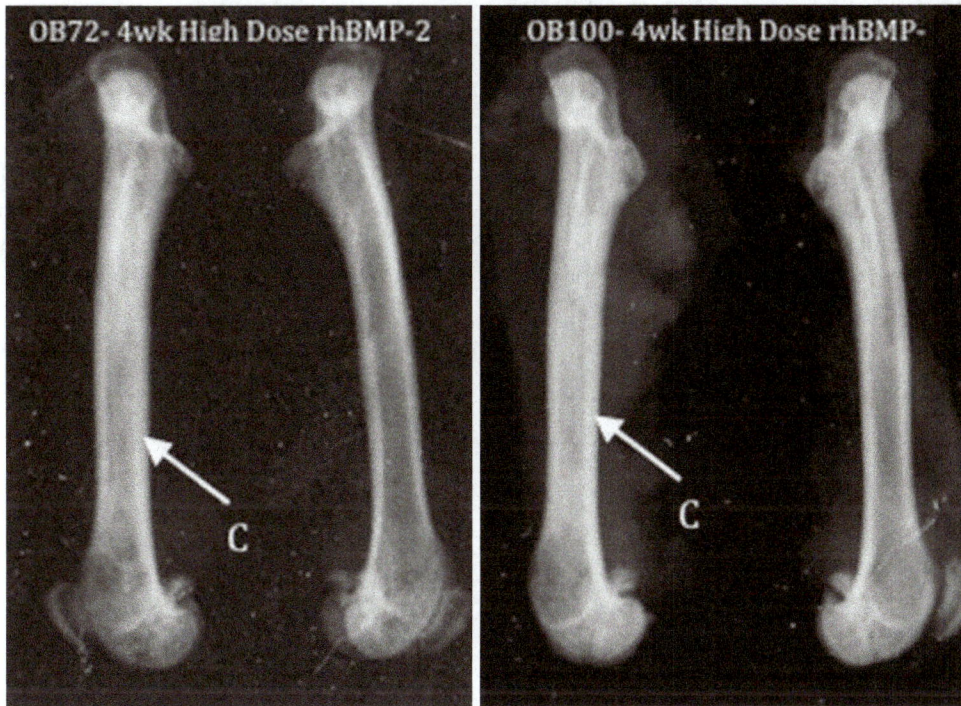

Fig. 1 Magnified lateral radiographs of re-sected femora at 4 weeks. *C* Qualitative observation of cortical thickening in rhBMP-2 treated femurs. Note: treated (right) femurs appear on the *left* in both radiographic images

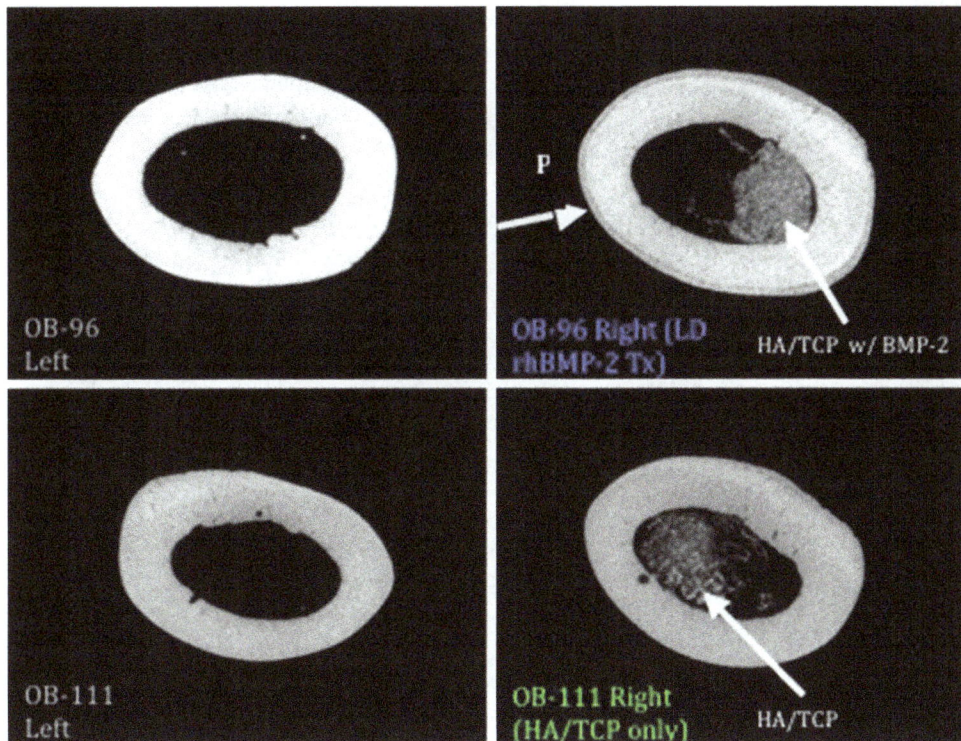

Fig. 2 MicroCT midshaft cortical scan: note new periosteal bone growth (*P*) in the LD rhBMP-2 treated femur on the *top right* compared to contralateral limb and HA/TCP-only treated sample

Based upon the proven osteogenic effects of rhBMP-2 and the theory of local growth factor deficiencies in DM-related osteoporosis, it was hypothesized that local delivery of rhBMP-2 via a HA/TCP carrier would improve the bone mineral density and biomechanical properties of intact, DM-induced osteoporotic bone in the DM BB Wistar rat. Bone mineral density of both LD and HD rhBMP-2 groups at 4 weeks and of the HD rhBMP-2 group at 8 weeks was significantly improved compared to the saline control group. However, while a

Table 3 Micro CT results at 4- and 8-week time-points

Groups	Bone mineral density*	p value
Saline		
4 weeks	0.951 ± 0.0179	–
8 weeks	1.01 ± 0.852	–
Buffer + HA/TCP		
4 weeks	1.43 ± 0.116	**0.0001**
8 weeks	1.15 ± 0.301	0.72
Low-dose rhBMP-2 + HA/TCP		
4 weeks	1.50 ± 0.0101	**0.007**
8 weeks	1.06 ± 0.0223	0.90
High-dose rhBMP-2 + HA/TCP		
4 weeks	1.59 ± 0.217	**0.002**
8 weeks	1.37 ± 0.271	**0.03**

* Values represent ratio of BMD on operative side to that on contralateral non-operative side (mean ± standard deviation)

p values represent comparison to control group. *Bold* indicates statistical significance

dose-dependent increasing trend in peak torque, torsional rigidity, shear stress, and shear modulus was noted in subsequent biomechanical testing, significance was not reached.

Since its discovery approximately 25 years ago, research has provided important insights into the role of BMPs and their effect on bone. Like most protein signaling substrates in the human body, their role is vast, diverse, and regulated in a complex manner, with both anabolic and catabolic effects. The BMP family, a subdivision of the TGF gene superfamily, exerts its effects on bone via several pathways, but in general by inducing the formation of extracellular matrix (cartilaginous scaffold), and later up- and down-regulating the promotion of osteoclasts and osteoblasts [22]. Often occurring via the promotion of angiogenesis, this pathway is affected by diabetes, and theoretically BMPs can improve bone rigidity and density via vascular regeneration [23–25]. Thus, delivering local BMP, even to intact bone, can help promote bone rigidity, and with an HA/TCP carrier a dose-dependent increase was noted. However, efficacy was lost after 8 weeks and this was likely due to the feedback control cited in the literature.

BMPs, in general, are only beneficial in specific dose ranges. Recent studies have demonstrated increased osteoclast activity and decreased anabolic effects in response to high-dose BMPs [26, 27]. Toth et al. [27] demonstrated concentration-dependent osteoclastic resorption of peri-implant bone associated with high levels of rhBMP-2. Furthermore, Vanketesh et al. hypothesized a

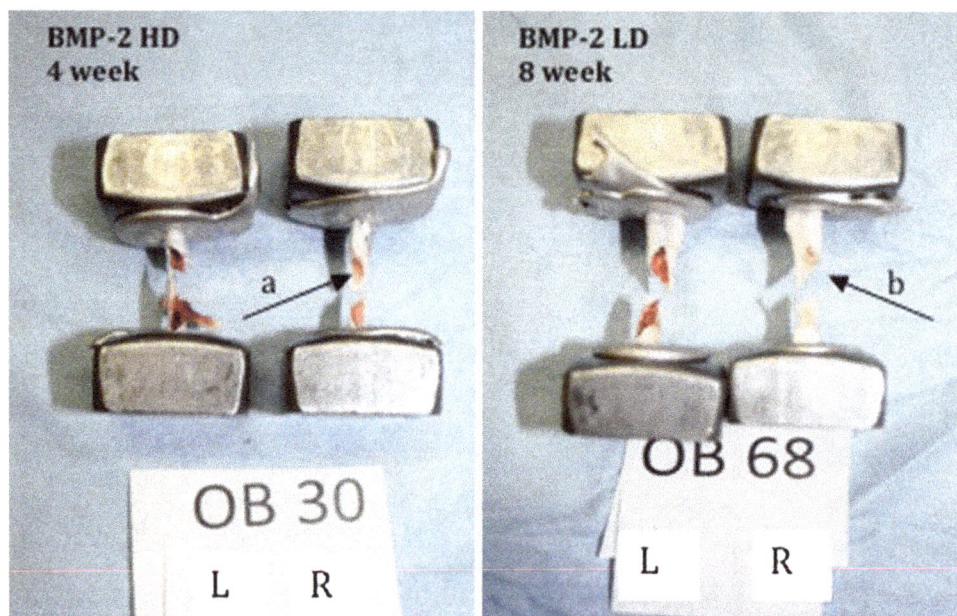

Fig. 3 Spiral fractures resulting from torsional testing. Pictures show mid-diaphyseal spiral fractures. Note that the IM canals of the treated right femora appear *lighter red* (**a**) and *white* (**b**) due to the presence of HA/TCP carrier

Table 4 4- and 8-week post-treatment mechanical testing

Groups	Maximum torque to failure (N m)	p value	Torsional rigidity (N m/rad)	p value	Maximum shear stress (MPa)	p value	Shear modulus (MPa)	p value
Saline								
4 weeks (n = 5)	728 ± 84	0.89	62,969 ± 12,195	0.77	210 ± 26.29	0.29	7,940 ± 1,158.95	0.70
8 weeks (n = 8)	647 ± 149	**0.04**	63,836 ± 18,828	0.89	210 ± 46	0.22	9,239 ± 2,554	0.69
Buffer + HA/TCP								
4 weeks (n = 6)	754 ± 144		57,740 ± 17,801		245.64 ± 36		8,306 ± 2,153.17	
8 weeks (n = 6)	828 ± 70		63,889 ± 10,177		258 ± 33		8,608 ± 1,088	
Low-dose rhBMP-2 + HA/TCP								
4 weeks (n = 5)	789 ± 104		65,992 ± 5,806		253 ± 46		9,030 ± 936	
8 weeks (n = 6)	765 ± 105		59,259 ± 14,865		234 ± 35		7,930 ± 1,914	
High-dose rhBMP-2 + HA/TCP								
4 weeks (n = 6)	740 ± 174		63,948 ± 14,238		223 ± 45		8,461 ± 1,164.52	
8 weeks (n = 6)	805 ± 130		65,437 ± 12,384		244 ± 52		8,517 ± 1,976	

Treated femur values; one-way ANOVA comparing all four groups at 4 and 8 weeks (mean ± standard deviation)

p value in *bold* indicates statistical significance

Table 5 4- and 8-week post-treatment mechanical testing (treated femur values normalized to normal (contralateral) side, one-way ANOVA to compare all four groups at 4 and 8 weeks)

Groups	Percent maximum torque to failure	p value	Percent torsional rigidity	p value	Percent maximum shear stress	p value	Percent shear modulus	p value
Saline								
4 weeks (n = 5)	107 ± 12	0.20	110 ± 29	0.12	100 ± 14	0.25	103 ± 29	0.53
8 weeks (n = 8)	83 ± 18	**0.01**	106 ± 25	0.85	82 ± 17	**0.02**	105 ± 34	0.73
Buffer + HA/TCP								
4 weeks (n = 6)	102 ± 17		85 ± 26		115 ± 21		95 ± 31	
8 weeks (n = 6)	117 ± 17		111 ± 18		106 ± 11		97 ± 15	
Low-dose rh-BMP-2 + HA/TCP								
4 weeks (n = 5)	116 ± 22*		118 ± 17*		117 ± 20*		115 ± 19*	
8 weeks (n = 6)	115 ± 24		98 ± 19		107 ± 22		89 ± 12	
High-dose rh-BMP-2 + HA/TCP								
4 weeks (n = 6)	123 ± 21*		116 ± 27*		124 ± 33*		118 ± 39*	
8 weeks (n = 6)	105 ± 19		102 ± 40		106 ± 12		100 ± 33	

Treated femur values normalized to untreated (contralateral) side; one-way ANOVA comparing all four groups at 4 and 8 weeks (mean ± standard deviation)

p value in *bold* indicates statistical significance

* Indicates a noticeable dose dependent trend in all four mechanical properties, although no statistical significance exists.

noggin-mediated negative feedback control mechanism which decreased anabolic activity at high doses of rhBMP-4 [26]. These findings introduce valid questions concerning dosage. It is possible that HD rhBMP-2, which showed improved BMD at both 4- and 8-week time points, may cause decreased anabolic responses at longer time-points.

Table 6 4-week mechanical testing

	Percent maximum peak torque	Percent torsional rigidity	Percent maximum shear stress	Percent shear modulus
Combined controls ($n = 11$)	104 ± 14	96 ± 30	108 ± 19	99 ± 0.287
rhBMP-2 (HD + LD) ($n = 11$)	120 ± 21 $p = 0.056$	117 ± 22 $p = 0.072$	121 ± 27 $p = 0.224$	117 ± 30 $p = 0.167$

4-week normalized ratio of right:left femur; combined treated vs. combined untreated (mean ± standard deviation)

Interestingly, the 8-week HA/TCP group performed better than the 4-week HA/TCP group in both peak torque and torsional rigidity and revealed similar trends to the 8-week LD rhBMP-2 group in peak torque. While BMP has been shown to lose its effect in the short term, it is reasonable to attribute the improved rigidity in the long term to the osteoconductivity of the carrier [28–31] as well as the stimulatory effect of the intramedullary reaming [32–35].

Wang et al. [36] conducted the only other study in intact bone, albeit in an osteonecrotic model. Examining the controlled localized release of rhBMP-2 in regeneration of osteonecrotic bone, rhBMP-2 was delivered via poly(lactic-glycolic acid) (PLGA)-HA microspheres to the site of necrotic bone utilizing an in vivo mouse model. Wang et al. reported improved osteogenesis and neo-vascularization at 2 and 4 weeks in rhBMP-2-treated groups.

DM-related osteoporosis fracture and segmental defect models inherently create greater differences between treated and untreated groups. Because this study dealt with intact bone, the differences in biomechanical properties of the bone were not as drastic and therefore required larger sample sizes for significance. In fact, drastic increases in certain properties would be detrimental in that they may create an imbalance between the rigid and flexible properties of bone. The consistency of increased strength and rigidity in both extrinsic and intrinsic properties in the experimental groups at 4 weeks suggests balanced improvement in the quality of the bone.

However, despite its limitations, this study sheds important light on the effect of rhBMP on diabetes-induced osteoporotic bone. Adding to the literature of utilizing HA/TCP as an important carrier could have important, immediate clinical translations. While improving overall BMD, further studies should look at the potential effects on angiogenesis and subsequent strengthening in diabetic bone. Future research to expand upon this specific study should include additional histological analysis as well as increasing animal numbers in order to obtain statistical significance. Additional studies in humans could be performed later to determine the benefit of rhBMP-2 in patients who are at risk of developing osteoporotic fractures, especially in the setting of diabetes.

Conflict of interest None.

Ethical standards All research protocols were approved by the Institutional Animal Care and Use Committee (IACUC) prior to the completion of this project.

References

1. McCabe LR (2007) Understanding the pathology and mechanisms of type I diabetic bone loss. J Cell Biochem 102(6):1343–1357. doi:10.1002/jcb.21573
2. Schneider LE, Schedl HP (1972) Diabetes and intestinal calcium absorption in the rat. Am J Physiol 223(6):1319–1323
3. Schneider LE, Wilson HD, Schedl HP (1977) Effects of diabetes and vitamin D-depletion on duodenal and ileal calcium transport in the rat. Acta Diabetol Lat 14(1–2):18–25
4. Weintroub S, Cohen DF, Salama R, Streifler M, Weissman SL (1980) Skeletal findings in human neutrolethyrism. Is there a human osteolathyrism? Eur Neurol 19(2):121–127
5. Kim SE, Jeon O, Lee JB, Bae MS, Chun HJ, Moon SH, Kwon IK (2008) Enhancement of ectopic bone formation by bone morphogenetic protein-2 delivery using heparin-conjugated PLGA nanoparticles with transplantation of bone marrow-derived mesenchymal stem cells. J Biomed Sci 15(6):771–777. doi:10.1007/s11373-008-9277-4
6. Wu X, Shi W, Cao X (2007) Multiplicity of BMP signaling in skeletal development. Ann N Y Acad Sci 1116:29–49. doi:10.1196/annals.1402.053
7. Garimella R, Tague SE, Zhang J, Belibi F, Nahar N, Sun BH, Insogna K, Wang J, Anderson HC (2008) Expression and synthesis of bone morphogenetic proteins by osteoclasts: a possible path to anabolic bone remodeling. J Histochem Cytochem 56(6):569–577. doi:10.1369/jhc.2008.950394
8. Zhao GQ (2003) Consequences of knocking out BMP signaling in the mouse. Genesis 35(1):43–56. doi:10.1002/gene.10167
9. Wan M, Cao X (2005) BMP signaling in skeletal development. Biochem Biophys Res Commun 328(3):651–657. doi:10.1016/j.bbrc.2004.11.067
10. Wang Y, Nishida S, Elalieh HZ, Long RK, Halloran BP, Bikle DD (2006) Role of IGF-I signaling in regulating osteoclastogenesis. J Bone Miner Res 21(9):1350–1358. doi:10.1359/jbmr.060610
11. Ishidou Y, Kitajima I, Obama H, Maruyama I, Murata F, Imamura T, Yamada N, ten Dijke P, Miyazono K, Sakou T (1995) Enhanced expression of type I receptors for bone morphogenetic proteins during bone formation. J Bone Miner Res 10(11):1651–1659. doi:10.1002/jbmr.5650101107
12. Zhang F, Qiu T, Wu X, Wan C, Shi W, Wang Y, Chen J, Wan M, Clemens TL, Cao X (2009) Sustained BMP signaling in osteoblasts stimulates bone formation by promoting angiogenesis and osteoblast differentiation. J Bone Miner Res. doi:10.1359/jbmr.090204

13. Autefage H, Briand-Mesange F, Cazalbou S, Drouet C, Fourmy D, Goncalves S, Salles JP, Combes C, Swider P, Rey C (2009) Adsorption and release of BMP-2 on nanocrystalline apatite-coated and uncoated hydroxyapatite/beta-tricalcium phosphate porous ceramics. J Biomed Mater Res B Appl Biomater 91(2):706–715. doi:10.1002/jbm.b.31447

14. Hannink G, Geutjes PJ, Daamen WF, Buma P (2013) Evaluation of collagen/heparin coated TCP/HA granules for long-term delivery of BMP-2. J Mater Sci Mater Med 24(2):325–332. doi:10.1007/s10856-012-4802-4

15. Hulsart-Billstrom G, Hu Q, Bergman K, Jonsson KB, Aberg J, Tang R, Larsson S, Hilborn J (2011) Calcium phosphates compounds in conjunction with hydrogel as carrier for BMP-2: a study on ectopic bone formation in rats. Acta Biomater 7(8):3042–3049. doi:10.1016/j.actbio.2011.04.021

16. Overman JR, Farre-Guasch E, Helder MN, ten Bruggenkate CM, Schulten EA, Klein-Nulend J (2013) Short (15 minutes) bone morphogenetic protein-2 treatment stimulates osteogenic differentiation of human adipose stem cells seeded on calcium phosphate scaffolds in vitro. Tissue Eng Part A 19(3–4):571–581. doi:10.1089/ten.TEA.2012.0133

17. Overman JR, Helder MN, ten Bruggenkate CM, Schulten EA, Klein-Nulend J, Bakker AD (2013) Growth factor gene expression profiles of bone morphogenetic protein-2-treated human adipose stem cells seeded on calcium phosphate scaffolds in vitro. Biochimie 95(12):2304–2313. doi:10.1016/j.biochi.2013.08.034

18. Tazaki J, Murata M, Akazawa T, Yamamoto M, Ito K, Arisue M, Shibata T, Tabata Y (2009) BMP-2 release and dose-response studies in hydroxyapatite and beta-tricalcium phosphate. Bio Med Mater Eng 19(2–3):141–146. doi:10.3233/BME-2009-0573

19. Khosla S, Westendorf JJ, Oursler MJ (2008) Building bone to reverse osteoporosis and repair fractures. J Clin Invest 118(2):421–428. doi:10.1172/JCI33612

20. Marliss EB, Nakhooda AF, Poussier P, Sima AA (1982) The diabetic syndrome of the 'BB' Wistar rat: possible relevance to type 1 (insulin-dependent) diabetes in man. Diabetologia 22(4):225–232

21. Verhaeghe J, Visser WJ, Einhorn TA, Bouillon R (1990) Osteoporosis and diabetes: lessons from the diabetic BB rat. Horm Res 34(5–6):245–248

22. Kamiya N (2012) The role of BMPs in bone anabolism and their potential targets SOST and DKK1. Curr Mol Pharmacol 5(2):153–163

23. Beam HA, Parsons JR, Lin SS (2002) The effects of blood glucose control upon fracture healing in the BB Wistar rat with diabetes mellitus. J Orthop Res 20(6):1210–1216. doi:10.1016/S0736-0266(02)00066-9

24. Gooch HL, Hale JE, Fujioka H, Balian G, Hurwitz SR (2000) Alterations of cartilage and collagen expression during fracture healing in experimental diabetes. Connect Tissue Res 41(2):81–91

25. Paglia DN, Wey A, Breitbart EA, Faiwiszewski J, Mehta SK, Al-Zube L, Vaidya S, Cottrell JA, Graves D, Benevenia J, O'Connor JP, Lin SS (2013) Effects of local insulin delivery on subperiosteal angiogenesis and mineralized tissue formation during fracture healing. J Orthop Res 31(5):783–791. doi:10.1002/jor.22288

26. Krishnan V, Ma Y, Moseley J, Geiser A, Friant S, Frolik C (2001) Bone anabolic effects of sonic/indian hedgehog are mediated by bmp-2/4-dependent pathways in the neonatal rat metatarsal model. Endocrinology 142(2):940–947. doi:10.1210/endo.142.2.7922

27. Toth JM, Boden SD, Burkus JK, Badura JM, Peckham SM, McKay WF (2009) Short-term osteoclastic activity induced by locally high concentrations of recombinant human bone morphogenetic protein-2 in a cancellous bone environment. Spine 34(6):539–550. doi:10.1097/BRS.0b013e3181952695

28. Urist MR, Lietze A, Dawson E (1984) Beta-tricalcium phosphate delivery system for bone morphogenetic protein. Clin Orthop Relat Res 187:277–280

29. Urist MR, Nilsson O, Rasmussen J, Hirota W, Lovell T, Schmalzreid T, Finerman GA (1987) Bone regeneration under the influence of a bone morphogenetic protein (BMP) beta tricalcium phosphate (TCP) composite in skull trephine defects in dogs. Clin Orthop Relat Res 214:295–304

30. Alam MI, Asahina I, Ohmamiuda K, Takahashi K, Yokota S, Enomoto S (2001) Evaluation of ceramics composed of different hydroxyapatite to tricalcium phosphate ratios as carriers for rhBMP-2. Biomaterials 22(12):1643–1651

31. Burg KJ, Porter S, Kellam JF (2000) Biomaterial developments for bone tissue engineering. Biomaterials 21(23):2347–2359

32. Bedi A, Karunakar MA (2006) Physiologic effects of intramedullary reaming. Instr Course Lect 55:359–366

33. Bhandari M, Schemitsch EH (2002) Bone formation following intramedullary femoral reaming is decreased by indomethacin and antibodies to insulin-like growth factors. J Orthop Trauma 16(10):717–722

34. Frolke JP, Nulend JK, Semeins CM, Bakker FC, Patka P, Haarman HJ (2004) Viable osteoblastic potential of cortical reamings from intramedullary nailing. J Orthop Res 22(6):1271–1275. doi:10.1016/j.orthres.2004.03.011

35. Niedziolka J (2000) Intramedullary osteosynthesis for treatment of pseudarthrosis. Chir Narzadow Ruchu Ortop Pol 65(4):427–430

36. Wang CK, Ho ML, Wang GJ, Chang JK, Chen CH, Fu YC, Fu HH (2009) Controlled-release of rhBMP-2 carriers in the regeneration of osteonecrotic bone. Biomaterials. doi:10.1016/j.biomaterials.2009.04.029

Vertebral body compression fracture after percutaneous pedicle screw removal in a young man

M. Cappuccio · F. De Iure · L. Amendola ·
A. Martucci

Abstract Hazards and potential complications associated with pedicle screw insertions have been reported. In contrast, complications due to implant removal are rarely described. An unreported case of acute vertebral body compression fracture following pedicle screw removal in a young man occurred during an episode of forceful coughing. Spinal implants need to be removed in cases of complications, pain or tissue irritation, and removal is mandatory when fixation involves L2 or the lower segments. Complications associated with spinal implant removal are rare but possible, and patients must be informed of this potential risk.

Keywords Complication · Compression fracture · Implant removal · Spine surgery

Introduction

In thoracolumbar fractures, the choice between conservative or surgical treatment and the final outcome depend on several factors: type of fracture, presence of neurological impairment, the patient's general condition and comorbidities, and associated injuries [1, 2].

Conservative treatment, especially bed rest, is not advisable in polytrauma patients, or in cases of claustrophobia, psychological disease, venous disease or previous deep venous thrombosis, obesity and bronchopulmonary diseases. In these situations percutaneous minimally invasive surgery can be an option [3]. This technique is used by the authors whenever conservative treatment is not advisable or when posterior open arthrodesis could represent an overtreatment.

Implant removal after percutaneous stabilization should restore a "normal" spine, provided screws are placed without damaging the facet joints, but this beneficial aspect has yet to be demonstrated. We report a case of acute vertebral body compression fracture of L1 following removal of pedicle screws previously placed to treat L2 fracture by means of percutaneous fixation. To the best of our knowledge, this type of fracture in a young man has not previously been reported.

Case report

A 29-year-old man was treated by percutaneous stabilization from L1 to L3 (pedicle screw diameter: 5.5 mm in L1 and 6.5 mm in L3) for a L2 burst fracture (type A3.1 according to Magerl's classification [1]) caused by a car accident (Fig. 1a).

After 6 months of follow-up the fracture was healed but the patient reported local pain, presumably due to mechanical irritation. Nine months after the first surgery, the spinal fixation was removed. No sign of implant failure or loosening was found on preoperative radiographs and on the operative field.

There were no intraoperative complications. The patient began to walk on the first post-operative day.

One month after the second surgery, the patient, suffering from bronchopneumonia, experienced a sharp pain in the upper lumbar spine during an episode of forceful coughing.

M. Cappuccio (✉) · F. De Iure · L. Amendola · A. Martucci
Department of Orthopedics and Traumatology - Spine Surgery,
Maggiore Hospital, Largo Nigrisoli, 2, 40100 Bologna, Italy
e-mail: m.cappuccio73@gmail.com;
michele.cappuccio@libero.it

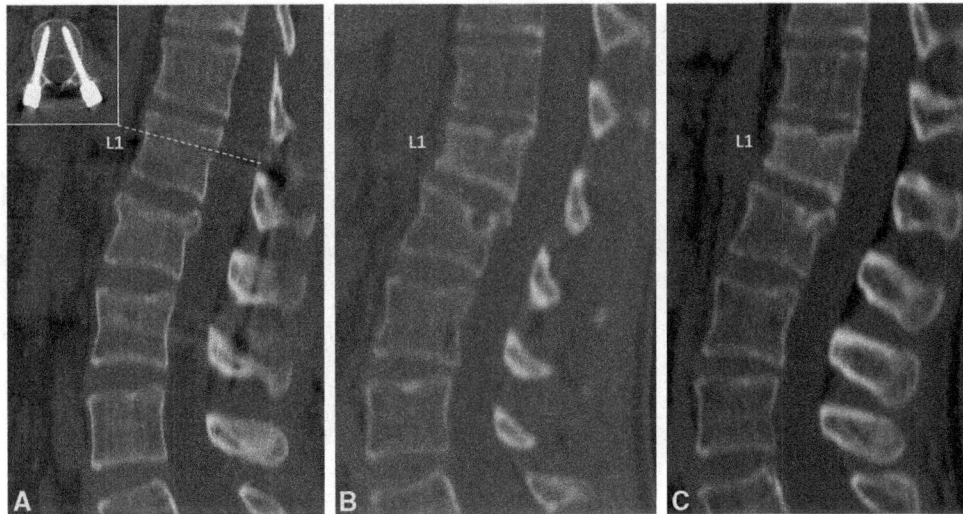

Fig. 1 a Postoperative CT scan showed a good reduction of the fracture with correct positioning of pedicle screw in L1 (in the *box*). **b** One month after implant removal, a CT scan showed an acute wedge fracture on L1. **c** Fracture healing after conservative treatment with 3-point brace for 3 months

X-ray, computed tomography (CT) scan and magnetic resonance imaging demonstrated an acute wedge fracture (A1.2) of the superior plate on L1 (Fig. 1b). No signs of spondylodiscitis were present.

Very precise peripheral measurements by quantitative CT for the evaluation of bone density showed normal cortical and cancellous bone density. The patient had never used steroids. Body mass index was below 25. Laboratory tests were in the normal range except for markers of inflammation (WBC and ESR). C-reactive protein was normal.

The fracture was treated conservatively by a 3-point brace and analgesics for 3 months and healed without further progression of the kyphotic deformity (Fig. 1c). The patient returned to his previous job after 4 months. At the time of last follow-up, 12 months after the second surgery, he was completely pain-free.

Discussion

In the management of thoracolumbar fractures, percutaneous pedicle screw fixation is used to reduce the approach-related morbidity of the open technique: iatrogenic muscle denervation, increased intramuscular pressures, ischemia, pain and functional impairment [4].

Hazards and potential complications associated with pedicle screw insertions have been reported [5].

In contrast, complications due to implant removal are rarely described. Vanichkachorn et al. [6] reported one case of potential large vessel injury during the removal of a broken pedicle screw. Waelchli et al. [7] showed two cases of acute vertebral compression fractures of the instrumented vertebral body adjacent to the fractured vertebra due to removal of pedicle screws. Both cases involved females who suffered from general osteoporosis and who had been previously treated for vertebral lumbar burst fracture. The authors assumed that the subcortical bone defect of the screw tracks was an important factor contributing to the additional weakening of the osteoporotic vertebral bodies.

To our knowledge, we describe the first acute vertebral compression fracture after percutaneous pedicle screw implant removal in a young man which occurred during an episode of forceful coughing.

Only one case of herniated lumbar disc associated with whooping cough is reported, probably as a result of the pressure effect from the tremendous force produced in the thoracic and abdominal cavity during a coughing access [8]. Vertebral fractures are reported in some cases associated with seizures in patients suffering from epilepsy [9, 10]. The authors assume that the forces generated during a tonic–clonic seizure can result in axial skeletal trauma, including thoracic or lumbar burst fractures. In the same way, the contraction force developed during a coughing access, although quantitatively lower, could result in a vertebral fracture if there is a subcortical bone defect of the screw tracks.

In the treatment of thoracolumbar fractures, percutaneous pedicle screw stabilization seems to be a good option.

Spinal implants need to be removed in cases of complications, pain or tissue irritations, and removal is mandatory when fixation involves L2 or the lower segments.

Complications associated with spinal implant removal are rare but possible, and patients must be informed of this potential risk.

Acknowledgments The authors thank Carlo Piovani for helpful collaboration in image storage and editing.

Conflict of interest None.

Ethical standards The patient provided his consent to the publication of this report.

References

1. Magerl F, Aebi M, Gertzbein SD et al (1984) A comprehensive classification of thoracic and lumbar injuries. Eur Spine J 3:184–201
2. Mumford J, Weinstein JN, Spratt KF, Goel VK (1993) Thoracolumbar burst fractures. The clinical efficacy and outcome of nonoperative management. Spine 18(8):955–970
3. Rampesaud YR, Annand N, Dekutoski MB (2006) Use of minimally invasive surgical technique in the management of thoracolumbar trauma. Spine 31(11 Suppl):S96–S102
4. Kim DY, Lee SH, Chung SK, Lee HY (2005) Comparison of multifidus muscle atrophy and trunk extension muscle strength: percutaneous vs open pedicle screw fixation. Spine 30(1):123–129
5. Verlaan JJ, Diekerhof CH, Buskens E et al (2004) Surgical treatment of traumatic fractures of the thoracic and lumbar spine: a systematic review of the literature on techniques, complications, and outcome. Spine 29:803–814
6. Vanichkachorn JS, Vaccaro AR, Cohen MJ, Cotler JM (1997) Potential large vessel injury during thoracolumbar pedicle screw removal. A case report. Spine 22:110–113
7. Waelchli B, Min K, Cathrein P, Boos N (2002) Vertebral body compression fracture after removal of pedicle screws: a report of two cases. Eur Spine J 11(5):504–506
8. Shvartzman P, Mader R, Stopler T (1989) Herniated lumbar disc associated with pertussis. J Fam Pract 28(2):224–225
9. McCullen GM, Brown CC (1994) Seizure-induced thoracic burst fracture: a case report. Spine 19(1):77–79
10. Grabe RP (1988) Fracture-dislocation of lumbar spine during a grand mal epileptic seizure. A case report. S Afr Med J 74:129–131

Risk factors for acute compartment syndrome of the leg associated with tibial diaphyseal fractures in adults

Babak Shadgan · Gavin Pereira · Matthew Menon ·
Siavash Jafari · W. Darlene Reid · Peter J. O'Brien

Abstract

Background We sought to examine the occurrence of acute compartment syndrome (ACS) in the cohort of patients with tibial diaphyseal fractures and to detect associated risk factors that could predict this occurrence.

Materials and methods A total of 1,125 patients with tibial diaphyseal fractures that were treated in our centre were included into this retrospective cohort study. All patients were treated with surgical fixation. Among them some were complicated by ACS of the leg. Age, gender, year and mechanism of injury, injury severity score (ISS), fracture characteristics and classifications and the type of fixation, as well as ACS characteristics in affected patients were studied.

Results Of the cohort of patients 772 (69 %) were male (mean age 39.60 ± 15.97 years) and the rest were women (mean age 45.08 ± 19.04 years). ACS of the leg occurred in 87 (7.73 %) of all tibial diaphyseal fractures. The mean age of those patients that developed ACS (33.08 ± 12.8) was significantly lower than those who did not develop it (42.01 ± 17.3, $P < 0.001$). No significant difference in incidence of ACS was found in open versus closed fractures, between anatomic sites and following IM nailing ($P = 0.67$). Increasing pain was the most common symptom in 71 % of cases with ACS.

Conclusions We found that younger patients are definitely at a significantly higher risk of ACS following acute tibial diaphyseal fractures. Male gender, open fracture and IM nailing were not risk factors for ACS of the leg associated with tibial diaphyseal fractures in adults.

Level of evidence Level IV.

Keywords Tibia fracture · Compartment syndrome · Fracture fixation intramedullary

B. Shadgan · P. J. O'Brien
Trauma Orthopaedic Division, Department of Orthopaedics, University of British Columbia, #110-828W 10th Ave, Vancouver, BC V5Z 1L8, Canada
e-mail: Peter.OBrien@vch.ca

B. Shadgan (✉)
5440-ICORD, Blusson Spinal Cord Centre, 818 West 10th Avenue, Vancouver, BC V5Z-1M9, Canada
e-mail: shadgan@alumni.ubc.ca

G. Pereira
University Hospital Coventry and Warwickshire, Clifford Bridge Road, Coventry CV2 2DX, UK
e-mail: GPer11@aol.com

M. Menon
Division of Orthopaedic Surgery, University of Alberta, 10150-121 Street, Edmonton, AB T5N 1K4, Canada
e-mail: mattmenon@hotmail.com

S. Jafari
School of Population and Public Health, Faculty of Medicine, University of British Columbia, 2206 East Mall, Vancouver, BC V6T 1Z3, Canada
e-mail: sjafarimd@yahoo.ca

W. Darlene Reid
Department of Physical Therapy, University of Toronto, 160-500 University Avenue, Toronto, ON M5G 1V7, Canada
e-mail: darlene.reid@ubc.ca

Introduction

Fracture of the tibia is the most common long-bone fracture worldwide [1]. Acute compartment syndrome (ACS) is considered to be one of the most serious complications of tibial fractures, and failure to diagnose and treat it in time can lead to catastrophic consequences that are devastating to patients, surgeons and health care providers. Giannoudis et al. [2] have shown that patients who sustained a tibial fracture followed by an ACS, performed worse on the EuroQol score than those who had uncomplicated fractures. Delayed or missed diagnosis of ACS following tibial shaft fracture negatively affects the health care team as well. In addition to the psychological stress for health care givers associated with poor patient outcome, the average indemnity paid for missed ACS is high and the rate of successful defence of cases is lower than with other orthopaedic medico legal cases [3, 4]. The cost of ACS is significant, resulting in prolonged hospital stays and charges that are more than doubled in patients with tibial fractures affected by ACS [5]. Physicians treating patients with traumatic injuries are normally aware of ACS. However, due to the low incidence of this condition, a high index of suspicion is usually required to initiate one's thought processes towards making a diagnosis of ACS. There has been no large-scale study on the epidemiology of lower leg compartment syndrome so far. It is therefore difficult to appreciate the burden of this problem.

The purpose of this study, therefore, was to examine the relationship between the development of ACS in the cohort of patients presenting to our hospital with tibial diaphyseal fractures and specific demographic, injury, and operative characteristics that could predict this occurrence. A thorough understanding of these risk factors and their relative influence on development of lower leg ACS may provide better insight into the recognition of high risk individuals, which is critical in an effort to optimize patient outcomes.

Materials and methods

This retrospective cohort study was conducted at a level-one trauma centre attended by five full-time orthopaedic trauma surgeons. All tibial diaphyseal fractures that were treated between January 1997 and December 2011 were retrieved from the orthopaedic trauma prospective data base. Patients developing ACS in this group were identified and relevant information on demographics and risk factors were collected.

ACS of the lower leg was defined for the purpose of this study as being an acute event following a tibial diaphyseal fracture diagnosed by clinical signs and symptoms and, where necessary, by intra-compartmental pressure measurements, using a handheld intra-compartmental pressure monitoring system (Stryker Surgical, Kalamazoo, MI), but confirmed at fasciotomy and entered prospectively into the data base as 'Acute Compartment Syndrome'. Patients who were treated with non-surgical fixation methods or primary amputation, or patients who had open fractures requiring vascular repair or intra-articular fractures, were excluded.

Information regarding gender, age, year of injury, mechanism of injury, injury severity score (ISS), fracture side, state of skin/soft tissue injury [6], site of fracture along the tibial shaft and method of fixation were abstracted from the data base. For the purpose of this study, mechanism of injury was subdivided into twisting, fall, direct blow, crushing injury, vehicle accident, bicycle accident, motorcycle accident, and pedestrian vs motor vehicle accident. The site of fracture was classified as being in the proximal, middle or distal third of the tibial diaphysis. When the fracture crossed 2 zones, it was entered as such. Extensive fractures were those that crossed all 3 zones. Methods of surgical fixation were classified into intramedullary (IM) nailing (dynamic locking nail, static locking nail, unlocked nail) and non-IM nailing (screw, plate, external fixator) methods. The choice of fixation was based on the pattern of fracture, the soft tissue involvement, and the general condition of the patient before and after the injury as well as surgeon's preference. The mean lengths of hospital stays of patients with and without ACS were also compared.

In addition we undertook a chart review of the 87 cases of ACS and recorded levels of consciousness, clinical symptoms and signs, intra-compartmental pressure measures as well as time interval between occurrence of tibial fracture and surgical fixation to fasciotomy.

The incidence of ACS following tibia diaphyseal fractures was determined from the data. Data on demographics, type of trauma, side of tibia fracture, year of fracture, open vs closed fracture, anatomical classification of the fracture, fracture pattern, mechanism of fracture, method of internal fixation, clinical symptoms at admission, and intra-compartmental pressure measures of all cases were collected. Student's t-test was used to compare the means of two groups. Pearson's chi square test or Fisher's exact tests were used to compare categorical variables. Relative risks and 95 % confidence interval (95 %CI) were calculated to assess the association between potential risks factors and development of ACS. Statistical significance at 5 % was selected in this study and the relative risk (RR) with 95 % confidence interval (CI) is reported where appropriate. STATA statistical software (StataCorp 2011. Stata Statistical Software: release 12. College Station, TX: StataCorp LP) was used for data analysis.

Results

For the 14-year period 1997–2011, inclusive, 1,125 tibial fractures were identified in 1,100 patients. Table 1 lists the characteristics of patients with tibia fractures included in this study. ACS of the leg occurred as an immediate or early complication in 87 limbs, 7.73 % of all tibia fractures. Henceforth in this paper, all statistics will refer to the tibial fractures and not patients. Characteristics of patients with tibial fractures and those who developed ACS are summarized in Tables 1 and 2, respectively.

The mean age of all participants was 41.32 ($\pm$17.2) with a range of 16–99 years. Male patients were overall younger than female patients with a mean age of 39.60 ($\pm$15.97) compared with 45.08 ($\pm$19.04) for female patients, and this difference was statistically significant ($t = 5.0143$;

Table 1 Characteristics of the patients included in the study

		N (1,125)	%
Age mean	41.32 ($\pm$17.2)		
Gender	Male	772	69
	Female	353	31
Trauma type	Single injury	662	58.84
	Multiple injury	179	15.91
	Multiple system trauma	284	25.24
Side of tibia fracture	Right	553	49.16
	Left	572	50.84
Skin	Close fracture	776	68.98
	Open fracture	349	31.02
Fracture classification	Proximal/3	147	13.07
	Middle/3	632	69.24
	Distal/3	265	23.56
	Extensive	81	7.2
Mechanism of fracture	Fall	399	35.47
	Pedestrian vs motor vehicle accident	305	27.11
	Motorcycle accident	188	16.71
	Twisting injury	80	7.11
	Direct blow	72	6.4
	Crushing injury	40	3.56
	Bicycle accident	23	2.04
	Motorized accident	18	1.6
Internal fixation method	Screw	21	1.87
	Plate	186	16.53
	External fixator	3	0.27
	Dynamic locking nail	22	1.96
	Static locking nail	886	78.76
	Unlocked nail	7	0.62
Early local complication	None	1,014	90.13
	Compartment syndrome	87	7.73
	Reduction/fixation failure	13	1.16
	Wound infection	7	0.62
	Neurovascular loss	4	0.36

Table 2 Characteristics of patients with tibial fractures who developed ACS

		N	%
Age mean	33.08 ($\pm$12.8)		
Gender	Male	66	76
	Female	21	24
Skin	Closed	66	75.86
	Open	21	24.14
Fracture classification	Proximal/3	11	12.64
	Middle/3	43	49.43
	Distal/3	25	28.74
	Extensive	8	9.2
Clinical signs and symptoms	Severe pain	31	35.23
	Paresthesia	7	7.95
	Motor weakness	4	4.55
	Unconscious	6	6.82
	Pain and paresthesia	17	19.32
	Pain and paresthesia and motor weakness	14	15.91
	Paresthesia + motor weakness	8	9.09
	Pressure	1	1.14
Mechanism of injury	Fall	26	29.89
	Pedestrian vs motor vehicle	22	25.29
	Motor accident	19	21.84
	Twisting injury	6	6.9
	Blow	6	6.9
	Crushing injury	5	5.75
	Motorized accident	2	2.3
	Bicycle	1	1.15
Fracture pattern	Comminuted	23	26.14
	Oblique	17	19.32
	Segmental	8	9.09
	Spiral	16	18.18
	Transverse	24	27.27
Involved compartments	Anterior	37	42.53
	Lateral	4	4.6
	Posterior	3	3.45
	Not specified	19	21.84
	Anterior + lateral	13	14.94
	All	11	12.64

Table 3 Comparison of patients with ACS with those without ACS

		Tibial fracture no ACS	Tibial fracture with ACS	Test statistics	P value
Age		42.01 (17.3)	33.08 (12.8)	$t = 4.7037; df = 1123$	<0.001
Gender	Male	706	66	$\chi^2 = 2.29; df = 1$	0.13
	Female	332	21		
Skin	Closed	710	66	$\chi^2 = 2.0884; df = 1$	0.148
	Open	328	21		
Fracture classification	Proximal/3	136	11	$\chi^2 = 2.3738; df = 3$	0.499
	Middle/3	589	43		
	Distal/3	240	25		
	Extensive	73	8		
Trauma type	Single injury	608	54	$\chi^2 = 1.0464; df = 2$	0.593
	Multiple system trauma	266	18		
	Multiple injury	164	15		
Fracture side	Left	529	43	$\chi^2 = 0.0760; df = 1$	0.783
	Right	509	44		
Fixation method	Static locking nail	812	74	$\chi^2 = 3.1695; df = 5$	0.674
Mechanism of injury	Plate	176	10		
	Dynamic locking nail	21	1		
	Screw	20	1		
	Unlocked nail	6	1		
	External fixator	3	0		
	Fall	399	26	$\chi^2 = 4.4011; df = 7$	0.733
	Pedestrian vs motor vehicle	305	22		
	Motor accident	188	19		
	Twisting injury	80	6		
	Blow	72	6		
	Crushing injury	40	5		
	Motorized accident	18	2		
	Bicycle	23	1		
ISS	01–10	802	76	$\chi^2 = 4.8735; df = 3;$	0.181
	11–20	109	5		
	21–30	74	4		
	>30	53	2		

$df = 1{,}123$, $P < 0.0001$). The mean age of those patients who developed ACS was 33.08 (± 12.8), which was much lower than the mean age of patients who did not develop ACS (42.01 $\pm$ 17.3) and this difference was statistically significant ($P < 0.001$). Of the 1,125 tibial fractures, 772 were in males and 353 in females. Sixty-six out of 772 men (8.55 %) and 21 out of 353 women (5.95 %) developed ACS. Male gender was found to be a risk factor for development of ACS (RR = 1.11; 95 %CI: 0.98–1.26) but this risk was not statistically significant (Pearson's $\chi^2 = 2.2971$, $df = 1$, $P = 0.130$) (Table 3).

In this study we did not find a significant relationship between type of fracture (open vs closed), anatomical site of tibia fracture, type of trauma, fixation method, or mechanism of injury and development of ACS. Although the relative risk of development of ACS was lower among patients with open fractures (RR = 0.76; 95 %CI: 0.52–1.12), this relationship was not statistically significant ($\chi^2 = 2.0884$; $df = 1$; $P = 0.148$). Among both groups, the distribution of the ISS was heavily influenced by the number of subjects with ISS 9. No difference could be found between these groups though.

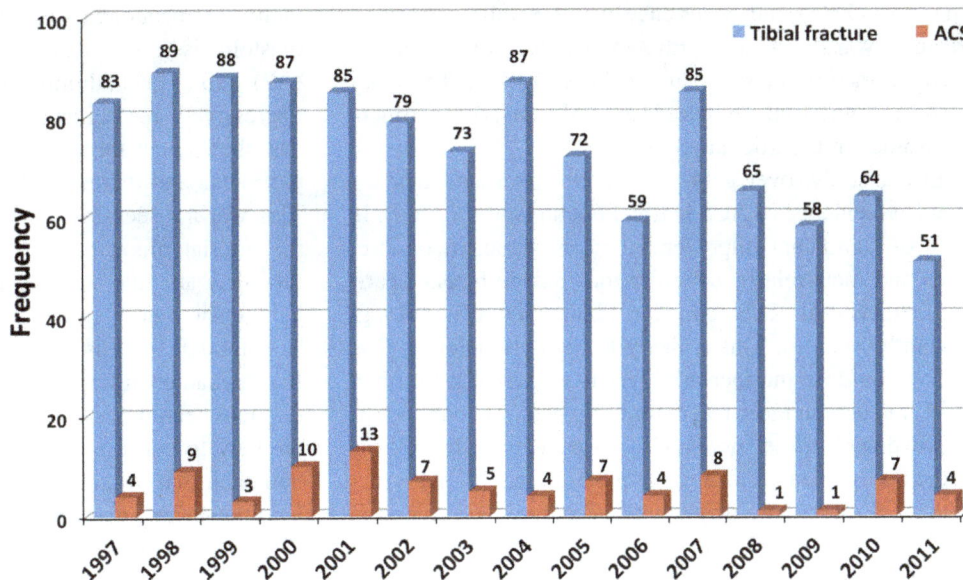

Fig. 1 Frequency distribution of tibial fractures and ACSs during the study period

The number of tibial fractures admitted to our hospital decreased over the 14-year period of observation. However, the incidence of ACS following tibial fractures did not show a significant decline (Fig. 1).

A retrospective review of the charts showed that 7 % of patients with ACS had an altered level of consciousness. The clinical features in the awake patients with ACS included increasing pain in 70 %, paresthesia in 52 %, motor weakness in 29 % and tense swelling of the calf in 1 %. Thirty-five percent of patients with ACS had pain as their only symptom, 8 % had only parasthesia, 4 % had only motor weakness and 1 % had only tense calf.

Out of 87 patients with ACS, 23 patients underwent fasciotomy at the time of fracture fixation, while 64 patients received fasciotomy as a second surgical procedure after initial fixation. The mean time interval between occurrence of tibia fracture and fasciotomy was 30.10 (±23.72) h. The mean time interval between surgical fixation of fracture and fasciotomy was 16.27 (22.58) h. The mean length of hospitalization of those patients who developed ACS was 14.88 (±11.80) days, which was higher than the mean length of hospitalization of patients who did not develop ACS (12.26 ± 10.28) and this difference was statistically significant ($P = 0.03$).

Using an intra-compartmental pressure monitoring instrument, compartment pressures were measured in 60 out of 87 patients with ACS and 92 % had an absolute reading of greater than 30 mmHg. This raised intra-compartmental pressure occurred in the anterior compartment in 87 %, lateral compartment in 35 % and posterior compartments in 37 % of cases. All patients with ACS have positive intra-operative findings.

Table 4 Summary of studies on ACS in tibial diaphyseal fractures

Author	Number of subjects	Number of ACS	Incidence (%)
DeLee (open) [38]	104	6	6
Blick SS [24]	198	18	9
McQueen (open) [33]	67	1	1.5
McQueen [23]	1,349	59	4.3
Mullett H [34]	626	17	2.7
Ogunlusi JD [39]	52	3	5.7
Park S [21]	173	14	8
Wind T [26]	626	34	5.4
This study	1,125	87	7.7

Discussion

Over the last four decades, much research has been published with regards to the pathophysiology [7–11], diagnosis [12–14], monitoring [13–15], and treatment of ACS [16–20]. However, there is little literature regarding the epidemiology of lower leg ACS and its associated risks factors [21, 22].

This epidemiological study on lower leg ACS is a retrospective cohort study, but we believe that the data quality is good, as the data was entered prospectively by the treating surgeons themselves and the data base was managed by a dedicated research staff. Our results are compared with other studies in Table 4.

Acute compartment syndrome from any cause occurs most commonly in the lower leg and most often follows a fracture of the tibia. McQueen et al. [23] reported in their epidemiological study that 36 % of all compartment syndromes occurred in association with a tibial shaft fracture.

They found that the occurrence of ACS following tibial fractures was 4.3 %. In North America, the prevalence has been reported in the range of 5.4–11 % [24–26]. There has been no other epidemiological study on compartment syndromes in a particular population.

In our study, over a 14-year period, we found that the average incidence of ACS in tibial fractures was 7.73 %. In spite of significant improvement in management of fractures and their related complications during recent years, the incidence of ACS following tibial fracture is not significantly reduced. This is likely to be multifactorial. One reason could be the increased trend to internally fix tibial shaft fractures in more recent times. In addition, continuous improvement in the survivability of patients with multiple injuries might lead to a larger number of patients surviving with ACS when they may have died before.

The popular belief is that ACS is more likely to occur in young males. In our study we found that women were just as likely as men to get ACS following their tibial fractures. However, we also found that ACS occurred more readily in younger patients. This we think is due to younger people having larger muscle bulk within a tight fascia with very little room to expand before the intra-compartmental pressure rises. Park et al. [21] also found age as a risk factor. They suggested that the young male is not only likely to have a larger muscle bulk, but the fascia and the inter-muscular septa are likely to be thicker, due to a larger collagen content. This can cause the pressure to rise rapidly within a compartment with a small increase in volume. We would agree with their hypothesis; however, we did not find a higher incidence of ACS in males. Therefore, we do not assume gender to be risk factor for ACS following tibial fracture.

Many physicians believe that high-energy trauma should be a risk factor for ACS. The perceived wisdom is that the soft tissue damage that occurs with a high energy transfer is likely to produce more necrosis, hypoxia, lactic acidosis, capillary leak and more interstitial fluid collection, leading to swelling of the compartment. However, this was not borne out in our study. This observation is similar to what Court-Brown et al. [27] reported.

There is no doubt that multiple injuries that affect a number of anatomical sites have a profound effect on the homeostasis of the body and the ensuing "chemical storm": systemic inflammatory response syndrome (SIRS) vs compensatory anti-inflammatory response syndrome (CARS) and endothelial damage is linked with occurrence of ACS [28]. However, ACS could be both one of the triggering factors for SIRS or indeed an effect of the endothelial damage and subsequent capillary leak. We assumed that those patients with a higher ISS score were more likely to get ACS. Polytrauma patients with high ISS scores are likely to be hypotensive and, theoretically, ACS

is likely to occur at a lower compartment pressure when the diastolic is lower: causing a lowered perfusion pressure (ΔP) [13]. In addition, polytrauma patients are often aggressively resuscitated with high volumes of fluid that can then enter the extravascular space in injured compartments and increases the intra-compartmental pressure. This was not seen in our study. In the study by Park et al., the arterial blood pressure of patients at admission was recorded and the authors found no correlation between hypotension and the incidence of ACS.

Although there is a risk of ACS with any type of tibia fracture, an open fracture is anecdotally considered to have de facto decompressed the compartments, and is therefore unlikely to cause an ACS. The auto decompression phenomenon that occurs with a high-grade open tibia fracture is hypothesized to cause an effect similar to a fasciotomy [23, 27]. Our study showed that ACS is just as likely to occur in open fractures as it is in closed fractures. These results are similar to those found by Park et al. [21].

We looked at the site of the fracture as a potential risk factor because the tibial shaft has various muscle attachments and varying bulk of muscle at different levels. The gastro-soleus complex is bulkier more proximally than distally. There is also less muscle and more tendinous structures more distally. If one considers that ACS can occur from bleeding alone, (as opposed to ischemic swelling), then it should be more common in more proximal fractures. In contrast, the peroneus tertius, whose muscle belly is alongside the distal third of the tibia, has a single arterial supply. It is conceivable that any fractures in the distal third of the tibia, which might damage the only blood supply to the muscle could cause ischemia, capillary leak and swelling followed by ACS. In this study, we could not show that the site of the fracture made any difference to the occurrence of ACS. Fractures that are more extensive along the length of the bone suggest a higher energy transfer. Similar to our findings for mechanism of injury, we did not find any correlation between 'extensive' fractures and ACS.

There are reports confirming a significant correlation between intramedullary nailing and ACS development [29–34]. These reports argue that: (1) the incidence of ACS in open reduction and internal fixation is likely to be lower due to the pari passu decompression of the compartment and evacuation of the fracture haematoma; (2) intramedullary nailing is known to increase the compartment pressures during reaming as well as insertion of the nail; and (3) the position of the limb during the procedure has shown to change the compartment pressures. Patients put on traction tables with traction applied to the limb during nailing have raised intra-compartmental pressures [35]. In this study we did not find a significantly higher rate of ACS development in those who were treated by intramedullary nailing, though.

Our data indicated that the length of hospital stays of patients with tibial fractures who were affected by ACS was higher than those without ACS. This finding supports previous reports of increased hospital stays up to 3 times longer in patients with ACS compared with uncomplicated tibia fractures [5]. This difference is likely due to at least two additional surgical procedures for wound closure in patients who are affected by this complication.

In our study, increasing leg pain was the main clinical symptom in patients with ACS, followed by paresthesia and motor weakness of leg muscles. Furthermore, the anterior compartment was the most involved compartment of the leg and absolute measures of intra-compartmental pressures of leg compartments were higher than 30 mmHg in 92 % of patients. These findings are in accordance with the literature [36].

There are shortcomings in this study. We did not collect data regarding some other potential risk factors such as a history of smoking prior to the injury. We were also not able to distinguish between cases of ACS that were diagnosed on the basis of a fasciotomy alone. O'Toole et al. [37] showed that within the same institution, the fasciotomy rate among surgeons varied. We did not analyse this. We also did not have records of patient consciousness levels in our data base, and hence we are unable to say whether ACS was more likely to occur in unconscious patients than conscious patients (who can complain of severe pain). However, we believe that consciousness levels are not variables that would directly influence the occurrence of ACS and therefore are not a direct risk factor.

This is one of the largest studies examining the possible risk factors that influence the occurrence of ACS in tibial diaphyseal fractures treated by surgical fixation. We found that younger patients are definitely at a significantly higher risk of ACS. Gender, mechanism of injury, Gustillo and anatomical classification, ISS and intramedullary nailing of tibial fracture did not influence ACS.

Conflict of interest None.

Ethical standards The study received institutional research ethics board approval and patients' informed consent was waived. All procedures complied with the Declaration of Helsinki.

References

1. Schmidt AH, Finkemeier CG, Tornetta P (2003) Treatment of closed tibial fractures. Instr Course Lect 52:607–622

2. Giannoudis PV, Nicolopoulos C, Dinopoulos H et al (2002) The impact of lower leg compartment syndrome on health related quality of life. Injury 33:117–121

3. Templeman D, Schmidt R, Varecka T (1993) The economic cost of missed compartment syndromes. Orthop Trans 17:989

4. Bhattacharyya T, Vrahas MS (2004) The medical-legal aspects of compartment syndrome. J Bone Joint Surg Am 86-A:864–868

5. Schmidt A (2011) The impact of compartment syndrome on hospital length of stay and charges among adult patients admitted with a fracture of the tibia. J Orthop Trauma 25:355–357

6. Gustilo RB, Anderson JT (1976) Prevention of infection in the treatment of one thousand and twenty-five open fractures of long bones: retrospective and prospective analyses. J Bone Joint Surg Am 58:453–458

7. Matsen FA 3rd, Mayo KA, Krugmire RB Jr et al (1977) A model compartmental syndrome in man with particular reference to the quantification of nerve function. J Bone Joint Surg Am 59:648–653

8. Whitesides TE, Haney TC, Morimoto K et al (1975) Tissue pressure measurements as a determinant for the need of fasciotomy. Clin Orthop Relat Res 113:43–51

9. Hargens AR, Schmidt DA, Evans KL et al (1981) Quantitation of skeletal-muscle necrosis in a model compartment syndrome. J Bone Joint Surg Am 63:631–636

10. Hargens AR, Romine JS, Sipe JC et al (1979) Peripheral nerve-conduction block by high muscle-compartment pressure. J Bone Joint Surg Am 61:192–200

11. Hargens AR, Mubarak SJ (1998) Current concepts in the pathophysiology, evaluation, and diagnosis of compartment syndrome. Hand Clin 14:371–383

12. Ulmer T (2002) The clinical diagnosis of compartment syndrome of the lower leg: are clinical findings predictive of the disorder? J Orthop Trauma 16:572–577

13. McQueen MM, Court-Brown CM (1996) Compartment monitoring in tibial fractures. The pressure threshold for decompression. J Bone Joint Surg Br 78:99–104

14. Shadgan B, Menon M, Sanders D et al (2012) Current thinking about acute compartment syndrome of the lower extremity. Can J Surg 53:329–334

15. McQueen MM, Christie J, Court-Brown CM (1996) Acute compartment syndrome in tibial diaphyseal fractures. J Bone Joint Surg Br 78:95–98

16. Ris HB, Furrer M, Stronsky S et al (1993) Four-compartment fasciotomy and venous calf-pump function: long-term results. Surgery 113:55–58

17. Mubarak SJ, Owen CA (1977) Double-incision fasciotomy of the leg for decompression in compartment syndromes. J Bone Joint Surg Am 59:184–187

18. Lagerstrom CF, Reed RL 2nd, Rowlands BJ et al (1989) Early fasciotomy for acute clinically evident posttraumatic compartment syndrome. Am J Surg 158:36–39

19. Nghiem DD, Boland JP (1980) Four-compartment fasciotomy of the lower extremity without fibulectomy: a new approach. Am Surg 46:414–417

20. Shadgan B, Menon M, O'Brien PJ et al (2008) Diagnostic techniques in acute compartment syndrome of the leg. J Orthop Trauma 22:581–587

21. Park S, Ahn J, Gee AO et al (2009) Compartment syndrome in tibial fractures. J Orthop Trauma 23:514–518

22. Frink M, Hildebrand F, Krettek C et al (2010) Compartment syndrome of the lower leg and foot. Clin Orthop Relat Res 468:940–950

23. McQueen MM, Gaston P, Court-Brown CM (2000) Acute compartment syndrome. Who is at risk? J Bone Joint Surg Br 82:200–203

24. Blick SS, Brumback RJ, Poka A et al (1986) Compartment syndrome in open tibial fractures. J Bone Joint Surg Am 68:1348–1353

25. Finkemeier CG, Schmidt AH, Kyle RF et al (2000) A prospective, randomized study of intramedullary nails inserted with and without reaming for the treatment of open and closed fractures of the tibial shaft. J Orthop Trauma 14:187–193

26. Wind TC, Saunders SM, Barfield WR et al (2012) Compartment syndrome after low-energy tibia fractures sustained during athletic competition. J Orthop Trauma 26:33–36

27. Court-Brown CM, McBirnie J (1995) The epidemiology of tibial fractures. J Bone Joint Surg Br 77:417–421

28. Keel M, Trentz O (2005) Pathophysiology of trauma. Injury 36:691–709

29. Heim D, Schlegel U, Perren SM (1993) Intramedullary pressure in reamed and unreamed nailing of the femur and tibia—an in vitro study in intact human bones. Injury 24(Suppl 3):S56–S63

30. Nassif JM, Gorczyca JT, Cole JK et al (2000) Effect of acute reamed versus unreamed intramedullary nailing on compartment pressure when treating closed tibial shaft fractures : a randomized prospective study. J Orthop Trauma 14:554–558

31. Tornetta P 3rd, French BG (1997) Compartment pressures during nonreamed tibial nailing without traction. J Orthop Trauma 11:24–27

32. Blachut PA, O'Brien PJ, Meek RN et al (1997) Interlocking intramedullary nailing with and without reaming for the treatment of closed fractures of the tibial shaft. A prospective, randomized study. J Bone Joint Surg Am 79:640–646

33. McQueen MM, Christie J, Court-Brown CM (1990) Compartment pressures after intramedullary nailing of the tibia. J Bone Joint Surg Br 72:395–397

34. Mullett H, Al-Abed K, Prasad CV et al (2001) Outcome of compartment syndrome following intramedullary nailing of tibial diaphyseal fractures. Injury 32:411–413

35. Kutty S, Laing AJ, Prasad CV et al (2005) The effect of traction on compartment pressures during intramedullary nailing of tibial shaft fractures. A prospective randomised trial. Int Orthop 29:186–190

36. Olson SA, Glasgow RR (2005) Acute compartment syndrome in lower extremity musculoskeletal trauma. J Am Acad Orthop Surg 13:436–444

37. O'Toole RV, Whitney A, Merchant N et al (2009) Variation in diagnosis of compartment syndrome by surgeons treating tibial shaft fractures. J Trauma 67:735–741

38. DeLee JC, Stiehl JB (1981) Open tibia fracture with compartment syndrome. Clin Orthop Relat Res (160):175–184

39. Ogunlusi JD, Oginni LM, Ikem IC (2005) Compartmental pressure in adults with tibial fracture. Int Orthop 29(2):130–133

5

Fracture pattern characteristics and associated injuries of high-energy, large fragment, partial articular radial head fractures: a preliminary imaging analysis

John T. Capo · Ben Shamian · Ramces Francisco ·
Virak Tan · Jared S. Preston · Linda Uko ·
Richard S. Yoon · Frank A. Liporace

Abstract

Background High-energy radial head injuries often present with a large partial articular displaced fragment with any number of surrounding injuries. The objective of the study was to determine the characteristics of large fragment, partial articular radial head fractures and determine any significant correlation with specific injury patterns.

Materials and methods Patients sustaining a radial head fracture from 2002–2010 were screened for participation. Twenty-five patients with documented partial articular radial head fractures were identified and completed the study. Our main outcome measurement was computed tomography (CT)-based analysis of the radial head fracture. The location of the radial head fracture fragment was evaluated from the axial CT scan in relation to the radial tuberosity used as a reference point. The fragment was characterized by location as anteromedial (AM), anterolateral (AL), posteromedial (PM) or posterolateral (PL) with the tuberosity referenced as straight posterior. All measurements were performed by a blinded, third party hand and upper extremity fellowship trained orthopedic surgeon. Fracture pattern, location, and size were then correlated with possible associated injuries obtained from prospective clinical data.

Results The radial head fracture fragments were most commonly within the AL quadrant (16/25; 64 %). Seven fracture fragments were in the AM quadrant and two in the PM quadrant. The fragment size averaged 42.5 % of the articular surface and spanned an average angle of 134.4°. Significant differences were noted between AM (49.5 %) and AL (40.3 %) fracture fragment size with the AM fragments being larger. Seventeen cases had associated coronoid fractures. Of the total 25 cases, 13 had fracture dislocations while 12 remained reduced following the injury. The rate of dislocation was highest in radial head fractures that involved the AM quadrant (6/7; 85.7 %) compared to the AL quadrant (7/16; 43.7 %). No dislocations were observed with PM fragments. Ten of the 13 (78 %) fracture dislocations had associated lateral collateral ligament (LCL)/medial collateral ligament tear. The most common associated injuries were coronoid fractures (68 %), dislocations (52 %), and LCL tears (44 %).

Conclusion The most common location for partial articular radial head fractures is the AL quadrant. The rate of elbow dislocation was highest in fractures involving the AM quadrant. Cases with large fragment, partial articular radial head fractures should undergo a CT scan; if associated with >30 % or >120° fracture arc, then the patient should be assessed closely for obvious or occult instability. These are key associations that hopefully greatly aid in the consultation and preoperative planning settings.

Level of evidence Diagnostic III.

Keywords Radial head fracture · Coronoid fracture · Radial head fragment · Elbow dislocation

J. T. Capo (✉)
Division of Hand Surgery, Department of Orthopaedic Surgery,
NYU Hospital for Joint Diseases, New York, NY 10009, USA
e-mail: john.capo@nyumc.org

B. Shamian · R. Francisco · V. Tan · J. S. Preston · L. Uko
Division of Hand and Microvascular Surgery, Department of
Orthopaedic Surgery, Rutgers New Jersey Medical School,
Newark, NJ, USA

R. S. Yoon · F. A. Liporace
Division of Orthopaedic Trauma, Department of Orthopaedic
Surgery, NYU Hospital for Joint Diseases, 301 E 17th Street
Suite 1402, New York, NY 10003, USA
e-mail: liporace33@gmail.com

Introduction

Radial head fractures commonly occur in the adult population and mostly affect active individuals between 20 and 60 years of age and account for one-third of all fractures of the elbow [1]. In the elbow, the radial head plays an important role as a secondary constraint during valgus stress in addition to its nearly circumferential articulation with the capitellum and the proximal radioulnar joint (PRUJ) [2, 3]. Thus, fractures of the radial head are at risk for elbow stiffness, decreased range of motion, decreased quality of life, and instability, either with or without surgery. While most minimally displaced fracture patterns are treated non-operatively and often do well, more complex fracture patterns, either with or without surgery, have produced mixed results, fueling continued controversy in this academic arena [4–6].

Proper function of the elbow joint is significantly dependent on the level of stability available along the full arc of motion. Identification of possible instability is of paramount importance in regard to operative decision making and pre-operative planning especially in regard to injuries sustained from more high-energy mechanisms. While previous studies have shown a correlation between instability of the elbow and the amount of displacement and the size of the radial head fracture, there are few reports on associated injuries, especially in regard to specific fracture location within the radial head [3, 7, 8]. Specifically, correlation between the position of the fracture fragment in the radial head and concomitant associated injuries of the elbow have not been investigated. Any associations found would prove valuable in the initial consultation and pre-operative setting in order to expect and rule out commonly associated ligamentous or soft tissue injuries that may or may not be the cause of elbow instability, especially in cases involving high-energy mechanisms. The purpose of this study was to evaluate high-energy, partial articular radial head fractures and identify any associated injuries of the elbow in reference to fracture location in the radial head. The objectives of this study were to provide radiographic pilot data for potential future correlation to operative and clinical outcomes in a larger, multi-center study setting.

Materials and methods

Between 2002 and 2010, 57 patients with documented radial head fractures seen at a level 1 trauma center were identified from the database of two attending orthopedic surgeons. Inclusion criteria for the study included acute injury, large fragment partial articular (AO/OTA 21B2) radial head fractures, high-energy mechanism (pedestrian

struck, motor vehicle accident (MVA), fall from above a standing height, etc.), skeletally mature individuals, and complete radiographic work-up including three adequate views of the elbow and computed tomography (CT) of the affected elbow. For those cases that were deemed operative, criteria included limited range of movement (ROM) secondary to block of motion or gross instability, gross instability at any point during the arc of motion, high degree of comminution, and/or >50 % radial head involvement [9, 10]. Exclusion criteria included those who sustained injuries from a gunshot wound, a low-energy fall, those without cortical contact with the radial neck/shaft, and those with incomplete clinical or radiographic medical records. Blinded, third party personnel collected demographic and operative data which was stored in a password-protected electronic database. The average age of the 25 patients was 43 years (range 19–72), with the injury involving the right side in 11 cases and the left side in 14 cases. Twenty-four cases were secondary to fall and one was due to an MVA (Table 1).

Imaging analysis

All imaging modalities were reviewed by a single fellowship-trained hand and upper extremity, attending physician (JTC). All radiographic data were de-identified prior to analysis, in an attempt to minimize bias. CT scans of the elbow with 1-mm slice thickness were evaluated for the position and size of the fracture fragment in the radial head. Of note, if involved with concurrent elbow dislocation, CT scans were obtained post-reduction and splinting. The axial cut that best revealed the largest diameter of the intact portion of the radial head and associated fracture defect was used to quantify the fracture (Fig. 1). The axial cut that best demonstrated the radial tuberosity was then used as a reference marker to determine the angular location of the fracture (Fig. 2a). The radial tuberosity, designated as the 6 o'clock position, was utilized as a bony marker that was deemed as the most consistent landmark that is least likely to change in the setting of high-energy trauma, which may obscure and change soft tissue position. These selected images were then placed in a Microsoft Powerpoint (Microsoft Corp., Redmond, WA, USA) file. A computer-generated calibrated dial was then created and used as a measurement guide (Fig. 2b). Using the radial tuberosity as a reference point, the calibrated dial was then superimposed on the CT scan cut that best depicted the radial head fracture (Fig. 2c). The radial head fractures were then quantified as an angular amount and as a range on the face of a clock. Fracture fragment anatomy was termed in a specific quadrant based on location on the clock face—fractures between the 12

Table 1 Demographic data of study cohort

Case	Age/sex	Mechanism of injury	Side affected	Associated injuries with radial head fracture	Treatment
1	37/M	Fall	Left	Radial shaft fx, elbow dislocation	ORIF (plate and screws), LCL/MCL repair
2	54/F	Fall	Right	Coronoid fx, elbow dislocation	Radial head arthroplasty, ORIF coronoid, MCL/LCL repair
3	33/M	Fall	Left	Monteggia fx	Open reduction, ORIF multiple screws
4	59/F	Fall	Right	Elbow dislocation	Hinged external fixator
5	37/M	Fall	Right	Coronoid fx	ORIF radial head with multiple screws
6	47/F	Fall	Right	Coronoid fx, LCL tear	Radial head arthroplasty, LCL repair
7	19/M	Fall	Left	Radial head fx, coronoid fx, elbow dislocation	ORIF radial head/neck fx with plate and screws, ORIF coronoid
8	46/F	Fall	Right	Elbow dislocation, distal radius fx	ORIF radial head w/plate and screws, application of external fixator, LCL repair, percutaneous pinning of distal radius fx
9	39/F	Fall	Right	Elbow dislocation	Elbow arthroscopy, LCL repair
10	28/M	Fall	Left	Coronoid fx	Manipulation under anesthesia, closed treatment
11	41/F	Fall	Left	None	Sling, early ROM
12	59/F	Fall	Left	LCL tear	ORIF radial head with multiple screws, LCL repair
13	60/F	Fall	Left	Capitellar fx, coronoid fx, chondral injury, elbow dislocation	Total elbow arthroplasty, ulnar nerve transposition
14	41/M	MVA	Right	Ulna fx, MC fx dislocation, elbow dislocation	ORIF radial head with multiple screws, LCL repair
15	53/M	Fall	Left	Elbow dislocation, scaphoid fx, distal radius fx	Radial head arthroplasty, ORIF coronoid fx, LCL repair, application of external fixator
16	39/M	Fall	Right	None	Cast
17	22/M	Fall	Left	Coronoid fx, LCL tear	Radial head arthroplasty, ORIF coronoid, LCL repair
18	33/M	Fall	Left	Capitellar fx	Radial head arthroplasty
19	58/M	Fall	Right	Elbow dislocation, coronoid fx, LCL/MCL tear	Radial head arthroplasty, ORIF coronoid, LCL/MCL repair, hinged external fixator
20	52/F	Fall	Right	LCL tear, coronoid fx	Radial head arthroplasty
21	20/M	Fall	Left	Elbow dislocation, LCL tear, coronoid fx	ORIF radial head, LCL repair
22	72/F	Fall	Left	Coronoid fx	Radial head arthroplasty
23	33/M	Fall	Left	Capitellar fx	Radial head arthroplasty
24	49/F	Fall	Right	Elbow dislocation, LCL tear	ORIF with external fixator, LCL repair
25	44/M	Fall	Left	Olecranon fx, coronoid fx	ORIF of radial head, coronoid, and olecranon

M male, *F* female, *MVA* motor vehicle accident, *fall* high-energy fall, *fx* fracture, *LCL* lateral collateral ligament, *MCL* medial collateral ligament, *MC* metacarpal, *ORIF* open reduction and internal fixation, *ROM* range of motion

o'clock and 3 o'clock position were referred to as anterolateral (AL) fragments, between 3 o'clock and 6 o'clock position as posterolateral (PL) fragments, between 6 o'clock and 9 o'clock as posteromedial (PM) fragment, and between 9 o'clock and 12 o'clock as anteromedial (AM) fragments (Fig. 3). Fracture fragments spanning two adjacent quadrants were reported based on the larger fracture fragment component, which was quantified via measurement and percentage comparison. The exact angle was measured using a picture archiving and communication systems (PACS, General Electric Company, Fairfield, CT, USA) angle measuring tool. The percent amount of articular surface involvement in the radial head, and the presence of associated elbow fractures, elbow dislocation/subluxation and other associated injuries were also noted and recorded. The percent amount of articular surface involved was estimated using computed measuring area software (Sky-Scan High-Resolution MicroCT System, Kontich, Belgium).

Statistical analysis was performed using Student's t test, and Fisher's exact test for categorical data. All statistics were analyzed via SPSS 18.0 (IBM Inc., Armonk, NY, USA); a p-value of ≤ 0.05 was considered significant.

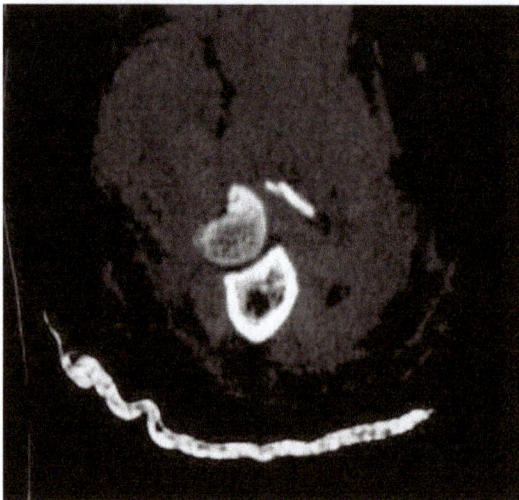

Fig. 1 CT scan of unicondylar radial head fracture. Example of an axial cut that best revealed the largest diameter of the intact portion of the radial head and associated fracture defect used to quantify the fracture

Results

Examination of the CT scans revealed fracture fragments in the AL (16), AM (7), and PM (2) quadrants. The average amount of radial head surface fractured was 42.5 % (10.8–58 %), spanning an average angle of 134.4° (65.7°–175°) from the center of the radial head. Cases with fracture dislocation (13/25) had an average radial head surface area involvement of 42.7 % while those that remained reduced (12/25) following the injury had 42.3 % ($p = 0.777$). Mean fracture fragment size of AM fractures were significantly larger than the AL and PM fragments (49.5 % vs 40.3 %; $p = 0.024$).

The incidence of dislocation among these various fracture fragments revealed that 6 out of 7 AM fragments had a dislocation (85.7 %) while only 7 of the 16 AL fragments had an associated dislocation (43.7 %; $p = 0.021$). No dislocations were observed with PM fragments. Posterior dislocations were observed in 11 cases while two had PL dislocations. Of the 23 operative cases, 11 had lateral collateral ligament (LCL) tears while 3 had combined LCL/ medial collateral ligament (MCL) tears. Of the eleven LCL tears, 7 had radial head fractures in the AL quadrant and 4 in the AM quadrant. The distribution of LCL/MCL injuries were two radial head fractures in the AM and one in the AL quadrant.

Twenty-three out of 25 cases had associated injuries. Seventeen cases had a coronoid fracture, with 12 of these cases having a type I coronoid fracture and five with a type II fracture. The group with fracture dislocations had a similar incidence of coronoid fractures (9/13; 70 %) compared to the non-dislocation group [9/12 (75 %)]. Coronoid fractures when correlated with the position of the radial

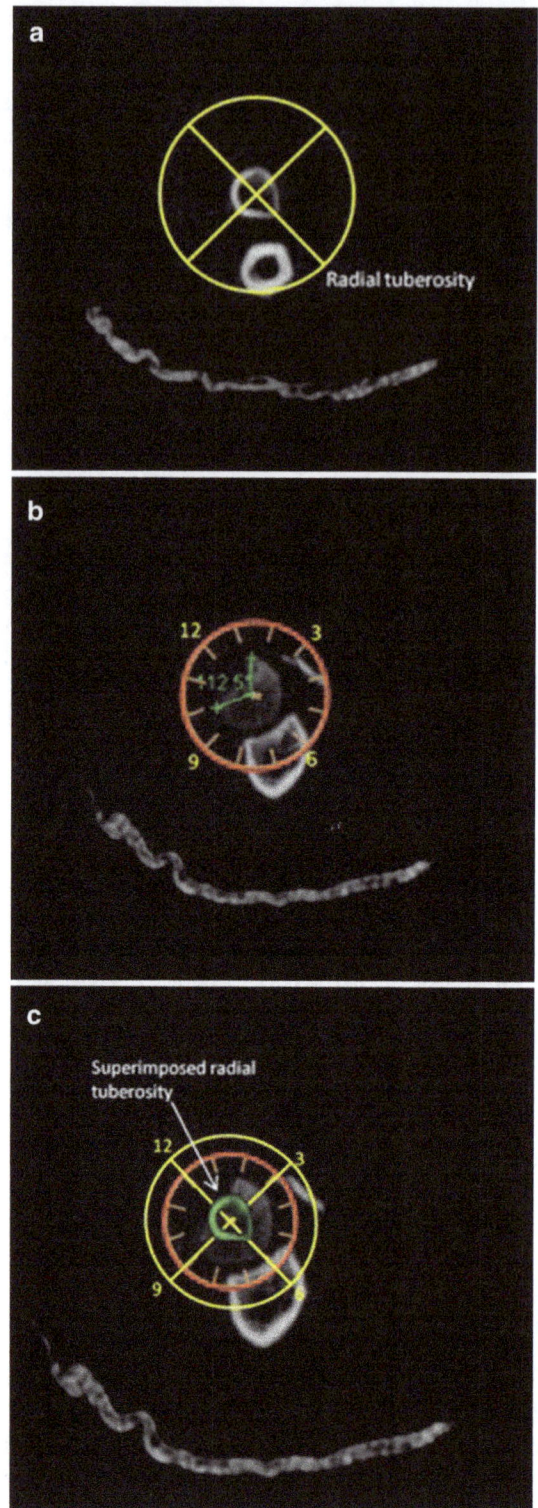

Fig. 2 a Axial CT scan best representing the radial tuberosity. **b** Axial CT scan of radial head with superimposed clock face and measured angles of missing radial head fracture. **c** Axial CT scan of radial head and superimposed radial tuberosity

head fracture fragment revealed that the highest incidence of radial head fragments were AL (12/16; 75 %) compared to AM (4/7; 57 %) and PM (1/2; 50 %) fragments. With

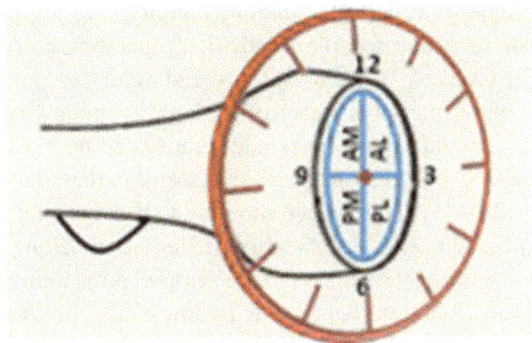

Fig. 3 Line drawing of a right radial head and tuberosity with overlaid clock face demonstrating the various locations of radial head fractures. Note that radial tuberosity is assigned as 6 o'clock. *AM* anteromedial; *AL* anterolateral; *PM* posteromedial; *PL* posterolateral

these small numbers, no statistical difference was noted between the incidence of coronoid fractures among the different fracture types—AM versus AL ($p = 0.409$), AL versus PM ($p = 0.499$), and AM versus PM ($p = 0.858$). No statistical difference was observed between the various fracture fragments and their association with LCL or MCL tears. Radial fracture fragment position, direction of dislocation and amount of surface area fractured are summarized in Table 2.

Discussion

Radial head fractures are common and may be associated with other injuries of clinical importance, especially when secondary to high-energy traumatic mechanisms. As well as the specific fracture pattern, associated humeroulnar dislocation, ligament disruption and other associated elbow fractures must be considered when evaluating fractures of the radial head. The extent of bony involvement, associated fractures and soft tissue injury helps to determine appropriate management of these complex injuries [11–13].

Kaas et al. evaluated 44 patients with 46 radial head fractures for associated soft-tissue injuries. The radial head injuries included 17 Mason type I fractures, 23 Mason type II fractures, and 6 Mason type III fractures. Using only magnetic resonance imaging (MRI), associated injuries were documented in 35 elbows—28 elbows had LCL lesions, 18 had capitellar injuries, 1 had a coronoid fracture, and 1 had an MCL injury [14]. In our series, documented injuries associated with radial head fractures were also high, exhibiting a high rate of both bony (coronoid) and soft tissue (MCL/LCL) injuries.

van Riet et al. [6] also evaluated the frequency of associated injuries in 333 radial head fractures. Two hundred and twenty-three (67 %) patients had Mason type I fractures, 46 had Mason type II (14 %) fractures, and 64

Table 2 Radial fracture fragment position, direction of dislocation and amount of surface area fractured

Case	Quadrant	Amount of articular surface fractured (%)	Arc of fracture fragment (°)	Direction of dislocation
1	AM	50.0	175	Posterior
2	AL	25.4	112.5	Posterior
3	AL	50.2	118.8	Posterior
4	AL	10.8	65.7	Posterior
5	AL	44.5	108.9	None
6	AL	40.0	131	None
7	AL	48.3	137.9	Posterolateral
8	AL	34.3	101.5	Posterolateral
9	AL	36.4	128.3	Posterior
10	AL	35.0	168.7	None
11	PM	31.7	151.5	None
12	AL	42.8	155.3	None
13	AM	42.1	146.2	Posterior
14	AM	40.7	141.2	Posterior
15	AM	55.5	126.3	Posterior
16	AL	33.3	114	None
17	PM	41.0	151.7	None
18	AM	50.2	162	None
19	AM	50.3	145	Posterior
20	AL	52.1	137.3	None
21	AM	58.1	157.6	Posterior
22	AL	50.2	167.3	None
23	AL	53.2	121.6	None
24	AL	53.2	111.2	Posterior
25	AL	35.2	124.7	None
Averages		42.5 %	134.4	

AM anteromedial, *AL* anterolateral, *PM* posteromedial, *PL* posterolateral

had Mason type III (19 %) fractures. One hundred and eighteen of 333 patients (39 %) had associated fractures or soft-tissue injury. Fifty-three (16 %) patients had coronoid fractures, and 45 patients (14 %) had elbow dislocations. Thirty-five LCL injuries (11 %), 5 MCL injuries (2 %), and 20 injuries involving both the LCL and MCL (6 %) were also reported. In the study by van Riet et al., the likelihood of associated elbow injuries increased ($p < 0.05$) with fracture severity. Additional injuries occurred in 8 % of patients with Mason type I radial head fractures (17/223 patients), in 50 % with Mason type II fractures (23/46 patients), and in 75 % with Mason type III fractures (48/64 patients). Our series revealed similar findings with the highest associated injury being coronoid fractures (68 %).

In another study by Beingessner et al. [7] the effect of radial head fracture size on radiocapitellar stability was examined. In their study, fractures were simulated in six fresh-frozen cadaveric radiocapitellar joints by sequential removal of 20° wedges from the AL aspect of each radial head until 140° of the radial head was removed. Decreased shear load at the radial head during joint loading was used as an indicator of decreased stability at the radiocapitellar joint. There was no difference in the shear load between the intact specimen and that with a 20° wedge removed ($p > 0.05$). However, stability decreased with each increase in wedge size between 20° and 120° ($p < 0.05$). Beyond 120° of wedge removal, which is one-third of the diameter of the radial head, the shear load was constantly low, indicating lower stability. They concluded that an inverse relationship exists between radiocapitellar joint stability and radial head fracture size [7]. In our series, regardless of fracture location, utilizing the aforementioned data provided by Beingessner et al., 18 fractures consisted of an arc >120°, of which 16 (89 %) were deemed unstable (i.e., concomitant dislocation, radiocapitallar instability, ligamentous injury, etc., (Tables 1, 2). While this correlation may be biased to the underpowered nature of our study, the trend is still worth noting that with a higher arc of fracture, a high incidence of concomitant instability is likely present.

In a study similar to ours, van Leeuwen investigated Mason type II fractures using 3-dimensional CT. Both studies showed fractures were most often found throughout the AL portion of the radial head. However, our study showed a wider distribution of fractures throughout the AM quadrant, whereas van Leeuwen conversely reported more patients with fractures through the AL portion. We found fractures to span a smaller arc, whereas van Leeuwen found the fractures to span 170°. van Leeuwen did not comment on injuries associated with Mason type II fractures or the percent involvement of the articular surface.

Radial head fractures can occur in isolation, or with associated ligament and bony injuries, which may further compromise elbow and forearm stability. Commonly, the amount of head involvement is used to determine the need for surgery in radial head fractures. Assessment of the size of the fragment must be combined with knowledge of associated injuries in planning appropriate treatment of these complex injuries. Associated injuries and their early knowledge may help guide treatment options that may vary from plate and screw fixation to prosthetic replacement [4, 15–18]. Furthermore, in the setting of the initial consultation, being aware of associated injuries that frequently occur has the potential to avoid missed injuries with a focus on looking for associated instability.

This study has several limitations. First and foremost, as a result of our strict inclusion and exclusion criteria, our overall number of study subjects is low and makes our study underpowered. This inhibited any type of regression analysis to notice specific trends (i.e., operative outcomes from associated fracture patterns and injuries). Furthermore, while the advantages of a single surgeon imaging analysis provides uniformity and removes some bias, lack of reliability calculations provides a scenario that may have provided lack of agreement should another observer have been possible. The aforementioned limitations along with the lack of impact on operative decision-making along with correlation with intraoperative findings also limited our study. However, the objectives of this study were to build upon the reliability findings determined by van Leeuwen et al. [19] and to provide initial preliminary data which we hope to utilize in a prospective, large-scale, multi-center study that will provide the ability to perform regression and obtain operative decision-making capacity and intraoperative correlation. Definitive assessment on a larger scale will provide important data, and this initial data provided here is the first step.

The findings in our study are consistent with the often-mentioned fact that the AL portion is the most common location of a high-energy, large fragment, partial articular radial head fracture. CT scans should be obtained and fractures associated with a >30 % or >120° fracture arc should be analyzed closely for occult or obvious instability. The most common associated injuries in our study include coronoid fractures, elbow dislocation and LCL tears. The size of an AM fragment was on average larger than an AL fragment. In addition, AM fractures had a higher association with elbow dislocation than AL fractures of the radial head. A better understanding of the characteristics of these unicondylar radial head fractures may assist in improved treatment of these injuries. Finally, knowledge of associated injuries will be valuable in the consultation setting, with a focus on not missing these crucially concomitant injuries of the elbow. Our objective is to utilize this preliminary data as the foundation for a larger, multi-center prospective study with intraoperative correlation to further assess and definitively determine associated fractures and instability patterns.

Conflict of interest None.

Ethical standards This study was authorized by the local ethical committee and was performed in accordance with the ethical standards of the 1964 Declaration of Helsinki as revised in 2000. Written informed consent was taken from all the patients prior to study execution.

References

1. Kaas L, van Riet RP, Vroemen JP, Eygendaal D (2010) The epidemiology of radial head fractures. J Shoulder Elbow Surg 19:520–523

2. Alcid JG, Ahmad CS, Lee TQ (2004) Elbow anatomy and structural biomechanics. Clin Sports Med 23:503–517 vii

3. Morrey BF, Tanaka S, An KN (1991) Valgus stability of the elbow. A definition of primary and secondary constraints. Clin Orthop Relat Res 265:187–195

4. Hotchkiss RN (1997) Displaced fractures of the radial head: internal fixation or excision? J Am Acad Orthop Surg 5:1–10

5. Rosenblatt Y, Athwal GS, Faber KJ (2008) Current recommendations for the treatment of radial head fractures. Orthop Clin North Am 39:173–185 vi

6. van Riet RP, Morrey BF, O'Driscoll SW, Van Glabbeek F (2005) Associated injuries complicating radial head fractures: a demographic study. Clin Orthop Relat Res 441:351–355

7. Beingessner DM, Dunning CE, Beingessner CJ, Johnson JA, King GJ (2003) The effect of radial head fracture size on radiocapitellar joint stability. Clin Biomech (Bristol, Avon) 18:677–681

8. Rineer CA, Guitton TG, Ring D (2010) Radial head fractures: loss of cortical contact is associated with concomitant fracture or dislocation. J Shoulder Elbow Surg 19:21–25

9. Ring D, Quintero J, Jupiter JB (2002) Open reduction and internal fixation of fractures of the radial head. J Bone Joint Surg Am 84(A):1811–1815

10. Duckworth AD, McQueen MM, Ring D (2013) Fractures of the radial head. Bone Joint J 95(B):151–159

11. Johnston GW (1962) A follow-up of one hundred cases of fracture of the head of the radius with a review of the literature. Ulster Med J 31:51–56

12. Katz MA, Beredjiklian PK, Bozentka DJ, Steinberg DR (2001) Computed tomography scanning of intra-articular distal radius fractures: does it influence treatment? J Hand Surg Am 26:415–421

13. Mason ML (1954) Some observations on fractures of the head of the radius with a review of one hundred cases. Br J Surg 42:123–132

14. Kaas L, Turkenburg JL, van Riet RP, Vroemen JP, Eygendaal D (2010) Magnetic resonance imaging findings in 46 elbows with a radial head fracture. Acta Orthop 81:373–376

15. Clembosky G, Boretto JG (2009) Open reduction and internal fixation versus prosthetic replacement for complex fractures of the radial head. J Hand Surg Am 34:1120–1123

16. Guitton TG, van der Werf HJ, Ring D (2010) Quantitative three-dimensional computed tomography measurement of radial head fractures. J Shoulder Elbow Surg 19:973–977

17. Guitton TG, van der Werf HJ, Ring D (2010) Quantitative measurements of the volume and surface area of the radial head. J Hand Surg Am 35:457–463

18. Ikeda M, Sugiyama K, Kang C, Takagaki T, Oka Y (2005) Comminuted fractures of the radial head. Comparison of resection and internal fixation. J Bone Joint Surg Am 87:76–84

19. van Leeuwen DH, Guitton TG, Lambers K, Ring D (2012) Quantitative measurement of radial head fracture location. J Shoulder Elbow Surg 21:1013–1017

6

Outcomes of dual-mobility acetabular cup for instability in primary and revision total hip arthroplasty

Riazuddin Mohammed · Keith Hayward ·
Sanjay Mulay · Frank Bindi · Murray Wallace

Abstract

Background The concept of a dual-mobility hip socket involves the standard femoral head component encased in a larger polyethylene liner, which in turn articulates inside a metal shell implanted in the native acetabulum. The aim of this study was to assess outcomes from using a Serf Novae® Dual Mobility Acetabular cup (Orthodynamics Ltd, Gloucestershire, UK) to address the problem of instability in primary and revision total hip arthroplasty (THA).

Materials and methods A retrospective review was carried out of all hip arthroplasties performed in a District General Hospital utilising the dual-mobility socket from January 2007 to December 2012. Clinical and radiological outcomes were analysed for 44 hips in 41 patients, comprising 20 primary and 24 revision THA. The average age of the study group was 70.8 years (range 56–84 years) for primary and 76.4 years (range 56–89 years) for revision arthroplasty. Among the primary THA, always performed for hip osteoarthritis or in presence of osteoarthritic changes, the reasons to choose a dual mobility cup were central nervous system problems such as Parkinson's disease, stroke, dementia (10), hip fracture (5), failed hip fracture fixation (2), severe fixed hip deformity (2) and diffuse peripheral neuropathy (1). The indications for revisions were recurrent dislocation (17), aseptic loosening with abductor deficiency (4), failed hemiarthroplasty with abductor deficiency (2) and neglected dislocation (1).

Results At a mean follow-up of 22 months (range 6–63 months), none of the hips had any dislocation, instability or infection and no further surgical intervention was required. Radiological assessment showed that one uncemented socket in a revision arthroplasty performed for recurrent dislocation had changed position, but was stable in the new position. The patient did not have complications from this and did not need any surgical intervention.

Conclusions Even though postoperative hip stability depends on several factors other than design-related ones, our study shows promising early results for reducing the risk of instability in this challenging group of patients undergoing primary and revision hip arthroplasty.

Level of evidence IV.

Keywords Hip arthroplasty · Dislocation · Instability · Dual-mobility socket

Introduction

Total hip arthroplasty (THA) is a very successful surgical intervention for advanced arthritis, but is a surgical challenge in patients with compromised abductor mechanism or systemic conditions that make them more prone to instability. Revision THA for recurrent dislocation is a significant challenge for both the patient and the surgeon to manage. Numerous surgical and patient-related factors have been implicated in the aetiology of prosthetic dislocation [1]. Various surgical options in dealing with instability include constrained liners, liner augments, trochanteric advancement, large-diameter prosthetic heads and dual articular sockets.

R. Mohammed (✉)
Wrightington Hospital, Appley Bridge, Wigan WN6 9EP, UK
e-mail: riaz22@hotmail.co.uk

K. Hayward · S. Mulay · F. Bindi · M. Wallace
Queens Hospital, Burton Hospitals NHS Foundation Trust,
Burton on Trent DE13 0RB, UK

The concept of a dual-mobility hip socket involves the standard femoral head component captured in a larger polyethylene liner, which in turn articulates inside a metal shell implanted in the native acetabulum. This large-diameter articulation increases the primary arc range and the lever range, thereby improving the range of movement and the stability. The aim of this study was to analyse the complications and outcomes of the Serf Novae® Dual Mobility Acetabular cup (Orthodynamics Ltd, Gloucestershire, UK) used to address the problem of instability in primary and revision THA (Fig. 1a, b).

Materials and methods

A retrospective review was carried out of all hip replacements performed from January 2007 to December 2012 in a District General Hospital in the United Kingdom utilising a dual-mobility socket. Patients were identified from the theatre database and their clinical data together with follow-up radiographs were analysed. All the procedures were performed under antibiotic prophylaxis and in a laminar flow operating theatre by experienced hip arthroplasty consultants. Depending on the surgeon's preference, a modified lateral approach or a posterior approach to the hip joint was used (Fig. 2a–c). All patients received prophylactic intravenous antibiotics for 24 h postoperatively. Venous thromboprophylaxis was with low-molecular-weight heparin in the hospital and discharge with rivaroxaban for 5 weeks. This regimen is based on a standardised departmental policy and is based on the guidelines issued by the National Institute for Health and Care Excellence, UK.

Standard postoperative rehabilitation as for any THA was followed. Patients were followed up at 6 weeks, 6 months, 1 year and then 3 yearly after the THA. Data was collected regarding patient demographics, indications for arthroplasty, complications and implant survival.

Primary outcome measures analysed the incidence of dislocation and the necessity for any surgical intervention

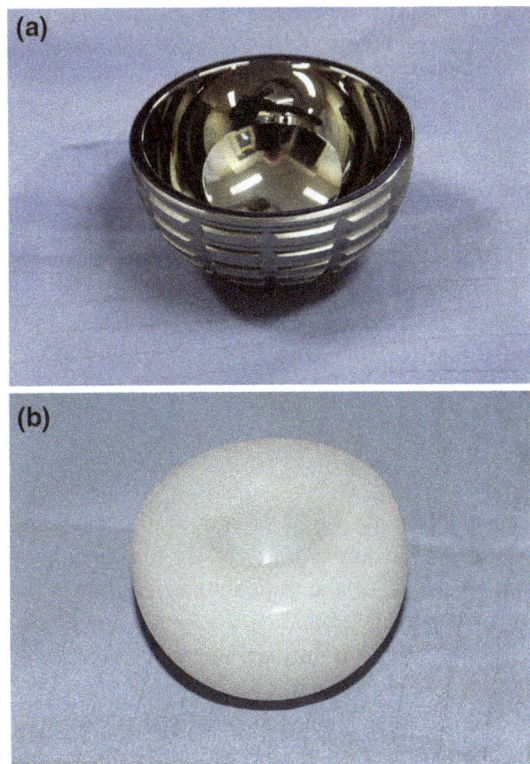

Fig. 1 a, b Serf Novae® Dual Mobility uncemented acetabular socket components

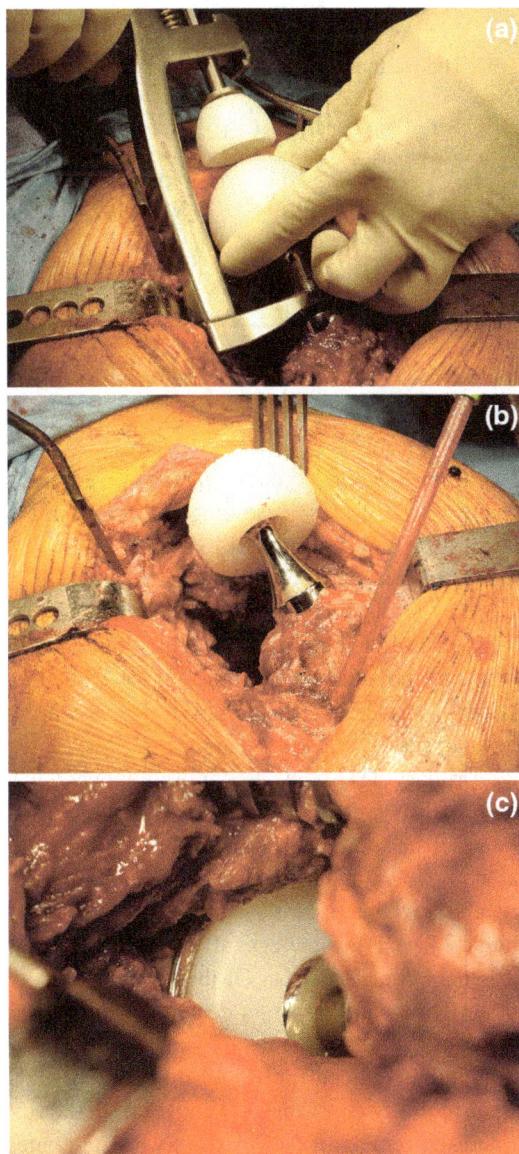

Fig. 2 a, b, c Intra-operative clinical photographs of socket-only revision being performed

Table 1 Details of patients included in the study

	Primary THA	Revision THA
Number of hips	20	24
Number of patients	17	24
Mean age in years (range)	70.8 years (56–84)	76.4 years (56–89)
Gender (M/F)	8/9	7/17
Right side/ left side	9/11	12/12
Indications for dual mobility socket use:		
	Central nervous system problems such as Parkinson's disease, stroke, dementia: 10	Recurrent dislocation: 17
	Hip fracture: 5	Aseptic loosening with abductor deficiency: 4
	Failed hip fracture fixation: 2	Failed hemiarthroplasty with abductor deficiency: 2
	Severe fixed hip deformity: 2	Neglected dislocation: 1
	Diffuse peripheral neuropathy: 1	

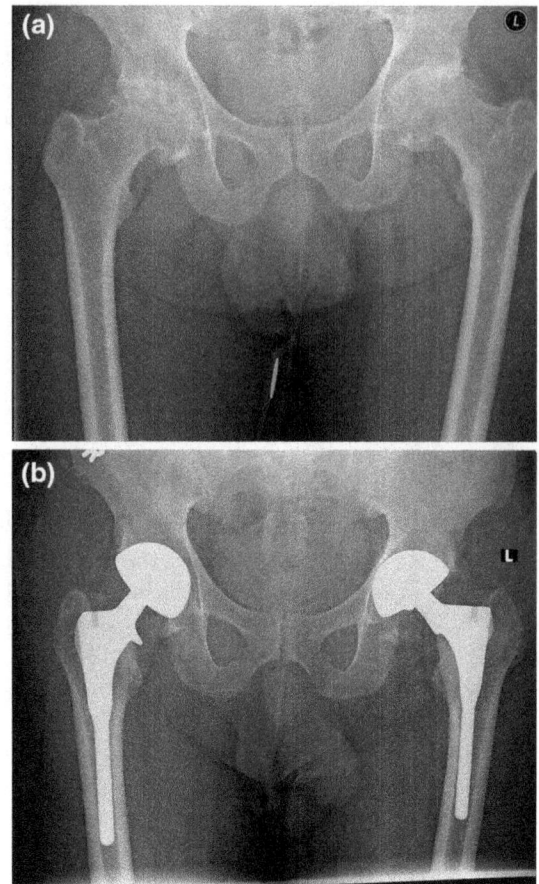

Fig. 3 a, b Pre- and post operative radiographs of staged bilateral dual-mobility socket primary THA in a 73-year-old male with severe Parkinson's disease

for dislocation. Secondary end-points included infection, peri-prosthetic fractures, radiological assessment of implant position and evidence of loosening.

Five patients were lost to follow-up. Two patients who underwent arthroplasty for proximal femur fracture died within 6 weeks after the procedure. Three patients did not attend the first post-discharge clinic. In total, 44 hips (20 primary and 24 revision THAs) in 41 patients were available for analysis.

In the primary THAs, the femoral component was un-cemented hydroxyapatite-coated modular titanium alloy stem in 8 hips and a polished double-tapered cemented femoral component in 12 hips. The mean time between primary and revision arthroplasty was 12.8 years (range 10 months–23 years). Nineteen of the 24 revision THAs involved socket-only revision. Of the five hips undergoing full revision, two hips had an un-cemented hydroxyapatite-coated modular titanium alloy stem and three had a polished double-tapered cemented femoral component. Seven of the dual-mobility cups were cemented (all in the revision group) and the remainder were hydroxyapatite-coated un-cemented cups. The details of the patient groups, indications and component sizes are depicted in Table 1.

Primary THA was performed in five patients leading active lifestyles with fracture of the neck of femur, who had coexistent arthritis in the hip. In two patients with failed internal fixation for proximal femur fracture and whose hip joints had secondary osteorthritis, primary THA with dual-mobility socket was performed to address potential instability, as would be anticipated in a hip fracture scenario.

Results

At a mean follow-up of 22 months (range 6–63 months) there were no dislocations in any of the hips in either group (Fig. 3a, b). None of the patients had any other complications such as infection, neuro-vascular injury or peri-prosthetic fracture. No further surgical intervention was required for any patient.

Radiological assessment showed that 42 hips (95 %) had an abduction angle in the acceptable range of 35°–50°. Anteversion was much more difficult to measure as the radiographs were not standardised. One uncemented socket in the revision group performed for recurrent dislocation had changed position at the 6-month review, but was stable in the new position (Fig. 4a–c). The patient did not have any complications from this and no intervention was necessary. No other radiographic complications were noted in any of the remaining acetabular components.

Discussion

The dual-mobility concept in THA was developed in the 1970s by Gilles Bousquet and André Rambert from France. The idea was to combine the "low-friction arthroplasty" principle of Charnley together with the advantage of a big femoral head principle of MacKee. The initial design of the cup had tripod fixation points on the rim of the shell along with an alumina ceramic outer coating. The newer-generation sockets have a dual-layer hydroxyapatite and alumina ceramic coating to enhance bony in-growth [2]. The shell is hemispherical with 0.5-mm polar effacement for better seating in the native acetabulum. The polyethylene insert is modified with a chamfer margin to reduce impingement on the neck of the femur prosthesis.

The Serf Novae® Dual Mobility Acetabular cup (Orthodynamics Ltd, Gloucestershire, UK) has the advantages of increased range of movement (up to 186°), better coaptation between the components and less stress on the bone implant interface, and is available in a range of sizes (43–69 mm for un-cemented, 43–63 mm for cemented fixation) and has options for cemented, cementless or reconstructive surgery. It can be used with either a 22.25-mm or a 28-mm femoral head.

One of the potential disadvantages levelled against dual-mobility articulation is the theoretical increased risk of polyethylene wear, because both the concave and convex surfaces of the polyethylene liner articulate with the metal components. However, a retrieval analysis study of 40 dual-mobility sockets showed that both the mean total wear (the sum of the wear on the convex and concave surfaces) as well as the mean annual total wear volume of the polyethylene liner was not more than that for conventional metal–polyethylene bearings [3].

A unique complication of the dual-mobility socket is intra-prosthetic dislocation (IPD) [4]. In this scenario, the femoral head dislodges from the mobile polyethylene liner. The metal head can then articulate with the metal socket, leading to devastating complications, including severe metallosis [5]. We did not encounter IPD in our series, probably because this complication is usually seen in the medium term, at about 8–10 years or more after the THA.

The indication for using a dual-mobility socket was quite varied in our series of patients and it was chosen for

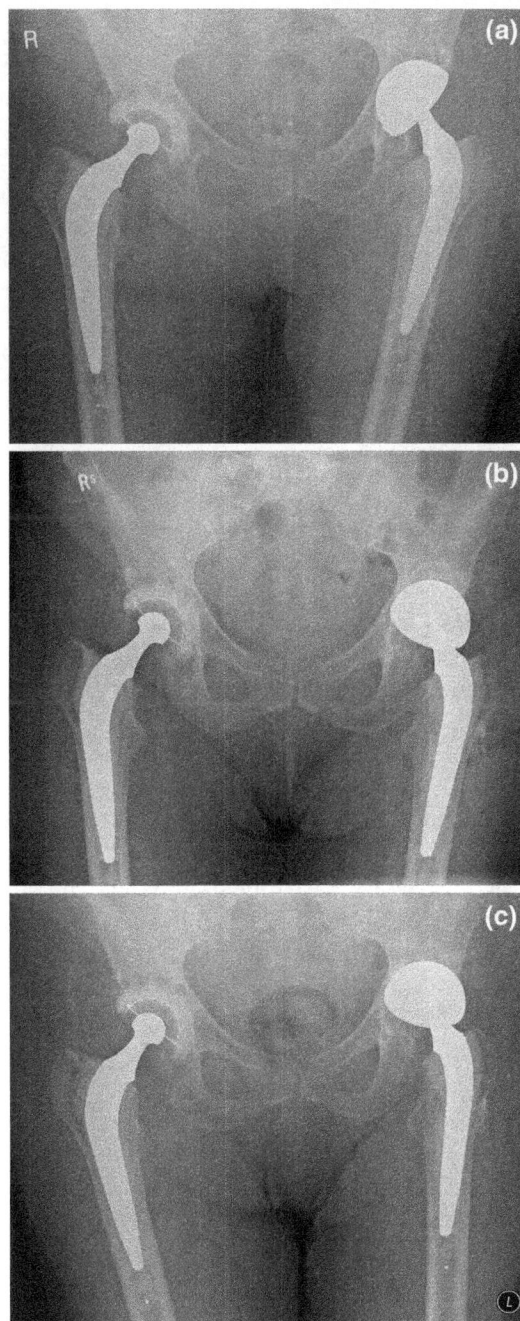

Fig. 4 a Immediate postoperative radiograph of an 86-year-old female's revision THA for recurrent dislocation showing satisfactory socket position. **b** 6 months postoperative radiographs depicting change in the socket orientation. **c** Radiograph at 30 months postoperative period with no further change in cup position

primary THA if the patient was deemed to have a higher risk of dislocation, supported by pre-operative clinical examination findings, or if an intra-operative query arose about potential instability. In the revision scenario, dual-mobility cups were used for established instability with or without aseptic loosening of the socket. The success of the socket in preventing dislocation in our series is in keeping with its versatility in various indications like hip trauma, primary hip arthroplasty and revision THA [6–8].

In our series, none of the patients had any subsequent instability or further surgical intervention. Similar short-term follow-up published evidence also supports very low dislocation rates and excellent implant survival rates [9–11]. Ten patients in our cohort had the procedure through a posterior approach to the hip joint. Studies have shown that meticulous surgical technique with careful soft tissue repair is essential to avoid instability, irrespective of the approach used [12].

Our study supports the concept of dual-mobility acetabular components in preventing the risk of dislocation for both revision THA, where instability is the main or associated reason for revision, and also in primary THA, where the dislocation can be a potential problem. The hip arthroplasty load in our centre is approximately 300–350 primary THAs and 10 revision THAs per year. The dual-mobility socket is currently the implant of choice and the only implant used in our unit in this challenging group of patients.

It is interesting that our cohort of 24 revision THAs included 19 hips with acetabular component-only revision. Revision involving the socket only can be utilised if the femoral component is well fixed and in satisfactory alignment, and thereby not a contributor to the instability. Civinini et al. [13] have shown that at 3-year mean follow-up, dual-mobility cups reduce dislocation for isolated acetabular revisions, without increased risk of loosening. Though limited by small numbers and short follow-up, our data show that one component-only revision can be successful in the management of prosthetic hip instability, thereby avoiding the complications of major revision hip surgery.

Our study is limited by being a retrospective series with a small number of patients and short follow-up. However, the study is an independent series from a heterogeneous district hospital setting outside mainland Europe.

Even though prosthetic hip stability depends on many factors other than the implant-related ones, the good results shown in our study reinforce the excellent outcomes reported in the literature, in both primary and revision THA, for the efficacy of dual-mobility cups in managing hip dislocation.

Acknowledgments The authors wish to acknowledge Paul D. Siney, Senior Research Fellow, The John Charnley Research Institute, Wrightington Hospital, Wigan, for help in the final preparation of the manuscript.

Conflict of interest None.

Ethical standards (1) The patients have given their informed consent prior to being included in the study; (2) the study was authorized by the local ethical committee as part of the Clinical Effectiveness & Audit Department (Registered number 2240) and was performed in accordance with the ethical standards of the 1964 Declaration of Helsinki as revised in 2000.

References

1. Hailer NP, Weiss RJ, Stark A, Kärrholm J (2012) The risk of revision due to dislocation after total hip arthroplasty depends on surgical approach, femoral head size, sex, and primary diagnosis. An analysis of 78,098 operations in the Swedish Hip Arthroplasty Register. Acta Orthop 83(5):442–448. doi:10.3109/17453674.2012.733919
2. Vielpeau C, Lebel B, Ardouin L, Burdin G, Lautridou C (2011) The dual mobility socket concept: experience with 668 cases. Int Orthop 35(2):225–230. doi:10.1007/s00264-010-1156-8
3. Adam P, Farizon F, Fessy MH. (2014) Dual mobility retentive acetabular liners and wear: surface analysis of 40 retrieved polyethylene implants. Orthop Traumatol Surg Res 18. doi: 10.1016/j.otsr.2013.12.011. [Epub ahead of print]
4. Philippot R, Boyer B, Farizon F (2013) Intraprosthetic dislocation: a specific complication of the dual-mobility system. Clin Orthop Relat Res 471(3):965–970. doi:10.1007/s11999-012-2639-2
5. Mohammed R, Cnudde P (2012) Severe metallosis owing to intraprosthetic dislocation in a failed dual-mobility cup primary total hip arthroplasty. J Arthroplast 27(3):e1–e3. doi:10.1016/j.arth.2010.11.019
6. Adam P, Philippe R, Ehlinger M, Roche O, Bonnomet F, Molé D, Fessy MH, French Society of Orthopaedic Surgery and Traumatology (SoFCOT) (2012) Dual mobility cups hip arthroplasty as a treatment for displaced fracture of the femoral neck in the elderly. A prospective, systematic, multicenter study with specific focus on postoperative dislocation. Orthop Traumatol Surg Res 98(3):296–300. doi:10.1016/j.otsr.2012.01.005
7. Combes A, Migaud H, Girard J, Duhamel A, Fessy MH (2013) Low rate of dislocation of dual-mobility cups in primary total hip arthroplasty. Clin Orthop Relat Res 471(12):3891–3900. doi:10.1007/s11999-013-2929-3
8. Langlais FL, Ropars M, Gaucher F, Musset T, Chaix O (2008) Dual mobility cemented cups have low dislocation rates in THA revisions. Clin Orthop Relat Res 466(2):389–395. doi:10.1007/s11999-007-0047-9
9. Tarasevicius S, Busevicius M, Robertsson O, Wingstrand H (2012) Dual mobility cup reduces dislocation rate after arthroplasty for femoral neck fracture. BMC Musculoskelet Disord 6(11):175
10. Hamadouche M, Biau DJ, Huten D, Musset T, Gaucher F (2010) The use of a cemented dual mobility socket to treat recurrent dislocation. Clin Orthop Relat Res 468(12):3248–3254. doi:10.1186/1471-2474-11-175
11. Guyen O, Pibarot V, Vaz G, Chevillotte C, Béjui-Hugues J (2009) Use of a dual mobility socket to manage total hip arthroplasty instability. Clin Orthop Relat Res 467(2):465–472. doi:10.1007/s11999-008-0476-0
12. Kwon MS, Kuskowski M, Mulhall KJ, Macaulay W, Brown TE, Saleh KJ (2006) Does surgical approach affect total hip arthroplasty dislocation rates? Clin Orthop Relat Res 447(6):34–38
13. Civinini R, Carulli C, Matassi F, Nistri L, Innocenti M (2012) A dual-mobility cup reduces risk of dislocation in isolated acetabular revisions. Clin Orthop Relat Res 470(12):3542–3548. doi:10.1007/s11999-012-2428-y

7

Hydroxyapatite and demineralized calf fetal growth plate effects on bone healing in rabbit model

Amin Bigham-Sadegh · Iraj Karimi ·
Mohamad Shadkhast · Mohamad-Hosein Mahdavi

Abstract

Background Synthetic hydroxyapatite (HA), beta-tricalcium phosphate (β-TCP) and their composite are promising biomaterials, specifically in the orthopedic and dental fields, as their chemical composition is similar to that of bone. Due to the need for safer bone graft applications, these bone graft substitutes are gradually gaining increased acceptability. To stimulate the process of bone healing, several methods have been used previously, including ultrasound, electrical stimulation, exposure to electromagnetic fields, bone grafts, interporous hydroxyapatite (as a bone graft substitute) and bone growth factors. The following study was designed to evaluate the effects of the concurrent usage of hydroxyapatite with demineralized calf fetal growth plate (DCFGP) on the bone healing process.

Materials and methods Fifteen female New Zealand white rabbits were used in this study. A mid-radius bone defect was created and in the first group ($n = 5$) was filled with hydroxyapatite, in the second group ($n = 5$) with hydroxyapatite and DCFGP, and finally in the third group ($n = 5$) with DCFGP alone. Radiological and histopathological evaluations were performed blindly and the results scored and analyzed statistically.

Results There was a significant difference for bone formation and remodeling at the 8th post-operative week radiographic assessment ($P < 0.05$), when the hydroxyapatite–DCFGP group was superior to other groups. On the contrary, macroscopical and histopathological evaluation did not revealed significant differences between the three groups

Conclusion Given the contrasting results of the radiographic assessment and the macro-/microscopic analysis of the healing response, further studies are needed before considering DCFGP-HA as a feasible alternative to HA alone, especially considering the potential hazards and costs of animal-derived biomaterials.

Level of evidence Not applicable.

Keywords Hydroxyapatite · Demineralized calf fetal growth plate · Bone healing · Rabbit

A. Bigham-Sadegh (✉)
Department of Veterinary Surgery and Radiology, Faculty of Veterinary Medicine, School of Veterinary Medicine, Shahrekord University, Shahrekord, Iran
e-mail: dr.bigham@gmail.com

I. Karimi
Veterinary Pathology, School of Veterinary Medicine, Shahrekord University, Shahrekord, Iran

M. Shadkhast
Veterinary Histology, School of Veterinary Medicine, Shahrekord University, Shahrekord, Iran

M.-H. Mahdavi
School of Veterinary Medicine, Shahrekord University, Shahrekord, Iran

Introduction

There is a continuing search for bone substitutes to avoid or minimize the need for autogenous bone grafts. The use of bone grafts in the management of nonunion cases is well accepted. These grafts act as scaffolds which provide the necessary biomechanical strength that is required to withstand the compressive forces involved during motion. They also promote the ingrowth of cells and other biological products, which eventually leads to the replacement of these grafts by bioactive tissues [1]. Autografts are most widely used by surgeons. These grafts contain viable cells such as bone marrow osteoprogenitor cells, a collagenous matrix and noncollagenous extracellular growth and differentiating factors. Consequently, the autograft is the pre-eminent therapy for bone repair, because it is capable of osteogenesis, osteoinduction and osteoconduction. However, a number of disadvantages such as morbidity in the donor site, the need for general anesthesia or sedation, and the occasional need for more than one surgical field have previously been described in the application of autografts. In addition, graft survival is unpredictable, its resorption cannot be foretold and its availability is limited [2, 3]. It is for these reasons that in recent years several biocompatible materials have emerged as substitutes for autologous bone. Biocompatible materials can be classified into two major organic and synthetic groups. Biological biomaterials can be allogeneic or homologous (human cortical bone and demineralized bone matrix or demineralized freeze-dried), heterologous or xenogeneic (organic bovine, porcine, caprine or coral-derived hydroxyapatite) and replicating (bone morphogenetic proteins; BMPs) [4]. Of the synthetic biomaterial applications of artificial or synthetic hydroxy-apatite, bioglasses and bioceramics are more common in orthopedic surgery [5].

Recently, BMPs have been used in clinical trials to enhance bone healing properties [6–8]. It has been stated that BMPs are able to stimulate local undifferentiated mesenchymal cells to transform into osteoblasts (osteoinduction), and lead to early bone formation [9–12]. More study is still necessary to identify which BMPs have higher osteoinductive properties and are more efficient in clinical application. Based on the recent literature, it seems that bone tissue engineering is the newest option for promoting and accelerating the healing potential of bone defects [13]. In bone tissue engineering, it is possible to combine synthetic scaffolds with biological biomaterials to stimulate cell infiltration and new bone formation and to enhance the healing process. In this regard, gene therapy (transfer of genes that code growth factors such as BMPs to target cells with the help of a plasmid or viral vector) may provide promising results, although concerns over trans-infection of the target cells with the gene are an unresolved issue [14–17].

Stem cells such as adipose-derived stem cells (ASCs) can differentiate into the osteogenic lineage. Furthermore, osteoid matrix formation has been observed when osteo-induced human ASCs were seeded onto hydroxyapatite/tricalcium phosphate scaffolds and implanted subcutaneously in nude mice [18]. Cowan et al. [19] demonstrated that osteo-induced ASCs along with the apatite-coated polylactic-coglycolic acid scaffold could repair a critical-sized calvarial defect of a mouse model. Meanwhile, Dudas et al. [20] showed that ASCs in combination with gelatin gel could repair a non-critical-sized defect in a rabbit

model with a follow-up of 6 weeks. All these results indicate that ASCs could be an alternative cell source for bone engineering [21].

Hydroxyapatite, a crystalline phase of calcium phosphate found naturally in bone minerals, has shown tremendous promise as a graft material. It exhibits initial mechanical rigidity and structure, and demonstrates osteoconductive as well as angiogenic properties in vivo [22]. Additionally, fabricated porous hydroxyapatite scaffolds have been reported to promote a strong mechanical inter-lock with the host bone tissue [22, 23]. Since the extent of bony ingrowth within the scaffold, the functionality of newly regenerated bone tissue, and the development of a vascularized network within the scaffold are dictated by the porous scaffold architecture, extensive studies have been performed to optimize new biomaterials needed for maximal bone tissue integration [24, 25].

The presence of transforming growth factor β (TGF-β) in growth plate [26] and BMPs 2 and 7 in human and rat fetal growth plate have been identified previously [27]. These proteins promote the chondroblastic differentiation of mesenchymal cells, followed by new bone synthesis by endochondral osteogenesis [28, 29]. A previous study proved that segmental bovine growth plate grafting has potential osteoinductive properties [30]. More recently, another study showed ectopic osteoinductive properties of calf fetal growth plate in a rat sub-muscular model [31] and bone healing enhancement in a rabbit bone defect model [32]. The present study was designed to evaluate the bone healing properties of demineralized calf fetal growth plate concurrent with hydroxyapatite in a critical-sized bone defect experimental rabbit model.

Materials and methods

Fifteen New Zealand white rabbits (12 months old, mixed sex, weighing 2.0 ± 0.5 kg) were kept in separate cages, fed a standard diet and allowed to move freely during the study. The animals were randomly divided into three equal groups: DCFGP group ($n = 5$), hydroxyapatite–DCFGP group ($n = 5$) and hydroxyapatite group ($n = 5$ group). All the animals were anesthetized by intramuscular administration of 40 mg/kg ketamine hydrochloride and 5 mg/kg xylazine. The right forelimb of all animals was prepared aseptically for operation. A 5-cm incision was made craniomedially in the skin of the forelimb and the radius was exposed by dissecting the surrounding muscles. An osteoperiosteal segmental defect was then created on the middle portion of each radius at least twice as long as the diameter of the diaphysis, for creation of a nonunion model [33]. As the diameter of the radius of the adult New Zealand albino rabbit is about 5–6 mm, the radial defect was

Table 1 Modified Lane and Sandhu radiological scoring system

Bone formation	
No evidence of bone formation	0
Bone formation occupying 25 % of the defect	1
Bone formation occupying 50 % of the defect	2
Bone formation occupying 75 % of the defect	3
Bone formation occupying 100 % of the defect	4
Union (proximal and distal evaluated separately)	
No union	0
Possible union	1
Radiographic union	2
Remodeling	
No evidence of remodeling	0
Remodeling of medullary canal	1
Full remodeling of cortex	2
Total points possible per category	
Bone formation	4
Proximal union	2
Distal union	2
Remodeling	2
Maximum score	10

10–12 mm long. Therefore, an approximately 10-mm segmental defect was created in the middle portion of each radius as a critical-sized bone defect. The defect in the animals in the hydroxyapatite group was filled with 1 mg of hydroxyapatite segments (OS Satura®, Isotis Co, Netherlands). In the hydroxyapatite–DCFGP group the bone defect was filled with 0.5 mg of hydroxyapatite segments and 0.5 mg of DCFGP powder, while the defects in the animals in the DCFGP group were filled with 1 mg of DCFGP powder. The animals were housed in compliance with our institution's guiding principles "on the care and use of animals". The local Ethics Committee for animal experiments approved the design of the experiment.

A 6-month old bovine fetus was collected from the local slaughter house. Metacarpal bones were dissected aseptically from the fetal calf (Holstein) and all soft tissues were removed. Radiographs were taken to determine the growth plate's margins and limitations. With an oscillating osteotome, proximal and distal growth plates were cut and retrieved under aseptic conditions. The retrieved growth plate was then sliced. The demineralization process was performed as described by Reddi and Huggins [34]. The harvested growth plates were cleaned of soft tissue and marrow, washed in sterile distilled water with continuous stirring, then washed three times in 95 % ethanol for 15 min, rinsed in ether for 15 min, and finally air-dried overnight. The cleaned and dried growth plates were milled (Universal Mill A-20; Tekmer Co, Cincinnati, OH, USA) to obtain 400–700-μm granules and then demineralized in

0.6-N HCl three times for 1 h (50 ml HCl per g of bone). The growth plate powder was rinsed with several changes of sterile distilled water to adjust the pH, three times in 95 % ethanol and once in ether. The growth plate powder was air-dried and stored in sterile plastic containers at 4 °C until being used for implantation. This entire process was performed under sterile conditions (except for the milling) and a sample was cultured to demonstrate that specimens contained no bacterial or fungal contamination.

To evaluate bone formation, union and remodeling of the defect, radiographs of each forelimb were taken postoperatively at the 2nd, 4th, 6th and 8th weeks post-injury. The results were scored using the modified Lane and Sandhu scoring system [35] (Table 1).

Animals were killed, and radius bones were explanted on the 56th postoperative day for gross and histopathological signs of healing. In gross evaluation, examination and blinded scoring of the specimens included presence of bridging bone, indicating a complete union (+3 score), presence of cartilage, soft tissue or cracks within the defect indicating a possible unstable union (+1 or +2 score), or complete instability at the defect site indicating no union (0 score).

For histopathological evaluation, sagital sections containing the defect were cut with a slow-speed saw from the harvested and dissected bones. Each slice was then fixed in 10 % neutral buffered formalin. The formalin-fixed bone samples were decalcified in 15 % buffered formic acid solution and processed for routine histological examination. Two sections 5 μm in thickness were cut from the centers of each specimen and were stained with hematoxylin and eosin. The sections were blindly evaluated and scored by two pathologists according to Emery's scoring system [36] and based on this scoring system the defects were evaluated as follows: if the gap was empty (score = 0), if the gap was filled with fibrous connective tissue only (score = 1), with more fibrous tissue than fibrocartilage (score = 2), more fibrocartilage than fibrous tissue (score = 3), fibrocartilage only (score = 4), more fibrocartilage than bone (score = 5), more bone than fibrocartilage (score = 6) and filled only with bone (score = 7).

Results

There was no intra-operative or postoperative death during the study. None of the rabbits sustained an ulna bone fracture at the radius bone defect.

At the 2nd, 4th and 6th postoperative weeks, the radiographs did not show any significant differences between any of the groups, whereas at the 8th postoperative week the radiographs showed significant differences

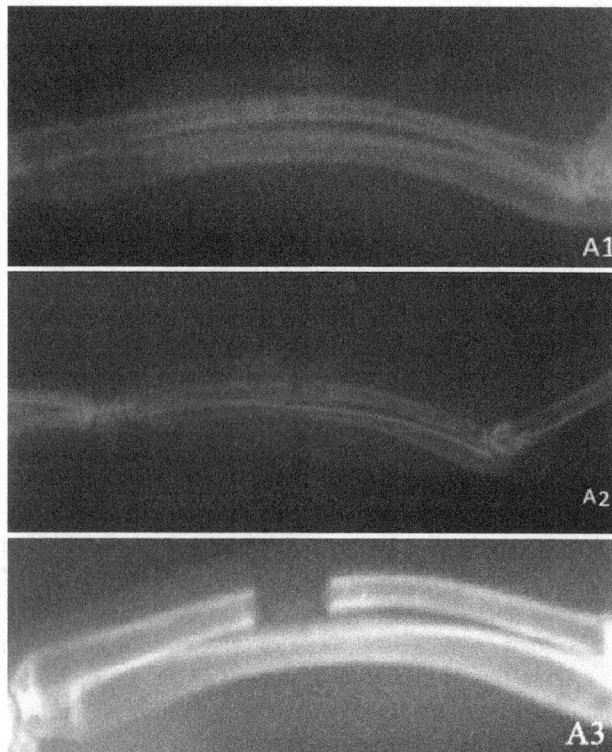

Fig. 1 Radiographs at 2nd week: **A1** hydroxyapatite group, **A2** hydroxyapatite–DCFGP group and **A3** DCFGP group

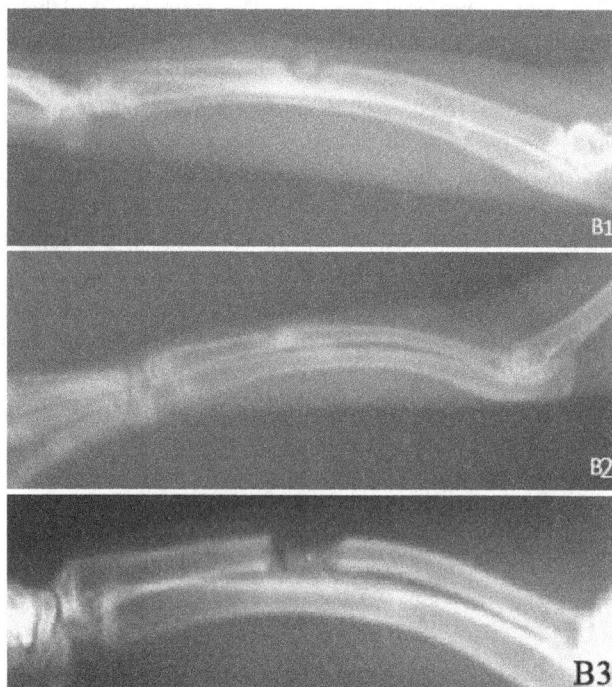

Fig. 3 Radiographs at 6th week, **C1** hydroxyapatite group, **C2** hydroxyapatite–DCFGP group and **C3** DCFGP group

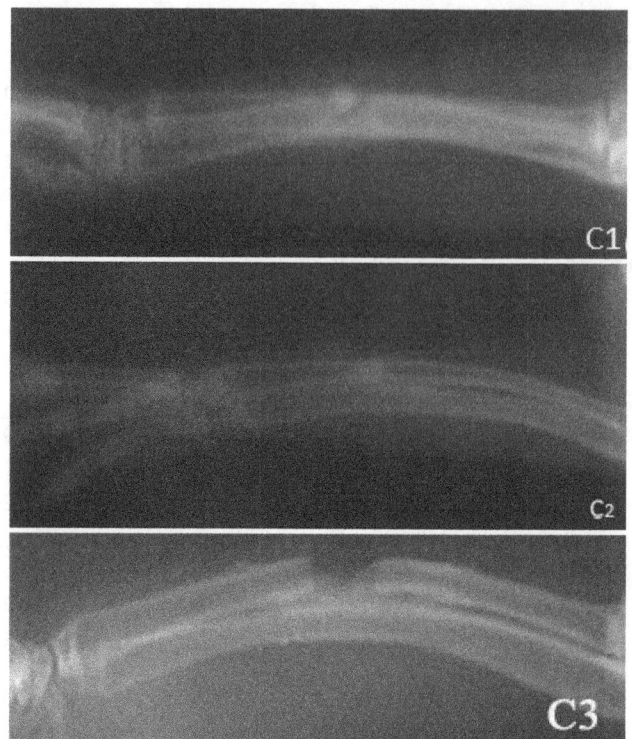

Fig. 2 Radiographs at 4th week, **B1** hydroxyapatite group, **B2** hydroxyapatite–DCFGP group and **B3** DCFGP group

groups. There were no significant differences between the DCFGP and hydroxyapatite groups on any postoperative day (Figs. 1, 2, 3, 4; Table 2).

The defect areas of the rabbits in all groups showed various amounts of new bone formation; the union scores of the rabbits in the hydroxyapatite–DCFGP group were not statistically superior to those of the animals in the hydroxyapatite and DCFGP groups (Table 3).

At the histopathological level, the defects in the animals in the hydroxyapatite–DCFGP and hydroxyapatite and DCFGP groups did not show significant differences on statistical analysis ($p > 0.05$) (Table 3).

The defects in all rabbits in the three groups were filled with mature cortical bone (Fig. 5). Normal trabecular and woven bone were uniformly formed within the defects and the regenerated bone completely spanned the defect and mostly produced full histological union (Fig. 5). No significant inflammatory response was evident in the lesions in the animals of different groups at 8 weeks post injury, although it may have been present earlier.

Discussion

To evaluate the bone healing potential of a combination of hydroxyapatite and DCFGP, a defect model was established in the radius bone of rabbits. This model has

between the groups ($p < 0.05$) (Figs. 1, 2, 3, 4; Table 2). The hydroxyapatite–DCFGP group was significantly ($p < 0.05$) superior to the hydroxyapatite and DCFGP

previously been reported suitable because there is no need for internal or external fixation which influences the healing process [37]. Chaubey et al., in a murine model, showed that bone defect healing occurred at 2 weeks and were completely healed by 5 weeks, with biomechanical properties not significantly different from normal controls. However, critical-sized defects showed no healing by histology or micro-computed tomography. These nonunion fractures also displayed no torsional stiffness or strength in

10 out of 12 cases [38]. In the present study the segmental defect was created in the middle portion of the radius, as long as 10 mm, for inducing a nonunion defect and to prevent spontaneous and rapid healing [33]. The hypothesis was on the basis that the addition of DCFGP to a mixture of particulate hydroxyapatite in a critical-sized defect in the radius bone of rabbit could have a positive effect on bone formation.

The results of the radiological examinations showed that bone healing was enhanced when DCFGP was used concurrently with hydroxapatite. Recently, a study indicated that satisfactory ectopic bone formation occurred in a submuscular rat model with xenogenic demineralized bovine fetal growth plate, and complications were not identified [31]. In addition, in two previous studies segmental calf fetal growth plate was grafted in the radial bone defect and a positive bone healing process was observed by investigators [30, 39]. A more recent study showed favorable bone defect healing with DCFGP in a rabbit model [32]. In our study too, the DCFGP group showed good bone healing the same as other groups on

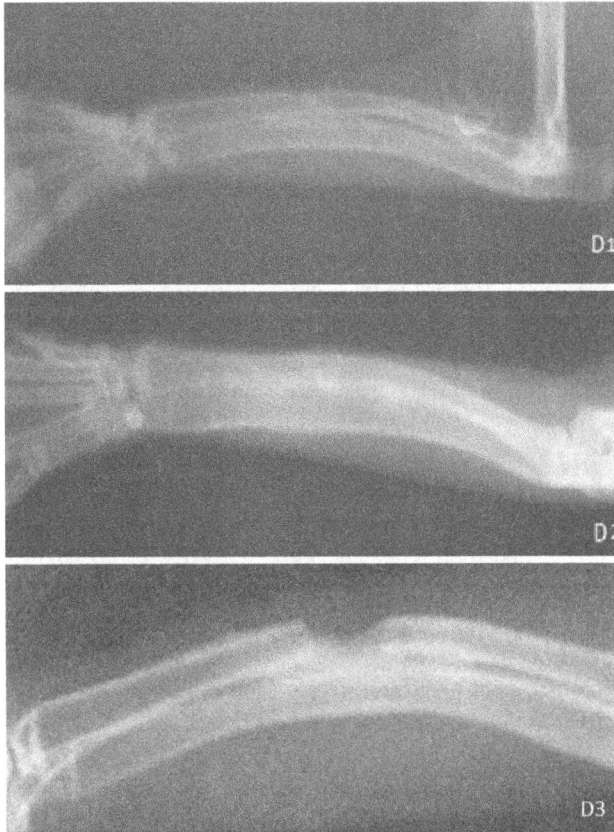

Fig. 4 Radiographs at 8th week, **D1** hydroxyapatite group, **D2** hydroxyapatite–DCFGP group and **D3** DCFGP group

Table 3 Bone measurements at macroscopic and microscopic level

Bone type evaluation	Median (min–max)			P^a
	Hydroxyapatite group ($n = 5$)	Hydroxyapatite–DCFGP group ($n = 5$)	DCFGP group ($n = 5$)	
Macroscopic union[a]	3 (2–2)	3 (2–3)	2 (2–2)	0.1
Microscopic evaluation[b]	6 (4–7)	7 (5–7)	5 (4–7)	0.1

[a] Complete union (+3 score), presence of cartilage, soft tissue or cracks within the defect indicating a possible unstable union (+ 1 or +2 score), complete instability at the defect site indicating nonunion (0 score)

[b] Empty (0 score), fibrous tissue only (1 score), more fibrous tissue than fibrocartilage (2 score), more fibrocartilage than fibrous tissue (3 score), fibrocartilage only (4 score), more fibrocartilage than bone (5 score), more bone than fibrocartilage (6 score) and bone only (7 score)

Table 2 Radiographical findings for healing of the bone defect (sum of the radiological scores) at various post-operative intervals

Postoperative weeks	Median (min–max)			P^a
	Hydroxyapatite group ($n = 5$)	Hydroxyapatite–DCFGP group ($n = 5$)	DCFGP group ($n = 5$)	
2	1 (0–3)	3 (1–4)	1 (0–3)	0.08
4	4 (3–8)	7 (4–10)	5 (3–6)	0.1
6	5 (2–8)	8 (6–10)	5 (4–7)	0.07
8	6 (4–9)	9 (8–10)[b]	5 (4–7)	**0.01**

Significant P values are shown in *bold face*

[a] Kruskal–Wallis non-parametric analysis of variance

[b] Compared with hydroxyapatite group ($p = 0.02$) and DCFGP group ($p = 0.008$) by Mann–Whitney U test. Hydroxyapatite–DCFGP group was significantly ($p < 0.05$) superior to hydroxyapatite and DCFGP groups

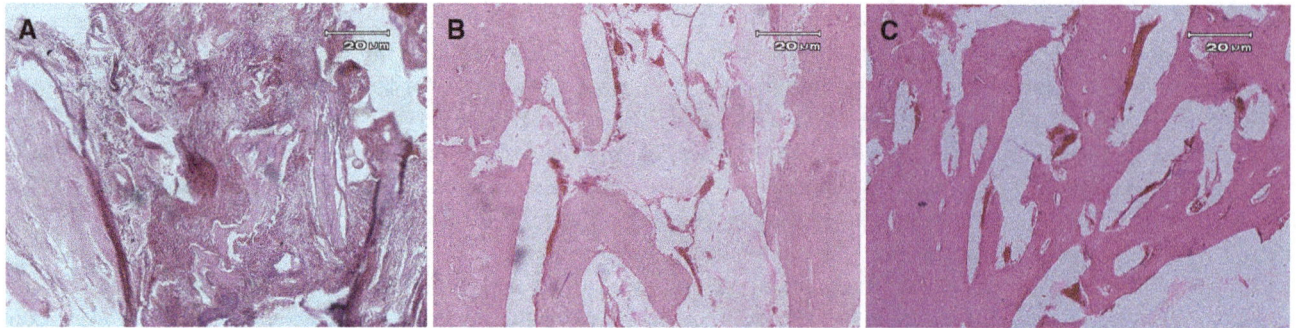

Fig. 5 Micrographs of the injured bones after 8 weeks. Regenerated bone with typical structure of trabecular bone is seen in the defect in the hydroxyapatite group (**a**, ×10), hydroxyapatite–DCFGP group (**b**, ×10) and DCFGP group (**c**, ×10) (hematoxylin and eosin staining)

histopathological evaluation. The presence of TGF-β in the growth plate [26] and BMPs 2 and 7 in human and rat fetal growth plate [27] has been identified. These proteins promote the chondroblastic differentiation of mesenchymal cells, followed by new bone synthesis by endochondral osteogenesis [29]. The primary osteoinductive component of demineralized bone matrix (DBM) is a series of low-molecular-weight glycoproteins that includes the BMPs. The decalcification of cortical bone exposes these osteo-inductive growth factors buried within the mineralized matrix, thereby enhancing the bone formation process. These proteins promote the chondroblastic differentiation of mesenchymal cells, followed by new bone synthesis by endochondral osteogenesis [29, 40]. We propose that in our study calf fetal growth plate demineralization led to the exposure of TGF-β and BMPs 2 and 7 in the injured site, and therefore the bone healing process in the DCFGP group was superior to the control group. In the present study DCFGP did not elicit any inflammatory reaction in the grafted site in the DCFGP and hydroxyapatite–DCFGP groups. It has been reported that the demineralization process destroys the antigenic materials in bone, so that the DBM becomes less immunogenic and does not induce an immunological reaction by the host [41]; we did not observe any inflammatory reaction throughout the histo-pathological evaluation.

Hydroxyapatite, a crystalline phase of calcium phosphate found naturally in bone minerals, has shown tremendous promise as a graft material. It exhibits initial mechanical rigidity and structure, and demonstrates osteoconductive as well as angiogenic properties in vivo [22, 42, 43]. In osteoperiosteal gaps bridged with hydroxyapatite only, the porosities were invaded with fibrous tissue or fibrocartilage tissues more than bone tissues. Occasionally, bone formation was observed in direct contact with hydroxyapatite, confirming its osteoconductive ability, but it was insufficient to allow union. These findings are similar to those reported using hydroxyapatite [25]. When the gap reaches a critical size, the osteoconductive properties

of the material are insufficient to fill the gap with formation of new bone [44]. This model therefore proved to be adequate for evaluating hydroxyapatite as a scaffold for DCFGP. More unexpected is the formation of the cortex and medullary canal together with mature lamellar bone observed in most of the cases. The previous in vitro studies have shown that artificial bone graft materials support the attachment, growth and differentiation of the bone-marrow stromal cells [45].

The rate of BMP release relies on its molecular weight, its conformation and its solubility [46]. Gene therapy-based strategies have also been introduced to improve BMP delivery and their effectiveness at the target site [47]. This technology provides the gene for the protein and results in a higher and more constant level of BMPs for a sustained time period [48]. To include the gene for BMPs into the target cell, a delivery vehicle or vector is needed, viral or non-viral [47].

Sohier et al. [49] investigated the efficiency of BMP-2 delivered by macroporous beta-tricalcium phosphate (β-TCP) scaffolds. The scaffolds, loaded with 15 and 30 μg of BMP-2, were implanted into the femoral defects and the back muscles of rabbits, respectively. Bone was formed within the BMP-2-loaded scaffold pores, both in the back muscles and bone defects, independent of the implant site effect. The results of that study indicated the efficacy and suitability of β-TCP scaffolds as BMP-2 carriers for bone regeneration. In another study, the in vitro and in vivo effectiveness of an absorbable collagen sponge (ACS) with 72 μg rhBMP-2 (BMPC) and fibrin matrix with 10 μg rhBMP-2 (BMPF) were compared with the ACS alone, fibrin alone, and empty groups. BMP-2 release was significantly higher in the BMPF group than in the BMPC group. The bone union of femoral defects and the bone volume were higher in the BMPC and BMPF groups than in other groups. Interestingly, fibrin matrix even with a seven-fold lower concentration of BMP-2 provided equivalent results to collagen sponge. According to those results, it seems that fibrin matrix could be an excellent carrier for BMP-2 [50].

Jun et al. [51] fabricated a silica xerogel–chitosan hybrid for incorporating BMP-2 onto a porous hydroxyapatite (HA) scaffold. They evaluated the biological properties of the hybrid coating incorporated with BMP-2, in terms of the release behavior of BMP-2, and also its in vivo performance on calvarial defects in rabbits. The BMP-2-loaded hybrids significantly enhanced new bone formation in comparison to the pure porous HA scaffolds without BMP-2. Indeed, the incorporation of BMP-2 into the hybrid promoted the osteoinductive properties of the HA scaffold. They introduced the silica xerogel–chitosan hybrid as a promising candidate for improving osteogenic properties of the HA scaffold with the constant and prolonged release of BMP-2.

The findings of the present study suggest that hydroxyapatite is a suitable resorbable carrier for DCFGP in vivo. It serves as a substrate to promote attachment and growth of the stem cells of the bone marrow, and as a template to guide bone morphogenesis in a clinically relevant volume. According to this phenomenon, in our study the hydroxyapatite–DCFGP group showed good enhancement of bone healing in comparison with hydroxyapatite and DCGP on radiological evaluation at the 8th postoperative week. Alper and colleagues [52] designed a study to identify the role of HA and DBM combination in fracture healing. After creating 5-mm segmental defects in the radii of the rats, defects were grafted using DBM, HA and DBM/HA mixture. After eight weeks of fracture healing, the radii were investigated histologically, and the HA group was found to have worse results when compared to the control group. They stated that DBM alone was an osteogenetic material for healing in non-union models of the rats, but that using HA in conjunction caused these effects to fade away. Moore and colleagues grafted wide ulnar defects of dogs with HA/TCP mixtures. They used a half-and-half mixture of autogenous cancellous bone and HA/TCP mixtures for one of the other groups, and pure autogenous cancellous bone for the control group. After six months, all groups were evaluated radiologically, mechanically and histhologically, and it was found that six dogs which were only grafted with the HA/TCP mixture showed fibrous nonunion, whereas other groups displayed union. As a result, they suggested that HA/TCP should be used as a mixture with autogenous grafts [53].

Hopp and colleagues [54] found similar results. They designed an experiment in which the ulnar defects of rats were grafted by HA, DBM, HA/DBM, autogenous bone graft and allogenic bone graft in five different groups. At the 6th week, they found that the plain HA group scored worse than the control group, whereas all other groups displayed better scores.

In our study, macroscopic and histopathological evaluation did not reveal any significant differences between the three groups after 8 weeks and showed favorable bone healing scores in the three groups. The authors proposed that there might be some differences during the earlier stages of the healing but by 8 weeks post-injury the three groups had reached almost the same level. As a result, similar macroscopic and microscopic healing responses were observed and further studies are needed before considering DCFGP-HA as an alternative to HA alone in clinical practice, especially considering the potential biological risks of animal-derived materials.

Conflict of interest   None.

Ethical standards   All the experimental procedures involving animals were conducted under a protocol reviewed and approved by the Ethics Committee of Shahrekord University (Permit Number: 930217).

References

1. Phieffer LS, Goulet JA (2006) Delayed unions of the tibia. J Bone Joint Surg Am 88:205–216
2. Bauer TW, Muschler GF (2000) Bone graft materials: an overview of the basic science. Clin Orthop Relat Res 371:10–27
3. Keating JF, McQueen MM (2001) Substitutes for autologous bone graft in orthopaedic trauma. J Bone Joint Surg Am 83(1):3–8
4. Bigham A, Dehghani S, Shafiei Z, Nezhad ST (2008) Xenogenic demineralized bone matrix and fresh autogenous cortical bone effects on experimental bone healing: radiological, histopathological and biomechanical evaluation. J Orthopaed Traumatol 9(2):73–80
5. Esposito M, Grusovin MG, Coulthard P, Worthington HV (2006) The efficacy of various bone augmentation procedures for dental implants: a Cochrane systematic review of randomized controlled clinical trials. Int J Oral Maxillofac Implants 21:696–710
6. Baltzer AW, Lattermann C, Whalen JD, Wooley P, Weiss K, Grimm M, Ghivizzani SC, Robbins PD, Evans CH (2000) Genetic enhancement of fracture repair: healing of an experimental segmental defect by adenoviral transfer of the BMP-2 gene. Gene Ther 7:734
7. Peng H, Usas A, Olshanski A, Ho AM, Gearhart B, Cooper GM, Huard J (2005) VEGF improves, whereas sFlt1 inhibits, BMP2-induced bone formation and bone healing through modulation of angiogenesis. J Bone Miner Res 20:2017–2027
8. Lee JY, Peng H, Usas A, Musgrave D, Cummins J, Pelinkovic D, Jankowski R, Ziran B, Robbins P, Huard J (2002) Enhancement of bone healing based on ex vivo gene therapy using human muscle-derived cells expressing bone morphogenetic protein 2. Hum Gene Ther 13:1201–1211
9. Bostrom MPG, Lane JM, Berberian WS, Missri AAE, Tomin E, Weiland A, Doty SB, Glaser D, Rosen VM (1995) Immunolocalization and expression of bone morphogenic proteins 2 and 4 in fracture healing. J Orthop Res 13:357–367
10. Cook SD, Baffes GC, Wolfe MW, Sampath TK, Rueger DC (1994) Recombinant human bone morphogenetic protein-7 induces healing in a canine long-bone segmental bone defects. J Bone Joint Surg Am 76:827–838

11. Kirker-Head AC (1995) Recombinant bone morphogenic protein: novel substancees for enhancining bone healing. Vet Surg 24:408–419

12. Reddi AH (1995) Bone morphogenetic proteins, bone marrow stromal cells, and mesenchymal stem cells. Maureen Owen revisited. Clin Orthop Relat Res 313:115–119

13. Bose S, Roy M, Bandyopadhyay A (2012) Recent advances in bone tissue engineering scaffolds. Trends Biotechnol 30(10):546–554

14. Kimelman-Bleich N, Pelled G, Zilberman Y, Kallai I, Mizrahi O, Tawackoli W, Gazit Z, Gazit D (2010) Targeted gene-and-host progenitor cell therapy for nonunion bone fracture repair. Mol Ther 19:53–59

15. Peterson B, Zhang J, Iglesias R, Kabo M, Hedrick M, Benhaim P, Lieberman JR (2005) Healing of critically sized femoral defects, using genetically modified mesenchymal stem cells from human adipose tissue. Tissue Eng 11:120–129

16. Pelled G, Ben-Arav A, Hock C, Reynolds DG, Yazici C, Zilberman Y, Gazit Z, Awad H, Gazit D, Schwarz EM (2009) Direct gene therapy for bone regeneration: gene delivery, animal models, and outcome measures. Tissue Eng Part B Rev 16(1):13–20

17. Egermann M, Baltzer A, Adamaszek S, Evans C, Robbins P, Schneider E, Lill C (2006) Direct adenoviral transfer of bone morphogenetic protein-2 cDNA enhances fracture healing in osteoporotic sheep. Hum Gene Ther 17:507–517

18. Hicok KC, Du Laney TV, Zhou YS, Halvorsen YDC, Hitt DC, Cooper LF, Gimble JM (2004) Human adipose-derived adult stem cells produce osteoid in vivo. Tissue Eng 10:371–380

19. Cowan CM, Shi YY, Aalami OO, Chou YF, Mari C, Thomas R, Quarto N, Contag CH, Wu B, Longaker MT (2004) Adipose-derived adult stromal cells heal critical-size mouse calvarial defects. Nat Biotechnol 22:560–567

20. Dudas JR, Marra KG, Cooper GM, Penascino VM, Mooney MP, Jiang S, Rubin JP, Losee JE (2006) The osteogenic potential of adipose-derived stem cells for the repair of rabbit calvarial defects. Ann Plast Surg 56:543

21. Bigham-Sadegh A, Mirshokraei P, Karimi I, Oryan A, Aparviz A, Shafiei-Sarvestani Z (2012) Effects of adipose tissue stem cell concurrent with greater omentum on experimental long-bone healing in dog. Connect Tissue Res 53:334–342

22. Appleford MR, Oh S, Oh N, Ong JL (2009) In vivo study on hydroxyapatite scaffolds with trabecular architecture for bone repair. J Biomed Mater Res A 89:1019–1027

23. Ohgushi H, Dohi Y, Tamai S, Tabata S (1993) Osteogenic differentiation of marrow stromal stem cells in porous hydroxyapatite ceramics. J Biomed Mater Res 27:1401–1407

24. Martin RB, Chapman MW, Sharkey NA, Zissimos SL, Bay B, Shors EC (1993) Bone ingrowth and mechanical properties of coralline hydroxyapatite 1 yr after implantation. Biomaterials 14:341–348

25. Parizi AM, Oryan A, Shafiei-Sarvestani Z, Bigham-Sadegh A (2013) Effectiveness of synthetic hydroxyapatite versus Persian Gulf coral in an animal model of long bone defect reconstruction. J Orthop Traumatol 14:259–268

26. Rosier RN, O'Keefe RJ, Hicks DG (1998) The potential role of transforming growth factor beta in fracture healing. Clin Orthop Relat Res 355:S294–S300

27. Anderson HC, Hodges PT, Aguilera XM, Missana L, Moylan PE (2000) Bone morphogenetic protein (BMP) localization in developing human and rat growth plate, metaphysis, epiphysis, and articular cartilage. J Histochem Cytochem 48:1493–1502

28. Urist MF, Sato K, Brownell AG (1983) Human bone morphogenetic protein. Proceedings of the Society for Experimental Biology and Medicine. Society for Experimental Biology and Medicine, New York, pp 194–199

29. Urist MR, Mikulski AJ, Lietz A (1979) Solubilized and insolubilized bone morphogenetic protein. Proc Natl Acad Sci USA 76:1828–1832

30. Dehghani SN, Bigham AS, Torabi Nezhad S, Shafiei Z (2008) Effect of bovine fetal growth plate as a new xenograft in experimental bone defect healing: radiological, histopathological and biomechanical evaluation. Cell Tissue Bank 9:91–99

31. Bigham AS, Shadkhast M, Bigham Sadegh A, Shafiei Z, Lakzian A, Khalegi MR (2011) Evaluation of osteoinduction properties of the demineralized bovine foetal growth plate powder as a new xenogenic biomaterial in rat. Res Vet Sci 91:306–310

32. Bigham-Sadegh A, Shadkhast M, Khalegi M-R (2013) Demineralized calf foetal growth plate effects on experimental bone healing in rabbit model. Veterinarski Arhiv 83:525–536

33. Bolander ME, Galian G (1983) The use of demineralize bone matrix in the repair of segmental defect. J Bone Joint Surg 68A:1264–1274

34. Reddi AH, Huggins C (1972) Biochemical sequences in the transformation of normal fibroblasts in adolescent rats. Proc Natl Acad Sci USA 69: 1601–1605

35. Lane JM, Sandhu HS (1987) Current approach to experimental bone grafting. Orthop Clin North Am 18:213–225

36. Emery SE, Brazinski MS, Koka A, Bensusan JS, Stevenson S (1994) The biological and biomechanical effects of irradiation on anterior spinal bone grafts in a canine model. J Bone Joint Surg 76:540

37. An YH, Friedman RJ (1999) Animal models in orthopedic research. CRC Press Inc., Boca Raton, Florida

38. Chaubey A, Grawe B, Meganck JA, Dyment N, Inzana J, Jiang X, Connolley C, Awad H, Rowe D, Kenter K (2013) Structural and biomechanical responses of osseous healing: a novel murine nonunion model. J Orthop Traumatol 14:247–257

39. Bigham AS, Dehghani SN, Shafiei Z, Torabi Nezhad S (2009) Experimental bone defect healing with xenogenic demineralized bone matrix and bovine fetal growth plate as a new xenograft: radiological, histopathological and biomechanical evaluation. Cell Tissue Bank 10:33–41

40. Oshin AO, Stewart MC (2007) The role of bone morphogenetic proteins in articular cartilage development, homeostasis and repair. Vet Comp Orthop Traumatol 20:151

41. Bauer TW, Muschler GF (2000) Bone graft materials: an overview of basic science. Clin Orthop Relat Res 371:10–27

42. Kilian O, Wenisch S, Karnati S, Baumgart-Vogt E, Hild A, Fuhrmann R (2008) Observations on the microvasculature of bone defects filled with biodegradable nanoparticulate hydroxyapatite. Biomaterials 29:3429–3437

43. Yoshikawa T, Ohgushi H, Nakajima H, Yamada E, Ichijima K, Tamai S (2000) In vivo osteogenic durability of cultured bone in porous ceramics: a novel method for autogenous bone graft substitution. Transplantation 69:128–134

44. Ohgushi H, Goldberg VM, Caplan AI (1989) Repair of bone defects with marrow cells and porous ceramic: experiments in rats. Acta Orthop Scand 60:334–339

45. Petite H, Kacem K, Triffitt JT (1996) Adhesion, growth and differentiation of human bone marrow stromal cells on non-porous calcium carbonate and plastic substrata: effects of dexamethasone and 1,25 dihydroxyvitamin D3. J Mater Sci Mater Med 7:665–671

46. Arrabal PM, Visser R, Santos-Ruiz L, Becerra J, Cifuentes M (2013) Osteogenic molecules for clinical applications: improving the BMP-collagen system. Biol Res 46:421–429

47. Menendez MI, Clark DJ, Carlton M, Flanigan DC, Jia G, Sammet S, Weisbrode SE, Knopp MV, Bertone AL (2011) Direct delayed human adenoviral BMP-2 or BMP-6 gene therapy for bone and cartilage regeneration in a pony osteochondral model. Osteoarthritis Cartilage 19:1066–1075

48. Wilson CG, Martn-Saavedra FM, Vilaboa N, Franceschi RT (2013) Advanced BMP gene therapies for temporal and spatial control of bone regeneration. J Dent Res 92:409–417

49. Sohier J, Daculsi G, Sourice S, De Groot K, Layrolle P (2010) Porous beta tricalcium phosphate scaffolds used as a BMP2 delivery system for bone tissue engineering. J Biomed Mater Res A 92:1105–1114

50. Schutzenberger S, Schultz A, Hausner T, Hopf R, Zanoni G, Morton T, Kropik K, van Griensven M, Redl H (2012) The optimal carrier for BMP-2: a comparison of collagen versus fibrin matrix. Arch Orthop Trauma Surg 132:1363–1370

51. Jun S-H, Lee E-J, Jang T-S, Kim H-E, Jang J-H, Koh Y-H (2013) Bone morphogenic protein-2 (BMP-2) loaded hybrid coating on porous hydroxyapatite scaffolds for bone tissue engineering. J Mater Sci Mater Med 24:773–782

52. Alper G, Bernick S, Yazdi M, Nimni ME (1989) Osteogenesis in bone defects in rats: the effects of hydroxyapatite and demineralized bone matrix. Am J Med Sci 298:371–376

53. Moore DC, Chapman MW, Manske D (1987) The evaluation of a biphasic calcium phosphate ceramic for use in grafting long-bone diaphyseal defects. J Orthop Res 5:356–365

54. Hopp SG, Dahners LE, Gilbert JA (1989) A study of the mechanical strength of long bone defects treated with various bone autograft substitutes: an experimental investigation in the rabbit. J Orthop Res 7:579–584

8

Vitamin D status in patients with knee or hip osteoarthritis in a Mediterranean country

Thomais Goula · Alexandros Kouskoukis · Georgios Drosos ·
Alexandros-Savvas Tselepis · Athanasios Ververidis · Christos Valkanis ·
Athanasios Zisimopoulos · Konstantinos Kazakos

Abstract

Background Vitamin D plays an important role in bone mineralization, remodeling, and maintenance and therefore its deficiency may be implicated in the pathogenesis of osteoarthritis (OA). Vitamin D status was evaluated in patients with knee or hip OA scheduled for joint replacement. The impact of anthropometric parameters such as gender, age, and body mass index on vitamin D levels was also examined. The study was conducted in a Mediterranean country (Greece).

Materials and methods We included 164 patients with knee or hip OA scheduled for joint replacement in this study. Serum levels of 25-hydroxyvitamin D (vitamin D) were measured in routine blood samples taken from the patients at their pre-admission visit, a week before the operation, using radioimmunoassay.

Results The majority of patients were vitamin D deficient (81.7 %); 15.2 % of them were vitamin D insufficient (hypovitaminosis). Only 3 % of patients were vitamin D sufficient. There was a significantly positive association between vitamin D levels and male gender.

Conclusion These findings indicate a large percentage of vitamin D deficient patients with knee or hip OA, which is unexpected considering the high annual insolation in northern Greece. Many other possible predisposing factors for OA should be taken into consideration. Whether treatment with vitamin D supplements may provide beneficial effects to these patients and the stage of disease in which this treatment should commence remains an issue for further scientific investigation.

Level of evidence Level IV.

Keywords Vitamin D · Osteoarthritis · Knee osteoarthritis · Hip osteoarthritis

T. Goula (✉) · G. Drosos · A. Ververidis · C. Valkanis ·
K. Kazakos
Department of Orthopaedics, Democritus University of Thrace,
University General Hospital of Alexandroupolis, Dragana,
Alexandroupolis 68100, Greece
e-mail: thetigoula@hotmail.com

G. Drosos
e-mail: drosos@otenet.gr

A. Ververidis
e-mail: averver@otenet.gr

C. Valkanis
e-mail: valkanisxr@yahoo.gr

K. Kazakos
e-mail: k.kazakos@med.duth.gr

A. Kouskoukis · A. Zisimopoulos
Department of Nuclear Medicine, Democritus University of
Thrace, University General Hospital of Alexandroupolis,
Alexandroupolis, Greece
e-mail: akouskoukis@gmail.com

A. Zisimopoulos
e-mail: azisimop@med.duth.gr

A.-S. Tselepis
Naval Hospital Of Athens, Athens, Greece
e-mail: savvalex@gmail.com

Introduction

Vitamin D deficiency is one of the most common and under-diagnosed medical conditions in the world, since a significant proportion of the population in many countries and regions around the world have low vitamin D levels [1–4]. The 25-hydroxyvitamin D level depends on various parameters, including the amount of solar ultraviolet B (UVB) irradiation (determined by the time of day, season [5–7] latitude, skin pigmentation, and use of sunscreen), age [7], dietary habits, gender, obesity [8], and many others [9].

Vitamin D plays an important role in bone mineralization, remodeling, and maintenance and therefore its deficiency may be implicated in the pathogenesis of osteoarthritis (OA) [10, 11]. Although the pathogenesis of OA is still unclear, recent evidence suggests that changes in subchondral bone remodeling—phases of bone absorption and of bone sclerosis—may be responsible for carti-lage damage. Vitamin D has been shown to modulate the activity of metalloproteinase enzymes. Low levels of 25(OH)D3 lead to an increased production of degradative enzymes [12]. The theory behind changes in the bone is that low levels of 25-hydroxyvitamin D slow the remodeling response of subarticular bone, resulting in thickening of the subchondral bone, osteophyte formation, and resultant cartilage damage [13].

Prospective epidemiological studies have found an association between dietary intake and serum levels of 25-hydroxyvitamin D and the development or progression of radiographic hip [14, 15] and knee OA [22]. Low serum levels of 25-hydroxyvitamin D have been reported in a significant proportion of patients with OA of hip and knee joints [14, 16–24]. Some authors suggest that achieving vitamin D sufficiency may prevent and/or delay cartilage loss in knee OA [15, 25]. In patients with hip OA who underwent total hip replacement, 25-hydroxyvitamin D levels were found to correlate positively with both pre- and post-operative Harris hip scores. Therefore, it seems that vitamin D deficiency in patients undergoing total hip replacement may be a risk factor for a suboptimal outcome [19].

However, results of other studies do not support an association between the low level of serum 25(OH)D and the development of OA [27–29]. An association of serum 25(OH)D levels with hip or knee OA has therefore not yet been fully established. The authors recommended serum 25(OH)D measurement in any patient with symptoms suggestive of knee OA, particularly at the initial stage of disease [23].

The main purpose of this study was to evaluate the vitamin D status in patients with knee or hip OA scheduled for joint replacement in a Mediterranean country. Associations between vitamin D serum levels and gender, age, and body mass index (BMI) were also investigated.

Materials and methods

This uncontrolled cohort study was conducted from December 2011 to October 2012 in a Mediterranean country. The study was approved by the hospital's scientific ethics committee and all patients provided informed consent.

Patients with hip or knee OA scheduled for hip or knee replacement were included in this study. Exclusion criteria were inflammatory arthritis, malignancy, renal failure, or anaemia.

The clinical examination of patients combined with a knee or hip plain radiograph set the diagnosis of OA. The Kellgren and Lawrence scale [26] was used and patients with grade 3 or 4 OA were scheduled for joint replacement. Age, gender, BMI, and co-morbidities were also recorded.

Blood samples were taken from the patients at their pre-admission visit by a resident orthopaedic surgeon, a week before the operation. The serum levels of 25-hydroxyvitamin D were measured by the Department of Nuclear Medicine, using radioimmunoassay (RIA) (radioactive material supplied by DiaSorin Inc., USA). The patients were categorized into three groups according to their vitamin D status. Vitamin D deficiency was defined as a 25-hydroxyvitamin D level below 20 ng/ml (50 nmol/L) and vitamin D insufficiency as a 25-hydroxyvitamin D level of 21–29 ng/ml (52.5–72.5 nmol/L) [30].

Clinical measurements were recorded by the biochemical laboratory of the Biopathology Department in order to exclude other bone disorders or systemic diseases. The following normal ranges were used: hematocrit (men, normal range: 40–54 %; women, normal range: 37–47 %), haemoglobin (men, normal range: 13.0–18.8 g/dL; women, normal range: 11.6–16.4g/dL), C-reactive protein (normal range: 0.07–8.2 mg/L), urea-BUN (normal range: 9–20 mg/dL), serum creatinine (men, normal range: 0.2-0.6 mg/dL; women, normal range: 0.6–1.0 mg/dL), serum glucose (normal range: 17–43 mg/dL), serum calcium (normal range: 8.1–10.4 mg/dL), and serum phosphorus (normal range: 2.5–4.5 mg/dL).

Results

In this study, 164 patients were included, 42 (25.6 %) of whom were men and 122 (74.3 %) were women. Age range was 48–86 years [mean = 68.9, standard deviation (SD) = 7.7 years]. All patients were Caucasian; 128 (78 %) of them suffered from knee OA and 36 (22 %) from hip OA. 19.5 % of patients belonged to the Muslim minority.

The levels of vitamin D ranged from 1.61 to 52.19 ng/ml (mean = 13.4, SD = 7.8 ng/ml). It is

Table 1 Patient groups according to gender, condition, BMI, and vitamin D serum levels

	Number	Percent
Gender		
Female	122	74.4
Male	42	25.6
Condition		
OA knee	128	78.0
OA hip	36	22.0
BMI groups		
<22 kg/m^2	1	0.6
22–24.9 kg/m^2	10	61
25–29.9 kg/m^2	60	36.6
>30 kg/m^2	93	56.7
Vitamin D groups		
Deficiency	134	81.7
Insufficiency	25	15.2
Normal	5	3.0
Total	164	100.0

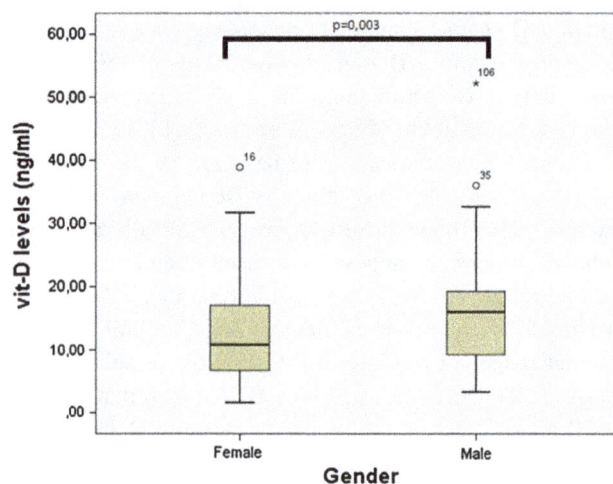

Fig. 1 Correlation of vitamin D serum levels and gender

A linear regression model was used to assess links between vitamin D levels and age, gender, and BMI. The regression equation was: VitD levels = 15.238 − (0.226 × BMI) + (0.005 × age) + (3.952 × gender), with $r^2 = 0.074$ and $p = 0.006$. Male gender had both the highest statistical significance ($p = 0.004$) and impact on the model ($\beta = 3.952$) in contrast to age ($p = 0.951$, $\beta = 0.005$). Male gender correlated positively with vitamin D serum levels ($p = 0.004$) (Fig. 1). BMI was borderline statistically insignificant ($p = 0.061$) and correlated negatively with vitamin D levels ($\beta = -0.226$).

Further analysis of vitamin D levels between men and women showed that, on average, men had levels higher by 4.12 ng/ml than women ($p = 0.003$). All analyses were undertaken using the statistical package SPSS for Windows (version 19.0; SPSS Inc., Chicago, USA).

Discussion

The most important finding of this study is the high prevalence (96.9 % deficiency and insufficiency) of low serum levels of 25-hydroxyvitamin D in a population with OA, in a sunny region of a Mediterranean country. Our study showed that over 4 out of 5 patients with knee or hip OA were vitamin D deficient with serum levels below 20 ng/ml. Several studies have shown a high incidence of vitamin D deficiency in patients with OA of hip or knee [17–19, 23, 24]. Considering the commonness of sunshine in Greece and in relation with existing studies [1–3], we had expected a higher vitamin D status in Greek patients with knee or hip OA. Moreover, the prevalence of vitamin D deficiency in patients with OA scheduled for total hip or knee replacement in our study was higher than the reported values of studies carried out in northern European countries such as Finland [17], Germany [18], and the UK [19] where annual insolation is significantly lower. However, in these countries consumption of vitamin D enriched foods is very common.

We also tried to correlate serum levels of vitamin D with related anthropometric predisposing factors such as age, gender, and BMI. A significant association with gender was observed, with female patients having lower serum levels of vitamin D. A higher prevalence of severe deficiency of vitamin D has also been demonstrated among US adult women compared to men [30]. In a study that took place in Quebec, Canada, gender was not associated with 25(OH)D concentration [31]. In addition, the same study showed that age and BMI were not correlated with 25(OH)D deficiency. This result corresponds to our findings regarding age and BMI. However, considering that BMI was a borderline insignificant predictor of vitamin D levels in our sample, it may be

noteworthy that most patients were vitamin D deficient (81.7 %). 15.2 % of patients were vitamin D insufficient (hypovitaminosis). Only 3 % of patients were vitamin D sufficient (Table 1). Regarding BMI, 6.1 % of patients had optimal weight (BMI range 22–24.9 kg/m^2), 36.6 % were overweight (BMI range 25–29.9 kg/m^2) and more than half of the patients (56.7 %) were obese (BMI over 30 kg/m^2) (Table 1). Additionally, 12 patients, all post-menopausal women, were under medication for osteoporosis with calcium and vitamin D supplements; 7 of them were vitamin D deficient, 4 were vitamin D insufficient and only 1 was vitamin D sufficient.

possible that other anthropometric obesity measurements may have stronger association with vitamin D levels. Such measurements could include waist-to-hip ratio and waist-to-height ratio. The notion of association of obesity with low vitamin D levels is supported by Lagunova et al. [32], who found that the prevalence of vitamin D deficiency is dependent on BMI and age separately. The results of that study suggested that 1 in 3 women and 1 in 2 men with BMI ≥ 40 kg/m^2 are vitamin D deficient.

The limitations of this study include a small sample size, particularly patients with hip OA. Another limitation is the absence of a control group and the scarcity of available data concerning the vitamin D status in the general population in our region. Despite the aforementioned limitations, the high prevalence of vitamin D deficiency in patients with knee or hip OA scheduled for joint arthroplasty is alarming.

Conflict of interest All named authors hereby declare that they have no conflicts of interest to disclose.

Ethical standards The study conforms to the Declaration of Helsinki [34]. An approval by the scientific ethical committee of our University General Hospital was obtained. All the patients provided informed consent prior to enrollment.

References

1. Endocrine Society Practice Guidelines JCEM (2011). Evaluation, treatement and prevention of vitamin D deficiency. http://www.endo-society.org/guidelines/final/upload/FINAL-Standalone-Vitamin-D-Guideline.pdf
2. Holick MF (2005) The vitamin D epidemic and its health consequences. J Nutr 135(11):2739S–2748S
3. Kull M Jr, Kallikorm R, Tamm A, Lember M (2009) Seasonal variance of 25-(OH) vitamin D in the general population of Estonia, a Northern European country. BMC Public Health 19(9):22
4. van der Wielen RP, Lφwik MR, van den Berg H, de Groot LC, Haller J, Moreiras O, van Staveren WA (1995) Serum vitamin D concentrations among elderly people in Europe. Lancet 346(8969):207–210
5. Holick MF (2007) Vitamin D deficiency. N Engl J Med 357(3):266–281
6. Holick MF, Chen TC, Lu Z et al (2007) Vitamin D and skin physiology: a D-lightful story. J Bone Miner Res 22(Suppl 2):V28–V33
7. Renier JC, Bernat M, Rebel A et al (1976) Study of circulating 25-hydroxyvitamin D. Rev Rhum Mal Osteoartic 43(7–9):481–489
8. Briot K, Audran M, Cortet B et al (2009) Vitamin D: skeletal and extraskeletal effects recommendations for good practice. Presse Med 38(1):43–54
9. Ovesen L, Andersen R, Jakobsen J (2003) Geographical differences in vitamin D status, with particular reference to European countries. Proc Nutr Soc 62(4):813–821
10. Samuels J, Krasnokutsky S, Abramson SB (2008) Osteoarthritis: a tale of three tissues. Bull NYU Hosp Jt Dis 66:244e50
11. Kwan Tat S, Lajeunesse D, Pelletier JP, Martel-Pelletier J (2010) Targeting subchondral bone for treating osteoarthritis: what is the evidence? Best Pract Res Clin Rheumatol 24:51–70
12. Dean DD, Schwartz Z, Schmitz J et al (1996) Vitamin D regulation of metalloproteinase activity in matrix vesicles. Connect Tissue Res 35:331–336
13. Radin EL, Rose RM (1986) Role of subchondral bone in the initiation and progression of cartilage damage. Clin Orthop 213:34–40
14. McAlindon TE, Felson DT, Zhang Y et al (1996) Relation of dietary intake and serum levels of vitamin D to progression of osteoarthritis of the knee among participants in the Framingham Study. Ann Intern Med 125:353–359
15. Bergink AP, Uitterlinden AG, Van Leeuwen JP, Buurman CJ, Hofman A, Verhaar JA, Pols HA (2009) Vitamin D status, bone mineral density, and the development of radiographic osteoarthritis of the knee: the Rotterdam Study. J Clin Rheumatol 15(5):230–237
16. Glowacki J, Hurwitz S, Thornhill TS, Kelly M, Leboff MS (2003) Osteoporosis and vitamin D deficiency among postmenopausal women with osteoarthritis undergoing total hip arthroplasty. J Bone Joint Surg Am 85-A:2371–2377
17. Makinen TJ, Alm JJ, Laine H, Svedstrφm E, Aro HT (2007) The incidence of osteopenia and osteoporosis in women with hip osteoarthritis scheduled for cementless total joint replacement. Bone 40(4):1041–1047
18. Breijawi N, Eckardt A, Pitton MB, Hoelzl AJ, Giesa M, von Stechow D, Haid F, Drees P (2009) Bone mineral density and vitamin D status in female and male patients with osteoarthritis of the knee or hip. Eur Surg Res 42(1):1–10
19. Nawabi DH, Chin KF, Keen RW, Haddad FS (2010) Vitamin D deficiency in patients with osteoarthritis undergoing total hip replacement: a cause for concern? J Bone Joint Surg Br 92(4):496–499
20. Chaganti RK, Parimi N, Cawthon P, Dam TL, Nevitt MC, Lane NE (2010) Association of 25-hydroxyvitamin D with prevalent osteoarthritis of the hip in elderly men: the osteoporotic fractures in men study. Arthritis Rheum 62(2):511–514
21. Bischoff-Ferrari HA, Zhang Y, Kiel DP, Felson DT (2005) Positive association between serum 25-hydroxyvitamin D level and bone density in osteoarthritis. Arthritis Rheum 53(6):821–826
22. Lane NE, Gore LR, Cummings SR, Hochberg MC, Scott JC, Williams EN, Nevitt MC (1999) Serum vitamin D levels and incidence changes of radiographic hip osteoarthritis: a longitudinal study: study of Osteoporotic Fractures Research Group. Arthritis Rheum 42:854–860
23. Heidari B, Heidari P, Hajian-Tilaki K (2011) Association between serum vitamin D deficiency and knee osteoarthritis. Int Orthop 35(11):1627–1631
24. Al-Jarallah KF, Shehab D, Al-Awadhi A, Nahar I, Haider MZ, Moussa MA (2012) Are 25(OH)D levels related to the severity of knee osteoarthritis and function? Med Princ Pract 21(1):74–78
25. Ding C, Cicuttini F, Parameswaran V, Burgess J, Quinn S, Jones G (2009) Serum levels of vitamin D, sunlight exposure, and knee cartilage loss in older adults: the Tasmanian older adult cohort study. Arthritis Rheum 60(5):1381–1389
26. Kellgren JH, Lawrence JS (1957) Radiological assessment of osteoarthrosis. Ann Rheum Dis 16:494–502
27. Felson DT, Niu J, Clancy M, Aliabadi P, Sack B, Guermazi A, Hunter DJ, Amin S, Rogers G, Booth SL (2007) Low levels of vitamin D and worsening of knee osteoarthritis: results of two longitudinal studies. Arthritis Rheum 56(1):129–136
28. Muraki S, Dennison E, Jameson K, Boucher BJ, Akune T, Yoshimura N, Judge A, Arden NK, Javaid K, Cooper C (2011)

Association of vitamin D status with knee pain and radiographic knee osteoarthritis. Osteoarthr Cartil 19(11):1301–1306

29. Konstari S, Paananen M, Helifvaara M, Knekt P, Marniemi J, Impivaara O, Arokoski J, Karppinen J (2012) Association of 25-hydroxyvitamin D with the incidence of knee and hip osteo-arthritis: a 22-year follow-up study. Scand J Rheumatol 41(2):124–131

30. Zadshir A, Tareen N, Pan D, Norris K, Martins D The prevalence of hypovitaminosis D among US adults: data from the NHANES III. Ethn Dis. 2005 Autumn;15(4 Suppl 5):S5-97-101

31. Barakı R, Weiler H, Payette H, Gray-Donald K (2010) Vitamin D status in healthy free-living elderly men and women living in Quebec, Canada. J Am Coll Nutr 29(1):25–30

32. Lagunova ZI, Porojnicu AC, Lindberg F, Hexeberg S, Moan J (2009) The dependency of vitamin D status on body mass index, gender, age and season. Anticancer Res 29(9):3713–3720

33. World Medical Association (2013) World medical association declaration of Helsinki: ethical principles for medical research-involving human. JAMA 310(20):2191–2194. doi:10.1001/jama. 2013.281053

9

Evaluations of guided bone regeneration in canine radius segmental defects using autologous periosteum combined with fascia lata under stable external fixation

Zhe Yu · Jie Geng · Haoran Gao · Xinwen Zhao · Jingyuan Chen

Abstract

Background Although bone defect is one of the most common orthopaedic diseases, treatment remains a challenge and an issue of debate. Guided bone regeneration (GBR) is primarily accompanied by barrier membranes; however, optional membranes show some inherent flaws in clinical application. The purpose of this study was to observe the healing velocity and quality of repairing canine radius segmental defect using transferred autologous periosteum combined with fascia lata, which can provide better biological safety than other materials.

Materials and methods Twenty adult male beagles weighing 11.45 ± 1.29 kg were used as animal models. The animals were randomly allocated into three groups, a blank control group, a fascia lata control group and a combined fascia lata and periosteum group. Standardised artificial bony defects were prepared at the radius and treated with autologous periosteum combined with fascia lata under stable external fixation. The newly formed bone-growth curve was made according to ultrasound (US) detection, and histopathologic and scanning electronic microscope (SEM) evaluations were also performed.

Results Bone union was seen in most individuals from the autologous periosteum combined with fascia lata group, within an average of 14.2 weeks. Histopathologic and SEM examinations both showed the different osteogenesis state between groups. Necropsy confirmed US findings with regard to distance of bone defects and location.

Conclusion These findings suggest that autologous periosteum combined with fascia lata is as effective as a GBR membrane, even in long tubular bone defects. With reliable biological safety, the autologous periosteum combined with fascia lata is expected to achieve increasing application in orthopaedic trauma patients.

Level of evidence Not applicable, animal study.

Keywords Guided bone regeneration · Periosteum · Bone defect · Bone formation

Abbreviations
BMT Barrier membrane technique
GBR Guided bone regeneration
GTR Guided tissue regeneration
SEM Scanning electronic microscope
ALP Alkaline phosphatase
OP   Osteopontin
OC   Osteocalcin

Z. Yu and J. Geng contributed equally to this study.

Z. Yu (✉) · H. Gao · X. Zhao
Department of Orthopedic Surgery, Tangdu Hospital, Fourth Military Medical University, Xi'an 710038, Shaanxi, People's Republic of China
e-mail: yuzhe19@gmail.com

J. Geng
Medical Department of Tangdu Hospital, Fourth Military Medical University, Xi'an 710038, Shaanxi, People's Republic of China

J. Chen
Faculty of Military Preventive Medicine, Fourth Military Medical University, 169 Changle West Road, Xi'an 710032, Shaanxi, People's Republic of China

Introduction

Bone healing is one of the most important processes in the orthopaedic clinical field, especially following osteomyelitis, nonunion, tumours and plastic surgery. In general, a major obstacle to bone healing and formation of new bone is the rapid formation of connective tissue, which prevents osteogenesis [1]. Since Gottlow et al. [2] successfully cured periodontal diseases by using the barrier membrane technique in 1982, guided tissue regeneration (GTR) [3, 4] and guided bone regeneration (GBR) [5, 6] have been successively applied in clinical settings. Both GTR and GBR use a barrier membrane to prevent epithelial migration and the appearance of connective tissue, and GBR also aims to promote bone regeneration. For more than a decade, this technique has been applied in clinical dentistry for various purposes, including dental implant therapy with an insufficient bone volume in the recipient site [7–9].

Since the GBR technique depends primarily on the use of barrier membranes, these membranes and their properties play an important role in outcomes. At present, nonbioresorbable and bioresorbable membranes are the two main types of barrier membranes available [10]. Expanded polytetrafluoroethylene (e-PTFE) is the most commonly used nonbioresorbable membrane [11], while collagen membrane is the most commonly used bioresorbable membrane [12]. However, neither is ideal for use in GBR. Although the e-PTFE membrane has been confirmed to have excellent biocompatibility in many studies, it requires a second surgical procedure for its removal because of its nonresorbability. On the other hand, the collagen membrane is resorbable, but it has inherent disadvantages, such as poor structural integrity, variable degradation rates and host immune reactivity [13]. Thus, in order to promote effective bone regeneration using the GBR approach, the barrier membrane used must have specific properties in terms of bioactivity (osteoconductivity) and bioresorption, as well as space-maintaining ability, which is related to its mechanical stability.

Periosteum can meet some prerequisites for tissue-engineered bone repair, as it contains pluripotential mesenchymal stem cells with the potential to form either cartilage or bone [14]. Periosteum has two discrete layers: an outer fibrous layer and an inner cambial layer. The fibrous layer appears to be composed of fibroblastic cells in a collagen and elastin fibre matrix, along with a nerve and microvascular networks. The cambium layer is highly cellular and contains numerous cell types, including fibroblasts, osteoblasts, and osteochondral precursor cells. Mesenchymal precursor cells in the periosteum differentiate into neochondrocytes, producing cartilage tissue during embryogenesis and contributing to bone apposition during intramembranous ossification by differentiating into osteoblasts [15]. Because it can be transplanted as a whole tissue, it can serve as its own scaffold or a matrix onto which other cells and/or growth factors can adhere. To further ensure the space-maintaining ability, we selected the fascia lata in order to increase supporting strength. This tissue is adjacent to the autologous periosteum donor organ of the femur and can provide considerable supporting effects that other soft tissue cannot.

According to the abovementioned principles, we proposed the use of autologous periosteum combined with fascia lata using a stable external fixation frame as a barrier membrane. The advantages of this membrane are that host immune reactivity need not be taken into consideration, and no surgery is required for its removal. To our knowledge, the effect of using autologous periosteum or fascia lata has not been examined previously in detail. Therefore, this study aimed to investigate local changes in new bone formation following bone defects in canine radii treated by the GBR technique with autologous periosteum combined with fascia lata under stable external fixation. We also wanted to identify local events occurring in response to the periosteum using imaging, histological examination, and scanning electron microscopy (SEM).

Materials and methods

All experimental procedures involving animals were conducted using a protocol reviewed and approved by the Ethics Committee of Tangdu Hospital, Fourth Military Medical University (Permit Number: 2012028). All work was carried out in accordance with national and international guidelines to minimise animal suffering. Adult male beagle dogs were purchased from the Laboratory Animal Research Centre of the Fourth Military Medical University of China. Animal experiments were conducted at the Orthopedics Oncology Institute of Chinese PLA. The dogs were housed in microisolator cages under specific pathogen-free conditions. The unilateral external fixation frame used in this study is commercially available. It is designed by Xia Hetao and is commonly used for upper-limb fractures in humans [16].

Twenty adult male beagle dogs weighing 11.45 ± 1.29 kg were randomly divided into three groups: A ($n = 6$), the blank control group, in which bone defects were fixed with a unilateral external frame and left to heal spontaneously; B ($n = 6$), the fascia lata control group, in which the externally fixed bone defects were covered and sutured with autologous fascia lata, without the periosteum; and C ($n = 8$), the periosteum combined with fascia lata group, in which the externally fixed bone defects were covered with autologous fascia lata to preserve the potential osteogenic area, following which the fascia lata was fixed with sutures to ensure adequate support and isolation. Surgical procedures were performed under aseptic conditions by the same surgical team and with the animals under general anaesthesia

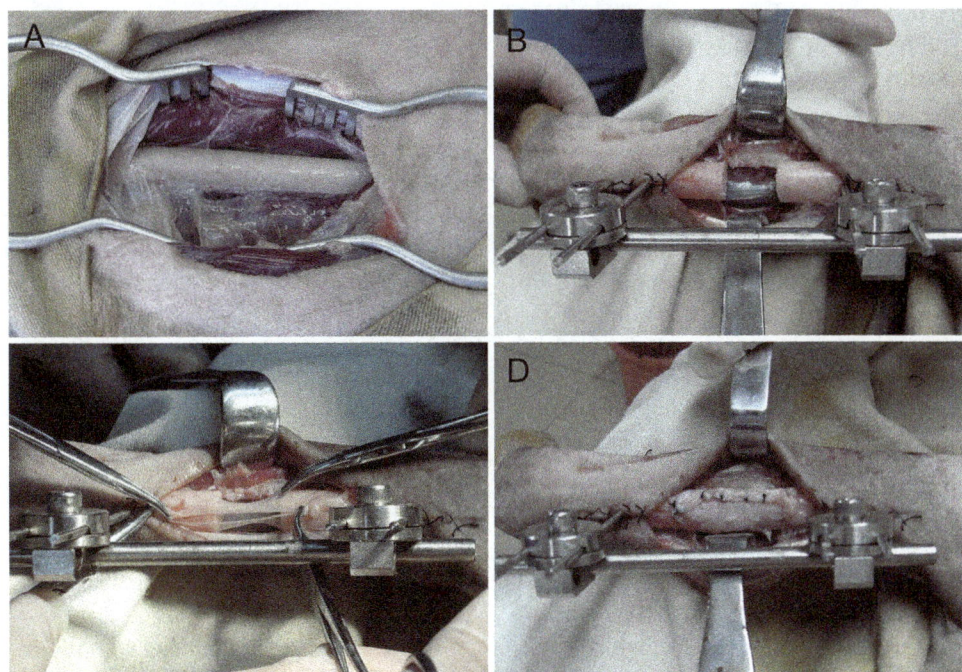

Fig. 1 Procedural steps: **a** exposure of canine radius; **b** unilateral external fixation and creation of a bone defect in the radius; **c** transplantation with autologous periosteum to preserve the osteogenic area; **d** suture fixation of the dissociated fascia lata

induced using isoflurane gas, in conjunction with endotracheal intubation. The experimental outline is illustrated in Fig. 1.

At the beginning of the experiment, a 15-mm defect was surgically created in a single radius (Fig. 1a, b). Simultaneously, the autologous periosteum and fascia lata were obtained from the left proximal femur and prepared for further transplantation. Unilateral external fixation was conducted according to biomechanical and humanitarian principles while minimising the time of the surgery to in turn minimise the animals' suffering.

In group C, the prepared autologous periosteum was sutured into the living periosteum at the fixed bone end of osteotomy to preserve the potential osteogenic area (Fig. 1c). To obtain adequate support and isolation, the dissociated fascia lata was fixed with sutures (Fig. 1d). In group B, the prepared fascia lata was transplanted into the segmental defects alone. In group A, the defects were left to heal spontaneously.

All incisions were closed using interrupted silk sutures. At this point, the process of surgical interference was complete. Postoperatively, the animals were administered 1 g of amoxicillin once daily for 5 days. Sutures were removed 14 days after surgery, and the animals were fed a soft laboratory diet for the study duration. Further, the operated areas and general conditions of the animals were checked daily according to standard veterinary postoperative care.

On a monthly basis, X-ray examination was conducted in live animals to study newly formed bone. Images were acquired such that they included the adjacent elbow and wrist joints. An X-ray microtomography (Micro CT SkyScan 1072; SkyScan, Kontich, Belgium) was used for this purpose, without any preparation. For ultrasound (US) imaging, a 5.0-MHz real-time scanner (SSA-550; Toshiba Medical Systems, Tokyo, Japan) was used. This procedure was conducted weekly, and a Doppler digital image optimiser (Toshiba Medical Systems, Tokyo, Japan) was used, which enables adaptive image processing for high sensitivity. The standard for bone healing was defined as disappearance of the defect area on US images, and then new bone growth curve was created.

After 20 weeks, the animals were sacrificed with an overdose of thiopental sodium. The radii were removed, block-resected using an oscillating saw and prepared for histological examination. The 20 bone blocks were immersed in a solution of 4 % formaldehyde, dehydrated in ethanol, and embedded in methyl methacrylate. Nondecalcified sections of ~ 300-mm thickness were obtained using a low-speed diamond saw with coolant. The sections were glued onto opalescent acrylic glass, ground to a final thickness of ~ 80 mm and surface stained with toluidine blue and basic fuchsin. To observe the morphology of the newly formed bone, sections were fixed with 1.5 % glutaraldehyde in 0.1 M phosphate-buffered saline (pH 7.4), passed through an alcohol gradient, dried in a Ladd Critical

Point Dryer and coated with platinum in a Polaron SEM coating system. The fixed sections were examined with a JEOL JSM-35CF SEM, and SEM studies were performed with backscattered electrons at 15 kV in conjunction with image analysis. The quantity of newly formed bone between the two ends of the osteotomy was analysed.

All samples were dehydrated in graded ethanol and acetone. Nondecalcified bone specimens were infiltrated and embedded in glycolmethacrylate resin. For each sample, 7-µm serial sections were cut perpendicular to the newly formed bone using a diamond saw (Reichert-Jung Supercut 2050) and fixed in buffered isotonic formaldehyde (100 ml 37 % formaldehyde solution, 900 ml distilled water, 4 g monobasic sodium phosphate, 6.5 g dibasic sodium phosphate) and embedded in paraffin. After 24 h, samples were immersed in 70 % alcohol, stained with hematoxylin–eosin (H&E) and examined histopathologically by a blinded pathologist using a light microscope (Leica DM-RBE microscope) equipped with a high-resolution video camera (Q-500 MC; Leica) coupled to a computer monitor. SPSS software (version 11.0; SPSS, Chicago, IL, USA) was used for data variation analysis. The length of the defect area measured from X-ray and ultrasound images and expressed as average ± standard error (SE) was compared among groups using Student's t test if the variables adjusted to a Gaussian distribution, with statistical significance set at $P < 0.05$. Means were compared using Kruskal–Wallis tests if data did not follow normal distribution. Bone healing rates were determined using the χ^2 test, for which $P < 0.05$ was again considered to indicate statistical significance.

Results

X-ray examination showed that in the blank control group, there was minimal proliferation at the end of the osteotomy surface immediately after the operation, and even 20 weeks later, bone defects showed minimal bone callus coverage with hardly distinguishable changes in length (Fig. 2a). Additionally, US images indicated that the distance between the two osteotomy ends also showed little change, and the final length of the defect area was 12.4 ± 2.43 mm (Table 1).

In the fascia lata control group, bone growth varied substantially among individual animals. Most bone defects showed a similar healing rate as the blank control group, showing callus abundance and reduced bone defect size (Fig. 2b). Only one animal showed rough bone union, in the 17th postoperative week, with proof of defect area disappearance on US imaging. The final length of the defect area in this group was 7.58 ± 3.74 mm.

In the periosteum combined with fascia lata group, bone union was observed in most individuals after an average period of 14.2 weeks (Fig. 2c). In fact, the newly formed bone was rebuilt in accordance with the original radius. Only two animals showed apparent bone defects on US imaging throughout the monitoring period. The final length of the defect area was 1.63 ± 3.2 mm.

US imaging showed persistent bone defect gaps in all animals in group A. In group B, only one animal showed a gradually reducing low-echo mass on uUS images. Then, rough bone union was observed after 17 weeks, and the low-echo area disappeared. Of the remaining five animals

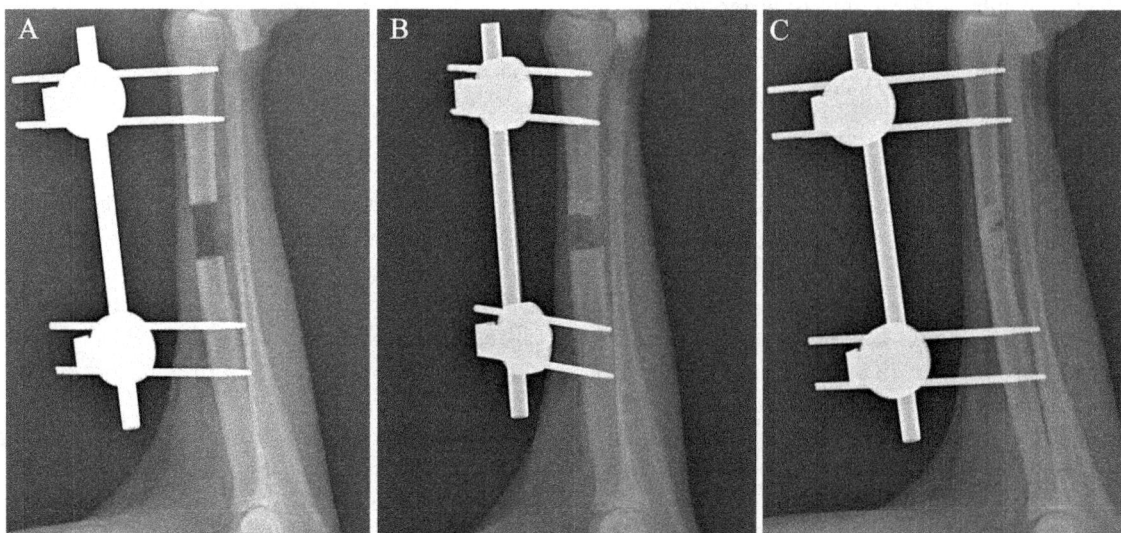

Fig. 2 X-ray comparison of union and nonunion: **a** group A showed minimal bone callus coverage and changes in defect lengths; **b** most bone defects in group B had a similar bone healing rate as group A, showing callus abundance and reduced bone defect size as changes; **c** complete bone healing in group C shows newly formed bone rebuilt in accordance with the original radius

Table 1 Bone healing rate and average bone defects

Groups	Intervention means	Animal numbers	Average bone defects (mm)	Average union time (weeks)	Animals with bone healing	Bone healing rate (%)
Group A	Blank control group	6	12.4 ± 2.43	0	0	0
Group B	Fascia lata control group	6	7.58 ± 5.38	17	1	16.7
Group C	Periosteum combined with fascia lata group	8	1.63 ± 3.2	14.2 ± 2.75	6	75

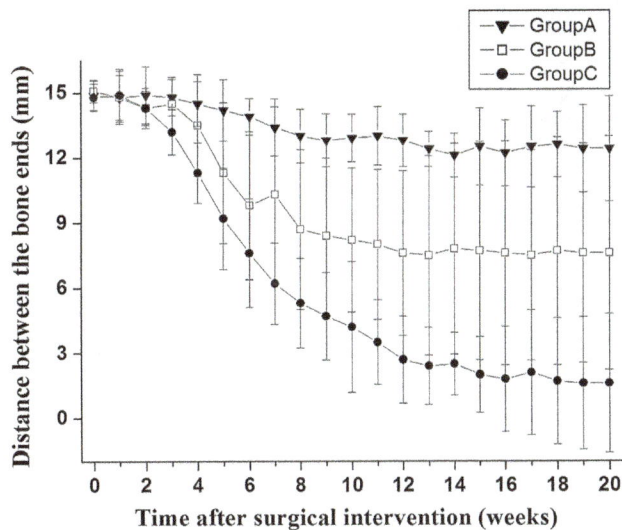

Fig. 3 Time course of new bone growth. Length of bone defect measured and calculated weekly after surgical intervention. Data represent mean distance ± standard deviation

in group B, neither apparent callus formation nor bone union was observed.

In general, 75 % of bone defects in group C healed within the 20-week study period; the median healing time was 14.2 ± 2.75 weeks (Fig. 3). The progress of bone healing was most evident during the 4–12 weeks after fracture. In two animals, bone defects were detected on US images throughout the monitoring period.

Histopathologic observation of the radii blocks showed that mostly fibrous connective tissue and a small amount of cartilaginous bone callus were present in the bone defect gaps in group A animals (Fig. 4a). However, in group C individuals showing bone healing, the presence of more abundant cartilaginous callus than the control group was histologically confirmed. Further, trabecular bone was tightly packed, and even the rebuilt Haversian canal system could be clearly distinguished (Fig. 4b). From one osteotomy end to the other, there was no visible defect gap in the newly formed bone area.

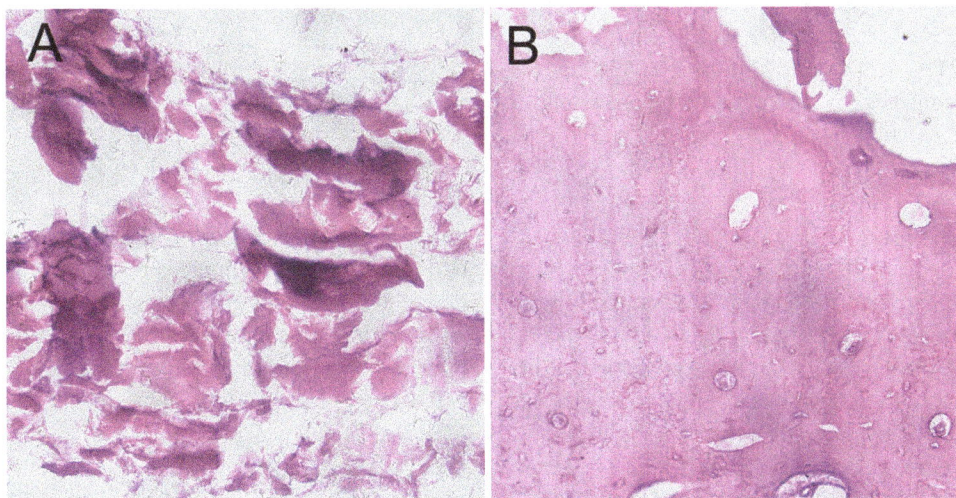

Fig. 4 Histopathological examination of radii blocks using hematoxylin & eosin staining: **a** fibrous connective tissue was observed in the bone defect gaps in group A; **b** group C individuals with bone healing showed abundant cartilaginous callus and tightly packed trabecular bone

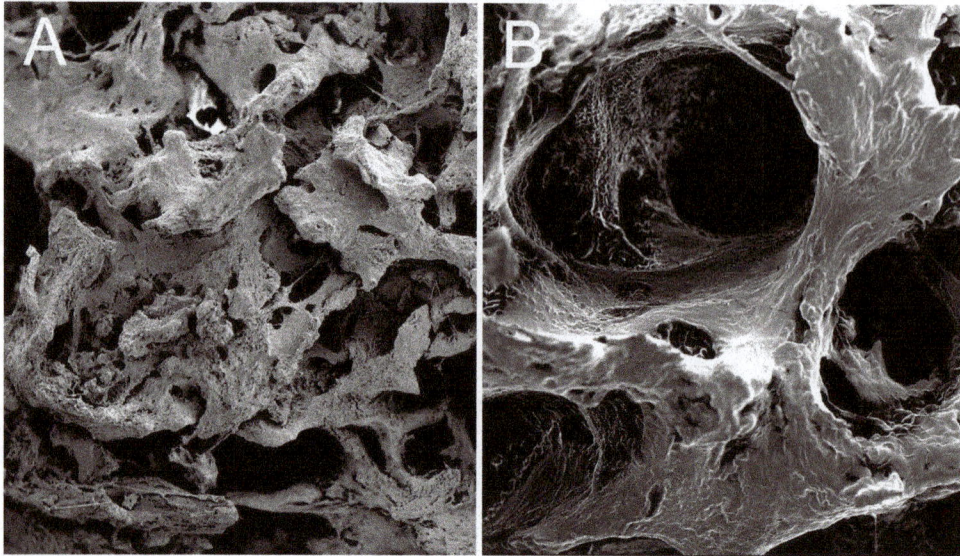

Fig. 5 Scanning electron microscopy (SEM) of radii blocks: **a** fibrous connective and muscle tissues were seen in the defect gaps in group A; **b** spongy newly formed bone was seen in group C, and the bone-forming surface had osteoblastic lacunae

SEM showed that the newly formed bone was connected to both osteotomy ends of the host bone by cartilaginous bone callus. The newly formed bone had a spongy appearance with many vascular spaces, and the bone-forming surface had osteoblastic lacunae (Fig. 5b). However, bone-defect gaps in group A were mostly filled with fibrous connective tissue and muscle tissue (Fig. 5a), and no signs of bone healing were detected between osteotomy ends.

On the day they were sacrificed, all animals was examined by Doppler US to obtain final values of bone-defect gaps. The animals were then necropsied, and the radii blocks were removed using a sliding calliper and examined histologically. Data of all 20 dogs were compared. A simple linear regression test showed a positive correlation between bone-defect length (mm) detected using US and necropsy ($r^2 = 0.924$; $P < 0.05$) (Fig. 6). Thus, necropsy confirmed US findings with regard to bone-defect length and location.

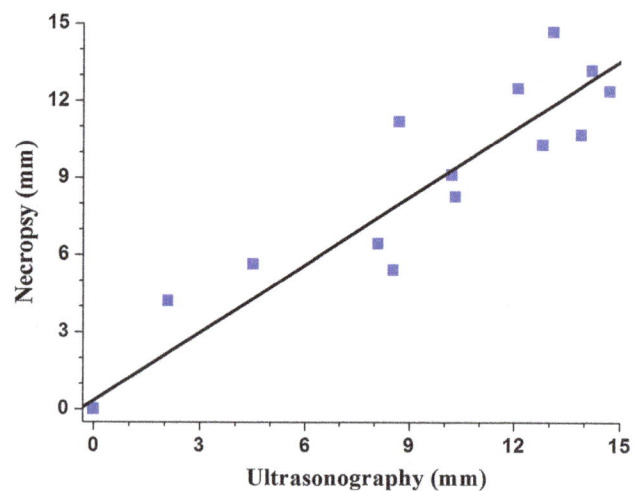

Fig. 6 Simple linear regression test showing a positive correlation between ultrasound and necropsy findings regarding length of bone defects (mm) ($r^2 = 0.924$; $P < 0.05$)

Discussion

Although bone defects are a common problem following injury, bone tumour or other pathologies, treating this disease remains a challenge and an issue of debate. With regard to treatment, the Ilizarov technique occupies an important position. This technique involves applying a stable external fixator made from thin wires and brackets and performing osteotomy with a minimal incision [17]. When connecting struts are moved toward the bone defect, new soft bone will stretch and form between osteotomy ends as a result of the stretch-stress stimulus, which promotes bone formation from fibroblast- and periosteum-derived bone [18]. Among the many steps of the Ilizarov procedure, preserving local blood supply and considerable integrity of periosteum probably play the most critical roles in bone formation. The periosteum not only preserves local osteogenesis but also acts as a barrier membrane combined with the fascia lata to prevent soft tissue invasion. Connective tissue formation is a major obstacle to bone healing and new bone formation. The presence of connective tissue at the bone defect site prevents osteogenesis, resulting in incomplete healing or nonunion [19]. If an enclosed space is created by periosteum, many growth factors, such as bone morphogenetic protein, alkaline phosphatase, osteopontin, osteocalcin, could be preserved to induce newly formed bone. The molecular mechanism of periosteum GBR probably resulted from the combined effects of the several factors mentioned earlier. Therefore, we developed an autologous periosteum transfer strategy wherein the periosteum combined with the fascia lata is applied directly to the osteotomy ends of the bone defect under stable external fixation. Membrane placement promotes osseous healing in bone defects by excluding competing nonosteogenic soft tissue cells from the bone-defect site. In addition, the space enclosed by the periosteum and fascia lata protects haematopoietic stem cells and bone progenitor cells from leakage or dilution and can provide considerable osteoblast activity and inductive capability with the collection of variable growth factors. In general, the principle of this technique is an extension of the barrier membrane technique, wherein a space protected from competing connective tissue invasion is provided in the defect gap to promote osteogenesis.

Compared with nonbioresorbable and bioresorbable membranes, the autologous periosteum combined with the fascia lata is a more natural alternative. Although nonbioresorbable membranes have been successfully used in several situations [20, 21], they usually cannot remain long in the living body with confirmed biological safety. Further, a second surgical procedure is required to remove these membranes because of their natural nonresorbability. In contrast, bioresorbable membranes do not require a secondary surgery, but they have weak structural integrity and variable degradation rates and show host immune reactivity [22]. Autologous periosteum combined with the fascia lata, which can be easily obtained from the adjacent bone surface, can be used to overcome these drawbacks. This alternative membrane is not associated with the risks of degradation, host rejection or biological toxicity and requires no secondary surgery. Thus, autologous periosteum combined with the fascia lata seems to have the greatest biological safety.

A significant finding in this study was the variation in growth rates of newly formed bone and bone-healing velocity amongst groups. Standardised artificial bony defects were created in the canine radius and covered with the periosteum combined with the fascia lata. In the first 3 weeks, no animal showed evident osteogenesis activity and only minimal bone callus formation adjacent to the osteotomy ends on US. Bone healing was most evident 4–12 weeks after fracture. In group C, most animals showed a gradually reducing defect gap on US monitoring, although the final average defect length was high, at 1.63 ± 3.2 mm, because two animals showed evident bone defects 8.53 and 4.51 mm long. Necroscopic examination in a nonunion animal model showed that the anastomotic

site of the periosteum and fascia lata failed to heal because of the presence of soft tissue at one osteotomy end, because of which the newly formed bone lost its union bridge. In group B, all anastomotic sites were confirmed for suture-assisted tissue healing.

Currently, the most commonly used technique for detecting bone defects and formation is X-ray examination. However, other techniques have also been used to characterise bone growth; for example, scintigraphy, micro-computed tomography-X, computed tomography and magnetic resonance imaging. Additionally, novel analytical tools are in development and may be adaptable to dogs. For instance, positron emission tomography can be performed with 2-[^{18}F]-fluoro-2-deoxy-D-glucose or 99mTc-bisphosphonate to detect the level of osteogenesis. Although Doppler US is not an emergent method, it is still valued by researchers in this field. It is convenient, noninvasive and can be used to visualise and measure bone growth at any stage, including growth of primary bone callus and the assessment of angiogenesis in the pathological region, even in living organisms.

In conclusion, to our knowledge, this is the first study to evaluate the efficacy of GBR treatment of long-bone defects by directly applying autologous periosteum combined with the fascia lata to the osteotomy ends under stable external fixation. It is also the first report confirming that the GBR technique could be effective for treating long tubular bone defects, which remains a challenge for orthopaedic surgeons, and it may enable superior bony union across a considerable bone defect gap of almost 15 mm. In our future research, we will conduct detailed immunocytochemical assays in order to determine the molecular mechanisms underlying GBR after autologous periosteum transplantation. Because of its reliable biological safety, we believe that autologous periosteum combined with the fascia lata will be applied more commonly in the orthopaedic trauma field.

Acknowledgments This study was supported by the Hong Kong Scholars Program (Grant No. HJ2012056), and China Postdoctoral Science Foundation (Grant No. 2013M542441 and 2014T70981, CHN). We thank Dr. Jiachang Wu for assistance with data processing.

Conflict of interest None.

Ethical standards All experimental procedures involving animals were conducted under a protocol reviewed and approved by the Ethics Committee of Tangdu Hospital, Fourth Military Medical University (Permit Number: 2012028). All animal work was carried out in accordance with national and international guidelines to minimise suffering to animals.

References

1. Lee EJ, Shin DS, Kim HE, Kim HW, Koh YH, Jang JH (2009) Membrane of hybrid chitosan–silica xerogel for guided bone regeneration. Biomaterials 30(5):743–750
2. Gottlow J, Nyman S, Lindhe J, Karring T, Wennström J (1986) New attachment formation in the human periodontium by guided tissue regeneration. Case reports. J Clin Periodontol 13(6): 604–616
3. Tsesis I, Rosen E, Tamse A, Taschieri S, Del Fabbro M (2011) Effect of guided tissue regeneration on the outcome of surgical endodontic treatment: a systematic review and meta-analysis. J Endod 37(8):1039–1045
4. Naylor J, Mines P, Anderson A, Kwon D (2011) The use of guided tissue regeneration techniques among endodontists: a web-based survey. J Endod 37(11):1495–1498
5. Buser D, Dula K, Belser U, Hirt HP, Berthold H (1993) Localized ridge augmentation using guided bone regeneration. 1. Surgical procedure in the maxilla. Int J Periodontics Restorative Dent 13(1):29–45
6. Hao J, Acharya A, Chen K, Chou J, Kasugai S, Lang NP (2013) Novel bioresorbable strontium hydroxyapatite membrane for guided bone regeneration. Clin Oral Implants Res. doi:10.1111/clr.12289
7. Schneider D, Weber FE, Grunder U, Andreoni C, Burkhardt R, Jung RE (2014) A randomized controlled clinical multicenter trial comparing the clinical and histological performance of a new, modified polylactide-co-glycolide acid membrane to an expanded polytetrafluorethylene membrane in guided bone regeneration procedures. Clin Oral Implants Res 25(2):150–158
8. Bottino MC, Thomas V, Schmidt G, Vohra YK, Chu TM, Kowolik MJ, Janowski GM (2012) Recent advances in the development of GTR/GBR membranes for periodontal regeneration–a materials perspective. Dent Mater 28(7):703–721
9. Yadav VS, Narula SC, Sharma RK, Tewari S, Yadav R (2011) Clinical evaluation of guided tissue regeneration combined with autogenous bone or autogenous bone mixed with bioactive glass in intrabony defects. J Oral Sci 53(4):481–488
10. Rakhmatia YD, Ayukawa Y, Furuhashi A, Koyano K (2013) Current barrier membranes: titanium mesh and other membranes for guided bone regeneration in dental applications. J Prosthodont Res 57(1):3–14
11. Carbonell JM, Martín IS, Santos A, Pujol A, Sanz-Moliner JD, Nart J (2014) High-density polytetrafluoroethylene membranes in guided bone and tissue regeneration procedures: a literature review. Int J Oral Maxillofac Surg 43(1):75–84
12. Taguchi Y, Amizuka N, Nakadate M, Ohnishi H, Fujii N, Oda K, Nomura S, Maeda T (2005) A histological evaluation for guided bone regeneration induced by a collagenous membrane. Biomaterials 26(31):6158–6166
13. Lee EJ, Shin DS, Kim HE, Kim HW, Koh YH, Jang JH (2009) Membrane of hybrid chitosan–silica xerogel for guided bone regeneration. Biomaterials 30(5):743–750
14. O'Driscoll SW, Fitzsimmons JS (2001) The role of periosteum in cartilage repair. Clin Orthop Relat Res (391 Suppl):S190–207
15. Ball MD, Bonzani IC, Bovis MJ, Williams A, Stevens MM (2011) Human periosteum is a source of cells for orthopaedic tissue engineering: a pilot study. Clin Orthop Relat Res 469(11): 3085–3093
16. Xia HT, Peng AM, Luo XZ, Qin SH, Han YL, Zhang BZ, Shi WY (2005) Combined external skeletal fixation instrumentation with locked intramedullary nailing for tibia lengthening. Zhonghua Wai Ke Za Zhi 43(8):495–498 (Chinese)
17. Borzunov DY, Chevardin AV (2013) Ilizarov non-free bone plasty for extensive tibial defects. Int Orthop 37(4):709–714
18. Feng ZH, Yuan Z, Jun LZ, Tao Z, Fa ZY, Long MX (2013) Ilizarov method with bone segment extension for treating large defects of the tibia caused by infected nonunion. Saudi Med J 34(3):316–318
19. Hu CT, Offley SC, Yaseen Z, O'Keefe RJ, Humphrey CA (2011) Murine model of oligotrophic tibial nonunion. J Orthop Trauma 25(8):500–505
20. Parrish LC, Miyamoto T, Fong N, Mattson JS, Cerutis DR (2009) Non-bioabsorbable vs. bioabsorbable membrane: assessment of their clinical efficacy in guided tissue regeneration technique. A systematic review. J Oral Sci 51(3):383–400
21. Jung RE, Fenner N, Hämmerle CH, Zitzmann NU (2013) Long-term outcome of implants placed with guided bone regeneration (GBR) using resorbable and non-resorbable membranes after 12–14 years. Clin Oral Implants Res 24(10):1065–1073
22. Stoecklin-Wasmer C, Rutjes AW, da Costa BR, Salvi GE, Jüni P, Sculean A (2013) Absorbable collagen membranes for periodontal regeneration: a systematic review. J Dent Res 92(9):773–781

10

Dual mobility acetabular component in revision total hip arthroplasty for persistent dislocation: no dislocations in 50 hips after 1–5 years

M. van Heumen · P. J. C. Heesterbeek ·
B. A. Swierstra · G. G. Van Hellemondt ·
J. H. M. Goosen

Abstract

Background A dual mobility cup has the theoretic potential to improve stability in primary total hip arthroplasty (THA) and mid-term cohort results are favorable. We hypothesized that use of a new-generation dual mobility cup in revision arthroplasty prevents dislocation in patients with a history of recurrent dislocation of the THA.

Materials and methods We performed a retrospective cohort study of patients receiving an isolated acetabular revision with a dual mobility cup for recurrent dislocation of the prosthesis with a minimum follow-up of 1 year. Kaplan–Meier survival analyses were performed with dislocation as a primary endpoint and re-revision for any reason as a secondary endpoint.

Results Forty-nine consecutive patients (50 hips) were included; none of the patients was lost to follow-up. The median follow-up was 29 months (range 12–66 months). Two patients died from unrelated causes. Survival after 56 months was 100 % based on dislocation and 93 % (95 % CI 79–98 %) based on re-revision for any reason. Radiologic analysis revealed no osteolysis or radiolucent lines around the acetabular component during the follow-up period.

Conclusion The dual mobility cup is an efficient solution for instability of THA with a favorable implant survival at 56 months.

Level of evidence Level 4, retrospective case series.

Keywords Revision hip arthroplasty · Dislocation · Dual mobility cup · Implant survival

M. van Heumen · B. A. Swierstra · G. G. Van Hellemondt ·
J. H. M. Goosen (✉)
Department of Orthopaedic Surgery, Sint Maartenskliniek,
PO Box 9011, 6500 GM Nijmegen, The Netherlands
e-mail: j.goosen@maartenskliniek.nl

P. J. C. Heesterbeek
Department of Research, Sint Maartenskliniek, Nijmegen,
The Netherlands

Introduction

The risk of dislocation after total hip arthroplasty (THA) varies from 0.4–8.7 % for primary procedures and from 5–20 % for revisions [1]. Many patient and surgical risk factors for dislocation are described including female gender, older age at the time of surgery, previous hip surgery and revision surgery, neuromuscular disorders, poor medical status/high American Society for Anesthesiologists score (ASA score) and a small diameter of the femoral head [2–5].

On-going research has led to the development of many different improvements in the design and technique of the THA in an attempt to reduce the rate of dislocation. If no clear malposition of prosthetic components was present, large femoral heads, acetabular augmentation rings and constrained tripolar prostheses could be used. Although all have shown a reduction in dislocation rates, the results were still unsatisfactory [5–9]. Another development was the dual mobility cup which was devised by Dr. Bousquet in the mid-1970s [10]. The dual mobility cup is a combination of two fundamental principles—(1) the smaller the head articulating against a polyethylene liner, the lower the wear rates because of low friction [11], and (2) the larger the diameter of the bearing, the greater the joint stability [12] (Fig. 1).

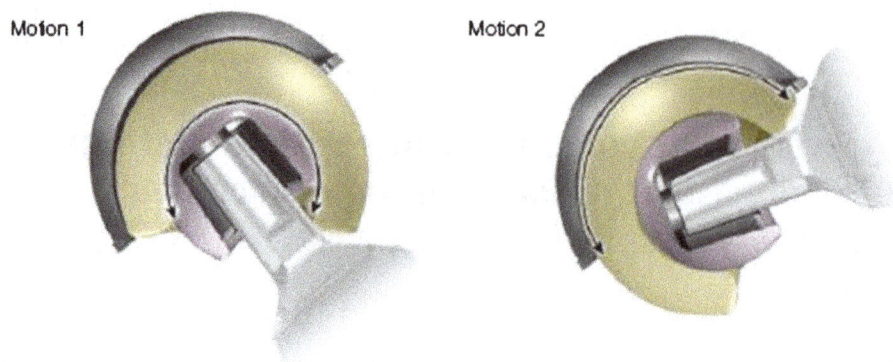

Fig. 1 The biomechanical concept of the dual mobility cup consists of a double articulation—between femoral head and liner and between liner and cup. The first motion occurs between the small femoral head and the inside of the polyethylene liner, until the neck of the femoral stem comes into contact with the liner. The secondary motion occurs between the outside of the polyethylene liner and the metal acetabular cup, when a larger range of motion is required. Here the polyethylene liner acts as a large femoral head

The application of a dual mobility cup has been described for both primary and revision THA, as well as without a reason for persistent dislocation [16, 17, 19–22] and high risk of dislocation [13, 14]. Furthermore, there are only a few reports concerning the use of this type of implant in revision cases for recurrent dislocation. Leiber-Wackenheim et al. [15] reported on a group of 59 patients with a mean follow-up of 8 years. There was one early dislocation without recurrence and all implants survived. Hailer et al. [18] described a series of 228 cases with a follow-up of 2 years. They observed a survival of 99 % (95 % CI 97–100) based on dislocation and 93 % (95 % CI 90–97) based on the revision rate for any reason.

In order to test this theoretic advantage in stability of the THA, we investigated the dislocation rate of a dual mobility cup used for revision in 49 patients (50 hips) with a history of recurrent dislocation of their THA. We hypothesized that use of this component in revision arthroplasty would decrease the risk of re-dislocation of the THA. A second aim of the study was to assess the survival of the component.

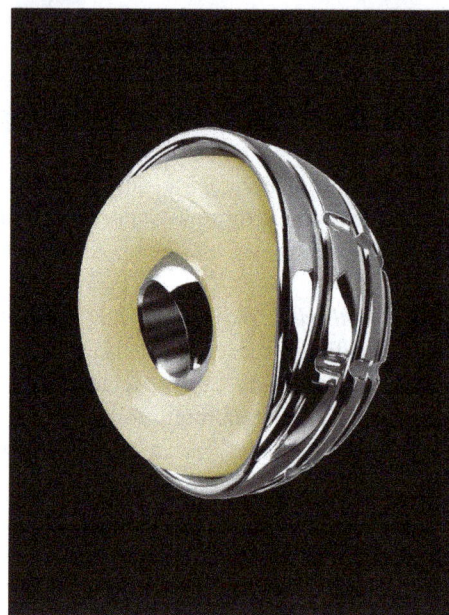

Fig. 2 The cemented version of the dual mobility cup (Avantage®)

Materials and methods

We performed a single-center retrospective study of patients who received an isolated acetabular revision with a dual mobility cup (Avantage®; Biomet, Warsaw, IN, USA) between January 2007 and June 2011. This cup has an uncemented shell design (coated with hydroxyapatite) or a polished shell for cementation (Fig. 2). The liner is made from argon-sterilized ultra-high molecular weight polyethylene (Arcom®; Biomet). Inclusion criteria were indication for revision with a dual mobility cup for recurrent dislocation or subluxation of the prosthesis (more than two episodes) and a minimum follow-up of 1 year after revision surgery. In total, 50 consecutive hips of 49 patients (one bilateral case) were included.

Surgery was performed using a posterolateral approach with the patient lying in a lateral decubitus position.

Postoperative management consisted of immediate full weight-bearing, using crutches for support, unless the intraoperative bone quality was poor and/or the surgeon used bone impaction grafting for reconstruction of the acetabulum. In these cases, partial weight-bearing over 3 months (15 % weight-bearing during the first 6 weeks, followed by 50 % for the next 6 weeks) was advised.

The clinical and radiologic data were retrieved from patient files. Demographic parameters included gender, age, height, weight, body mass index (BMI), ASA score,

Table 1 Patient characteristics

Characteristics	N
Gender	
Male	10
Female	39
Mean height	170 cm (range 153–195 cm)
Mean weight	79 kg (range 40–120 kg)
Mean BMI	27.17 kg/m^2 (range 16.6–43.0 kg/m^2), with 34 patients overweight (BMI >25)
Mean age at operation	67 years (range 32–90 years)
Mean ASA-score	2.02 (range 1–3)

Table 2 Indication primary THA

Diagnosis	N	%
Osteoarthritis	31	62
Congenital hip dysplasia with secondary osteoarthritis	12	24
Medial collum fracture	3	6
Femoral head necrosis (after medial collum fracture/ acetabular fracture with central luxation of the femoral head)	4	8

Table 3 Surgical history

No. of surgical procedures of the affected hip before revision with the dual mobility cup	No. of patients	%
1	20	40
2	14	28
3	6	12
4	5	10
5	3	6
6	0	0
7	1	2
8	0	0
9	0	0
10	0	0
11	1	2

Table 4 Revision surgery for any reason

No. of revisions for any reason, before revision with the dual mobility cup	No. of patients	%
0	23	46
1	17	34
2	4	8
3	4	8
4	2	4

Table 5 Revision surgery for instability

No. of revisions for instability, before revision with the dual mobility cup	No. of patients	%
0	29	58
1	17	34
2	2	4
3	2	4

Table 6 Operative characteristics

Characteristic	N
Operated side	
Left	24
Right	26
Size of acetabular cup	
48	5
50	19
52	7
54	14
56	3
58	1
60	1
Femoral head size	
22	5
28	45
Fixation	
Cemented	46
Uncemented	4
Bone impaction grafting	
Yes	6
No	44

medical and surgical history, and side of planned surgery (Table 1). Primary indication and surgical history of the patients are presented in Tables 2 and 3. One patient with a history of seven surgeries prior to the revision had some traumatic dislocations of the hip prosthesis, requiring several open re-position revision surgeries. Another patient with a history of 11 surgeries prior to revision underwent several operations because of congenital hip dysplasia, followed by surgical lavage and a two-stage revision due to a joint infection of the primary THA, which was postoperatively complicated by persistent dislocation, leading to re-revision surgery. Thirty of the 50 cases had undergone two or more previous surgeries to the affected hip. In 23 cases, no previous revision surgery had been performed prior to the revision with the dual mobility cup; therefore, 27 of the procedures were re-revisions (Tables 4, 5). No additional pathologies with impact on the dislocation rate, like neurologic disorders, were found.

Data regarding the type and size of implant, fixation method, technical details (Table 6) and complications, as well as information on any other occurring complications during the entire hospitalization, including infection, thrombosis, pulmonary embolism, hematoma, skin necrosis, nerve injury and/or death were obtained.

Postoperatively, outpatient clinic visits were routinely scheduled for radiologic (acetabular inclination angle and loosening of the cup) and clinical follow-up at 6 weeks, 3 months, and 1 year and were continued annually. Follow-up endpoints were dislocation of the THA, re-revision of the THA or death for any reason. Patients who did not attend the outpatient clinic visits for more than 1 year were contacted by telephone to ask for any dislocations or re-revisions postoperatively. When patients died, the general practitioner was contacted to obtain information on dislocations and implant re-revisions.

Descriptive statistics were presented as frequencies, and median values with ranges. Two Kaplan–Meier survival analyses were performed; one to estimate the cumulative probability of remaining free of dislocation, and the other to estimate the cumulative probability of remaining free of revision. The survival analysis was truncated when the number of patients remaining in the sample reached ten percent of the initial population. All statistical analyses were performed using STATA version 10.1 for Windows.

Results

None of the 49 patients (50 hips) were lost to follow-up. Two patients died (of unrelated causes) before final analysis. The median time from revision surgery to evaluation was 29 months (range 12–66 months).

No postoperative dislocations were observed during follow-up. At final follow-up, three of the hips revised with a dual mobility cup had been re-revised. In one case, a two stage re-revision took place because of a postoperative joint infection 7 months after surgery. The second case was also a postoperative joint infection where the prosthesis was removed and left with a Girdlestone procedure. In the third case, there was a cup loosening based on an undersized uncemented shell (technical/surgical failure) directly after the revision and this was re-revised on the same day. In addition, three patients required re-operation with retention of the prosthesis—two of these patients required a wound revision, following debridement and early antibiotic treatment due to prolonged effusion of the wound. Tissue cultures showed a postoperative joint infection, which was managed by continuing antibiotic treatment for 3 months. During follow-up, the prosthesis could be retained and there were no signs of persistent infection. The third patient underwent re-operation due to sciatic nerve palsy. Drainage of a compressive hematoma was performed and the patient fully recovered after 4 months. Radiographic analysis

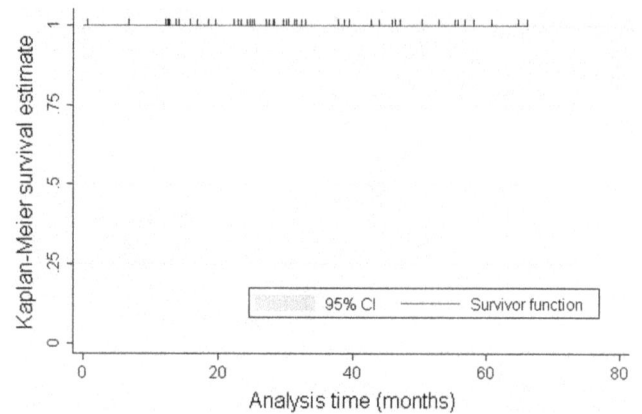

Fig. 3 Cumulative survival of 50 prostheses with dislocation defined as failure event. The small vertical spikes represent censored data

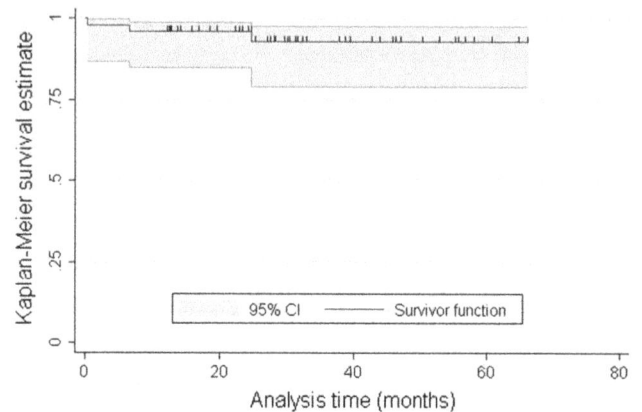

Fig. 4 Cumulative survival of 50 prostheses with revision for any reason defined as failure event. The small vertical spikes represent censored data

revealed a mean acetabular inclination of 49° (range 31–65°). No osteolysis or radiolucent lines occurred around the acetabular component during the follow-up period.

The mean cumulative survival for remaining free of dislocation after 56 months was 100 % (Fig. 3). The mean cumulative survival for remaining free of revision for any reason after 56 months was 93 % (95 % CI 79–98) (Fig. 4).

Discussion

Implant survival in our study (93 %) was comparable with other reports in the literature [13–20].

The current study population consisted of patients with an isolated acetabular revision due to recurrent dislocation of their THA. Most previous reports show comparable favorable results [13–18]. Langlais et al. [13] reviewed the results of 88 isolated acetabular revisions (82 patients at high risk of dislocation) using cemented dual mobility cups with a mean follow-up of 3 years (range 2–5 years). There was one dislocation (1.1 %) and survival was 94.6 % (two cases of aseptic loosening). Götze et al. [14] described their experience with an acetabular or total hip revision with a dual mobility cup (as used in our study) in 27 patients with a high risk of dislocation (14 cases) or a history of recurrent dislocation (13 cases). At a mean follow-up of one and a half years, there had been one dislocation of the polyethylene liner and the implant survival rate was 100 %. Leiber-Wackenheim et al. [15] are one of the few who reported on a series of isolated acetabular revisions with an uncemented dual mobility cup in a group of 59 patients with a history of recurrent dislocations. There was one early dislocation without recurrence after a mean follow-up of 8 years. All implants survived, and no component explantations were required. Civinini et al. [16] performed a prospective study of 33 patients (33 hips) with isolated acetabular revision with a dual mobility implant as used in the current study. Indication for revision was aseptic loosening (32 cases) or malposition of the cup (one case). At a mean follow-up of 3 years, no dislocations had occurred and survival rates were 97 % (95 % CI 82–98). Philippot et al. [17] showed the results of 163 acetabular revisions with a dual mobility cup. At a mean follow-up of 5 years, there were six cases (3.7 %) of dislocation and two cases of acetabular loosening; cup survival was 96.1 % (95 % CI 93–99). Recently, Hailer et al. [18] identified 228 THA cup revisions from the Swedish Hip Arthroplasty Register in patients with persistent dislocations with a dual mobility component as used in our study. They were only able to detect re-operations. At 2-year follow-up, they observed a survival of 99 % (95 % CI 97–100) based on dislocation and 93 % (95 % CI 90–97) based on the revision rate for any reason.

In contrast with the favorable results described above and the results found in the present study, Massin and Besnier [19] performed acetabular revisions using an uncemented dual mobility cup in 23 patients and reported a re-dislocation rate of 8.7 % at a mean follow-up of 4.5 years (range 2–10 years). Guyen et al. [20] reported on a series of 54 patients operated with a dual mobility cup at revision THA. At a mean follow-up of 3.9 years (range 2–6), the redislocation rate was 5.5 %.

In primary THA, survival rates after use of a dual mobility component were comparable [21–23] to the results of the present study. Philippot et al. [21] reported on a large series of 384 patients operated on with a dual mobility cup at primary THA. At a mean follow-up of 15 years (range 12–20), there were 14 cases (3.6 %) of dislocation (intra-prosthetic dislocation: femoral head dislocates from liner) with an overall survival of 97 %. Bouchet et al. [22] performed a case–control study of primary THAs with use of a dual mobility cup in 105 patients, compared with the use of conventional implants in a matched group of 106 patients.

At a mean follow-up of 4.3 years (range 3.2–5.6 years) there had been no dislocations in the dual mobility group versus five dislocations (4.6 % dislocation rate) in the matched group. Survival was 100 %. In a case series of ten THA patients with cerebral palsy no dislocations were observed at 39-month follow-up [23].

The main limitations of our study are the retrospective design and the lack of long-term follow-up (median 29 months; range 12–66 months). However, most dislocations occurred in the first 3 months postoperatively [24] and most re-revisions due to re-dislocation should have been performed during the first 2 years postoperatively [25]. We truncated the survival analysis at 56 months when only five patients remained.

Another limitation of the study is the absence of detailed functional results of the THA according to a clinical scale. These data would have provided more information about the functional performance of the implant. The study also included only a relatively small number of patients (49 patients, 50 hips). However, large series of isolated acetabular revisions concentrated on patients with recurrent dislocations are relatively uncommon in the literature. The strength of our study is the well-described homogeneous patient group. The results are comparable with the few other reports on this topic. This reinforces the favorable results of this type of implant in difficult revision cases.

In conclusion, the present study demonstrates an excellent 5-year survival rate with respect to the occurrence of postoperative dislocation with a dual mobility cup in revision THA due to instability. The re-revision rate for any reason is also promising. Thus, the dual mobility cup seems to be an efficient solution in revision cases for persistent dislocation of the THA. However, longer follow-up of a larger study population is required to confirm these relatively short-term findings and before firm conclusions can be drawn.

Conflict of interest   None.

Ethical standards   All patients gave informed consent before inclusion into the study; the study was authorized by the institutional review board and was performed in accordance with the ethical standards of the 1964 Declaration of Helsinki as revised in 2000.

References

1. van der Grinten M, Verhaar JAN (2003) Dislocation of total hip prostheses: risk factors and treatment. Ned Tijdschr Gen 147:286–290

2. Khatod M, Barber T, Paxton E, Namba R, Fithian D (2006) An analysis of the risk of hip dislocation with a contemporary total joint registry. Clin Orthop Relat Res 447:19–23

3. Byström S, Espehaug B, Furnes O, Havelin LI (2003) Femoral head size is a risk factor for total hip luxation: a study of 42,987 primary hip arthroplasties from the Norwegian Arthroplasty Register. Acta Orthop Scand 74:514–524

4. Jolles BM, Zangger P, Leyvraz PF (2002) Factors predisposing to dislocation after primaru total hip arthroplasty: a multivariate analysis. J Arthroplasty 17:282–288

5. Alberton GM, High WA, Morrey BF (2002) Dislocation after revision total hip arthroplasty: an analysis of risk factors and treatment options. J Bone Joint Surg (Am) 84:1788–1792

6. Beaule PE, Schmalzried TP, Udomkiat P, Amstutz HC (2002) Jombo femoral head for the treatment of recurrent dislocation following total hip replacement. J Bone Joint Surg (Am) 84:256–263

7. Bosker BH, Ettema HB, Verheyen C, Castelein RM (2009) Acetabular augmentation ring for recurrent dislocation of total hip arthroplasty: 60% stability rate after an average follow-up of 74 months. Int Orthop 33(1):49–52

8. Williams JT Jr, Ragland PS, Clarke S (2007) Constrained components for the unstable hip following total hip arthroplasty: a literature overview. Int Orthop 31(3):273–277

9. Della Valle CJ, Chang D, Sporer S, Berger RA, Rosenberg AG, Paprosky WG (2005) High failure rate of a constrained acetabular liner in revision total hip arthroplasty. J Arthroplasty 20:103–107

10. Farizon F, de Lavison R, Azoulai JJ, Bousquet G (1998) Results with a cementless alumina-coated cup with dual mobility. A twelve-year follow-up study. Int Orthop 22:219–224

11. Charnley J (1972) Long term results of low friction arthroplasty of hip as primary intervention. J Bone Joint Surg (Br) 54:61–76

12. McKee G, Farrar J (1966) Replacement of arthritic hips by the McKee-Farrar prosthesis. J Bone Joint Surg (Br) 48:245–259

13. Langlais FL, Ropars M, Gaucher F, Musset T, Chaix O (2008) Dual mobility cemented cups have low dislocation rates in THA revisions. Clin Orthop Relat Res 466:389–395

14. Götze C, Glosemeyer D, Ahrens J, Steens W, Gosheger G (2010) Die bipolare pfanne avantage in der hüftrevisionschirurgie. Z Orthop Unfall 148:420–425

15. Leiber-Wackenheim F, Brunschweiler B, Ehlinger M, Gabrion A, Mertl P (2011) Treatment of recurrent THR dislocation using of a cementless dual-mobility cup: a 59 cases series with a mean 8 years follow-up. Orthop Traumatol Surg Res 97:8–13

16. Civinini R, Carulli C, Matassi F, Nistri L, Innocenti M (2012) A dual-mobility cup reduces risk of dislocation in isolated acetabular revisions. Clin Orthop Relat Res 470:3542–3548

17. Philippot R, Adam P, Reckhaus M, Delangle F, Verdot FX, Curval G, Farizon F (2009) Prevention of dislocation in total hip revision surgery using a dual mobility design. Orthop Traumatol Surg Res 95:407–413

18. Hailer NP, Weiss RJ, Stark A, Kärrholm J (2012) Dual-mobility cups for revision due to instability are associated with a low rate of re-revisions due to dislocation: 228 patients from the swedish hip arthroplasty Register. Acta Orthop 83:556–571

19. Massin P, Besnier L (2012) Acetabular revision using a press-fit dual mobility cup. Orthop Traumatol Surg Res 96:9–13

20. Guyen O, Pibarot V, Vaz G, Chevillotte C, Bejui-Hugues J (2009) Use of a dual mobility socket to manage total hip arthroplasty instability. Clin Orthop Relat Res 467:465–472

21. Philippot R, Camilleri JP, Boyer B, Adam P, Farizon F (2009) The use of a dual-articulation acetabular cup system to prevent dislocation after primary total hip arthroplasty: analysis of 384 cases at a mean follow-up of 15 years. Int Orthop 33:927–932

22. Bouchet R, Mercier N, Saragaglia D (2011) Posterior approach and dislocation rate: a 213 total hip replacements case–control study comparing the dual mobility cup with a conventional 28 mm metal head/polyethylene prosthesis. Orthop Traumatol Surg Res 97:2–7

23. Sanders RJ, Swierstra BA, Goosen JH (2013) The use of a dual mobility concept in total hip arthroplasty patients with spastic disorders. No dislocations in a series of ten cases at midterm follow-up. Arch Orthop Trauma Surg 133:1011–1016

24. Blom AW, Astle L, Loveridge J, Learmonth ID (2005) Revision of an acetabular liner has a high risk of dislocation. J Bone Joint Surg (Br) 87:1636–1638

25. Phillips CB, Barrett JA, Losina E, Mahomed NN, Lingard EA, Guadagnoli E, Baron JA, Harris WH, Poss R, Katz JN (2003) Incidence rates of disloation, pulmonary embolism, and deep infection during the first six months after elective total hip replacement. J Bone Joint Surg (Am) 85:20–26

11

Complications of calcific tendinitis of the shoulder: a concise review

Giovanni Merolla · Mahendar G. Bhat ·
Paolo Paladini · Giuseppe Porcellini

Abstract Calcific tendinitis (CT) of the rotator cuff (RC) muscles in the shoulder is a disorder which remains asymptomatic in a majority of patients. Once manifested, it can present in different ways which can have negative effects both socially and professionally for the patient. The treatment modalities can be either conservative or surgical. There is poor literature evidence on the complications of this condition with little consensus on the treatment of choice. In this review, the literature was extensively searched in order to study and compile together the complications of CT of the shoulder and present it in a clear form to ease the understanding for all the professionals involved in the management of this disorder. Essentially there are five major complications of CT: pain, adhesive capsulitis, RC tears, greater tuberosity osteolysis and ossifying tendinitis. All the above complications have been explained right from their origin to the control measures required for the relief of the patient.
Level of evidence 5.

Keywords Calcific tendinitis · Shoulder · Rotator cuff · Complications

G. Merolla (✉) · M. G. Bhat · P. Paladini · G. Porcellini
Unit of Shoulder and Elbow Surgery, D. Cervesi Hospital,
Cattolica, AUSL della Romagna Ambito Territoriale di Rimini,
Rimini, Italy
e-mail: giovannimerolla@hotmail.com;
giovanni.merolla@auslrn.net

G. Merolla
Biomechanics Laboratory "Marco Simoncelli", D. Cervesi
Hospital, Cattolica, AUSL della Romagna Ambito Territoriale di
Rimini, Rimini, Italy

Introduction

Calcifying tendinitis (CT) of the shoulder is a frequently occurring painful disorder characterized by the presence of calcified deposits in the tendons of the rotator cuff (RC) mainly affecting the supraspinatus tendon but occasionally is seen in the infraspinatus and subscapularis [1–5].

The prevalence has been reported to be 2.7 percent in asymptomatic individuals, more common in females between the 4th and 6th decades of life and in sedentary workers [6, 7]. Two speculative hypotheses have been introduced to explain the etiology of CT [8]. The first one was proposed by Codman as an initial degeneration within the tendon fibers which is followed by calcification [9]. Moseley expanded on this further by defining a "critical zone" in the tendon-bone insertion area [10]. The second one was proposed by Uhthoff who considered CT as a reactive calcification within a healthy tendon [11]. CT is a disabling clinical condition that in the acute phase induces severe pain and limitation of shoulder function. Although most cases of CT elapse almost asymptomatically, it is not uncommon that some of them present in an emergency or with frequent outpatient office visits due to the ineffectiveness of the various conservative treatment modalities. CT heals either spontaneously or by conservative methods such as nonsteroidal anti-inflammatory drugs (NSAIDs), physiotherapy, subacromial injections, bursal lavage and extracorporeal shock-wave therapy (ESWT) (Fig. 1a–c) [3, 12–21]. In cases resistant to non operative measures, surgical removal of the calcium deposits is recommended [11, 22–25].

To our knowledge no review articles have been elaborated on the complications of CT. Hence, in this paper a literature review has been done on the various complications or sequelae of the CT of the shoulder preceded by a

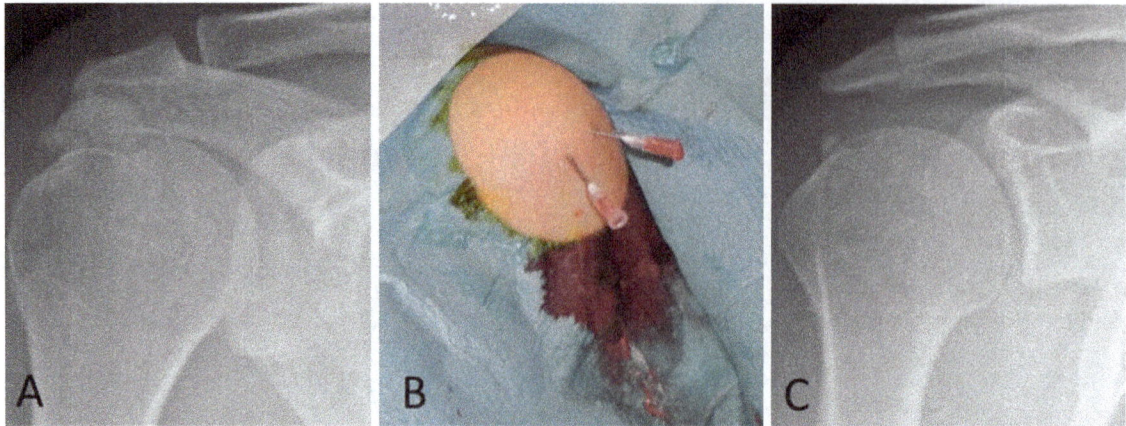

Fig. 1 **a** AP view radiograph shows a big calcium deposit (>1 cm) of the supraspinatus (SS) tendon in a case with acute phase, **b** image of the same case who underwent ultrasound guided needling and bursal lavage of the subacromial space with leakage of copious amounts of semisolid calcium deposits, **c** X-ray performed after 2 months from bursal lavage showed almost complete resorption of the calcium deposit

brief overview on its histopathology, classification and diagnostic imaging.

Histopathology and classification

The evolution of CT essentially passes through 3 distinct stages: pre-calcific, calcifying and post-calcific [26]. In the pre-calcific stage, numerous factors stimulate a metaplastic change of the tenocytes into chondrocytes. This is followed by the calcific stage which is subdivided into three phases—formation, resting and resorption—characterized by deposition of amorphous calcium phosphate followed by vascularisation and finally by resorption which coincides with significant clinical pain. The post calcific stage is demonstrated by the collagenisation of the lesion by fibroblasts [26]. Intra-operatively, the gross specimens of CT can be either in the form of a sandy tough mass or a toothpaste-like fluid or an amorphous mass composed of many small round or ovoid bodies [27]. The material of these deposits has been identified to be calcium carbonate apatite [28]. This carbonate apatite has been further classified as an A and B-type apatite [29]. Chiou et al. [30] studied the chemical components in CT and found that both types of the carbonate apatite varied in quantities during the formative, resting and resorption phases. Histochemical studies have demonstrated the presence of extracellular matrix vesicles near calcified deposition of the RC [26, 31, 32] and the authors have tried to correlate this finding in the pathogenesis of CT. Normally, the vesicles are inhibited from mineralization but in the presence of any pathology, the inhibitory stimulus may be lost leading to vesicles getting mineralized.

Radiographically, these deposits have been classified by different authors as described in Table 1.

Maier M et al. [36] assessed the intra- and interobserver reliability of the various classification systems using plain radiographs and CT scans and concluded that all the scores showed insufficient reliability and reproducibility. Although marginal improvement could be seen using CT scans it still remained statistically insignificant to be recommended as a routine investigation.

Diagnostic imaging

The first imaging modalities to identify CT were X-ray and ultrasound, as calcium deposits are readily identifiable on both. Radiograms should be performed in anterior-posterior (AP)—neutral, internal rotation and external rotation—axillary and outlet view. On radiographs calcific deposits appear homogeneous, amorphous densities without trabeculation, which allows a differentiation from heterotopic ossification or accessory ossicles [37]. Most of calcifications are ovoid, and the margins may be smooth or ill-defined. Ultrasound (US) is advantageous in the diagnosis of CT as it helps to detect other associated conditions as well such as rotator cuff tears and long head of the biceps (LHB) pathologies [38]; moreover, it also characterizes deposit consistency, their tendon location, and can be helpful to assist injections and bursal lavage [39]. According to the morphology of the calcium deposit, US has been used to classify the different type of CT due to its ability to discriminate between well defined calcifications with strong shadowing, and those with faint or absent shadowing. Chiou et al. [40] classifies calcific depositions into four shapes: an arc shape (echogenic arc with clear shadowing), a fragmented or punctate shape (at least two separate echogenic spots or plaques, with or without

Table 1 Radiological classification of the calcific tendinitis of the shoulder according to the current literature evidence

References	Radiographic criteria	Classification
Bosworth et al. [7]	Size	Large (>1.5 cm)
		Medium (in between)
		Small (rarely seen)
Depalma et al. [3]	Morphologic features	Type I (fluffy, amorphous and ill defined)
		Type II (defined and homogeneous)
Gartner et al. [33, 34]	Morphologic features	Type I (well demarcated, dense)
		Type II (soft contour and dense or sharp contours and transparent)
		Type III (soft contours, translucent and cloudy)
Mole' et al. [35]	Morphologic features	Type A (dense, rounded, sharply delineated)
		Type B (multilobular, radiodense, sharp)
		Type C (radiolucent, heterogeneous, irregular outline)
		Type D (dystrophic calcific deposits)

shadowing), a nodular shape (echogenic nodule without shadowing), and a cystic shape (a bold echogenic wall with an anechoic area, weak internal echoes or layering content). Conditions associated with non arc-shape calcifications include hypervascularity, widening of subacromial-subdeltoid bursa and the large size of calcifications. High resolution US in combination with color Doppler can differentiate between formative or resorptive status. In the resorptive phase, the deposits are nearly liquid and can be successfully aspirated. US has been also used with success in overhead athletes to identify CT showing a prevalence greater than that reported in the general population and that the presence of calcific tendinopathy correlates positively with age [41]. CT scan and MRI should be reserved for doubtful cases [42]. Computed tomography has an excellent resolution to detect calcium deposit as high density foci of solid stippled or amorphous character, but the cost and the exposure to radiation limit its use. MRI should not be used as a first line imaging modality, because deposits appear as vague regions of low signal on T1 and T2, and can be missed. Some enhancement around the deposit can be seen after contrast, and surrounding areas of hyperintensity on T2, due to peripheral edema or subacromial-subdeltoid bursal fluid are possible. MRI is advisable when the deposit is so large as to produce a strong shadow on US thus confusing it with RCTs.

Complications

Pain

The reason why pain has been considered as a complication in this review is due to the fact that this condition remains primarily asymptomatic in most of the patients [6]. When CT becomes symptomatic, the pain is extremely severe and is typically shooting type in the area of the shoulder with no radiation to elbow or hand [43]. In the acute phase, the pain tends to be so severe so as to allow only limited shoulder motion with marked tenderness. In the chronic or subacute phase, pain can be severe but generally shoulder motion is allowed [44]. The cause of occurrence of pain in CT is either due to an inflammatory response to the local chemical pathology or to direct mechanical irritation [45]. Neer classically described four types of pain peculiar to calcium deposition. First is the pain that is caused by the chemical irritation of the tissue by calcium. The second is the pain caused by tissue pressure due to its swelling. The third is an impingement-like pain caused by bursal thickening or irritation by the deposit itself. The fourth is the pain caused by a chronic stiffening of the glenohumeral joint due to voluntary prolonged immobilization by the patient to avoid possible irritation by the deposits with abduction or overhead activities [46]. Substance P is involved in the pain transmission caused by the stimulation of A delta/C fibers by certain noxious stimuli in the dorsal horn of the spinal cord. It is also contained in the small sensory neurons of the peripheral tissue. It's release from the sensory neurons play a significant role in mediating neurogenic inflammation [47]. Gotoh M et al. [47] studied the relation of the amount of substance P in the subacromial bursa and the shoulder pain in patients with rotator cuff diseases with radioimunoassay and immunohistochemistry. He found an increase in the number of immunoreactive nerve fibres in the synovial tissue of patients with rotator cuff diseases. These fibres were predominantly located around the blood vessels, suggesting an active role in its regulation and subsequent inflammation. He also hypothesized that certain mechanical (impingement) and chemical (bursitis) factors could be a source for the noxious stimuli inducing increased amounts of substance P in the afferent nerves. The conclusion of his study was that the subacromial bursa was the site associated with shoulder pain caused by rotator cuff disease.

We suggest to pay special attention to patients with persistent pain due to chronic CT. This subpopulation requires periodical outpatient visit (every 4 months) to exclude stiffness and monitor the evolution of calcium deposit with ultrasound; in addition, radiograms should be performed annually to assess the morphology of the deposit and its relationship with the underneath bone. NSAIDs are recommended when the pain score is more than 5 on a Visual Analogic scale (0–10). A standard program of physiotherapy including self aided mobilization and home exercises are prescribed to prevent stiffness. ESWT may be advised to foster calcium resorption, while other physical therapies (Laser, Transcutaneous electrical nerve stimulation) may help to treat associated LHB tendinopathies.

In addition, we do believe that some of the other complications listed below could be an important source of chronic and resistant pain in CT.

Adhesive capsulitis

Although the etiology of adhesive capsulitis is still not well understood, the pathophysiology has been much better explained over the years [48]. Two forms are commonly described: primary and secondary forms. While immobility is an important factor in the etiology, some case series have shown no predisposing factors for the primary form [49–52]. The secondary form is the more common type and can be precipitated by extrinsic factors or systemic diseases [53–58] or from intrinsic diseases in which CT is an important cause [59, 60]. Despite the efforts in elucidating this condition, there is still difficulty in deciding if the capsule abnormalities have resulted from inflammation of the surrounding structures or vice versa [48]. The amorphous calcium deposits lead to pain and dysfunction in the shoulder. The physical characteristics of these deposits influence the clinical presentation of the patient. If the calcium is in liquid state, an acute process is generally manifested with severe pain being the most important symptom. But if the deposit is dry and hard, a chronic form is usually seen in which the pain is superseded by a limited range of shoulder motion with a secondary frozen shoulder being the most important sequela (Fig. 2a–c) [61]. Shoulder stiffness is not well tolerated by patients with CT and must be treated with standard manual therapies to gain a complete recovery of shoulder mobility. Shoulder stiffness associated with CT is not easy to resolve and may require long-term rehabilitation, NSAIDs consumption and articular steroid injections in resistant cases. Therefore, we recommend to each physician who deals with cases of CT to precociously recognize any case of stiffness and address it appropriately.

Another interesting association of stiffness and CT is found in the post operative phase in arthroscopy. In a study by Jacobs et al. [62] the incidence of frozen shoulder after surgery was 18 % and the cause was considered to be the irritation of the glenohumeral capsule by residual calcium debris and hence thorough lavage was recommended to avoid such a possibility. Although he did not have literature evidence to support his claim, this assumption may not be entirely misplaced. In the section on pain previously described, one cause for it was considered to be stiffening due to voluntary prolonged immobilization. Conversely, the pain produced could further limit the compliance of the patient with respect to physiotherapy and rehabilitation thus producing a vicious cycle. Overall this association would usually lead to a prolonged recovery phase with regards to strength and motion.

Rotator cuff tears

This pathology can coexist either pre-operatively or intra-operatively. In the pre-operative setting, in the earlier times it was strongly believed that there could not be a coexistence of both the entities [63] but with time this theory

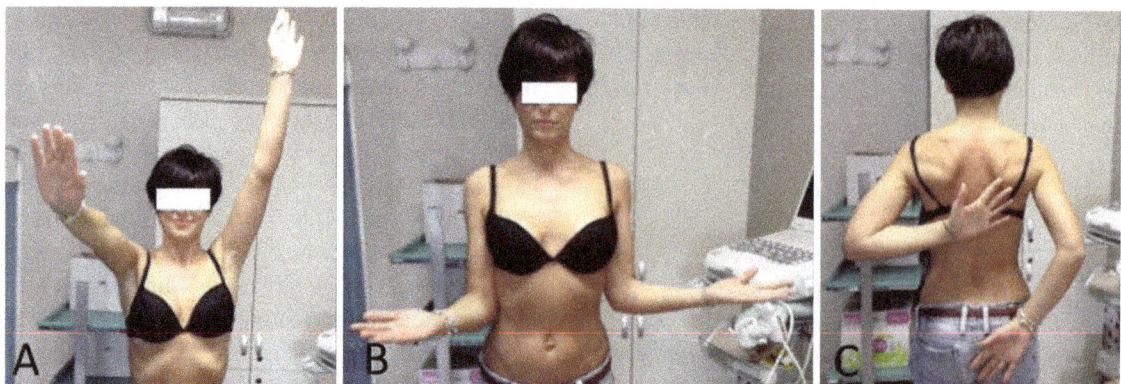

Fig. 2 **a–c** Active range of motion in a young lady with chronic calcifying tendinitis of the SS. At 2 months from the onset of pain she developed a stiff shoulder that required 6 months of manual physiotherapy for full recovery of shoulder motion

became disputed. Kernwein showed with arthrography a 90 % probability to reveal a rotator cuff tears (RCTs) in a patient older than 40 years with CT. He explained that large calcium deposits can rupture thus leading to complete RCTs [64]. Wolfgang reported an incidence of 23 % of CT in his subjects who underwent surgical repairs of RC tear [65]. Hsu also studied the relationship between these 2 pathologies and finally summarized his findings into 12 observations. His study showed a 28 % probability of coexistence of CT and RCTs. He observed the tears to be associated with smaller sized deposits and that the integrity of the cuff, the tear pattern, the shape, site and sex were significantly related to the texture of the calcific deposit [66]. Progression from calcifying tendinitis to RCTs has been also reported by Gotoh et al. [67]. On the basis of these research findings we may speculate that inflammation following a cuff tear can lead to resolution of the calcium

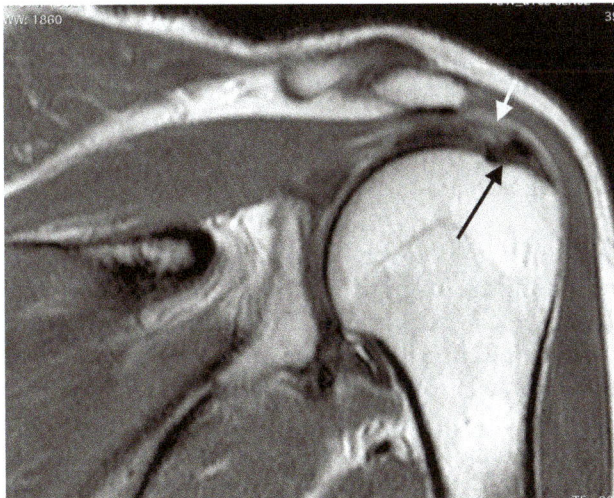

Fig. 3 T1-weighted coronal oblique MRI shows a solid calcium deposit at the insertion of the SS (*black arrow*) with partial tear of the related tendon on the bursal side (*white arrow*)

deposits and hence may produce a radiographic picture of a small sized deposit (Fig. 3). However, there is no literature evidence to support this belief.

The second association of RC tears with CT is in the intra-operative findings. Usually, removal of the calcium deposits leaves various degrees of RC defects which depend on the amount of the deposit present and the extent of re-section. If the defects are full thickness or large partial thickness then intra-operative repair is recommended (Fig. 4). There is no general consensus in the current literature regarding the extent of the resection of the deposits to be done. Some authors have suggested complete removal of the deposits with repair of the rotator cuff if necessary as it is believed that there is an inverse relation between clinical outcomes and any residual calcium deposits [22, 68–70]. In contrast, other researchers have reported good clinical outcomes with minimal tendon damage [1, 24, 62, 71, 72]. These studies were based on the hypothesis that the pain in CT is due to edema and increased intratendinous pressure as a result of calcification and thus just tendon decompression would suffice. Also, the same authors asserted that most of the patients with remnant deposits tended to show progressive resorption over time. Balke M et al. [1] in a mid term follow up study (2–13 years) reported worse clinical outcomes in the operated cases of CT, who also showed a high rate of partial supraspinatus tears. Nevertheless this study was the object of criticism for the involvement of multiple surgeons and lack of account for residual calcifications in the follow up [73]. Seil R et al. [72] in a follow up of over 24 months found complete resolution of residual calcium in all his cases except 2 along with an excellent clinical score in more than 90 % of the patients. Conversely, Porcellini et al. [22] in a follow up of over 36 months found that the Constant score was significantly lesser in those patients with persistent calcium deposits. Yoo et al. [69] noticed significant pain relief in 30 out of 35 patients at 6 months after surgery which was considered to

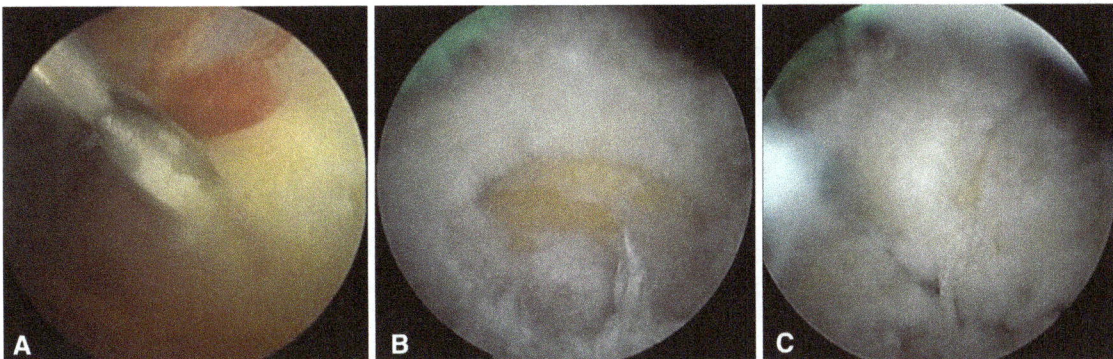

Fig. 4 Arthroscopic steps in a patient with chronic calcific deposit of the SS tendon. **a** Intraoperative needling to identify the site of deposit and delimit the amount of tendon to be removed, **b** full thickness insertional SS tear produced after complete removal of calcium deposit, **c** SS reattached on its footprint using a suture anchor (Cross FT 4.5 mm, Linvatec, Largo, FL—USA)

be due to aggressive surgical debridement; furthermore it was interesting to note that the residual calcium deposits in 6 patients showed complete resolution with time.

Greater tuberosity osteolysis

This is an extremely uncommon complication of CT. Sometimes, the classical course of CT may be altered leading to a longer duration of symptoms and greater functional impairment [74]. Osteolytic lesions (OL) of the tuberosities can be one of such causes [22, 42, 75]. Flemming G et al. [42] described a diffuse form of heterogeneous calcification, deep within the tendon near its insertion as a reason for the worst and most persistent symptoms. Seil R et al. [72] tried to correlate the persistent pain experienced by some patients to the penetration of calcium into bone as a result of the cortical erosion and the biochemical effects of bone lysis. Porcellini G et al. [75]

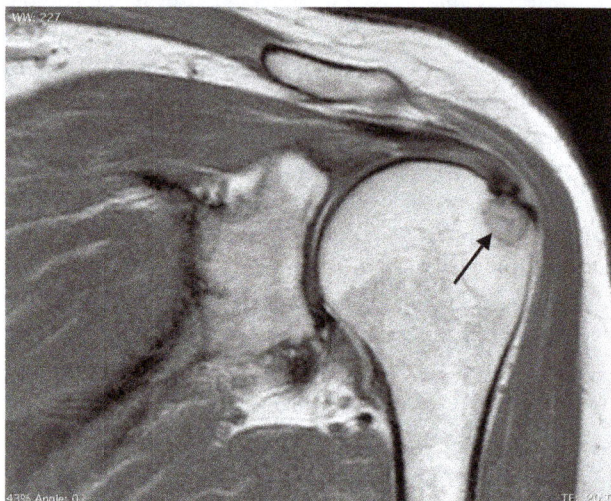

Fig. 5 T1-weighted coronal oblique MRI highlights a greater tuberosity osteolysis (*black arrow*) in a case with a calcium deposit of the SS in contact with the bone

studied a large series of such patients. MRI was used as the imaging modality of choice for detection of osteolysis as it was shown to be more reliable in demonstrating contact between the deposit and the bone (Fig. 5). He found that those calcium deposits which were in contact with the tuberosities consistently produced cortical lesions. These lesions were not related to the shape and size of the deposits or to the sex, age and occupation of the patients. Also, he found a significant correlation between clinical and imaging findings i.e. the more severe the osteolytic lesions, especially those extending to the lateral facet, the less improvement noticed at the final follow-up. Finally, he concluded that this subset of patients had less favorable outcomes with respect to the degree and time of functional recovery. Overall, in presence of OL the prognosis of patients with CT is worse and may be particularly resistant to the common conservative therapies. Although this subset of patients gain lower postoperative clinical scores, surgical approach should be considered in case of severe pain when all the other non-operative treatment fails; arthroscopic approach allow to identify the site of OL and to perform an accurate cleaning of the bone that is useful to reduce pain and improve shoulder function.

Ossifying tendinitis

This is an extremely rare complication of CT and to date only one article has been found to be published in a broad based literature search [6]. This is a type of heterotopic ossification characterized by deposition of hydroxyapatite crystals in a histologic pattern of mature lamellar bone [76]. It is usually associated with surgical intervention or trauma with the Achilles tendon, distal biceps and in gluteus maximus tendons. Merolla G et al. [6] studied two such cases in shoulder who had an arthroscopic removal of CT and subsequently was histologically proved to be ossifying tendinitis (OT) (Fig. 6a, b). Incidentally, both the

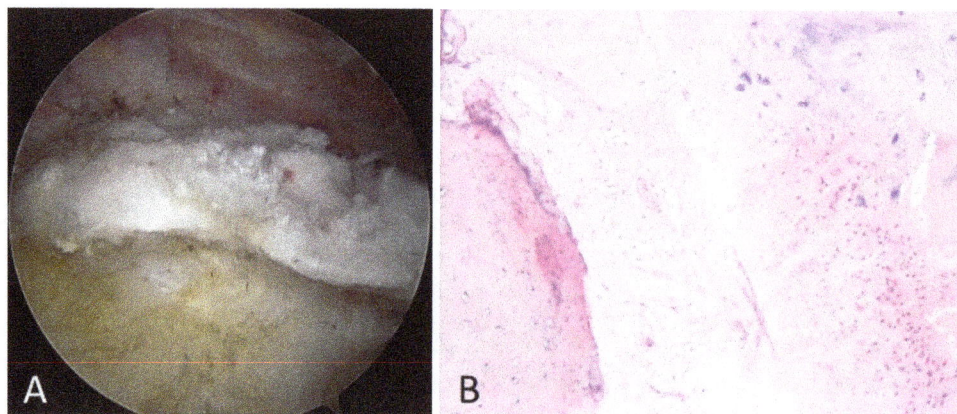

Fig. 6 a Arthroscopic finding of recurrence of calcific tendinitis of the rotator cuff in the form of ossifying tendinitis, **b** histologic examination confirmed the diagnosis showing tendinous tissue mixed with areas of chondroid and bone metaplasia

cases had an initial arthroscopic removal of a routine CT with subsequent recurrence which manifested itself as ossifying tendinitis. He hypothesized that the ossifications found could have been the result of a transformation of mesenchymal cells to bone-forming cells in response to the surgical excision of calcium deposit and suturing of the tendon during the index arthroscopic procedure. He recommended to consider arthroscopic excision of calcium deposits with caution and to be meticulous during the subacromial debridement of calcific foci to minimize the risk of recurrence. OT is a very rare complication of CT but the actual rate is unknown because of the very few patients have who undergone arthroscopic second-look in presence of radiographic evidence of recurrence of CT. We do believe that the number of cases with this complication is underestimated and we advise to be cautious in dealing with such cases and to refer the doubtful cases with persistent pain for more than a year to the surgeon.

Conclusions

The ideal treatment for the CT of the shoulder is not well established and for some aspects still controversial. The clinical course may be complicated by several conditions that should be diagnosed and treated when we manage a patient with CT of the RC. Whereas pain and stiffness are generally recognized and treated, the risk of RC tears is not well considered and the related surgical approach is a concern. Greater tuberosity osteolysis is less known and often not identified on radiograms or ultrasound, therefore, we would suggest to investigate with MRI in those patients with persistent chronic pain and doubtful standard X-ray. Finally, ossifying tendinitis is very rare and only recently reported as complication of CT that should be considered and investigated with X-ray in subjects with CT already treated with conservative or operative measures. We do believe that this review gives a quick summary of the potential complications of the CT, inviting all professionals (orthopaedic surgeons, physiatrists, radiologists and physiotherapists) who deal with this disease to consider not only the regular course of the CT but also the complications that must be identified and treated as well as possible.

Conflict of interest None.

Ethical standards The patients represented in this study provided informed consent to the publication of their clinical cases.

References

1. Balke M, Bielefeld R, Schmidt C, Dedy N, Liem D (2012) Calcifying tendinitis of the shoulder: midterm results after arthroscopic treatment. Am J Sports Med 40(3):657–661. doi:10.1177/0363546511430202
2. Cho NS, Lee BG, Rhee YG (2010) Radiologic course of the calcific deposits in calcific tendinitis of the shoulder: does the initial radiologic aspect affect the final results? J Shoulder Elb Surg 19:267–272. doi:10.1016/j.jse.2009.07.008
3. DePalma AF, Kruper JS (1961) Long term study of shoulder joints afflicted with and treated for calcific tendinitis. Clin Orthop Relat Res 20:61–72
4. Lippmann RK (1961) Observations concerning the calcific cuff deposit. Clin Orthop Relat Res 20:49–60
5. Rowe CR (1985) Calcific tendinitis. Instr Course Lect 34:196–198
6. Merolla G, Dave AC, Paladini P, Campi F, Porcellini G (2014) Ossifying tendinitis of the rotator cuff after arthroscopic excision of calcium deposits: two case reports and literature review. J Orthop Traumatol 15 [Epub ahead of print]
7. Bosworth B (1941) Calcium deposits in the shoulder and subacromial bursitis: a survey of 12122 shoulders. JAMA 116:2477–2482
8. El Shewy MT (2011) Arthroscopic removal of calcium deposits of the rotator cuff: a 7-year follow-up. Am J Sports Med 39(6):1302–1305. doi:10.1177/0363546510396320
9. Codman EA (1906) On stiff and painful shoulders. Boston Med Surg J 154:613–620
10. Moseley HF, Goldie I (1963) The arterial pattern of the rotator cuff of the shoulder. J Bone Joint Surg Br 45:780–789
11. Uhthoff HK, Loehr JW (1997) Calcific tendinopathy of the rotator cuff: pathogenesis, diagnosis and management. J Am Acad Orthop Surg 5:183–191
12. Plenk HP (1952) Calcifying tendinitis of the shoulder. Radiology 59:384–389
13. Re LP, Karzel RP (1993) Management of rotator cuff calcifications. Orthop Clin North Am 24:125–132
14. Friedman MS (1957) Calcified tendinitis of the shoulder. Am J Surg 94(1):56–61
15. Pfister J, Gerber H (1997) Chronic calcifying tendinitis of the shoulder-therapy by percutaneous needle aspiration and lavage: a prospective open study of 62 shoulders. Clin Rheumatol 16(3):269–274
16. Lee KS, Rosas HG (2010) Musculoskeletal ultrasound: how to treat calcific tendinitis of the rotator cuff by ultrasound-guided single-needle lavage technique. AJR Am J Roentgenol 195(3):638. doi:10.2214/AJR.10.4878
17. Serafini G, Sconfienza LM, Lacelli F, Silvestri E, Aliprandi A, Sardanelli F (2009) Rotator cuff calcific tendonitis: short-term and 10-year outcomes after two-needle US-guided percutaneous treatment. Nonrandomized controlled trial. Radiology 252(1):157–164. doi:10.1148/radiol.2521081816
18. Sabeti-Aschraf M, Dorotka R, Goll A, Trieb K (2005) Extracorporeal shock wave therapy in the treatment of calcific tendinitis of the rotator cuff. Am J Sports Med 33:1365–1368
19. Loew M, Daecke W, Kusnierczak D, Rahmanzadeh M, Ewerbeck V (1999) Shock wave therapy is effective for chronic calcifying tendonitis of the shoulder. J Bone Joint Surg Br 81:863–867
20. Loew M, Jurgowski W, Mau HC, Thomsen M (1995) Treatment of calcifying tendinitis of rotator cuff by extracorporeal shock waves: a preliminary report. J Shoulder Elb Surg 4:101–106
21. Rompe JD, Zoellner JZ, Nafe B (2001) Shock wave therapy versus conventional surgery in treatment of the calcifying tendonitis of the shoulder. Clin Orthop Relat Res 387:72–82

22. Porcellini G, Paladini P, Campi F, Paganelli M (2004) Arthroscopic treatment of calcifying tendinitis of the shoulder: clinical and ultrasonographic follow-up findings at two to five years. J Shoulder Elb Surg 13:503–508

23. McLaughlin HL (1963) The selection of calcium deposit for operation: the technique and results of operation. Surg Clin North Am 43:1501–1504

24. Ark JW, Flock TJ, Flatow EL, Bigliani LU (1992) Arthroscopic treatment of calcific tendonitis of the shoulder. Arthroscopy 8:183–188

25. Ellman H (1987) Arthroscopic subacromial decompression: analysis of one to three year results. Arthroscopy 3:173–181

26. Uhthoff HK, Sarkar K, Maynard JA (1976) Calcifying tendinits: a new concept of its pathogenesis. Clin Orthop Relat Res 118:164–168

27. Oliva F, Via AG, Maffulli N (2012) Physiopathology of intratendinous calcific deposition. BMC Med 10:95. doi:10.1186/1741-7015-10-95

28. Hamada J, Tamai K, Ono W, Saotome K (2006) Does the nature of deposited basic calcium phosphate crystals determine clinical course in calcific periarthritis of the shoulder? J Rheumathol 33:326–332

29. Penel G, Leroy G, Rey C, Bres E (1998) MicroRaman spectral study of the PO4 and CO3 vibrational modes in synthetic and biological apatites. Calcif Tissue Int 63:475–481

30. Chiou HJ, Hung SC, Lin SY, Wei YS, Li MJ (2010) Correlations among mineral components, progressive calcification process and clinical symptoms of calcific tendonitis. Rheumatology 49:548–555. doi:10.1093/rheumatology/kep359

31. Archer R, Bayley J, Archer C, Ali S (1993) Cell and matrix changes associated with pathological calcification of the human rotator cuff tendons. J Anat 182:1–12

32. Gohr CM, Fahey M, Rosenthal AK (2007) Calcific tendonitis: a model. Connect Tissue Res 48:286–291

33. Gartner J, Heyer A (1995) Calcific tendinitis of the shoulder. Orthopade 24(3):284–302

34. Gartner J, Simons B (1990) Analysis of calcific deposits in calcifying tendinitis. Clin Orthop 254:111–120

35. Molé D, Kempf JF, Gleyze P, Rio B, Bonnomet F, Walch G (1993) Results of endoscopic treatment of non-broken tendinopathies of the rotator cuff. Calcifications of the rotator cuff [in French]. Rev Chir Orthop 79:532–541

36. Maier M, Schmidt-ramsin J, Glaser C, Kunz A, Küchenhoff H, Tischer T (2008) Intra- and interobserver reliability of classification scores in calcific tendinitis using plain radiographs and CT scans. Acta Orthop Belg 74:590–595

37. Gosens T, Hofstee DJ (2009) Calcifying tendinitis of the shoulder: advances in imaging and management. Curr Rheumatol Rep 11(2):129–134

38. Le Goff B, Berthelot JM, Guillot P, Glémarec J, Maugars Y (2010) Assessment of calcific tendonitis of rotator cuff by ultrasonography: comparison between symptomatic and asymptomatic shoulders. Joint Bone Spine 77:258–263. doi:10.1016/j.jbspin.2010.01.012

39. Martinoli C, Bianchi S, Prato N, Pugliese F, Zamorani MP, Valle M, Derchi LE (2003) US of the shoulder: non-rotator cuff disorders. RadioGraphics 23:381–401

40. Chiou HJ, Chou YH, Wu JJ, Hsu CC, Huang DY, Chang CY (2002) Evaluation of calcific tendonitis of the rotator cuff—role of color doppler ultrasonography. J Ultrasound Med 21:289–295

41. Monteleone G, Tramontana A, Mc Donald K, Sorge R, Tiloca A, Foti C (2014) J Sports Med Phys Fitness 27 [Epub ahead of print]

42. Flemming DJ, Murphey MD, Shekitka KM, Temple HT, Jelinek JJ, Kransdorf MJ (2003) Osseous involvement in calcific tendinitis: a retrospective review of 50 cases. AJR Am J Roentgenol 181:965–972

43. Bayam L, Ahmad MA, Naqui SZ, Chouhan A, Funk L (2011) Pain mapping for common shoulder disorders. Am J Orthop 40(7):353–358

44. Spivey JL, Carrell TM (2009) Severe pain in the shoulder with no history of trauma. Calcific tendinitis. JAAPA 22(4):59–60

45. Hurt G, Baker CL Jr (2003) Calcific tendinitis of the shoulder. Orthop Clin North Am 34:567–575

46. Neer CS II (1990) Less frequent procedures. In: Neer CS II (ed) Shoulder reconstruction. WB Saunders, Philadelphia, pp 421–485

47. Gotoh M, Hamada K, Yamakawa H, Inoue A, Fukuda H (1998) Increased substance P in subacromial bursa and shoulder pain in rotator cuff diseases. J Orthop Res 16(5):618–621

48. Chen SK, Chou PH, Lue YJ, Lu YM (2008) Treatment for frozen shoulder combined with calcific tendinitis of the supraspinatus. Kaohsiung J Med Sci 24:78–84. doi:10.1016/S1607-551X(08)70101-3

49. Anton HA (1993) Frozen shoulder. Can Fam Physician 39:1773–1778

50. Cutts S, Clarke D (2002) The patient with frozen shoulder. Practitioner 246:730, 734–736,738–739

51. Harryman DT 2nd (1993) Shoulders: frozen and stiff. Instr Course Lect 42:247–257

52. Neviaser TJ (1987) Adhesive capsulitis. Orthop Clin North Am 18:439–443

53. Minter WT III (1967) The shoulder-hand syndrome in coronary disease. J Med Assoc Ga 56(2):45–49

54. Wohlgethan JR (1987) Frozen shoulder in hyperthyroidism. Arthritis Rheum 30(8):936–939

55. Cheville AL, Tchou J (2007) Barriers to rehabilitation following surgery for primary breast cancer. J Surg Oncol 95(5):409–418

56. Bowman CA, Jeffcoate WJ, Pattrick M, Doherty M (1988) Bilateral adhesive capsulitis, oligoarthritis and proximal myopathy as presentation of hypothyroidism. Br J Rheumatol 27(1):62–64

57. Ogilvie-Harris DJ, Myerthall S (1997) The diabetic frozen shoulder: arthroscopic release. Arthroscopy 13(1):1–8

58. Arkkila PE, Kantola IM, Viikari JS, Rönnemaa T (1996) Shoulder capsulitis in type I and II diabetic patients: association with diabetic complications and related diseases. Ann Rheum Dis 55(12):907–914

59. Rokito AS, Loebenberg MI (1999) Frozen shoulder and calcific tendonitis. Curr Opin Orthop 10:294–304

60. Neviaser RJ (1983) Painful conditions affecting the shoulder. Clin Orthop Relat Res 173:63–69

61. Noel E (1997) Treatment of calcific tendinitis and adhesive capsulitis of the shoulder. Rev Rhum Engl Ed 64:619–628

62. Jacobs R, Debeer P (2006) Calcifying tendinitis of the rotator cuff: functional outcome after arthroscopic treatment. Acta Orthop Belg 72:276–281

63. Mclaughlin HL, Asherman EG (1951) Lesions of the musculotendinous cuff of the shoulder. J Bone Joint Surg Am 33:76–86

64. Kernwein GA (1965) Roentgenographic diagnosis of shoulder dysfunction. JAMA 194:1081–1085

65. Wolfgang GL (1974) Surgical repair of tears of the rotator cuff of the shoulders: factors influencing the result. J Bone Joint Surg Am 56:14–26

66. Hsu HC, Wu JJ, Jim YF, Chang CY, Lo WH, Yang DJ (1994) Calcific tendinitis and rotator cuff tearing: a clinical and radiographic study. J Shoulder Elb Surg 3:759–764. doi:10.1016/S1058-2746(09)80095-5

67. Gotoh M, Higuchi F, Suzuki R, Yamanaka K (2003) Progression from calcifying tendinitis to rotator cuff tear. Skelet Radiol 32(2):86–89

68. Jerosch J, Strauss JM, Schmiel S (1998) Arthroscopic treatment of calcific tendinitis of the shoulder. J Shoulder Elb Surg 7:30–37

69. Yoo Jh, Park WH, Koh KH, Kim SM (2010) Arthroscopic treatment of chronic calcific tendinitis with complete removal and

rotator cuff tendon repair. Knee Surg Sports Traumatol Arthrosc 18:1694–1699. doi:10.1007/s00167-010-1067-7

70. Kayser R, Hampf S, Seeber E, Heyde CE (2007) Value of pre-operative ultrasound marking of calcium deposits in patients who require surgical treatment of calcific tendinitis of the shoulder. Arthroscopy 23:43–50

71. Ozkoc G, Akpinar S, Hersekli MA, Ozalay M, Tandogan RN (2002) Arthroscopic treatment of rotator cuff calcifying tendinitis. Acta Orthop Traumatol Turc 36:413–416

72. Seil R, Litzenburger H, Kohn D, Rupp S (2006) Arthroscopic treatment of chronically painful calcifying tendinitis of the supraspinatus tendon. Arthroscopy 22:521–527

73. Maier D, Balke M, Jaeger M, Izadpanah K, Suedkamp NP, Ogon P, Liem D (2012) Arthroscopic treatment of calcific tendinitis of

the shoulder: Letter to the Editor. Am J Sports Med 40(7): NP12-13. doi:10.1177/0363546512453459

74. Chan R, Kim DH, Millett PJ, Weissman BN (2004) Calcifying tendinitis of the rotator cuff with cortical bone erosion. Skelet Radiol 33:596–599

75. Porcellini G, Paladini P, Campi F, Pegreffi F (2009) Osteolytic lesion of greater tuberosity in calcific tendinitis of the shoulder. J Shoulder Elb Surg 18:210–215. doi:10.1016/j.jse.2008.09.016

76. Ozaki J, Kugai A, Tomita Y, Tamai S (1992) Tear of an ossified rotator cuff of the shoulder. A case report. Acta Orthop Scand 63:339–340

12

Midfoot reconstruction with serratus anterior–rib osteomuscular free flap following oncological resection of synovial sarcoma

Bruno Battiston[1] · Stefano Artiaco[2] · Raimondo Piana[3] · Elena Boux[3] ·
Pierluigi Tos[4]

Abstract During recent decades, the concept of surgical treatment of malignant bone and soft tissue sarcomas has evolved, with the aim of preserving limb function. In this paper we report a case of metatarsal reconstruction by means of serratus and rib free flap after excision of a synovial sarcoma located in the dorsal aspect of the midfoot. Five years after the operation, the patient was free from recurrence and recovered full foot function. Amputation has been widely used in the past and this procedure still remains a valuable option when limb salvage is not possible. Nevertheless, in selected cases, reconstruction by means of composite free flaps may be successfully used for limb preservation in the treatment of malignant foot tumors after surgical excision.

Keywords Microsurgery · Serratus anterior rib composite flap · Foot sarcoma

✉ Stefano Artiaco
stefartiaco@libero.it

[1] III Orthopaedic Division, Department of Orthopaedics and Traumatology, Orthopaedic and Trauma Center, Turin, Italy

[2] IV Orthopaedic Division, Department of Orthopaedics and Traumatology, Orthopaedic and Trauma Center, Via Zuretti 29, 10126 Turin, Italy

[3] Oncologic Orthopaedic Division, Department of Orthopaedics and Traumatology, Orthopaedic and Trauma Center, Turin, Italy

[4] Microsurgery Unit, Department of Orthopaedics and Traumatology, Orthopaedic and Trauma Center, Turin, Italy

Introduction

During recent decades the concept of surgical treatment of malignant bone and soft tissue sarcomas has progressively evolved, and the preservation of the uninvolved parts of the extremities and the achievement of an acceptable limb function have become a major goal of oncological and reconstructive surgery [1].

The foot is a very difficult site for limb salvage surgery because bone, tendons and neurovascular structures are present in close proximity. Anatomical compartments may be therefore difficult to isolate and preserve during oncological excision. Furthermore, this area does not offer opportunities for performing local flaps effective for covering and reconstructing complex tissue defects.

Amputation has been widely used in the past and this procedure still remains a valuable option in order to eradicate the tumor and preserve an overall good prognosis for the patient in many cases. However, free flaps have now become a possible solution for limb salvage and functional preservation.

Until now the use of free flaps for the treatment of complex defects of the foot, secondary to oncological excision of bone and soft tissue tumors, was limited to a small number of patients. It has been described in the literature by a few authors, who reported isolated clinical cases or small clinical series [1–4].

In this paper we report a case of metatarsal reconstruction by means of free serratus and rib flap after excision of a synovial sarcoma located in the dorsal aspect of the midfoot. This flap was previously used in a few cases reported in the literature for traumatic defect of the lower extremities [5–8]. To our knowledge, this is the first case in which this kind of flap has been used for the functional reconstruction of the foot in a patient affected by a malignant disease.

Case report

Clinical history

A 42-year-old woman came to our attention after two previous operations performed in another hospital for excision of a tumor mass located in the dorsal aspect of the midfoot. The patient presented 1 year after the second excisional biopsy which reported a diagnosis of neurinoma because of the recurrence of the tumor that was clinically located on the dorsal aspect of the foot in the 3rd metatarsal space (Fig. 1). No bone resection was performed during prior surgery. Magnetic resonance scanning confirmed the recurrence and defined the tumor extent, which did not involve neurovascular structures. Except for oncological disease, the patient was healthy and her clinical history was unremarkable. The specimens obtained during previous surgery were re-examined by a pathologist specialized in musculo-skeletal oncology, revealing a synovial sarcoma. The patient was then informed about the diagnosis and further surgical procedure was discussed in a consultation with oncological, orthopaedic, microsurgical and reconstructive staff. The operation was planned according to an oncological resection of the sarcoma including the 3rd and 4th metatarsal bones followed by reconstruction with osteomuscular serratus anterior and rib free flap in order to fill the defect and restore bone continuity for functional preservation. This flap was preferred to a vascularized fibular flap in order to avoid donor site morbidity because of the characteristics of the patient (highly active woman practising climbing and running).

En bloc tumor resection with wide margins, including the proximal and medial thirds of the 3rd and 4th metatarsal bone, was performed (Fig. 2). The plantar surface was disease-free, so the sensitivity of the foot was preserved. After tumor excision, a serratus anterior osteomuscular free flap including the 7th rib was transferred by

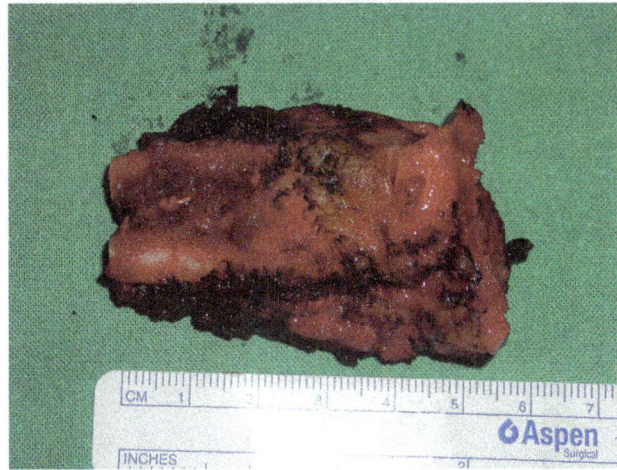

Fig. 2 En-bloc resected tumor

means of termino-lateral suture to the dorsalis pedis artery and vein (Fig. 3). The rib was fixed to the distal third of the 3rd and 4th metatarsal bones and to the base of the fifth metatarsal bone by means of K-wires (Fig. 4). Skin grafting was used to cover the flap and a temporary short leg splint was applied. The specimen was sent to the pathologist for histological examination. The tumor had a diameter of 1 cm and was located in the central part of the specimen with wide resection margins. Macroscopically, bone and surrounding soft tissues were not infiltrated. Microscopically, the tumor was immune-reactive to vimentin. The final histological diagnosis confirmed the preoperative suspicion of biphasic synovial sarcoma.

Postoperative course

The postoperative course was regular. K-wires were removed 2 months after the procedure. The vascularized rib graft healed with metatarsal bones and a progressive remodeling of the bones in the site of conjunction of the distal aspect of the transferred rib and proximal aspect of the 3rd and 4th metatarsal bones was observed (Fig. 5). No adjuvant therapy was performed. No donor site morbidity was observed due to rib resection. Partial and then full weight bearing were allowed in 2 and 3 months, respectively. Radiological healing was observed in 3 months. The patient returned to activities of daily life without limitation in 5 months and to sports activity (running and climbing) in 6 months. She did not show limitation of ankle or foot range of motion. Ambulation was physiological without limp and distance limitation. She had a periodical follow-up every 6 months, with clinical examination and magnetic resonance scan which did not show tumor recurrence. At last follow-up, 5 years after tumor excision and reconstructive procedure, the patient was free of recurrence and full functional recovery of the foot was observed (Fig. 6).

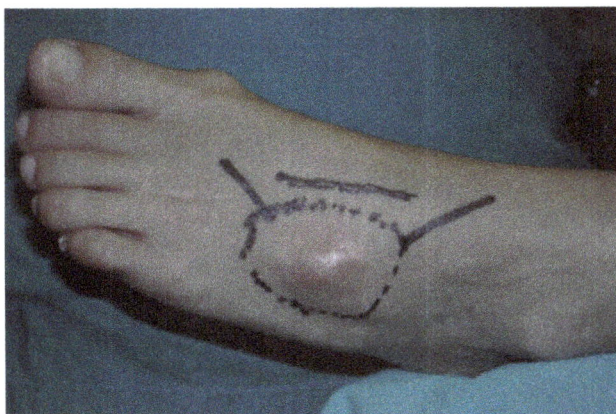

Fig. 1 Preoperative clinical view

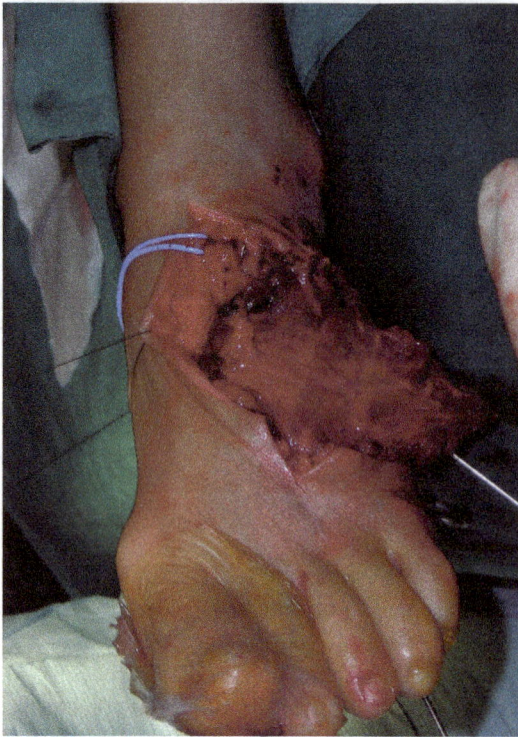

Fig. 3 Serratus anterior–rib composite flap transferred and fixed on the foot

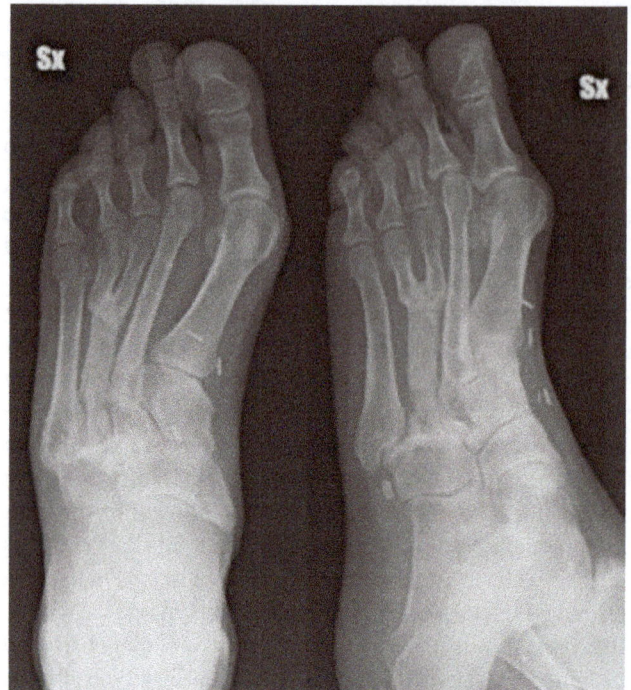

Fig. 5 Radiographic oblique and antero-posterior view at follow-up

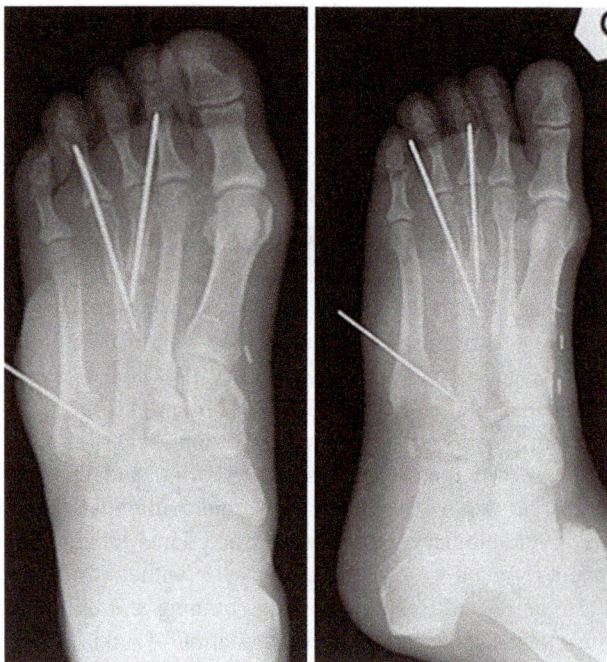

Fig. 4 Postoperative radiographic oblique and antero-posterior view

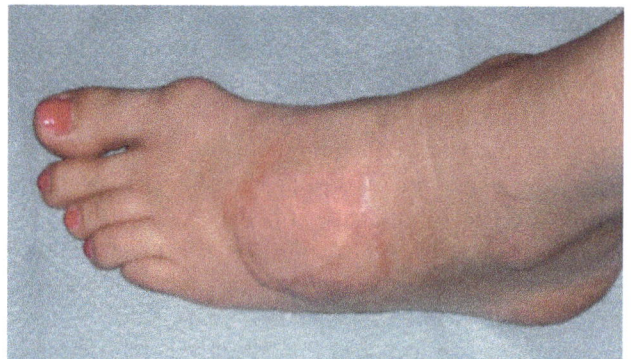

Fig. 6 Clinical view at follow-up

Discussion

Serratus anterior and rib free flap based on the serratus branches of the thoracodorsal artery was described by Richards et al. [9]. Anatomical studies demonstrated that the serratus muscle has a consistent anatomy, a long pedicle and an excellent malleability, and that the anastomosis around the rib between its vessels and those arising from the intercostal artery allows harvesting of composite muscle and rib flap useful for covering complex defects [10].

Metatarsal and soft tissue reconstruction with serratus anterior and rib flap has been rarely described in sequelae of traumatic injuries of the foot. Kurokawa repaired four metatarsal bones in the same foot, transferring a flap which included the 5th and 7th ribs into the flap and Kitsiou used the serratus anterior and rib flap in three further cases without complications, achieving positive clinical results [6–8].

In our case we performed the reconstruction after excision of synovial sarcoma involving the dorsal aspect of the midfoot. To our knowledge, this is the first case in which the serratus anterior and rib free flap was used for the reconstruction of defect following excision of foot sarcoma.

As reported by Toma et al. [1], limb salvage surgery may be an alternative to amputation in the treatment of malignant bone and soft tissues tumors involving the extremities but it is not an option for all malignant tumors of the foot. Optimal reconstruction requires resistance to mechanical stresses and intact sensation of the plantar surface which is essential for foot function and skin integrity [1]. Thus, this surgery is a valuable option in the case of tumors with dorsal extension, as observed in our case. Metatarsal reconstruction is particularly important when the first and second metatarsal rays are involved by the sarcoma. In these cases, weight bearing and foot propulsion on the first and second metatarsal ray should be preserved in order to avoid postoperative sequelae including painful overuse syndrome, transfer metatarsalgia and osteoarthritis of tarsal–metatarsal joints. If reconstruction of the foot after wide resection does not allow for functionality, or requires continuous medical care, sparing surgery of the foot would be burdensome for the patient. In these cases amputation followed by prosthetic fitting would be the optimal choice of treatment.

Conflict of interest The authors received no financial support for the research, authorship, and/or publication of this article. All authors disclose no financial or personal relationships with other people or organizations that could inappropriately influence their work.

Ethical standards All procedures performed in studies involving human participants were in accordance with the ethical standards of the institutional and/or national research committee and with the 1964 Helsinki declaration and its later amendments or comparable ethical standards. The patient gave informed consent to the publication of this article.

References

1. Toma CD, Dominkus M, Pfeiffer M, Giovanoli P, Assadian O, Kotz R (2007) Metatarsal reconstruction with use of free vascularized osteomyocutaneous fibular grafts following resection of malignant tumor of the midfoot. A series of six cases. J Bone Joint Surg 89-A:1553–1564
2. Tomczak RL, Johnson RE, Hamilton J (1993) The treatment of monostotic fibrous dysplasia of the first metatarsal with free vascularized fibular bone grafts. J Foot Ankle Surg 32:604–610
3. Exner GU, Jacob HA, Middendorp J (1998) Reconstruction of the first and second metatarsals with free microvascular fibular bone graft after resection of a Ewing sarcoma. J Pediatr Orthop B 7:239–248
4. Mochizuki K, Ishii Y, Yamaguchi H, MInabe T (1999) Vascularized tissue transplantation in limb salvage procedure for musculoskeletal sarcoma. J Orthop Surg 7:23–32
5. Duteille F, Waast D, Perrot P, Cronier P, Hubert L, Pannier M (2005) The serratus anterior free flaps in limb reconstruction. About 30 cases. Ann Chir Plast Est 50:71–75
6. Kitsiou C, Perrot P, Duteille F (2013) Reconstruction of complex foot defects by serratus anterior osteomuscular free flap: about four cases. Ann Chir Plast Est 58:321–326
7. Kurokawa M, Muneuchi G, Hamagami H, Fujita H (1998) Reconstruction of four metatarsal bone and soft tissue defects using a serratus anterior muscle rib osteomyocutaneous free flap. Plast Rec Surg 101:1616–1619
8. Kurokawa M, Yamada M, Suzuki S, Muneuchi G (2004) Long term follow-up of reconstruction of four metatarsal bone and soft tissue defects using a serratus anterior muscle rib osteomyocutaneous free flap. Plast Rec Surg 114:1553–1555
9. Richards MA, Poole MD, Godfrey AM (1985) The serratus anterior rib composite flap in mandibular reconstruction. Br J Plast Surg 38:466–477
10. Sabri F, Leclerq A, Vanwicik R (1993) Surgical anatomy of the serratus anterior-rib composite flap. Acta Ortho Belg 93:271–275

13

All-inside meniscal repair surgery: factors affecting the outcome

Haroon Majeed · SaravanaVail Karuppiah ·
Kohila Vani Sigamoney · Guido Geutjens ·
Robert G. Straw

Abstract

Background Meniscal injury is currently a well-recognized source of knee dysfunction. While it would be ideal to repair all meniscus tears, the failure rate is significantly high, although it may be reduced by careful selection of the patients. Our objective was to assess the outcome of meniscal repair surgery and the role of simultaneous reconstruction of the anterior cruciate ligament (ACL).

Materials and methods Retrospectively, all consecutive patients between January 2008 and 2011 who underwent meniscal repair were included. Patients were identified using the hospital database with diagnosis and procedure codes. Patient notes were reviewed, including details of the type of tear, chronicity, location, and surgery. We used symptomatic resolution as the outcome measure.

Results 136 Meniscal repairs were performed in 122 patients with a mean age of 26.8 years. Mean follow-up duration was 9 months. 63 % of the patients underwent medial and 37 % underwent lateral meniscal repair, with failure rates of 19 % for medial and 12 % for lateral menisci. Ligament injuries were found in 61 % of the patients ($n = 83$). Failure of meniscal repair occurred in 14.5 % ($n = 12$) of the patients who had early ACL reconstruction and in 27 % ($n = 22$) of the patients who had delayed ACL reconstruction ($p = 0.0006$). The failure rate was found to be 13 % in patients who were younger than 25 years (61 %) and 15 % in patients who were older than 25 years (39 %).

Conclusion The success rate of meniscal repair was found to be significantly better when ACL reconstruction was performed simultaneously with meniscal repair.

Level of evidence Level IV.

Keywords Meniscal preservation · Meniscal anchors · Knee meniscus · Knee arthroscopy · Failure of meniscal repair

H. Majeed (✉)
University Hospital of North Staffordshire,
Stoke-on-Trent ST4 6QG, UK
e-mail: haroonmajeed@gmail.com

S. Karuppiah · K. V. Sigamoney
Trauma and Orthopaedics, Royal Derby Hospital, Derby, UK
e-mail: saravanavail@gmail.com

K. V. Sigamoney
e-mail: kohilavani_sigamoney@yahoo.com

G. Geutjens · R. G. Straw
Royal Derby Hospital, Derby, UK
e-mail: guido.geutjens@derbyhospitals.nhs.uk

R. G. Straw
e-mail: robert.straw@derbyhospitals.nhs.uk

Introduction

Meniscal injury is currently a well-recognized source of knee dysfunction, and its arthroscopic treatment has become one of the most commonly performed orthopedic procedures around the world [1]. Meniscal resection is usually performed more commonly than repair, but there has been a shift in focus from meniscal resection to meniscal preservation and repair in recent years [1]. The meniscus withstands different forces, including shear, tension, and compression, and plays a crucial role in load-bearing, load transmission, and shock absorption. The contact area of a tibiofemoral joint surface may decrease by up to 20 % following a partial meniscectomy and by 50–70 % following a total meniscectomy. Hence, the resultant increase in contact stresses accelerates the progression of degenerative arthritis following a meniscectomy [2]. The development of arthritis following meniscal resection surgery may take up to 10–15 years in the case of a medial meniscus, but it may happen within 2 years in the case of a lateral meniscus [3].

The techniques employed for meniscal repair have also evolved in recent years. First-generation techniques for meniscal repair were based on Henning's technique (first inside-out repair, 1980) [4], but the potential risk of neurovascular damage has been a major concern for this type of repair. Russell Warren [5] introduced an outside-in technique which aimed at reducing neurovascular complications. In recent years, an all-inside technique has been introduced, which is widely used currently (Figs. 1, 2) [6].

It would be ideal to repair all meniscus injuries; however, the failure rate has been found to be significantly high and the implant costs considerable, requiring careful consideration and selection of the patients. Some studies have reported success rates for meniscal repair to be up to 60–90 % depending on the region of meniscal repair [7–10]. Meniscal repairs performed in conjunction with ACL reconstruction are generally thought to have a better healing rate than meniscal repair in knees with intact ACLs [7]. The objective of our study was to assess the outcome of meniscal repair surgery, focusing in particular on meniscal

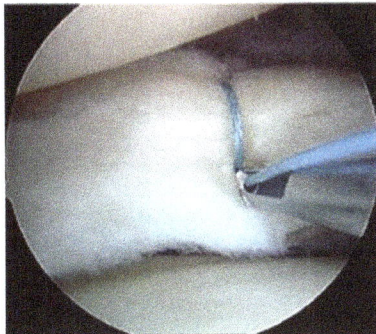

Fig. 1 Meniscal repair using the vertical mattress technique

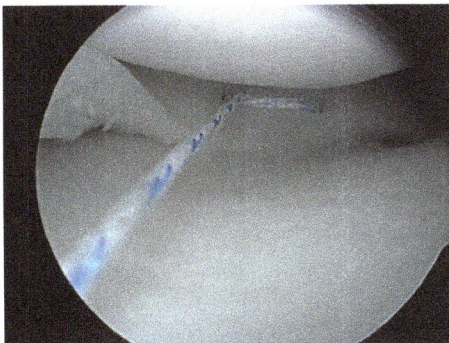

Fig. 2 Meniscal repair using the horizontal mattress technique

healing when the surgery is performed in conjunction with ACL reconstruction.

Materials and methods

We performed a retrospective review covering 3 years (January 2008–2011) in a large teaching hospital. All consecutive patients who underwent meniscal repair were included. The data were collected through patients' case notes and included demographic details, mechanism of injury, symptoms and their durations, details of the meniscal tear (type, location, size, age), postoperative rehabilitation regimen, concurrent surgical procedure, recurrent symptoms, and subsequent surgeries performed. We analyzed the data from different perspectives, comparing the outcomes for medial and lateral menisci, tears of different ages (more than 6 weeks and less than 6 weeks old), different age groups of patients (over 25 and under 25 years); menisci repaired with and without ACL reconstruction, and repairs in different zones of menisci.

All of our patients underwent arthroscopic meniscal repair performed using FasT-Fix anchors (Smith & Nephew®). The all-inside technique was used in all our patients. Postoperatively, the range of knee flexion was limited from 0 to 90° using an off-the-shelf knee brace for 6–8 weeks in order to protect the repaired menisci, followed by gradual rehabilitation with physiotherapy. Weight-bearing was allowed as tolerated, except in those patients who had multiligament reconstruction. This regime was followed in all our patients after surgery. We used symptomatic resolution (pain, swelling, and locking) as the outcome measure in order to assess the success rate. Statistical analysis was done using Fisher's exact test (two-tailed) for categorical variables and Student's t test (two-tailed) for numerical variables.

Results

One hundred thirty-six meniscal repairs were performed in 122 patients during our study period. The male to female ratio was 4:1. Age ranged from 11 to 58 years (mean 26.8 years). In male patients, age ranged from 11 to 49 years (mean 25 years), and in female patients it ranged from 20 to 58 years (mean 35.6 years). Mean follow-up duration was 9 months (1–26 months). The emergency department was the main source of referrals (53 %), followed by primary care (25 %) and the physiotherapy department (14 %). Main symptoms included pain (94 %), swelling (68 %), and mechanical locking (38 %). Instability (47 %) was seen predominantly in patients with associated ligament injuries. Plain X-rays were performed in

47 % of the patients and MRI scans in 86 % of the patients during the initial assessment of their injuries. Sixteen patients (11 %) were lost to follow-up 6–12 weeks after their surgery.

Mechanisms of injury included sports-related accidents in 58 % of the cases (football, rugby, cricket), falls (26 %), and road traffic accidents (5 %), while 5 % had no definite history of any specific trauma. Our patients belonged to three main categories of occupations: manual workers (28 %), office workers (23 %), and students (23 %), while 4 % of the patients were professional sportsmen. Indeed, most (79 %) of the patients included regular sporting activities in their daily routine (football, rugby, cricket, and gym exercises).

We used clinical symptomatic resolution as the outcome measure in our patients to assess the failure rate. Based on this assessment, 83 % ($n = 113$) of the meniscal repairs were assumed to have healed, as the patients had complete or significant resolution of their symptoms on subsequent regular follow-up. 17 % ($n = 23$) of the meniscal repairs were considered to have failed to heal due to ongoing or recurrent symptoms in these patients (pain, swelling, locking) (Table 1).

Medial vs. lateral meniscal tears

63 % of the tears were present in medial and 37 % in lateral menisci. The failure rate was found to be 19 % in cases of medial and 12 % in cases of lateral meniscal repair

($p = 1.00$). 33 % of the tears ($n = 45$) were found to be present in the white-white zone, 48 % ($n = 66$) in the red-white zone, and 9 % ($n = 12$) in the red-red zone. The failure rate of meniscal repairs in the white-white zone was 20 % ($n = 9$), that in the red-white zone was 14 % ($n = 9$), and that in the red-red zone was 16 % ($n = 2$). Bucket handle tears comprised the majority of the tears (70 %), followed by transverse (5 %), radial (4 %), and longitudinal (3 %) tears.

Associated ligament injuries

Ligament injuries were found in 83 patients (61 %) along with meniscal tears. These included acute ACL ruptures in 71 (52 %) patients, old ACL ruptures in 4 (3 %) patients, and recurrent ACL ruptures (which had been previously reconstructed) in 2 (1.5 %) patients. Six (4 %) patients had multiligament injuries. Of these 83 patients with ruptured ligaments, 55 (66 %) had simultaneous ACL reconstruction or reconstruction performed within 6 weeks of injury, while 26 (32 %) had their ACL reconstructed at a later stage following an initial meniscal repair (after 6 weeks of injury), and 2 (2.5 %) patients did not require reconstruction (no instability symptoms). Comparison of the results for the patients with an intact ACL with those for the patients with a reconstructed ACL (combined early and delayed) showed failure rates of meniscal repair of 16 % for the intact ACL group and 14 % for the reconstructed ACL

Table 1 Summary of outcomes for patients who underwent meniscal repair

	Number of meniscal repairs	Percentage success (%)	Failed repairs (%)	p Value
Age				
<25 years	83	87	13	0.80
>25 years	53	85	15	
Time of repair				
Early (<6 weeks)	82	91	9	0.49
Late (>6 weeks)	50	87	13	
ACL reconstruction				
With	81	86	14	0.20
Without (intact ACL)	53	84	16	
ACL reconstruction				
Simultaneous ACL	55	86	14	0.0006
Delayed ACL	26	77	27	
Zone of repair				
W/W	45	80	20	0.75
R/W	66	86	14	
R/R	12	84	16	
Side				
Medial	50	81	19	1.00
Lateral	86	88	12	

group. In the reconstructed ACL group, further analysis revealed that patients who had ACL reconstruction performed early (at the same time as meniscal repair or within 6 weeks of injury) had a meniscal repair failure rate of 14.5 % ($n = 12$). In comparison, patients who had delayed ACL reconstruction (after an initial meniscal repair and after 6 weeks of injury) had a meniscal repair failure rate of 27 % ($n = 22$; $p = 0.0006$). The difference between these two groups was found to be statistically significant.

Timing of surgery

60 % of the patients had meniscal repair surgery within 6 weeks after sustaining the injury (defined as "early repairs") and 37 % had surgery more than 6 weeks after the injury due to their delayed presentation (defined as "late repairs"). The failure rate was found to be 9 % in early repairs and 13 % in late repairs ($p = 0.49$). This difference was not statistically significant.

Young vs. old

In patients who were younger than 25 years (61 %), the failure rate was found to be 13 %, in comparison with a 15 % failure rate in patients who were older than 25 years (39 %; $p = 0.80$).

No evidence of degenerative changes was seen in 79 % cases, while 19 % showed pre-existing grade I/II changes and 2 % showed grade III/IV changes in articular cartilage. Two patients (1.6 %) had postoperative complications, including 1 patient with tense hemarthrosis requiring further washout and 1 patient who developed DVT in the operated leg (calf) and was treated with warfarin. The number of FasT-Fix anchors ranged from 2 to 7 for each meniscal repair (mean 2.7) (Fig. 3).

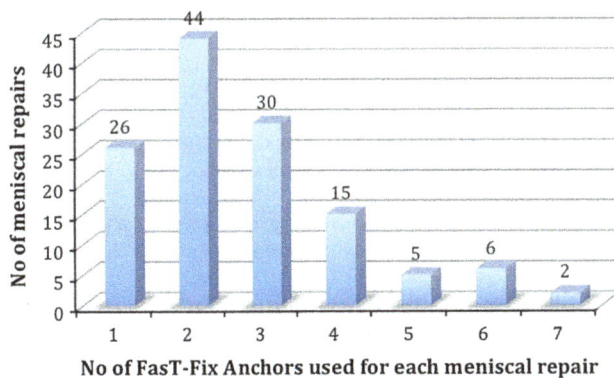

Fig. 3 Locations of tears in different zones of menisci

Failed meniscal repairs

The patients who were considered to have failed meniscal repairs (17 %, $n = 23$) underwent further investigations (MRI or CT arthrograms) and subsequently had repeat arthroscopy, which resulted in partial meniscal resection in 11 patients and re-repairs of the tears in 6 patients (the other 6 patients were lost to follow-up). The average age of the patients with failed repairs was 25.8 years (15–45 years). Another 10 % of the patients ($n = 14$) presented with recurrence of symptoms after initial resolution, with the recurrence occurring on average 5 months after surgery. Five of these patients had a history of recurrent trauma. Due to the persistence of their recurrent symptoms, after MRI or CT arthrograms, these patients underwent repeat arthroscopy which showed satisfactory healing of the menisci (complete or partial healing), without a new tear. On further follow-up, the symptoms in these patients gradually improved with physiotherapy within a few months.

Discussion

No single accepted definition for failure of meniscal repair exists in the current literature. Noyes et al. [11] defined failure of the repair as the "persistence of symptoms (swelling, locking, or joint pain) and/or the requirement for repeat knee arthroscopy and meniscectomy." There are three possible ways of identifying the healing (or failure) status of the repaired meniscus: repeat arthroscopy, repeat MRI scan, and correlation with clinical symptoms. Some studies have found that, on repeat arthroscopy after previous meniscal repair, the menisci were partially healed in the absence of ongoing clinical symptoms [12]. Muellner [13] showed that MRI does not have the ability to differentiate whether a meniscus has healed or not. Using clinical symptoms as a tool to assess the healing status provides only indirect evidence of successful healing. However, this is still to be accepted as an assessment tool because routine repeat arthroscopy in every patient to assess meniscal healing is not feasible in routine clinical practice. In addition, the patients may not want to be followed up once their symptoms have settled down after successful surgical management [11].

In young patients, sports-related injuries are usually the most common cause of a meniscal tear, accounting for more than one-third of all cases [14, 15]. The underlying mechanism of these injuries usually involves cutting or twisting movements and hyperextension [16]. Meniscal tears during these sports injuries have been reported to be accompanied by the rupture of the ACL in more than 80 % of cases [17]. In their study, Warren et al. [5] reported that the success rate of meniscal repair with ACL reconstruction can be up to 90 %, while the failure rate was 30–40 % when the knee remained unstable due to the ruptured ACL.

Our results showed that the failure rate was lower in cases of lateral meniscal repair. Previous studies have shown failure rates of 10 % for lateral and up to 40 % for medial meniscal repairs [18]. Our patients who had delayed ACL reconstruction had double the meniscal repair failure rate of the patients who had early ACL reconstruction along with meniscal repair ($p = 0.0006$). This is consistent with previous studies suggesting that 90 % of meniscal repairs are successful if the ACL is reconstructed at the same time as the meniscal repair, whereas failure rates of 30–40 % are seen if the knee remains unstable [5]. In addition to stability, ACL reconstruction is also considered to provide a favorable environment for meniscal repair healing due to intra-articular bleeding.

In our patients, the failure rate was only slightly better if meniscal tears were repaired within 6 weeks of injury. The available literature also does not suggest that the outcome changes depending on the age of the tear [19]. No major difference in the outcome was seen between different age groups of patients. The available literature does not suggest that the failure rate varies with patient age; however, in younger patients, meniscal preservation should be the preferred option in order to reduce the risk of subsequent arthritis, particularly for lateral meniscal tears. In our patients, the failure rate of meniscal repairs in the white-white zone was higher; this is consistent with previous studies which have suggested failure rates of up to 32 % in this zone [3].

Our study has a few limitations. It was a retrospective study. We used symptomatic resolution as the outcome measure in order to assess the success rate, and did not use objective scoring to accurately analyze our results. Our follow-up duration was short, and 11 % of the patients were lost to follow-up.

Our results have shown that the outcome of meniscal repair is statistically significantly better if ACL reconstruction is performed simultaneously with the meniscal repair ($p = 0.0006$). No significant dependence of the outcome on the age of the patient or the age or location of the tear was found ($p > 0.05$). However, considering the important role of the meniscus in maintaining knee function and preventing arthritis, meniscal preservation surgery should be considered whenever possible, especially in younger patients and cases of lateral meniscal tear.

Acknowledgments No financial support was received from any source for this study.

Conflict of interest None.

Ethical standards As this was a retrospective clinical audit, it did not require informed consent from the patients or Institutional Review Board approval under the regulations of the National Patient Safety Agency in the United Kingdom. The study conforms to the Declaration of Helsinki. All procedures were in accordance with ethical standards of the institutional and/or national research committee.

References

1. Tuckman DV et al (2006) Outcomes of meniscal repair: minimum of 2-year follow-up. Bull Hosp Jt Dis 63(3–4):100–104
2. McDermott ID, Amis AA (2006) The consequences of meniscectomy. J Bone Joint Surg Br 88(12):1549–1556
3. Gallacher PD et al (2010) White on white meniscal tears: to fix or not to fix? Knee 17(4):270–273
4. Henning CE (1983) Arthroscopic repair of meniscal tears. Orthopaedics 6:1130–1132
5. Warren RF (1985) Arthroscopic meniscus repair. Arthroscopy 1(3):170–172
6. Haas AL et al (2005) Meniscal repair using the FasT-Fix all-inside meniscal repair device. Arthroscopy 21(2):167–175
7. Ahn JH et al (2010) Clinical and second-look arthroscopic evaluation of repaired medial meniscus in anterior cruciate ligament-reconstructed knees. Am J Sports Med 38(3):472–477
8. DeHaven KE (1999) Meniscus repair. Am J Sports Med 27(2):242–250
9. Scott GA, Jolly BL, Henning CE (1986) Combined posterior incision and arthroscopic intra-articular repair of the meniscus. An examination of factors affecting healing. J Bone Joint Surg Am 68(6):847–861
10. Arnoczky SP, Warren RF (1982) Microvasculature of the human meniscus. Am J Sports Med 10(2):90–95
11. Noyes FR, Barber-Westin SD (2010) Repair of complex and avascular meniscal tears and meniscal transplantation. J Bone Joint Surg Am 92(4):1012–1029
12. Rodeo SA (2000) Arthroscopic meniscal repair with use of the outside-in technique. Instr Course Lect 49:195–206
13. Muellner T et al (1999) Open meniscal repair: clinical and magnetic resonance imaging findings after 12 years. Am J Sports Med 27(1):16–20
14. Baker BE et al (1985) Review of meniscal injury and associated sports. Am J Sports Med 13(1):1–4
15. Steinbruck K (1999) Epidemiology of sports injuries: 25-year-analysis of sports orthopedic-traumatologic ambulatory care. Sportverletz Sportschaden 13(2):38–52
16. Greis PE et al (2002) Meniscal injury: I. Basic science and evaluation. J Am Acad Orthop Surg 10(3):168–176
17. Rubman MH, Noyes FR, Barber-Westin SD (1998) Arthroscopic repair of meniscal tears that extend into the avascular zone. A review of 198 single and complex tears. Am J Sports Med 26(1):87–95
18. Logan M et al (2009) Meniscal repair in the elite athlete: results of 45 repairs with a minimum 5-year follow-up. Am J Sports Med 37(6):1131–1134
19. Kalliakmanis A et al (2008) Comparison of arthroscopic meniscal repair results using 3 different meniscal repair devices in anterior cruciate ligament reconstruction patients. Arthroscopy 24(7):810–816

14

A comparison of lateral release rates in fixed- versus mobile-bearing total knee arthroplasty

K. B. Ferguson · O. Bailey · I. Anthony ·
P. J. James · I. G. Stother · M. J. G. Blyth

Abstract

Background With increasing functional demands of patients undergoing total knee arthroplasty, mobile-bearing (MB) implants were developed in an attempt to increase the functional outcome of such patients. In theory, with MB implants, the self-alignment should reduce the rate of lateral release of the patella, which is usually performed to optimise patellofemoral mechanics. This study reports on the lateral release rates for the P.F.C. Sigma® MB posterior-stabilised total knee replacement (TKR) implant compared with its fixed-bearing (FB) equivalent.

Materials and methods A total of 352 patients undergoing TKR were randomly allocated to receive either MB (176 knees) or FB (176 knees) posterior-stabilised TKR. Further sub-randomisation into patellar resurfacing or retention was performed for both designs. The need for lateral patellar release was assessed during surgery using a 'no thumb technique', and after releasing the tourniquet if indicated.

Results The lateral release rate was the same for FB (10 %) and MB implants (10 %) ($p = 0.9$). However, patellar resurfacing resulted in lower lateral release rates when compared to patellar retention (6 vs 14 %; $p = 0.0179$) especially in MB implants (3 %).

Conclusions It has been previously reported that alterations to the design of the P.F.C. system with a more anatomical trochlea in the femoral component improved patellar tracking. The addition of a rotating platform tibial component to the P.F.C. Sigma system has, on its own, had no impact on the lateral release rate in this study. Optimising patellar geometry by patellar resurfacing appears more important than tibial-bearing design. Although MB implants appear to reduce the need for lateral release in the P.F.C. Sigma Rotating Platform, this only occurs when the patellar geometry has been optimised with patellar resurfacing.

Level of evidence Level 2.

Keywords Knee arthroplasty · Lateral release · Mobile bearing

Introduction

Fixed-bearing (FB) total knee arthroplasty is a successful operation with well-documented excellent long-term results [1, 2]. However, because of changing demographics in patients who require total knee arthroplasty, i.e., shifting to a younger population with higher functional demands, newer designs have been developed to achieve greater survivorship and clinical outcomes.

Mobile bearings (MBs) were designed to reduce the peak loading stress and backside wear observed as a cause of aseptic loosening in FB designs [3]. To achieve this, they have a more conforming superior articular surface which, in theory, reduces the contact stresses [1, 4–8]. The introduction of a second bearing interface results in a decoupling of the complex multidirectional motions which occur in FB designs producing unidirectional motion at the two bearing interfaces of the MB implant which, in theory, should reduce polyethylene wear. There have been concerns raised, however, about the risk of MB dislocation and

K. B. Ferguson (✉) · O. Bailey · I. Anthony ·
I. G. Stother · M. J. G. Blyth
Department of Orthopaedics and Trauma, Glasgow Royal Infirmary, 84 Castle Street, Glasgow G4 0SF, Scotland, UK
e-mail: kimbferguson@gmail.com

P. J. James
Department of Orthopaedics and Trauma, Nottingham City Hospital, Nottingham, UK

some reports of early backside wear in some clinical studies [1, 7].

In addition, MB designs have the potential to correct any rotational malalignment of the femoral and tibial components by allowing the patellar tendon to self-align throughout a range of motion, enhancing both patellofemoral and tibiofemoral mechanics [9]. Little attention has been given to the potential effects that this decoupling may have on the patellofemoral joint portion of the articulation. In theory, the self-alignment seen with MB designs should reduce the rate of lateral release of the patella, which is usually performed to optimise patellofemoral mechanics. This study reports on the lateral release rates for P.F.C.® Sigma MB posterior-stabilised TKR compared with its FB equivalent.

Materials and methods

Three hundred and fifty-two patients were randomised to receive a PFC Sigma© total knee replacement (TKR) with either FB or MB implants. The randomisation occurred at the pre-operative assessment stage with the inclusion of patients who had a pre-operative diagnosis of osteoarthritis. Patients who had undergone previous knee surgery, inflammatory arthropathy or had a significant co-morbidities were excluded from the trial.

The study was granted full ethical approval from the Multisite Research Ethics Committee and the Local Research Ethics Committee. Informed consent was obtained from each patient following a full explanation and provision of all necessary patient information.

A single knee design was used in this study (PFC Sigma® Posterior Stabilised; DePuy Inc., Warsaw, IN, USA) with all components being cemented using Palacos®cement. The femoral component was constant for all patients with the tibial component being randomised into two main groups (MB vs FB) using a third party computerised randomisation process.

Each patient was randomised into receiving either FB or MB prosthesis, and sub-randomisation was performed to determine whether the patella would be resurfaced or not. The need for lateral release was determined at the time of surgery using a 'no thumb technique' and releasing the tourniquet if required. Lateral release was performed where tilting or subluxation of the patella occurred as the knee was taken through a range of motion, before retinacular closure. There was no difference between lateral release rates between surgeons (Fig. 1).

The surgical details of the 352 patients recruited into the trial were used. The two groups were matched for age, sex and body mass index (Table 1). Statistical analysis of the data was performed by an independent statistician. For normally distributed data, the two-sample t-test was used. Where the data had unequal variance or was not normally distributed, the Wilcoxon rank sum test was used.

Results

The lateral release rate was the same for both the FB and MB designs with 17 patients in each group requiring lateral release (10 %) ($p = 0.9$) (Table 2).

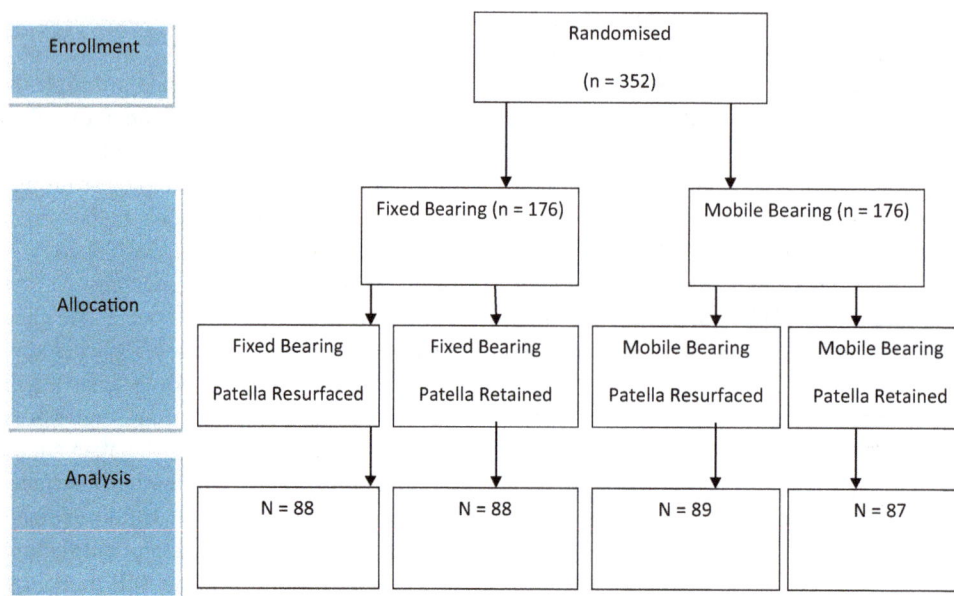

Fig. 1 CONSORT diagram

Table 1 Cohort demographics

	Fixed-bearing implants	Mobile–bearing implants	p value
Patients (n)	176	176	
Age			
Mean (years) (SD)	69.8 (8.16)	70.2 (7.60)	0.70*
Range	42–89	52–89	
Gender			
Female (n) (%)	94 (53 %)	93 (53 %)	1.0+
Male (n) (%)	82 (47 %)	83 (47 %)	
ASA			
I (n) (%)	66 (38 %)	47 (27 %)	0.03!
II (n) (%)	100 (57 %)	111 (63 %)	
III (n) (%)	9 (5 %)	18 (10 %)	
No data (n)	1 (1 %)	0	
Body mass index			
Mean (kg/m²) (SD)	29.7 (4.9)	31.1 (5.0)	0.28*

* p value based on a two-sample t-test with unequal variance

! p value based on chi-squared test

+ p value based on Fisher's exact test

There was a statistically significant difference, however, in the lateral release rates between the patients who had their patella resurfaced and those who did not (6 vs 14 %) (p = 0.0179) (Table 3).

Closer analysis of the data including sub-randomisation of the bearing type, revealed an insignificant difference in the lateral release rates between those who had patellar resurfacing and those who did not in the FB group (8 vs 11 %) (p = 0.4). However, there was a significantly lower rate of lateral release in the patients in the MB group who had patellar resurfacing compared to those who did not (3 vs 16 %) (p = 0.009) (Table 4).

Discussion

Lateral release has been performed with FB TKA to optimise patellar tracking [10]; however, it is not without complications by jeopardising soft tissue and wound healing [10, 11]. Lateral release has also been proposed as a cause of avascular necrosis of the patella by interrupting the blood supply [11, 12]. Scuderi et al. demonstrated a higher incidence of vascular compromise to the patella when lateral release was performed [12]. If MB reduces the lateral release rate it may therefore reduce the rate of these complications.

In MB total knee arthroplasty there is potential for self-alignment of the bearing with the femoral component [13]. In an FB design that is inserted with internal rotation of the tibial component, the tibial tubercle becomes lateralized; however, with an MB design the self-alignment potentially permits correction in this circumstance [9, 13]. Rees et al. [14] provided evidence in support of this theory with in vivo fluoroscopic studies. Sawaguchi et al. [13] demonstrated in an intra-operative kinematic study that there was significantly improved patellar tracking with decreased patellofemoral contact stresses. Despite this theoretical advantage, there is no evidence as yet to demonstrate better clinical outcomes [9].

Design improvements of the femoral component of the PFC Sigma® system created a more anatomic trochlear groove that has favourably enhanced patella tracking [15]. In this study, Ballantyne et al. demonstrated a lateral release rate of 15.1 % for the newer FB PFC Sigma® design [15] compared to the older press-fit condylar prosthesis in prospective groups of patients. The addition of a rotating platform tibial component had no impact on the lateral release rate in our study; however, there was a statistically significant positive advantage for patellar resurfacing. This suggests that it is patellofemoral congruency rather than patellofemoral alignment that determines the need for lateral release in TKR.

Table 2 Lateral release rates of fixed versus mobile bearings

	No release n (%)	Lateral release n (%)	Medial release n (%)	Other n (%)
Fixed (n = 176)	159 (90)	17 (10)	0 (0)	0 (0)
Mobile (n = 176)	158 (90)	17 (10)	0 (0)	1 (<1)*
p value		p = 0.9		

* Posterior release

Table 3 Lateral release rates of patella resurfacing versus retention

	No release n (%)	Lateral release n (%)	Medial release n (%)	Other n (%)
Patella resurfaced (n = 176)	166 (94)	10 (6)	0 (0)	0 (0)
Patella retained (n = 176)	151 (86)	24 (14)	0 (0)	1 (<1)*
p value		p = 0.0179		

Table 4 Lateral release rates of fixed versus mobile versus patella

Bearing	Patella	No release n (%)	Lateral release n (%)	Medial release n (%)	Other n (%)
Fixed	Resurfaced ($n = 89$)	81 (92)	7 (8)	0 (0)	0 (0)
	Retained ($n = 88$)	78 (89)	10 (11)	0 (0)	0 (0)
p value			$p = 0.44$		
Mobile	Resurfaced ($n = 88$)	85 (96)	3 (3)	0 (0)	0 (0)
	Retained ($n = 89$)	73 (84)	14 (16)	0 (0)	1 (<1)
p value			$p = 0.009$		

The data also show the positive effects of patellar resurfacing and MB TKR which together gave the lowest lateral release rates of all groups. Perhaps the benefits offered by the rotating platform design which allows self-alignment of the patella are only realised once the patellofemoral geometry has been optimised. We believe that patellar resurfacing may therefore reduce the need for lateral release in MB knees and should be considered when tracking is suboptimal at the time of assessment with trial components in situ.

Acknowledgments The authors would like to thank Pauline May and Wendy Gerrard-Tarpey for their contribution.

Conflict of interest The authors declare that institutional support was received from DePuy. One of the senior authors is a paid consultant of DePuy.

Ethical standards The study was subjected to full ethical approval through both the Multisite Research Ethics Committee and the Local Research Ethics Committee and was performed in accordance with the ethical standards of the 1964 Declaration of Helsinki as revised in 2000. All patients provided informed consent prior to enrolment within the trial.

References

1. Bhan S, Malhotra R, Kiran EK, Shukla S, Bijjawara M (2005) A comparison of fixed-bearing and mobile-bearing total knee arthroplasty at a minimum follow-up of 4.5 years. J Bone Joint Surg Am 87(10):2290–2296
2. Kim YH, Kim JS, Choe JW, Kim HJ (2012) Long-term comparison of fixed-bearing and mobile-bearing total knee replacements in patients younger than fifty-one years of age with osteoarthritis. J Bone Joint Surg Am 94(10):866–873
3. Ball ST, Sanchez HB, Mahoney OM, Schmalzried TP (2011) Fixed versus rotating platform total knee arthroplasty: a prospective, randomized, single-blind study. J Arthroplast 26(4):531–536
4. Argenson JN, Parratte S, Ashour A, Saintmard B, Aubaniac JM (2012) The outcome of rotating-platform total knee arthroplasty with cement at a minimum of ten years of follow-up. J Bone Joint Surg Am 94(7):638–644
5. Jolles BM, Grzesiak A, Eudier A, Dejnabadi H, Voracek C, Pichonnaz C et al (2012) A randomised controlled clinical trial and gait analysis of fixed- and mobile-bearing total knee replacements with a five-year follow-up. J Bone Joint Surg Br 94(5):648–655
6. Watanabe T, Tomita T, Fujii M, Hashimoto J, Sugamoto K, Yoshikawa H (2005) Comparison between mobile-bearing and fixed-bearing knees in bilateral total knee replacements. Int Orthop 29(3):179–181
7. Bhatt H, Rambani R, White W, Chakrabarty G (2012) Primary total knee arthroplasty using the P.F.C Sigma®-rotating platform cruciate retaining endoprosthesis—a 6 year follow up. Knee 19(6):856–859
8. Stukenborg-Colsman C, Ostermeier S, Hurschler C, Wirth CJ (2002) Tibiofemoral contact stress after total knee arthroplasty: comparison of fixed and mobile-bearing inlay designs. Acta Orthop Scand 73(6):638–646
9. Pagnano MW, Trousdale RT, Stuart MJ, Hanssen AD, Jacofsky DJ (2004) Rotating platform knees did not improve patellar tracking: a prospective, randomized study of 240 primary total knee arthroplasties. Clin Orthop Relat Res 428:221–227
10. Laskin RS (2001) Lateral release rates after total knee arthroplasty. Clin Orthop Relat Res 392:88–93
11. Lewonowski K, Dorr LD, McPherson EJ, Huber G, Wan Z (1997) Medialization of the patella in total knee arthroplasty. J Arthroplast 12(2):161–167
12. Scuderi G, Scharf SC, Meltzer LP, Scott WN (1987) The relationship of lateral releases to patella viability in total knee arthroplasty. J Arthroplast 2(3):209–214
13. Sawaguchi N, Majima T, Ishigaki T, Mori N, Terashima T, Minami A (2010) Mobile-Bearing total knee arthroplasty improves patellar tracking and patellofemoral contact stress. In vivo measurements in the same patients. J Arthroplast 25(6):920–925
14. Rees JL, Beard DJ, Price AJ, Gill HS, McLardy-Smith P, Dodd CA et al (2005) Real in vivo kinematic differences between mobile-bearing and fixed-bearing total knee arthroplasties. Clin Orthop Relat Res 432:204–209
15. Ballantyne A, McKinley J, Brenkel I (2003) Comparison of the lateral release rates in the press fit condylar prosthesis and the PFC Sigma prosthesis. Knee 10(2):193–198

15

Relationship between the Charlson Comorbidity Index and cost of treating hip fractures: implications for bundled payment

**Daniel J. Johnson · Sarah E. Greenberg · Vasanth Sathiyakumar ·
Rachel Thakore · Jesse M. Ehrenfeld · William T. Obremskey ·
Manish K. Sethi**

Abstract

Background The aim of this study is to investigate how the Charlson Comorbidity Index (CCI) scores contribute to increased length of stay (LOS) and healthcare costs in hip fracture patients.

Materials and methods Through retrospective analysis at an Urban level I trauma center, charts for all patients over the age of 60 years who presented with low-energy hip fracture were evaluated. 615 patients who underwent operative fixation of hip fracture or hemiarthroplasty secondary to hip fracture were identified using Current Procedural Terminology (CPT) codes search and included in the study. Data was collected on patient demographics, medical comorbidities, and hospitalization length; from this, the CCI score and the cost to the institution (with an average cost/day of inpatient stay of $4,530) were calculated.

Results Multivariate linear regression analysis modeled the length of stay as a function of CCI score. Each unit increase in the CCI score corresponded to an increase in length of hospital stay and hospital costs incurred [effect size = 0.21; (0.0434–0.381); $p = 0.014$]. Patients with a CCI score of 2 (compared to a baseline CCI score of 0), on average, stayed 1.92 extra days in the hospital, and incurred $8,697.60 extra costs.

Conclusions The CCI score is associated with length of stay and hospital costs incurred following treatment for hip fracture. The CCI score may be a useful tool for risk assessment in bundled payment plans.

Level of evidence Level III.

Keywords Charlson Comorbidity Index · Costs · Length of stay (LOS)

Institutuional Review Board approval: this study has approval from the Vanderbilt IRB JORT-D-14-00156.

D. J. Johnson · S. E. Greenberg · V. Sathiyakumar · R. Thakore
· J. M. Ehrenfeld · W. T. Obremskey · M. K. Sethi (✉)
The Vanderbilt Orthopaedic Institute Center for Health Policy,
Vanderbilt University, Suite 4200, South Tower, MCE,
Nashville, TN 37221, USA
e-mail: manish.sethi@vanderbilt.edu;
Manish.K.Sethi@Vanderbilt.edu

D. J. Johnson
e-mail: Daniel.j.johnson@vanderbilt.edu

S. E. Greenberg
e-mail: Sarah.e.greenberg@Vanderbilt.edu

V. Sathiyakumar
e-mail: Vasanth.sathiyakumar@vanderbilt.edu

R. Thakore
e-mail: Rachelvthakore@gmail.edu

J. M. Ehrenfeld
e-mail: Jesse.ehrenfeld@vanderbilt.edu

W. T. Obremskey
e-mail: William.obremskey@vanderbilt.edu

Introduction

Hip fracture procedure volumes have risen in recent years, largely due to an aging population, and this trend is expected to increase dramatically in the coming decades, from 250,000 procedures annually to 500,000 by 2040 [1]. With current estimates of treating a hip fracture averaging $11,844–13,805, bundled payments have been proposed to contain costs without sacrificing quality in hip fracture treatment [2–4]. Bundled payments, otherwise known as episode-of-care payments, set a fixed reimbursement amount that collectively holds all providers responsible for patient outcomes. A key component of episode-based payment is that it attributes an episode of care as the length of time that an "average" patient would need for a certain intervention, and any increase in cost due to an unplanned prolonged length of stay (LOS) may have a significant negative financial impact on any institution caring for a hip fracture patient [5]. To protect the institution from incurring such costs, it is imperative to identify the patient factors that are associated with increased costs, and to develop methods to standardize their weighting and quantify their economic impact.

A number of scoring systems which summarize the patient's overall health status have been developed, including the American Society of Anesthesiologist's score (the ASA score), the Elixhauser score, and the Charlson Comorbidity Index (CCI). Higher ASA scores have been shown to be associated with increased hospital costs secondary to increased LOS in hip fracture patients [6]. Similarly, work by Nikkel et al. [2] demonstrated that higher Elixhauser scores are correlated with increased length of hospitalization and hospital costs incurred in hip fracture patients. Higher Charlson Comorbidity Index scores have been shown to correlate with increased 30-day mortality after hip fractures [7], increased 90-day mortality after hip fractures [8], increased in-hospital mortality in patients with hip fractures [9], and readmission rates after orthopedic procedures, including treatment of hip fractures [10]. Data about the relationship between CCI and LOS following hip fracture is limited, and at the present time, there are no studies to our knowledge, looking at the relationship between CCI scores and length of hospitalization in the United States; therefore, this study assesses the relationship between CCI, as a useful indicator of patient health and LOS following hip fracture, and estimates additional hospital costs that may be used to weight bundled payments.

Materials and methods

Institutional review board approval was obtained for this study. This was a retrospective cohort study that included all patients who underwent operative fixation of hip fracture or hemiarthroplasty secondary to hip fracture, including both femoral neck fractures and intertrochanteric fractures, at Vanderbilt University Medical Center, a level one trauma center, from January 2000 to December 2009. Current Procedural Terminology (CPT) codes were used to find patients who had experienced a hip fracture from a low-energy fall and received an intervention of cephalomeduallary nailing (CMN), closed reduction and percutaneous pinning (CRPP), total hip arthroplasty (THR), hemiarthroplasty (hemi), or open reduction internal fixation (ORIF). All patients over the age of 60 years with acetabular, proximal femoral, femoral neck, and

trochanteric fractures were selected. Patients with incomplete medical records were excluded. Additional demographic and clinical covariates were collected from our institution's electronic medical records database. Medical comorbidities were documented preoperatively by routine preoperative assessment, and, from this data, the Charlson Comorbidity Index was calculated according to Deyo's description [11].

The average total cost to the hospital of an inpatient day ($4,530 per day) was obtained from the institution's financial services and the average cost was treated as a unit cost per inpatient day. All fractional LOS values were rounded to the nearest whole number and multiplied by the per day cost.

The primary outcome of interest was the relationship between the CCI and the length of hospitalization. Risk of the occurrence of the outcome of interest (i.e. LOS) was modeled as a function of the preoperative CCI using multivariable linear regression. The multivariate linear regression model controlled for confounders (gender, ASA, body mass index, race, smoking status, anesthesia type and comorbidities) previously found to be associated with the outcome (i.e. prolonged LOS). Statistical significance was set at $p = 0.05$.

Results

Six hundred and fifteen complete records were obtained for isolated low-energy hip fractures in patients 60 years or older who were treated at our Level 1 trauma center. The average age of the hip fracture patient was 78.4 years and 51.7 % of our patients were aged 75–89 years. Caucasians comprised the majority of our patient cohort (84.7 %), followed by African-Americans (7.3 %). Nearly three-quarters of our patient cohort had a CCI score less than 3, and more than half of the cohort had a CCI score of either 0 or 1. Patient characteristics and demographic data are summarized in Table 1.

The different surgical procedures performed, classified by CPT codes, and the average LOS and hospital costs incurred for the inpatient stay are summarized in Table 2. The three most common procedures, representing 52.7 % of the procedures performed, were partial hip hemiarthroplasty (CPT code 7125; 19.7 %), open reduction and internal fixation of inter/per/subtrochanteric fracture with plate or screw, with/without cerclage (CPT 27244; 19.0 %), and open reduction and internal fixation of femoral neck fracture (CPT 27236; 14.0 %). These three procedures had an average LOS of 7.37 days with an average cost of $33,401. Overall, for all the procedures, the average LOS was 5.84 days and the average cost was $26,470 with a median of $27,180.

Table 1 Demographic information

	N	%
Age (years)		
60–64	76	12.4
65–69	67	10.9
70–74	77	12.5
75–79	107	17.4
80–84	106	17.2
85–89	105	17.1
>90	77	12.5
Gender		
Male	201	32.7
Female	414	67.3
Race		
African-American	45	7.3
Asian	3	0.5
Caucasian	521	84.7
Hispanic/Latino	2	0.3
Declined to volunteer	44	7.2
Current smoker		
No	599	97.4
Yes	16	2.6
CCI Score		
0	179	29.1
1	165	26.8
2	110	17.9
3	58	9.4
4	37	6.0
5	13	2.1
6	13	2.1
7	11	1.8
8	11	1.8
9	10	1.6
10	3	0.5
11	3	0.5
12	1	0.2
13	0	0.0
14	1	0.2

Male gender (which represented 33 % of our cohort) was also significantly associated with an additional 1.12 (95 % CI 0.375–1.865) days in hospital ($p = 0.003$); the financial implication of this finding is that each male patient costs the hospital an additional $5,073.60 as compared to a female patient (see Table 1). There was also an association between smoking status and hip fractures, but this did not reach statistical significance, probably due to the lack of power as there were only 16 current smokers, representing 2.6 % of our patient cohort.

There was an association between CCI score and LOS [effect size: 0.21 (0.0434–0.381); $p = 0.014$] with higher CCI scores having an increased likelihood of longer hospital LOS, and consequently higher costs, as summarized in Figs. 1 and 2. The average LOS for our patients with a CCI score of 0 was 5.8 days ($26,274.00); patients with a CCI score of 1 had an average LOS of 6.5 days ($30,577.50); patients with a CCI score of 2 had an average LOS of 7.72 days ($34,971.60); patients with a CCI score of three or greater had an average LOS of 7.77 days ($35,175.45). Therefore, the financial difference between treating a patient with a CCI score of 0 as compared to a patient with a CCI score of 2 was an additional $8,697.60 per patient.

Discussion

We found that increasing CCI scores are associated with longer LOS following hip fracture, and we quantified the cost burden attributable to this prolonged LOS. Our finding supports the work of other authors who have noted a relationship between comorbidities and prolonged LOS and increased hospital costs following hip fracture [2]; however, our study is the first to assess this relationship using the CCI.

Because there are currently no other published studies examining the relationship between the CCI score and LOS and hospital costs following hip fractures, we compared our findings with those reported for total joint arthroplasty. In the Tien et al. [12] study of total joint arthroplasty in Taiwan, a CCI score of 1 or higher correlated well with length of hospitalization and higher hospital costs. In parallel, our study is the first to suggest that an increased CCI score is associated with a prolonged LOS and increased hospital costs after hip fracture treatment. The relationship between the CCI score and LOS following different procedures implies that the CCI score can succinctly summarize a patient's overall health status, and therefore makes it a versatile tool to use for risk stratification in negotiating bundled payments. The CCI score has also been shown to be associated with short-term mortality following hip fractures [7–9] and a relationship between higher CCI scores and readmission rates following any orthopedic procedure has also been identified [10].

There are several factors to consider in the interpretation of our results. First, the comorbidities of our patient population and the cost of inpatient care reflect the practice of a single, tertiary care, academic medical center, and further analysis is necessary to determine whether our findings are applicable to other surgical settings. Secondly, we only evaluated bundled payments that were related to the inpatient cost from the index procedure, and although this limitation does not affect our findings regarding the association between the CCI score and increased hospital

Table 2 Procedures

CPT code	Procedure	Number of cases	Percentage (%)	Average LOS (days)	Average cost ($4530 per day)
75.35	Insertion of intramedullary nail – femur	6	1.0	6.00	$27,180.00
78.59	Percutaneous pinning of hip	14	2.3	5.36	$24,280.80
79.352	Open reduction internal fixation of femoral neck	1	0.2	3.00	$13,590.00
79.353	Open reduction internal fixation of femoral head	2	0.3	3.00	$13,590.00
79.783	Percutaneous pinning of lower extremity	2	0.3	5.50	$24,915.00
79.855	Open reduction internal fixation of hip with compression screw and plate	3	0.5	6.00	$27,180.00
79.857	Open reduction internal fixation of intertrochanteric fx	20	3.3	5.05	$22,876.50
81.6	Arthroplasty of hip – total primary	2	0.3	6.50	$29,445.00
846	Hemiarthroplasty of hip	29	4.7	5.95	$26,953.50
7125	Hemiarthroplasty hip – partial	121	19.7	7.72	$34,971.60
27130	Arthroplasty, acetabular and proximal femoral prosthetic replacement with or without autograft/allograft	37	6.0	8.41	$38,097.30
27130A	Arthroplasty, acetabular and proximal femoral prosthetic replacement with or without autograft/allograft, anterior	5	0.8	9.00	$40,770.00
27235	Percutaneous skeletal fixation, femoral fx, proximal, neck	45	7.3	5.67	$25,685.10
27236	Treatment, open femoral fx, proximal end, neck, internal fixation/prosthetic replacement	86	14.0	7.12	$32,253.60
27244	Treatment, inter/per/subtrochanteric femoral fx, with plate/screw type implant,with or without cerclage	117	19.0	7.28	$32,978.40
27245	Open treatment, inter/per/subtrochanteric femoral fx, with intermedullary implant, with or without screw/cerclage	82	13.3	6.95	$31,483.50
27248	Open treatment, greater trochanteric fx, with or without internal or external fixation	5	0.8	4.40	$19,932.00
27254	Open treatment, hip dislocation, traumatic, with acetabular wall/femoral head fx, with or without internal or external fixation	1	0.2	7.00	$31,710.00
27506	Open treatment, femoral shaft fx, with insertion, intramedullary implant, with or without screw/cerclage	30	4.9	6.30	$28,539.00
27507	Open treatment, femoral shaft fx, with plate/screws, with or without cerclage	6	1.0	3.50	$15,855.00
27509	Percutaneous skeletal fixation, femoral fx, distal end	1	0.2	3.00	$13,590.00

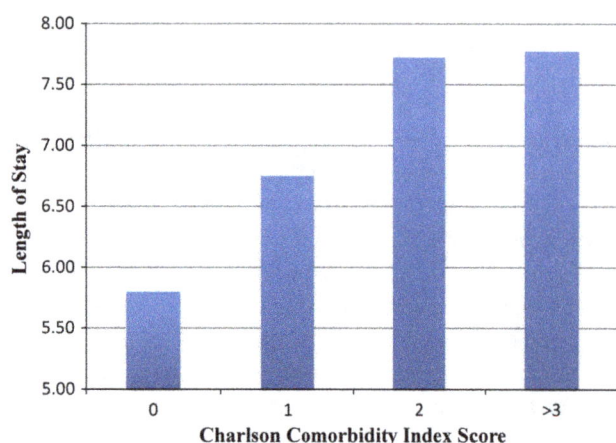

Fig. 1 Mean length of stay per CCI score calculated from patient's medical comorbidities found in charts

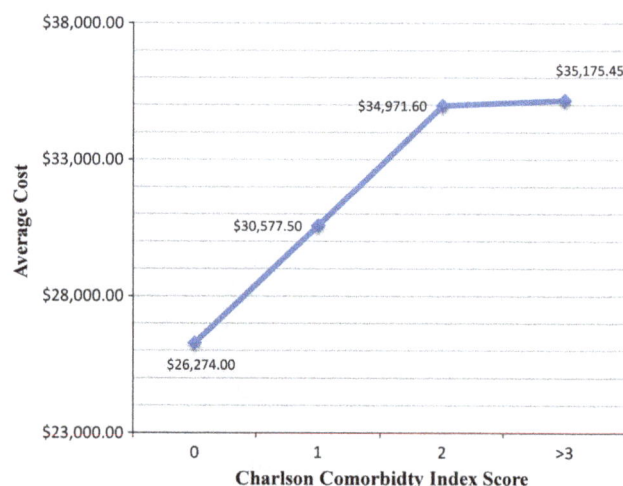

Fig. 2 Mean cost of stay per CCI score

costs, it is important to recognize that the cost burden we found represents the minimum additional cost incurred, and more research is needed to quantify the relationship between the CCI score and other factors which would affect hospital costs in a bundled payment model.

The rationale for bundled payments is to incentivize various providers to collaboratively deliver high-quality care at the lowest possible cost, but several authors have noted potential downsides of this payment model, both for the patients and the providers. With respect to the former, Bozic et al. [13] noted that bundled payment models simultaneously create the incentive to withhold care, and because of this, there is a growing awareness that institutions need methods to calculate the specific cost burden of patient factors associated with a particular procedure prior to entering into a bundled payment reimbursement agreement [5]. This is not only imperative for the financial solvency of the institution [5], but it is also necessary to ensure that more complex patients with multiple comorbid conditions receive the care they need. The results of our study, which show the impact of increasing CCI scores on hospital LOS and its financial implications further highlight the importance of quantifying the specific cost burden of patient factors, both to protect the financial interests of the institution and to ensure that funds are allotted to meet the needs of medically complex patients. In summary, the results of our study suggest that the CCI score may have a role in predicting hospital costs and negotiating reimbursement rates for the treatment of hip fractures, and, based on our results, more research is warranted to evaluate the impact of the CCI score on other costs included in bundled payments.

Conflict of interest   Author William Obremskey has previously consulted for biometrics; provided expert testimony in legal matters, and received a grant from the Department of Defense. For the remaining authors no conflicts of interest are declared.

Ethical standards   This study was authorized by the local ethical committee (Vanderbilt IRB) with a waiver of informed consent and was performed in accordance with the Ethical standards of the 1964 Declaration of Helsinki as revised in 2000. All procedures were in accordance with the ethical standards of the institutional and/or national research committee.

References

1. Braithwaite RS, Col NF, Wong JB (2003) Estimating hip fracture morbidity, mortality and costs. J Am Geriatr Soc 51(3):364–370
2. Nikkel LE, Fox EJ, Black KP et al (2012) Impact of comorbidities on hospitalization costs following hip fracture. J Bone Joint Surg Am 94(1):9–17
3. Birkmeyer JD, Gust C, Baser O et al (2010) Medicare payments for common inpatient procedures: implications for episode-based payment bundling. Health Serv Res 45(6 Pt 1):1783–1795
4. Sood N, Huckfeldt PJ, Escarce JJ et al (2011) Medicare's bundled payment pilot for acute and postacute care: analysis and recommendations on where to begin. Health Aff (Millwood) 30(9): 1708–1717
5. Bosco JA 3rd, Karkenny AJ, Hutzler LH et al (2014) Cost burden of 30-day readmissions following medicare total hip and knee arthroplasty. J Arthroplast 29(5):903–905
6. Garcia AE, Bonnaig JV, Yoneda ZT et al (2012) Patient variables which may predict length of stay and hospital costs in elderly patients with hip fracture. J Orthop Trauma 26(11):620–623
7. Kirkland LL, Kashiwagi DT, Burton MC et al (2011) The Charlson Comorbidity Index score as a predictor of 30-day mortality after hip fracture surgery. Am J Med Qual 26(6):461–467
8. Souza RC, Pinheiro RS, Coeli CM et al (2008) The Charlson Comorbidity Index (CCI) for adjustment of hip fracture mortality in the elderly: analysis of the importance of recording secondary diagnoses. Cad Saude Publica 24(2):315–322
9. Neuhaus V, King J, Hageman MG et al (2013) Charlson comorbidity indices and in-hospital deaths in patients with hip fractures. Clin Orthop Relat Res 471(5):1712–1719
10. Voskuijl T, Hageman M, Ring D (2014) Higher Charlson Comorbidity Index Scores are associated with readmission after orthopaedic surgery. Clin Orthop Relat Res 472(5):1638–1644
11. Deyo RA, Ciol MA (1992) Adapting a clinical comorbidity index for use with ICD-9-CM administrative databases. J Clin Epidemiol 45:613–619
12. Tien WC, Kao HY, Tu YK et al (2009) A population-based study of prevalence and hospital charges in total hip and knee replacement. Int Orthop 33(4):949–954
13. Bozic KJ, Ward L, Vail TP et al (2014) Bundled payments in total joint arthroplasty: targeting opportunities for quality improvement and cost reduction. Clin Orthop Relat Res 472(1): 188–193

16

A prospective randomized radiographic and dual-energy X-ray absorptiometric study of migration and bone remodeling after implantation of two modern short-stemmed femoral prostheses

Volker Brinkmann · Florian Radetzki ·
Karl Stefan Delank · David Wohlrab ·
Alexander Zeh

Abstract

Background The aim of this prospective randomized study was to analyze migration and strain transmission of the Metha^{TM} and Nanos^{TM} femoral prostheses.

Materials and methods Between 1 January 2011 and 2 April 2013, 50 patients were randomized to receive short-stemmed femoral prostheses. Metha^{TM} stems were implanted in 24 patients (12 female, 12 male; mean age 58.7 years; mean body mass index [BMI] 27.4) and Nanos^{TM} stems in 26 patients (10 female, 16 male; mean age 59.7 years; mean BMI 27.1). Longitudinal stem migration, varus–valgus alignment, changes of center of rotation (COR), femoral offset and caput-collum-diaphyseal angle, leg length discrepancy, periprosthetic radiolucent lines incidence, and dual-energy X-ray absorptiometry (DEXA) scans were analysed after an average of 98 and 381 days.

Results There was no significant change of varus–valgus alignment or clinically relevant migration of the Metha^{TM} or Nanos^{TM} prostheses during postoperative follow-up. After 12.3 months, the DEXA scans showed small but significant differences of bone mineral density in Gruen zones 1 (minus $\sim$8 %) and 6 (plus $\sim$9 %) for the Metha^{TM} and in Gruen zone 1 (minus $\sim$14 %) for the Nanos^{TM} (paired t test). Visual analog scale (VAS) and Harris Hip Score (HHS) improved significantly for both implants (Nanos^{TM}/Metha^{TM} 12.3 months postoperatively HSS 96.5/96.2; VAS 0.7/0.8, respectively). COR or offset did not change significantly after surgery.

Conclusions Neither implant showed signs of impaired osseointegration. DEXA demonstrated proximally located load transfer with only moderate proximal stress shielding. *Level of evidence* II.

Keywords Metha^{TM} · Nanos^{TM} · Short-stemmed prosthesis · DEXA · Stress shielding

Introduction

The use of short-stemmed femoral prostheses in total hip arthroplasty (THA) has increased considerably with the development of several such stems by different manufacturers [1].

There are numerous studies reporting excellent short- and medium-term clinical and radiological results [2–7]. Short-stemmed femoral implants were designed to achieve proximal load transfer in the femoral metaphysis in order to prevent stress shielding and preserve metaphyseal bone. Because of their shape and short design, they are particularly suitable for less invasive approaches [8].

Investigations of load transfer after femoral stem implantation have generally been performed using dual-energy X-ray absorptiometry (DEXA) measurements [2, 3, 5–7, 9, 10], although other study groups favor computed tomography scans [11]. Studies examining strain distribution after implantation of short-stemmed femoral prostheses have yielded conflicting results regarding the achievement of selectively proximal load transfer [5, 6, 12, 13]. Proximal load transfer is considered one major advantage compared to conventional stems, which typically produce clinically relevant stress shielding. It is thus conjectured that short-stemmed prostheses should preserve metaphyseal bone and, in this way, facilitate the eventual exchange

V. Brinkmann · F. Radetzki · K. S. Delank · D. Wohlrab ·
A. Zeh (✉)
Department of Orthopaedics and Traumatology, Faculty
of Medicine, Martin-Luther-University of Halle-Wittenberg,
Ernst-Grube-Strasse 40, 06120 Halle/Saale, Germany
e-mail: alexander.zeh@uk-halle.de

to conventional prostheses, e.g., in cases of aseptic loosening [1]. In addition, there is evidence that bone loss around femoral stems might be associated with an increased risk of aseptic loosening [14].

To date, no single published study has concluded that short-stemmed femoral implants show the same excellent long-term survival as conventional cementless stems and/or lead to improved options for revision THA.

The Metha^{TM} (Aesculap AG, Tuttlingen, Germany) non-cemented stem is anchored in the metaphysis within the closed ring of the femoral neck. The conical shape promotes primary stability and proximal force transfer. The good primary stability is further enhanced by the rounded tip of the stem along the dorsolateral cortex. The Plasmapore$^®$μ-CaP coating of the entire proximal surface encourages rapid secondary osseointegration. In this study, the Metha^{TM} stem was implanted as a monoblock, which is available with neck angles of 125, 130, and 135° (courtesy of Aesculap AG).

The Nanos^{TM} (Smith & Nephew GmbH, Marl, Germany) prosthesis is designed to affix in the calcar region to ensure optimum load transfer, and to bind along the distal lateral cortex to support and compensate varus loading. The implant is made of a titanium forged alloy (ISO 5832-3), with an osteoconductive proximal coat. The roughness of the titanium plasma surface both increases surface area and ensures superior primary stability. The additional calcium phosphate (BONIT$^®$) allows acceleration of the osseointegration process (courtesy of Smith & Nephew GmbH).

This study investigated osseointegration and bone remodeling after implantation of the Metha^{TM} or Nanos^{TM} prostheses, to analyze whether proximal load transfers could be achieved and whether there are differences between the two implants.

Materials and methods

Between 1 January 2011 and 2 April 2013, 50 patients undergoing THA for severe primary coxarthrosis (Kellgren III or IV) and failed conservative treatment were randomized to receive short-stemmed femoral prostheses. Metha^{TM} stems were implanted in 24 patients (12 female, 12 male)

and Nanos^{TM} stems were implanted in 26 patients (10 female, 16 male) (Table 1). Patients >70 years, those receiving cortisone therapy, and those with cancer, rheumatoid arthritis, osteoporosis, and/or other bone or connective tissue diseases were excluded from the study.

Postoperatively, all patients were mobilized with full weightbearing. Study follow-up visits were scheduled at 3 months (FU1; mean 98 days, SD 10 days) and 1 year (FU2; mean 381 days, SD 23 days).

Longitudinal migration and varus−valgus alignment of the femoral stem were analyzed on anteroposterior (AP) radiographs taken immediately after surgery and at FU1 and FU2 by a single examiner using Wristing$^®$ software and the associated technique described in a recent study [7].

Since these measurements can be influenced by rotational positioning of the proximal femur during AP radiographs and DEXA, hip joint positioning aids were routinely used.

According to the systemic measurement error defined by the Wristing$^®$ digital software, significant migration or tilt change of the femoral stem was defined as a difference of at least 2 mm or 3°, respectively [15].

AP radiographs of the affected hip taken preoperatively and at FU1 were evaluated to compare caput-collum-diaphyseal (CCD) angle, center of rotation (COR), and offset according to the method described by Lecerf et al. [16].

To evaluate leg length discrepancy (LLD), AP whole pelvis films taken preoperatively were compared with postoperative films (taken prior to hospital discharge). The distance from the tip of the lesser trochanter to the line between the ischial spines (perpendicular) was measured and the difference was calculated. An increased postoperative length value was marked with a plus and a decrease with a minus [17].

AP radiographs were used to evaluate the incidence of periprosthetic radiolucent lines (RL), which were then correlated with Gruen zones at FU2 [18]. RLs were defined as areas of radiolucency at least 1 cm long and 1 mm wide between the prosthesis and the surrounding bone [19].

DEXA scans with Gruen zone analysis were performed immediately after THA and at FU1 and FU2 (Lunar DPX-L Fa; Lunar Corp., Wisconsin, USA) (Fig. 1).

Table 1 Antropometric data	Parameter	Metha^{TM} group (SD) [min−max]	Nanos^{TM} group (SD) [min−max]
	Age (years)	58.7* (7.9) [43/70]	59.7* (6.5) [48/70]#
* Mean	Height (cm)	172.9* (6.7) [163/189]	172* (8) [156/190]#
SD = standard deviation, min−max = minimum−maximum	Weight (kg)	81.4* (13.1) [56/105]	80.3* (11.5) [60/108]#
	BMI (kg/m^2)	27.4* (4.5) [19/39]	27.1* (2.4) [21/33]#
# Not significant (unpaired t-test, p > 0.05)	OP-time (min)	75* (23) [35/111]	69* (23) [30/115]#

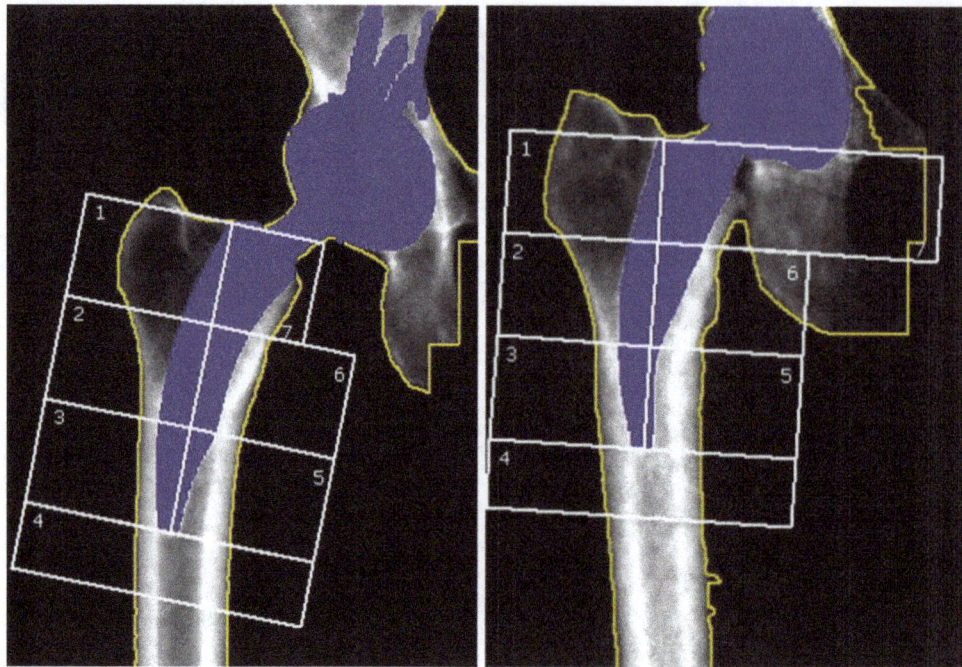

Fig. 1 Example of DEXA of the Nanos[TM] (*right*) and Metha[TM] (*left*) prosthesis with defined modified Gruen zones

Clinical results were evaluated using a visual analog scale (VAS) and the Harris Hip Score (HHS) preoperatively and at FU1 and FU2.

For statistical analysis, unpaired and paired t-tests as well as the chi-squared test were used (SPSS 19.0, IBM Company).

Results

The Metha[TM] and Nanos[TM] groups did not significantly differ according to demographic and perioperative data (Table 1).

Significant longitudinal migration was evident in both groups after 3 months, with no significant differences evident between 3 and 12 months postoperatively (paired t-test) (Table 2).

CCD measurements showed statistically significantly differences measured pre- and postoperatively (Metha[TM] = 131° vs 127°; Nanos[TM] = 130° vs 136°; paired t-test,

$p = 0.001$). Measurements of COR and off-set did not significantly differ, and were thus regarded as clinically irrelevant.

In addition, both groups exhibited minimal and clinically irrelevant LLDs between the operated and contralateral hips postoperatively. For the Nanos[TM] group, LLD in the operated contralateral hip averaged 1 mm (min −10 mm, max +6 mm), and for the Metha[TM] group, the mean LLD measured 0.8 mm (min −2 mm, max +5 mm).

One case in the Nanos[TM] group resulted in a LLD of 1.0 cm. This is explained by a stem migration of 10 mm at FU1. No further migration occurred between FU1 and FU2. No other radiological or clinical signs of aseptic loosening were present.

Tilt did not significantly change for either Nanos[TM] or Metha[TM] stems over follow-up (paired t-test, $p > 0.05$).

Areas of radiolucency were detected in 11 cases in the Metha[TM] group and 8 cases in the Nanos[TM] group. None of these exceeded a width of 2 mm or length of 1 cm. Therefore, these findings were not considered signs of aseptic loosening [19] and statistical analysis evaluating differences between the groups was not performed.

After 12 months, the DEXA scans showed a very small but significant difference of bone mineral density (BMD) in Gruen zones 1 (approximately −9 %) and 6 (approximately +8 %) for the Metha[TM] prosthesis (Table 3). For the Nanos[TM] prosthesis, a significant decrease of BMD was detected in Gruen zone 1 (approximately −14 %; Table 4).

Table 2 Longitudinal migration

	Mean	SD	min–max	*paired t*-test
Metha[TM] group FU 1	1.87 mm	2.25 mm	0–7 mm	$p < 0.01$
Nanos[TM] group FU 1	1.96 mm	2.65 mm	0–10 mm	$p < 0.01$
Metha[TM] group FU 2	1.96 mm	2.37 mm	0–7 mm	$p = 0.16$
Nanos[TM] group FU 2	2.04 mm	2.65 mm	0–10 mm	$p = 0.18$

SD = standard deviation, min–max = minimum–maximum

Significant and adequate improvements on VAS and HHS were observed for both implants at 12 months post-surgery. HHS and VAS were 96.5 and 0.7 for the Nanos[TM] group and 96.2 and 0.8 for the Metha[TM] group, respectively.

In summary, there was no evidence for aseptic loosening during follow-up.

No intra- or postoperative complications were observed in this study.

Discussion

The implantation of short-stemmed prostheses has notably increased over the past few years [1–4, 20–25]. In Germany, approximately 15–20 % of primary THAs are now performed using short-stemmed femoral implants.

Possible advantages of short-stemmed femoral prostheses are the reduction of bone loss compared to conventional implants [9, 10, 26–28], their suitability for less invasive surgery, the potential to avoid stress shielding, and theoretically to enable easier revision surgery [1].

Another major point of interest is strain distribution, as this is a precondition for understanding bone remodeling and its impact on the bone quality of the proximal femur. In order to investigate the strain distribution of short-stemmed implants, several studies have been performed, generally based on DEXA scan evaluations. DEXA scans are widely used to evaluate stress shielding and thus indirectly, the force transmission of the prosthetic stem on femoral bone [2, 5, 6, 9, 11–13].

This method is considered an effective way to evaluate BMD over postoperative follow-up, allowing conclusions regarding load transfer induced by the femoral implant [29]. In addition, the reliability of differentiated analysis of BMD according to seven modified Gruen zones after implantation of a femoral implant has been verified [30].

In a prospective randomized trial, Hube et al. (2004) [31] used DEXA scans to compare the osseointegration of the Mayo[TM] Stem (Zimmer, Warsaw, USA) to that of the ABG[TM] Prosthesis (Stryker GmbH & Co.KG, Duisburg, Germany) in 93 patients. Approximately 12 months after implantation of the Mayo[TM] Stem, BMD in the calcar region was increased.

Logroscino et al. (2011) [13] used DEXA scans to evaluate osseointegration of Proxima[TM] (De-Puy-J&J) and Nanos[TM] (Smith & Nephew) prostheses. Metaphyseal bone stock was preserved by both implants. Significantly higher BMD values were observed within the metaphysis of the femur with the Nanos[TM] prosthesis.

In a previous study with a different study group, we investigated bone remodeling and osseointegration of the Nanos[TM] short-stemmed prosthesis in 25 patients. There were significant decreases of BMD in zones 1, 2, and 7 of 15, 5, and 12 %, respectively, and a significant increase of BMD in Gruen zone 6 of 12 %, which was interpreted as a result of a distally located load transfer and moderate proximally located stress shielding [7].

Lerch et al. (2012) used DEXA scans to validate their finite element (FE) model of strain distribution for the Metha[TM] stem. To develop the FE model, the law of bone adaptation was used to calculate changes of apparent bone density (ABD) under simulation of physiological loading. They found no difference in ABD or BMD in the distal femur while applying their FE and analyzing the DEXA scans. This finding was interpreted as an absence of stress shielding, which is characteristically found in conventional stems [9].

However, a moderate decrease of BMD was found in the proximal portion of the femur, which was attributed to

Table 4 Nanos[TM] group: results of Dexa

Gruen zone	Postoperative g/cm² (SD)	FU 1 g/cm² (SD)	FU 2 g/cm² (SD)
1	0.91 (0.18)	0.83 (0.17)$^{p=0.001}$	0.80 (0.17)$^{p=0.005}$
2	1.53 (0.32)	1.52 (0.28)#	1.48 (0.23)#
3	2.26 (0.28)	2.23 (0.25)#	2.27 (0.26)#
4	2.14 (0.27)	2.15 (0.36#	2.14 (0.4)#
5	2.17 (0.24)	2.14 (0.38)#	2.15 (0.3)#
6	1.59 (0.3)	1.59 (0.42)#	1.57 (0.37)#
7	1.44 (0.2)	1.31 (0.3)$^{p=0.02}$	1.37 (0.3)#

SD = standard deviation

Not significant (paired t-test, $p > 0.05$)

Table 3 Metha[TM] group: results of Dexa

Gruen zone	Postoperative g/cm² (SD)	FU 1 g/cm² (SD)	FU 2 g/cm² (SD)
1	0.86 (0.23)	0.79 (0.26)$^{p=0.001}$	0.79 (0.27)$^{p=0.004}$
2	1.36 (0.26)	1.42 (0.3)#	1.31 (0.34)#
3	2.22 (0.33)	2.24 (0.33)#	2.13 (0.36)#
4	2.08 (0.35)	2.07 (0.32)#	2.03 (0.36)#
5	1.92 (0.48)	1.94 (0.31)#	1.92 (0.3)#
6	1.5 (0.33)	1.49 (0.31)#	1.62 (0.35)$^{p=0.012}$
7	1.28 (0.3)	1.13 (0.28)$^{p=0.004}$	1.14 (0.28)#

SD = standard deviation

Not significant (paired t-test, $p > 0.05$)

stress shielding. The considerable remodeling in Gruen zone 6, which contrasts with findings of other study groups [2, 3], was explained by design differences of short-stemmed implants and varying primary rotational stability [6].

In a study examining osseointegration of the Nanos™ prosthesis, Götze et al. (2010) [5] identified bone loss of approximately 7 % in the calcar region and 6 % at the greater trochanter. In contrast to the above-mentioned studies, BMD was significantly increased in Gruen zones 2 and 3, by approximately 10 %. Significant lateral load transfer was present. Thus, the authors concluded that proximal force transmission is not achieved with the Nanos™ prosthesis.

Unfortunately, Götze et al. (2010) did not report on postoperative stem position. According to a previous study, one must consider that valgus positioning of the stem leads to more lateral load transfer and pattern changes of the DEXA. Thus, DEXA results can be affected by different stem positions. The average stem position in the study by Götze et al. (2010) was probably in valgus, which might explain the distal load transfer. To our mind, DEXA results in combination with the Nanos™ stem should particularly be discussed with consideration of the stem position, because the concept of this implant involves an off-set modulation by different implant angulation [5, 7].

In general, studies report decreased BMD of the proximal femur within Gruen zones 1, 2, and 7, and less than what one would expect in conventional THA [9, 10]. This is considered evidence for a moderate distal load transfer.

We found a small to moderate decrease of BMD in Gruen zone 1 for the Metha™ (minus ∼9 %) as well as for the Nanos™ stem (minus ∼14 %) which supports the conclusion that proximal load transfer occurs for both implants. The Metha™ prosthesis showed an additional increase of BMD in zone 6 (plus ∼9 %) that indicates a relevant distal strain distribution. This specific result agrees with the findings of Lerch et al. (2012) [6] who identified a significant BMD loss in Gruen zones 1 and 7 (∼10 %), and a BMD increase in Gruen zone 6 for the Metha™ stem (∼10 %) after 2 years.

In summary, our study results confirm the conclusions of other investigators who postulated a significant and clinically relevant proximal load transfer for both the Metha™ and Nanos™ stems [3, 6].

These findings suggest only moderate bone loss in the calcar region after implantation of the Metha™ or Nanos™ stems approximately one year postoperatively. For the Mayo™ short-stemmed prosthesis, for instance, a bone loss between 15 % and 18 % has been previously described (4). For conventional THA, proximal BMD loss has been quoted as high as 30 % [10].

The migration of approximately 2 mm after 96 days is not interpreted as a sign of instability of the implants as there was no further migration at the latest follow-up and because of the absence of other signs of aseptic loosening. Furthermore, migration of an implant should not be assumed before a determined difference of 2 mm [32].

We cannot confirm the conclusions in the prospective DEXA study by Goetze et al. (2010) who reported a significant distal load transfer for the Nanos™ implant [5, 7].

In our previous study, we found significant and constant decreases of BMD in zones 1, 2, and 7, of 15, 5, and 12 %, respectively, after 12 months, and a significant increase of BMD in Gruen zone 6 of 12 % [7]. In the current study, there was a significant decrease of BMD of ∼10 % in Gruen zone 1 only. There is no plausible explanation for these differences, as the study groups are in the same age group (59.9 [7] vs. 59.8 years), have similar stem position (CCD = 133° [7] vs. 136°), and underwent follow-up DEXA scans at the same time postoperatively (368 [7] vs 381 days). The current study also identified a significant change in BMD in Gruen zone 7 at FU1 (98 days); however, this was not present at FU2.

Lerch et al. described the finding of an increased BMD in Gruen zone 6 for the Metha™ stem as a well-known phenomenon explained by the 'vast proximal cross section' of this implant and others like the Mayo™ prosthesis. This circumstance would lead to stress shielding of the proximal portion of the calcar and the greater trochanter, resulting in bone mass decrease. We are convinced that rather than stress shielding, a substantial distally located load transfer is responsible for the moderate loss of BMD in the femoral metaphysis. This conclusion is implied by the interpretation of the law of bone adaptation also used by Lerch et al. [6] for their calculations. In addition, the Mayo™ conservative hip does not feature a 'vast proximal cross section'. The double-wedge shape of the Mayo™ prosthesis shows a large proximal sagittal diameter compared with other short-stemmed implants such as the Metha™ [33].

Kress et al. [11] suggested that quantitative computed tomography (QCT)-assisted osteodensitometry might be helpful for three-dimensional analysis of the particular remodeling of cortical and cancellous bone around femoral stems. In their study of stress shielding of the C.F.P™ stem (Waldemar Link, Hamburg, Germany), the authors focused on differentiated analyses of BMD changes within cortical and cancellous bone. Because of the different elastic modules of cortical and cancellous bone, they concluded that new prosthetic designs should be validated by in vivo QCT data investigating strain distribution. On the other hand, they conceded that the clinical relevance of such measurements remains to be proven.

The accuracy of DEXA, and its relevance for the assessment of load transfer around femoral implants, has been reported by many others. Lerch et al. [6] pointed out that based on their study results DEXA is an excellent method to analyze bone remodeling after the implantation of short-stemmed prostheses. Cohen et al. [34] concluded that DEXA is a precise method for measurement of small changes in BMD around femoral implants. They indicated that femoral rotation is one of the main causes of failure, and therefore, correct positioning of patients is essential to obtain reliable results. In addition, many other authors have underscored the reliability of DEXA to analyze periprosthetic mineralization processes as a consequence of bone remodeling [9–11, 26–28, 35] or other influences [36]. According to our study protocol, which included the use of positioning aids for DEXA scans, we conclude that the preconditions for precise measurement were present.

One might assume that different stem positions could affect DEXA results. Unfortunately exact stem position has not been reported by other investigators [2, 3, 5, 6, 11, 13]. The law of bone adaptation [37] implies that a particular strain situation induced by different stem positions with variations of off-set and CCD would have consequences regarding the reaction of bone. For example, the Nanos^{TM} short-stemmed prosthesis allows reconstruction of off-set and CCD by different implant positioning, so that bone remodeling should be regarded not only as a prosthesis-specific pattern, but also according to implant position. Therefore, we firmly believe that for short-stemmed implants particularly, the comparability of DEXA studies is limited if stem position is not reported.

The current study has several limitations. One might speculate that follow-up was sufficient to detect changes of BMD. On the other hand, previous studies of conventional stems have concluded that maximum bone remodeling takes place 6 months after surgery and reaches a plateau after ~ 1 year. Further changes are due to long-term biomechanical adaptation and occur for another 1–2 years. Such changes are minor and show no substantial variation [10, 26]. The size of the study groups is comparable with others [2, 5, 6, 9, 11]. In addition, DEXA measurements are regarded as extremely reliable and unaffected by subjective errors [29].

The radiological measurement of stem migration and angulation was not performed using an established method like EBRA [38]. However, the method used in this study has been validated and successfully performed in other similar investigations [15, 39, 40].

In summary, we conclude that the Nanos^{TM} and Metha^{TM} prostheses show no substantial or clinically relevant differences regarding the reduction or loss of bone in the proximal aspect of the femur. Both stems show excellent clinical results and reliable osseointegration over a short follow-up period.

The moderate BMD changes of the femoral metaphysis are interpreted as a result of the presence of physiological strain distribution [37, 41]. Thus, the concept of a short-stemmed femoral implant with proximal strain distribution is confirmed for both implants.

However, neither of the prostheses was able to completely prevent a certain amount of stress shielding in the calcar and major trochanter regions, which is interpreted as moderate underloading and distal load transfer, respectively. Furthermore, one must consider that evidence is still pending regarding the clinical value of the preservation of proximal bone mass in terms of long-term survival or improved options for revision surgery for these kinds of implants.

Conflict of interest No benefits or funds were received in support of the study.

Ethical standards In all cases, the indication for implantation of a THA was severe primary coxarthrosis (Kellgren III or IV) and unsuccessful conservative treatment. All patients gave informed consent prior to inclusion in the study. The study was approved by the local ethics committee in accordance with the ethical standards of the 1964 Declaration of Helsinki as revised in 2000. The authors certify that they have no affiliations with or involvement in any organization or entity with any financial interest or non-financial interest in the subject matter or materials discussed in this manuscript.

References

1. Gulow J, Scholz R, von Freiherr S-S (2007) Short-stemmed endoprostheses in total hip arthroplasty. Orthopade 36:353–359
2. Chen HH, Morrey BF, An KN, Luo ZP (2009) Bone remodeling characteristics of a short-stemmed total hip replacement. J Arthroplasty 24:945–950
3. Falez F, Casella F, Panegrossi G, Favetti F, Barresi C (2008) Perspectives on metaphyseal conservative stems. J Orthop Traumatol 9:49–54
4. Gilbert RE, Salehi-Bird S, Gallacher PD, Shaylor P (2009) The mayo conservative hip: experience from a district general hospital. Hip Int 19:211–214
5. Gotze C, Ehrenbrink J, Ehrenbrink H (2010) Is there a bone-preserving bone remodelling in short-stem prosthesis? DEXA analysis with the Nanos total hip arthroplasty. Z Orthop Unfall 148:398–405
6. Lerch M, der Haar-Tran A, Windhagen H, Behrens BA, Wefstaedt P, Stukenborg-Colsman CM (2012) Bone remodelling around the Metha short stem in total hip arthroplasty: a prospective dual-energy X-ray absorptiometry study. Int Orthop 36:533–538
7. Zeh A, Pankow F, Rollinhoff M, Delank S, Wohlrab D (2013) A prospective dual-energy X-ray absorptiometry study of bone remodeling after implantation of the Nanos short-stemmed prosthesis. Acta Orthop Belg 79:174–180
8. Von Salis-Soglio G, Gulow J Große Gelenke: Hüfte: Kurzstiel. In: Gradinger H, Gollwitzer H (Hrsg) Össäre Integration. Springer, S116–S119
9. Albanese CV, Rendine M, De Palma F, Impagliazzo A, Falez F, Postacchini F, Villani C, Passariello R, Santori FS (2006) Bone

remodelling in THA: a comparative DXA scan study between conventional implants and a new stemless femoral component. A preliminary report. Hip Int 16(Suppl 3):9–15

10. Boden HS, Skoldenberg OG, Salemyr MO, Lundberg HJ, Adolphson PY (2006) Continuous bone loss around a tapered uncemented femoral stem: a long-term evaluation with DEXA. Acta Orthop 77:877–885

11. Kress AM, Schmidt R, Nowak TE, Nowak M, Haeberle L, Forst R, Mueller LA (2012) Stress-related femoral cortical and cancellous bone density loss after collum femoris preserving uncemented total hip arthroplasty: a prospective 7-year follow-up with quantitative computed tomography. Arch Orthop Trauma Surg 132:1111–1119

12. Hube R, Hein W Die Mayo-Hüfte—eine neue Philosophie zur proximalen Femurverankerung. In: Perka C, Zippel H (Hrsg) Trends und Kontroversen in der Endoprothetik

13. Logroscino G, Ciriello V, D'Antonio E, De TV, Piciocco P, Magliocchetti LG, Santori FS, Albanese CV (2011) Bone integration of new stemless hip implants (proxima vs. nanos). A DXA study: preliminary results. Int J Immunopathol Pharmacol 24:113–116

14. Furnes O, Lie SA, Espehaug B, Vollset SE, Engesaeter LB, Havelin LI (2001) Hip disease and the prognosis of total hip replacements. A review of 53,698 primary total hip replacements reported to the Norwegian Arthroplasty Register 1987–99. J Bone Joint Surg Br 83:579–586

15. Schönrath F Digitale Migrationsmessung in der Hüftendoprothetik am Beispiel der ABG-Prothese

16. Lecerf G, Fessy MH, Philippot R, Massin P, Giraud F, Flecher X, Girard J, Mertl P, Marchetti E, Stindel E (2009) Femoral offset: anatomical concept, definition, assessment, implications for preoperative templating and hip arthroplasty. Orthop Traumatol Surg Res 95:210–219

17. Konyves A, Bannister GC (2005) The importance of leg length discrepancy after total hip arthroplasty. J Bone Joint Surg Br 87:155–157

18. Gruen TA, McNeice GM, McNeice GM, Amstutz HC (1979) "Modes of failure" of cemented stem-type femoral components: a radiographic analysis of loosening. Clin Orthop Relat Res 141:17–27

19. Zweymuller KA, Schwarzinger UM, Steindl MS (2006) Radiolucent lines and osteolysis along tapered straight cementless titanium hip stems: a comparison of 6-year and 10-year follow-up results in 95 patients. Acta Orthop 77:871–876

20. Fottner A, Schmid M, Birkenmaier C, Mazoochian F, Plitz W, Volkmar J (2009) Biomechanical evaluation of two types of short-stemmed hip prostheses compared to the trust plate prosthesis by three-dimensional measurement of micromotions. Clin Biomech (Bristol, Avon) 24:429–434

21. Ghera S, Pavan L (2009) The DePuy Proxima hip: a short stem for total hip arthroplasty. Early experience and technical considerations. Hip Int 19:215–220

22. Gill IR, Gill K, Jayasekera N, Miller J (2008) Medium term results of the collum femoris preserving hydroxyapatite coated total hip replacement. Hip Int 18:75–80

23. Rohrl SM, Li MG, Pedersen E, Ullmark G, Nivbrant B (2006) Migration pattern of a short femoral neck preserving stem. Clin Orthop Relat Res 448:73–78

24. Synder M, Drobniewski M, Pruszczynski B, Sibinski M (2009) Initial experience with short Metha stem implantation. Ortop Traumatol Rehabil 11:317–323

25. Westphal FM, Bishop N, Honl M, Hille E, Puschel K, Morlock MM (2006) Migration and cyclic motion of a new short-stemmed

hip prosthesis—a biomechanical in vitro study. Clin Biomech (Bristol, Avon) 21:834–840

26. Brodner W, Bitzan P, Lomoschitz F, Krepler P, Jankovsky R, Lehr S, Kainberger F, Gottsauner-Wolf F (2004) Changes in bone mineral density in the proximal femur after cementless total hip arthroplasty. A five-year longitudinal study. J Bone Joint Surg Br 86:20–26

27. Reiter A, Sabo D, Simank HG, Buchner T, Seidel M, Lukoschek M (1997) Periprosthetic mineral density in cement-free hip replacement arthroplasty. Z Orthop Ihre Grenzgeb 135:499–504

28. Sabo D, Reiter A, Simank HG, Thomsen M, Lukoschek M, Ewerbeck V (1998) Periprosthetic mineralization around cementless total hip endoprosthesis: longitudinal study and cross-sectional study on titanium threaded acetabular cup and cementless Spotorno stem with DEXA. Calcif Tissue Int 62:177–182

29. Roth A, Richartz G, Sander K, Sachse A, Fuhrmann R, Wagner A, Venbrocks RA (2005) Periprosthetic bone loss after total hip endoprosthesis. Dependence on the type of prosthesis and preoperative bone configuration. Orthopade 34:334–344

30. Naal FD, Zuercher P, Munzinger U, Hersche O, Leunig M (2011) A seven-zone rating system for assessing bone mineral density after hip resurfacing using implants with metaphyseal femoral stems. Hip Int 21:463–467

31. Hube R, Zaage M, Hein W, Reichel H (2004) Early functional results with the Mayo-hip, a short stem system with metaphyseal-intertrochanteric fixation. Orthopade 33:1249–1258

32. Bieger R, Cakir B, Reichel H, Kappe T (2014) Accuracy of hip stem migration measurement on plain radiographs: reliability of bony and prosthetic landmarks. Orthopade 43:934–939

33. Morrey BF, Adams RA, Kessler M (2000) A conservative femoral replacement for total hip arthroplasty. A prospective study. J Bone Joint Surg Br 82:952–958

34. Cohen B, Rushton N (1995) Accuracy of DEXA measurement of bone mineral density after total hip arthroplasty. J Bone Joint Surg Br 77:479–483

35. Lazarinis S, Mattsson P, Milbrink J, Mallmin H, Hailer NP (2013) A prospective cohort study on the short collum femoris-preserving (CFP) stem using RSA and DXA. Primary stability but no prevention of proximal bone loss in 27 patients followed for 2 years. Acta Orthop 84:32–39

36. Hennigs T, Arabmotlagh M, Schwarz A, Zichner L (2002) Dose-dependent prevention of early periprosthetic bone loss by alendronate. Z Orthop Ihre Grenzgeb 140:42–47

37. Behrens BA, Nolte I, Wefstaedt P, Stukenborg-Colsman C, Bouguecha A (2009) Numerical investigations on the strain-adaptive bone remodelling in the periprosthetic femur: influence of the boundary conditions. Biomed Eng Online 8:7

38. Krismer M, Bauer R, Tschupik J, Mayrhofer P (1995) EBRA: a method to measure migration of acetabular components. J Biomech 28:1225–1236

39. Zeh A, Weise A, Vasarhelyi A, Bach AG, Wohlrab D (2011) Medium-term results of the Mayo short-stem hip prosthesis after avascular necrosis of the femoral head. Z Orthop Unfall 149:200–205

40. Zeh A, Radetzki F, Diers V, Bach D, Rollinghoff M, Delank KS (2011) Is there an increased stem migration or compromised osteointegration of the Mayo short-stemmed prosthesis following cerclage wiring of an intrasurgical periprosthetic fracture? Arch Orthop Trauma Surg 131:1717–1722

41. Kuiper JH, Huiskes R (1997) The predictive value of stress shielding for quantification of adaptive bone resorption around hip replacements. J Biomech Eng 119:228–231

17

Triceps-sparing approach for open reduction and internal fixation of neglected displaced supracondylar and distal humeral fractures in children

Ahmed Shawkat Rizk

Abstract

Background Supracondylar humeral fractures are one of the most common skeletal injuries in children. In cases of displacement and instability, the standard procedure is early closed reduction and percutaneous Kirschner wire fixation. However, between 10 and 20 % of patients present late. According to the literature, patients with neglected fractures are those patients who presented for treatment after 14 days of injury. The delay is either due to lack of medical facilities or social and financial constraints. The neglected cases are often closed injuries with no vascular compromise. However, the elbow may still be tense and swollen with abrasions or crusts. In neglected cases, especially after early appearance of callus, there is no place for closed reduction and percutaneous pinning. Traditionally, distal humeral fractures have been managed with surgical approaches that disrupt the extensor mechanism with less satisfactory functional outcome due to triceps weakness and elbow stiffness. The aim of this study is to evaluate the outcome of delayed open reduction using the triceps-sparing approach and Kirschner wire fixation for treatment of neglected, displaced supracondylar and distal humeral fractures in children.

Materials and methods This prospective study included 15 children who had neglected displaced supracondylar and distal humeral fractures. All patients were completely evaluated clinically and radiologically before intervention, after surgery and during the follow-up. The follow-up period ranged from 8 to 49 months, with a mean period of 17 months. Functional outcome was evaluated according to the Mayo Elbow Performance Index (MEPI) and Mark functional criteria.

Results All fractures united in a mean duration of 7.2 weeks (range 5–10 weeks) with no secondary displacement or mal-union. Excellent results were found at the last follow-up in 13 of the 15 patients studied (86.66 %), while good results were found in two patients (13.33 %) according to the MEPI scale. According to the Mark functional criteria, there was one patient with a fair result (6.66 %).

Conclusion The results were very satisfactory if compared with traditional operative techniques, with many advantages including anatomical reduction and fixation of the fractures, avoidance of ulnar nerve injury, preservation of the extensor mechanism, decrease in incidence of myositis ossificans around the elbow and decrease in postoperative stiffness.

Level of evidence IV.

Keywords Neglected distal humeral fractures · Children · Triceps-sparing approach · Kirschner wire fixation

A. S. Rizk (✉)
Orthopaedics and Traumatology Department,
Faculty of Medicine, Benha University, Benha, Egypt
e-mail: drahmadshawkat@gmail.com

A. S. Rizk
Shebeen el-kanater, Qualiobia, Egypt

Introduction

Supracondylar humeral fractures (SCHF) are common pediatric injuries [1] representing about 3 % of all fractures, and are the most common elbow fractures in children [2]. Over the past several decades there has been a shift from non-operative management to surgical stabilization for these fractures [3].

SCHF are classified using the modified Gartland classification and most of them are of extension type [4].

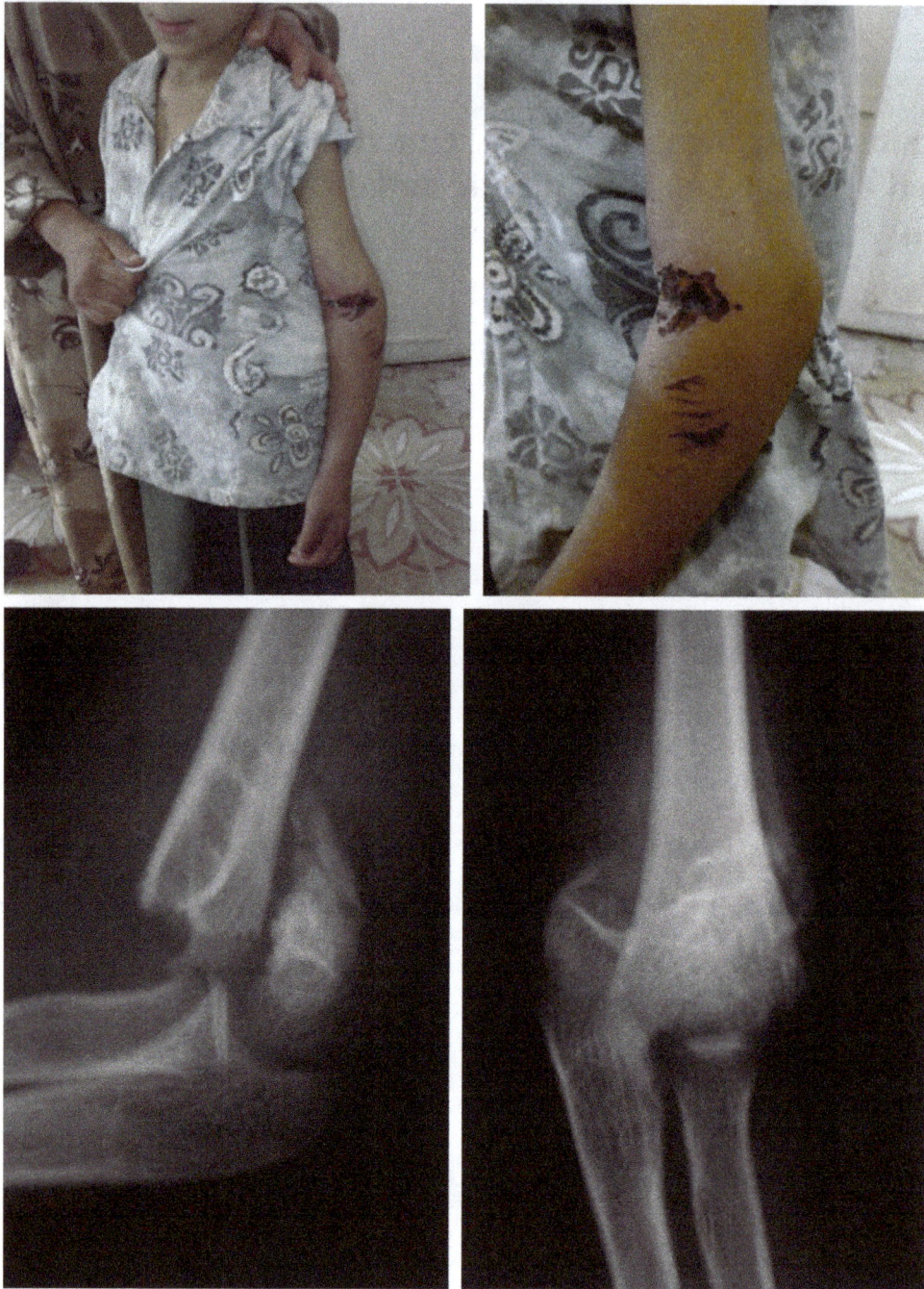

Fig. 1 (*Top*) clinical photograph showing elbow swelling, deformity with sagging and crusts in a case of extension supracondylar fracture humerus neglected for 27 days. (*Bottom*) X-ray showing off-ending of the fragments with marked posterior displacement with early callus formation. Nerve conduction study showed incomplete radial nerve involvement (patient 1)

Displaced SCHF are challenging injuries to treat and entail technically difficult procedures for orthopedic surgeons [5, 6]. Supracondylar humeral fractures are usually treated as an emergency in children [3].

Currently, the preferred approach for the treatment of displaced pediatric supracondylar fractures is closed reduction and percutaneous pinning; this technique requires experience and is not free of complications or partial failure [7]. It fails in up to 25 % of patients [8], and requires remanipulation because of inadequate reduction or malpositioning of wires in 1–7 % of patients [9].

If attempts at closed reduction fail, then open reduction of the fracture followed by cross-pinning should be considered. Open reduction may also frequently be required in late-presented SCHF [3]. Severe swelling or skin problems around the elbow are the universally accepted indications for delaying surgical intervention following a SCHF in children. In developing countries, problems relating to disorganized health insurance systems and some traditional incorrect interventions (by non-medical personnel) unique to that specific country can also significantly influence the time interval between the injury and the definitive treatment. Under these circumstances, management of a late-presented SCHF becomes inevitable for the orthopedic surgeon [3].

Surgical exposure can be accomplished by a variety of approaches [10, 11]. A surgical approach should permit a safe and rapid reduction, with full anatomical alignment, obtaining adequate functional and cosmetic outcomes, as well as fewest complications. There is no clear evidence in the literature regarding which of the surgical approaches brings about the best functional and cosmetic outcomes, as well as minimizing complications [2].

Materials and methods

This prospective study was carried out in the Orthopaedic Department at Benha University Hospital, Benha, Egypt from March 2007 to April 2013, and comprised 15 patients, all male. Their ages ranged from 6 to 11 years (mean 8.6 years). All patients had an initial treatment in the form of closed reduction and above elbow slab in private clinics or local hospitals and presented to the author late. The duration between their initial injury and presentation ranged from 16 to 34 days (mean 19 days). Twelve patients (80 %) had neglected extension type supracondyar fractures, two patients (13.33 %) had neglected flexion-type supracondylar fractures, while the last patient (6.67 %) had a neglected lower fourth humeral fracture. At the time of presentation, two patients (13.33 %) had skin abrasions and crusts with signs of radial nerve involvement in one patient and ulnar nerve involvement in the other. No patients had vascular involvement. No patients had open supracondylar fractures. No patients had any previous trial of surgical intervention in the form of closed reduction with percutaneous pinning.

Any case of acute displaced supracondylar fracture or supra-intercondylar fracture of the humerus or supracondylar fracture of the humerus after closure of the epiphysis was excluded. Only patients with neglected, displaced, supracondylar or lower humeral fractures with no previous operative intervention were included in this study.

Careful evaluation of the patients was made pre-operatively; a complete history of the initial trauma was taken, with the associated injuries, the initial management done, and the reason why the parents sought advice. The interval between initial injury and presentation was recorded.

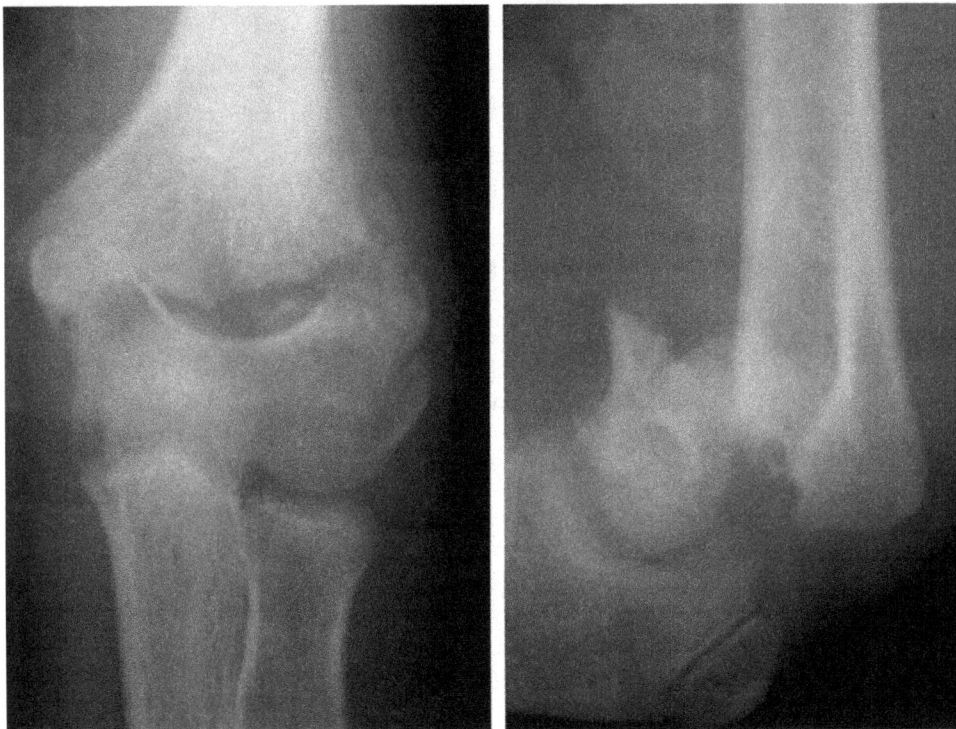

Fig. 2 X-ray of a patient with flexion-type supracondylar fracture humerus neglected for 22 days showing off-ending of the fragments with marked anterior displacement of the distal stump with early callus formation (seen in antero-posterior view) (patient 14)

Examination included careful inspection of the skin and soft tissue envelope around the elbow, deformity or sagging at the elbow region (Fig. 1) and active finger movements. Palpation was performed for distal pulse and tenderness over the elbow. Pre-operative radiographs were evaluated for the presence of comminution, other associated injuries around the elbow that may affect the treatment or the prognosis, early callus formation, the site of the fracture and its type as extension- or flexion-type injuries (Figs. 1, 2, 3).

Nerve conduction studies were done to document neural insult prior to intervention in any patient suspected to have nerve injury. All the patients in this study were treated by open reduction and internal fixation (ORIF) through a posterior triceps-sparing approach using at least two crossing wires depending on the size of the distal fragment and the intra-operative stability.

The procedure was done under general anesthesia, with tourniquet applied. All the patients were in the prone position with their arms supported on a side post with the elbow semi-flexed to relive tension on the ulnar and radial nerves. A midline straight skin incision was made with the proximal two-thirds of the incision above the tip of the olecranon while the remaining one-third was over the back of the forearm from the tip of the olecranon. The distal part

facilitates exposure and isolation of the ulnar nerve which is critical for the safe exposure of the distal humerus.

After exposure and isolation of the ulnar nerve, the scalpel was used to sharply separate the anterio-medial border of the triceps muscle from the medial intermuscular septum down to the bone.

Sharp dissection down to the bone was also done laterally between the anterio-lateral border of the triceps muscle and the lateral intermuscular septum with the radial nerve and the profunda brachii artery passed within it from the back of the arm anteriorly [12], so that the back of the humerus could be safely reached without endangering these vital structures.

By elevation and retraction of the whole bulk of the muscle, the posterior surface of the humerus could be safely reached without interruption or violation of the integrity of the triceps muscle and its tendon.

Manipulation and reduction of the displaced bony fragments, whatever the level of the fracture (supracondylar or lower fourth humeral fractures) or the direction of displacement (anterior or posterior displacement of the distal fragment), could now be done easily and safely.

Anatomical reduction could easily be done and assessed both by palpation and by direct vision of the fracture with no need for image intensification. Fixation could then be

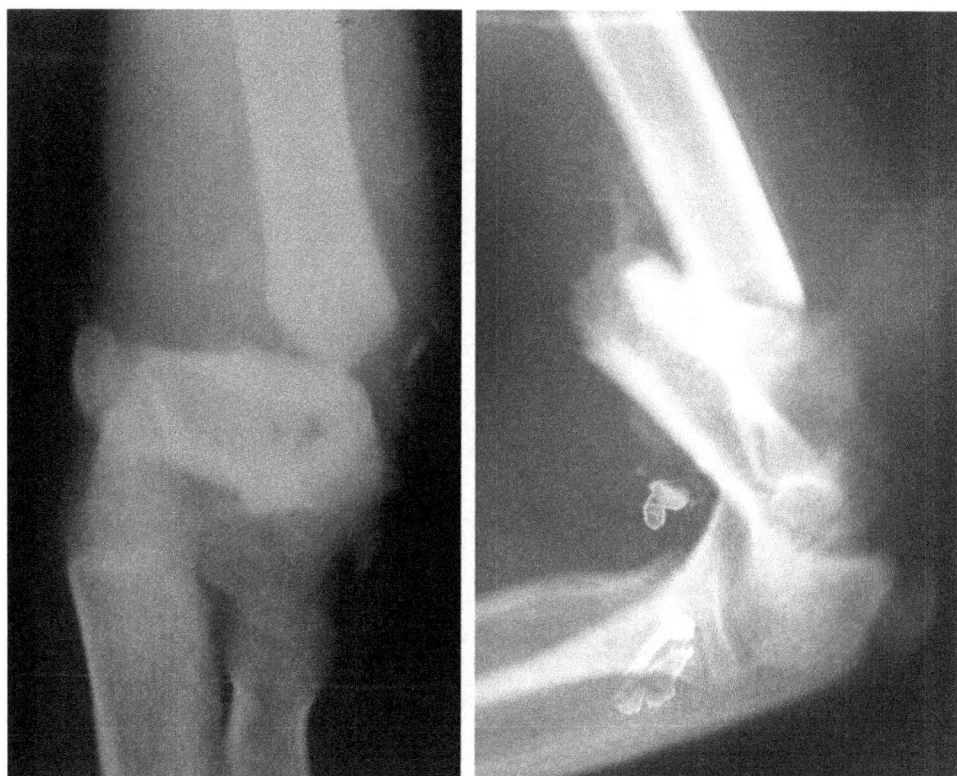

Fig. 3 X-ray of a patient with displaced lower fourth fracture humerus neglected for 34 days showing off-ending of the fragments with visible callus formation in the lateral view (patient 8)

achieved by at least two crossing Kirschner wires inserted under direct vision, avoiding the ulnar nerve and engaging the opposite cortex.

In all the patients with neglected supracondylar fractures, the wires were left protruding from the skin for easy removal as an outpatient procedure (Fig. 4a). In the case of lower fourth humeral fracture and due to the location of the fracture and age of the patient, the wires were impeded and kept within the wound to be left safely for a longer duration until union (Fig. 4b).

The tourniquet was removed before wound closure with good hemostasis, then the wound closed in layers (the subcutaneous and skin layers) with no need to insert a suction drain. An above elbow slab in 90° flexion was applied with no risk of edema or compartmental syndrome, as all patients were neglected for more than 2 weeks and there was no vascular insult in any patient; in addition a good hemostasis was achieved after torniquet removal before closure of the wound.

Post-operative care started immediately after recovery from anesthesia by evaluating the movements of all fingers and the neurovascular condition of the patient. Post-operative X-rays were taken to evaluate the result of intervention and to be used as a reference in the follow-up period to detect any position change or re-displacement. The above elbow slab and sutures were removed 2 weeks after the operation with active range of motion (ROM) started with the wires in place. Regular follow-up (clinical and radiological) was done every 2 weeks until complete union and wire removal, then monthly until complete restoration of the ROM and every 6 months subsequently until the last visit. The functional results were assessed according to Mark et al. [13] and the Mayo Elbow Performance Index (MEPI), which comprises four parameters: pain, arc of motion, stability, and activities of daily living.

Functional outcome was evaluated according to the MEPI as described by Turchin et al. [14]. MEPI is a four-part scale where clinical information is rated based on a 100-point scale, as follows:

- 90–100: excellent
- 75–89: good
- 60–74: fair
- Below 60: poor

1. Pain: The therapist asks the patient how severe the pain is and how frequently the pain appears. 45 points are for patients who do not have pain, 30 points are given to patients who have mild pain, and moderate pain results in 15 points; patients with severe pain get 0 points.
2. The arc of elbow motion: 20 points are given when the arm reaches more than 100° flexion; when the angle is between 100° and 50° the patient is given 15 points. When the maximum flexion is no more than 50°, then 5 points are given.
3. Stability: When the elbow is considered stable, 10 points are scored. A mildly unstable elbow results in 5 points. An unstable elbow receives 0 points.
4. ADL (Activities of Daily Living): five ADLs are each given 5 points, viz. combing hair, performing personal hygiene, eating, and putting on shirt and shoes.

The Mark et al. [13] scale also has four parts rated as excellent/good/fair/poor based on the following items: loss of motion, loss of the carrying angle and pain/neurovascular lesion.

Statistical analysis was done using a two-tailed Student t test; $p < 0.05$ was considered significant.The correlations between various categories were investigated.

Fig. 4 a The reduced fracture under the completely undisturbed triceps muscle was fixated by two crossing wires with the medial one distant from the identified ulnar nerve. After torniquet release, good hemostasis was achieved with the wires left outside the skin for easy removal. b The same procedure was done with the wires bent and kept inside the wound in the case of neglected displaced lower fourth humeral fracture

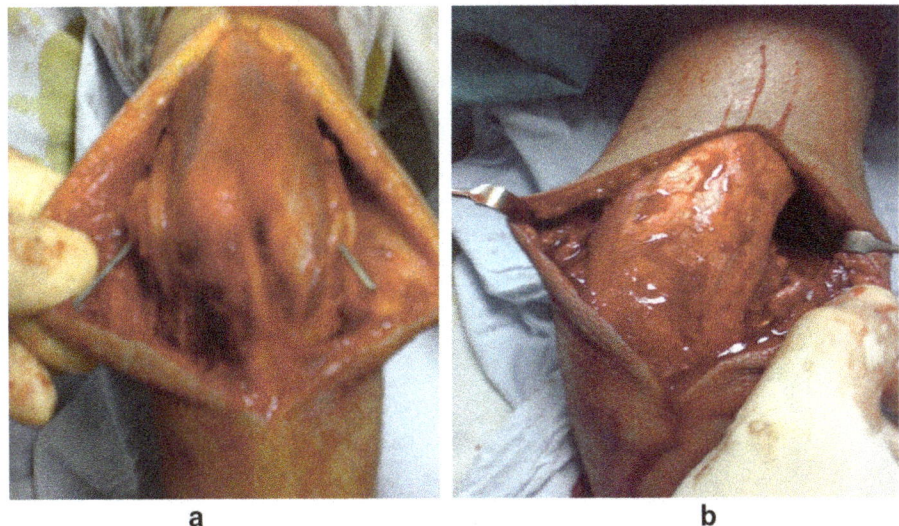

a   b

Using the Pearson product-moment correlation coefficient, values less than 0.25 indicated a weak correlation, between 0.25 and 0.50 mild, between 0.50 and 0.75 moderate and greater than 0.75 good.

Results

The points to be considered when assessing and analyzing the results in this study included the adequacy of the initial reduction, radiological union of the fracture and any loss of reduction or mal-union with any deformity, other possible complications such as loosening or osteolysis around the wires, myositis ossificans formation and the functional outcome of the injured elbow.

Radiological results

All fractures (100 % of patients) united (Figs. 5, 6, 7) in a mean duration of 7.2 weeks (range 5–10 weeks), as shown in Table 1. In one patient, the anterior humeral line, as a radiological sign of anatomical reduction, was not restored due to non-anatomical reduction in the lateral view X-ray (Fig. 5). In three patients, Baumann's angle could not be measured radiologically in the antero-posterior view due to imperfect radiographic projections. Although in a number of patients (four) the anatomical radiographic parameters of the elbow (Baumann's angle—anterior humeral line) were not measurable or not perfect, patients had no axial deviation or deformity.

Variation in the union time could be due to different factors such as the site of fracture (supracondylar or lower humeral fracture), the degree of displacement and the need for much dissection, the presence of comminution, the different ages of the patients studied, and the time interval between fracture and ORIF. Statistical analysis of the results showed that the younger the patient (age) the faster the union (time needed for union), and the earlier the intervention (injury–surgery interval) the faster the union (time needed for union), as shown in Table 2.

The fracture type (extension or flexion), the direction of displacement (postero-lateral or postero-medial) and the number of wires (two or four) or the wires being hidden or protruding from the skin had no influence on the healing time.

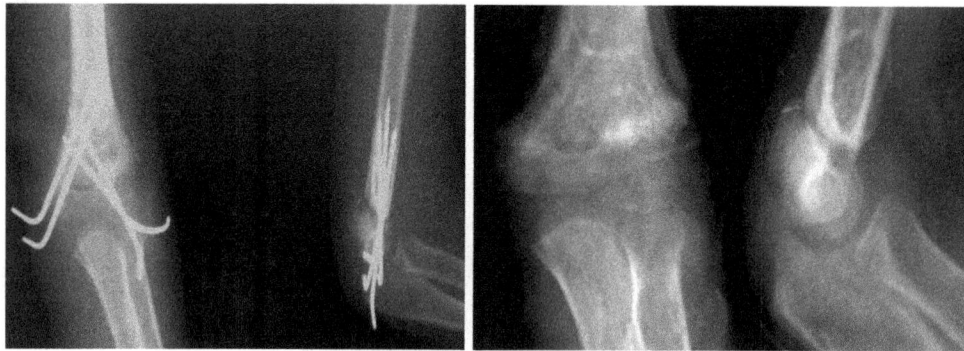

Fig. 5 Fixation by four crossing wires and after complete union and removal of wires (patient 1)

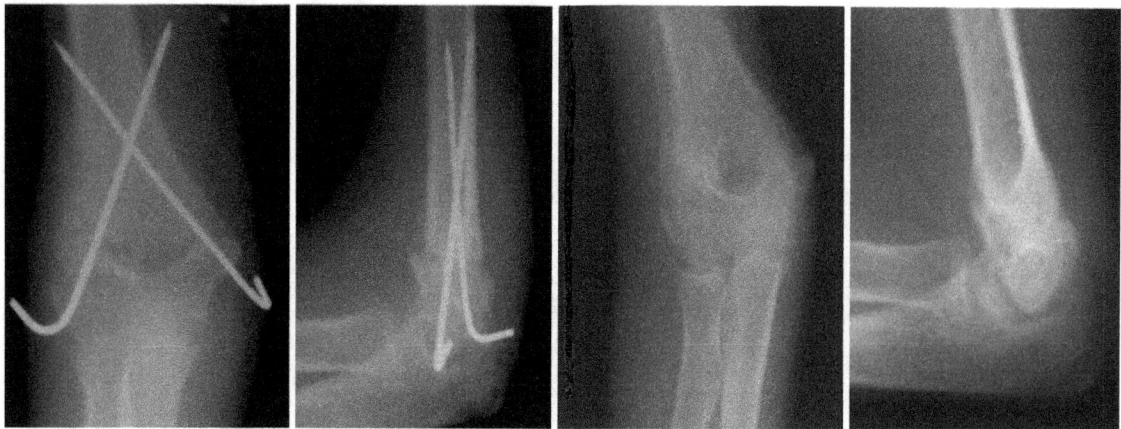

Fig. 6 Fixation by two crossing wires and after complete union in excellent position and wire removal (patient 14)

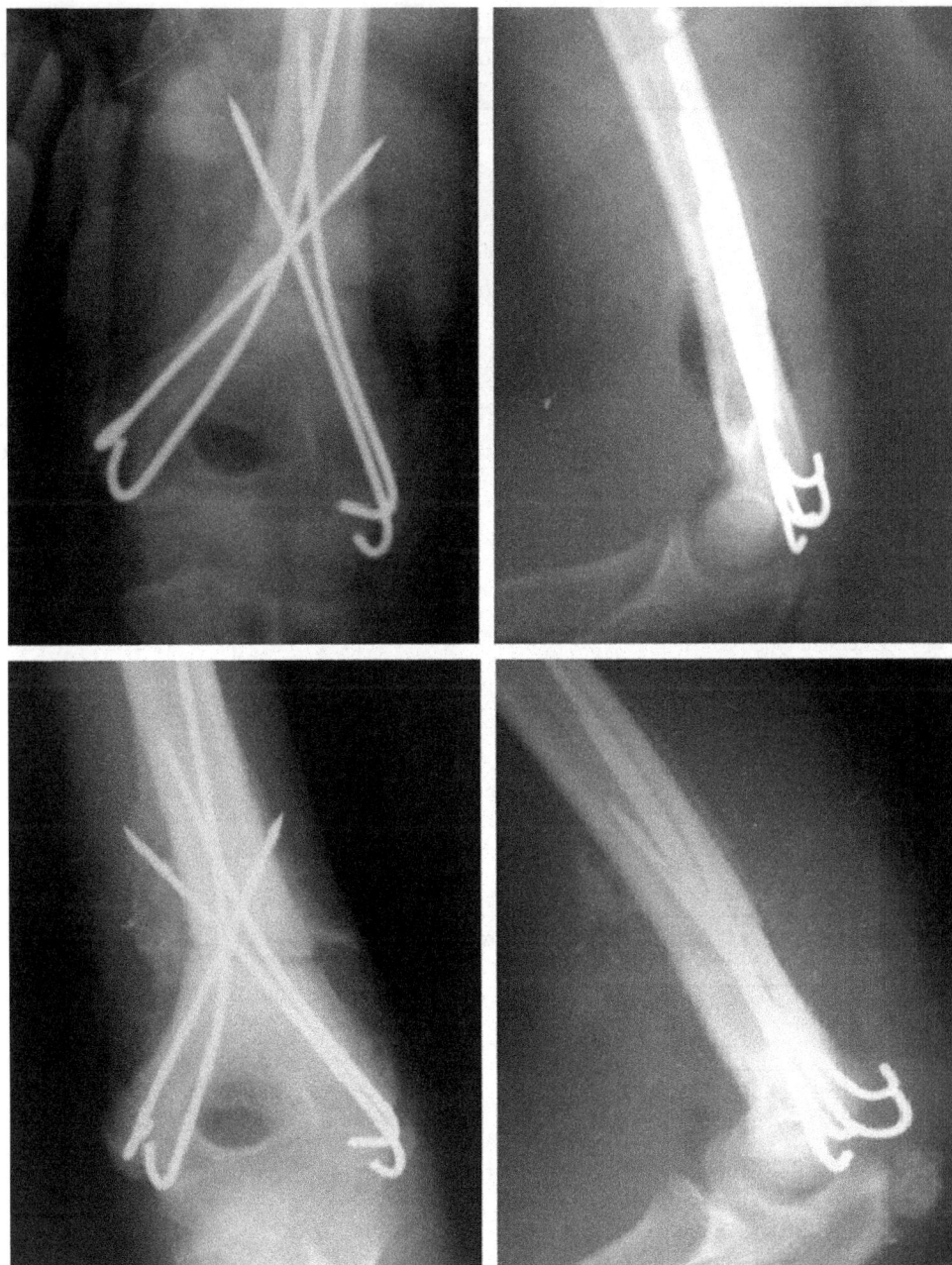

Fig. 7 Fixation by four crossing wires immediately post-operatively and after union with visible callus (patient 8)

Up to complete radiological union and removal of wires, there was no loss of reduction or secondary displacement, no mal-union, and no loosening or osteolysis around the wires. There was no myositis ossificans at the last follow-up (Table 1).

Functional results

All patients and parents expressed appreciation and satisfaction with the outcome, especifically functional recovery, except for two patients. The time to regain the normal ROM ranged from 8 to 20 weeks with a mean of 13 weeks, as shown in Table 1.

Excellent results were found in 13 patients (86.66 %) (Figs. 8, 9). Good results were found in two patients (13.33 %) at the last follow-up according to MEPI (Table 3). According to the Mark functional criteria, there was one patient with a fair result (6.66 %) (Table 4). The MEPI is much more forgiving than the criteria given by Mark et al., due to the difference in rating the amount of loss of motion in the elbow joint. This explains the difference in results using the two systems for evaluation.

Table 1 Characteristics of the presented patients

Cases	Age (years)	Type of fracture	Time needed for union (weeks)	Injury/surgery interval (days)	Surgery/full ROM interval (weeks)	Follow-up period (months)	Complications
1	10.00	Extension-type	10	27	Not fully restored	10	Re-fracture
2	6.00	Extension-type	5	16	10	17	Superficial pin track infection
3	9.20	Flexion-type	7	18	15	18	No complications
4	9.90	Extension-type	7	18	16	14	No complications
5	8.10	Extension-type	6	16	12	15	No complications
6	7.00	Extension-type	5	16	8	8	No complications
7	8.00	Extension-type	9	17	13	14	Superficial pin track infection
8	10.00	Lower 1/4 humerus	10	34	19	49	No complications
9	8.00	Extension-type	6	16	12	12	Superficial pin track infection
10	9.20	Extension-type	7	17	14	15	No complications
11	8.00	Extension-type	6	18	10	22	No complications
12	10.00	Extension-type	9	19	Not fully restored	17	Superficial pin track infection
13	9.00	Extension-type	6	17	14	13	Superficial pin track infection
14	11.00	Flexion-type	10	22	20	17	No complications
15	6.20	Extension-type	5	16	8	16	No complications
Mean ± SD	8.6 ± 1.3		7.2 ± 1.9	19 ± 5	13 ± 3.8	17 ± 9.4	

Table 2 Correlation between the ages of the patients, the injury–surgery intervals and the time needed for union

Time needed for union	Pearson correlation	P value	Significance
Age	0.835	0.001	HS
Injury–surgery interval	0.749	0.001	HS

HS highly significant

Five patients (33.33 %) developed superficial pin track infections that started 1 week after slab removal and at the beginning of active ROM; this was managed simply by pure alcohol and oral antibiotics, as shown in Table 1.

No patients had iatrogenic nerve injury or vascular insult. No patients developed deep wound infection or wire loosening or migration. No patients developed physeal arrest or deformity up to the last follow-up.

Re-fracture occurred in one patient (6.66 %) with incomplete restoration of the ROM. In this patient, the time to union was about 10 weeks and after wire removal there was inadequate callus formation in the lateral view. The patient was again put in above elbow slab for another 2 weeks for protection. There was marked limitation of the ROM, mostly due to volar skin abrasions with contracted elbow flexors due to the prolonged immobilization period. The patient was referred for physiotherapy, and after 2 weeks presented with a swollen tender elbow. X-ray

revealed re-fracture; he was put in a slab for 3 weeks, the slab was removed after the pain completely disappeared and X-ray showed dependable callus formation. He was sent back for gentle physiotherapy and followed up monthly until improvement. After 6 months, there was complete union and remodeling of the fracture to an accepted position denoted by the anterior humeral line cutting the capitulum as a radiological sign of good reduction with improved ROM (Fig. 10).

Discussion

It is clear that the goal of treatment of any fracture is to obtain consolidation without complications.

According to the literature, children with neglected supracondylar humeral fractures are those who presented for treatment after 14 days of injury and had already started the biological process of healing with early callus formation.

There are various factors leading to delayed treatment following supracondylar humeral fractures in children. Inability to achieve a satisfactory closed reduction of the fracture due to continued swelling and/or skin problems is the main concern. The need for ORIF increases as the time to surgery increases. The rate of conversion to open reduction has been reported as ranging from less than 3 % to about 46 % [15].

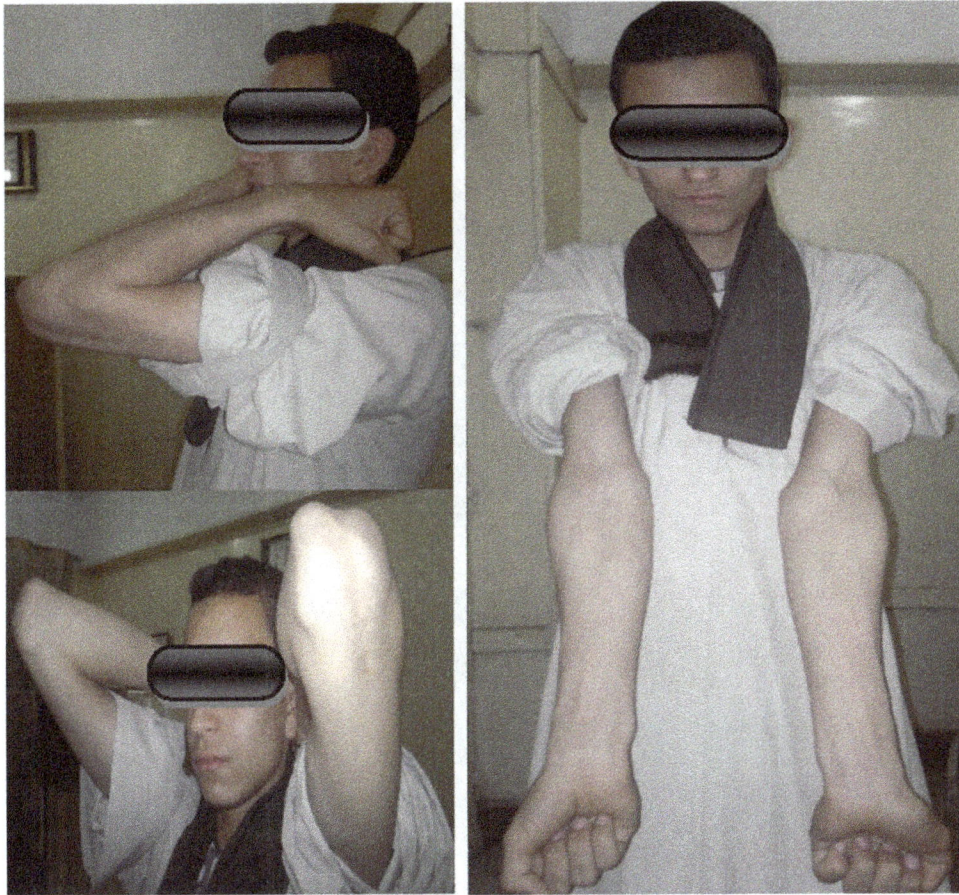

Fig. 8 Full ROM of the elbow at the last follow-up 4 years post-operatively (patient 8)

Tiwari et al. [16] consider operative treatment the best option for such late-presenting fractures. In the past, open reduction led to concerns regarding elbow stiffness, myositis ossificans, unsightly scarring and iatrogenic neurovascular injury. However, several studies [17] have recently demonstrated a low rate of complications associated with open reduction. Some authors have demonstrated no correlation between stiffness and the type of surgical approach used, especially regarding the posterior approach [18].

All patients in this study presented after more than 2 weeks, with a mean duration between their presentation and the initial injury of 19 days (range 16–34 days).

A study by Lal and Bhan [19] included 20 children with delayed open reduction by means of a posterior approach for supracondylar humeral fractures. The delay time ranged from 11 to 17 days. In another study by Eren et al. [3] the average delay time was 6 days (range 2–19 days).

The average time for complete union in the current study was 7.2 weeks (range 5–10 weeks). In a study by Dehao et al. [20], all fractures healed within 6–8 weeks. The difference in healing time could be due to the fact that the mean age of the patients in the present study and the

interval between injury and presentation for surgery were larger than in the study by Dehao et al. [20].

Nerve injuries associated with displaced supracondylar humeral fractures may be separated into those associated with the injury itself and those associated with treatment of the injury [21]. A literature review demonstrated iatrogenic nerve injury in 3.6 % of patients, with the ulnar nerve being involved in 81 % of these cases [22]. In the current study, and due to fact that the fixation was done after open reduction with exposure and identification of the ulnar nerve, there was no iatrogenic nerve injury and the two patients with radial and ulnar nerve involvement preoperatively resolved spontaneously within 3 months postoperatively with no need for nerve conduction studies.

In this study, the time to regain the normal ROM ranged from 8 to 20 weeks with a mean duration of 13 weeks, with faster recovery in patients with less immobilization. In the study by Eren et al. [3], full functional recovery was achieved within 3 months in 29 patients (93.5 %), and there was no evidence of a correlation between duration of immobilization and delay in ROM recovery.

Regarding complications such as pin track infection, deep infection, compartment syndrome, mal-union and

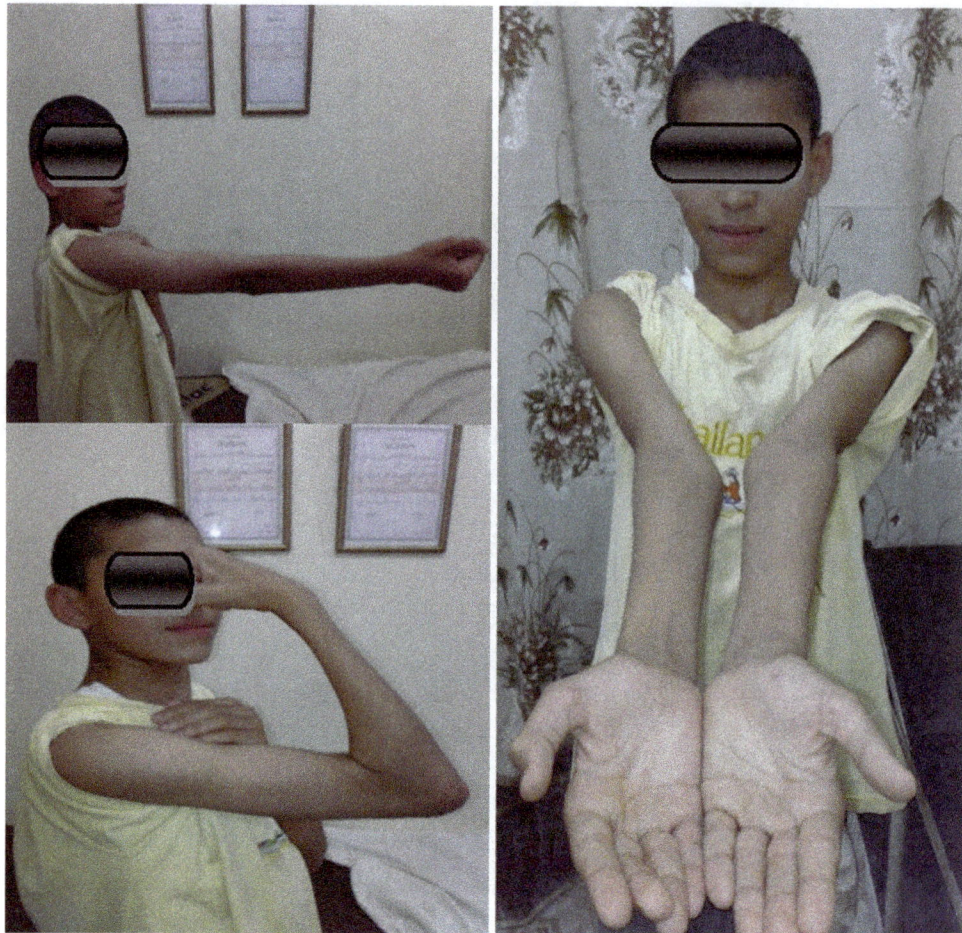

Fig. 9 Nearly full ROM of the elbow at the last follow-up 1 year post-operatively (patient 14)

Table 3 Results of the patients studied according to Mayo Elbow Performance Index (MEPI)

Result grade	Points	No. of cases	
Excellent	90–100	13	Mean MEPI 96.6
Good	75–89	2	–
		MEPI 86 MEPI 80	–
Fair	60–74	0	–
Poor	Below 60	0	–

deformities, the results of the present study are comparable with other studies by Lal and Bhan, Dehao et al., Eren et al. and Tiwari et al. [19, 20].

Another study by Jason et al. [12] preserved triceps integrity and function using an extensor mechanism-on approach for fixation of distal humeral fractures. They documented that there is limited literature regarding elbow motion, functional outcomes and objective strength assessment following the extensor mechanism-on approach; although the age group and mode of fixation were different from that in the current study, the results could be matched regarding the functional recovery of the elbow.

Jason et al. [12] documented that open treatment of distal humeral fractures with an extensor mechanism-on approach results in excellent healing, a mean elbow

Table 4 Results of the patients studied according to Mark criteria

Result grade	Loss of motion	Loss of carrying angle	Pain/neurovascular lesion	No. of cases
Excellent	None	None	None	13
Good	<20°	<10°	None	1
Fair	20–50°	10–20°	Minimal pain with excessive use No neurovascular lesion	1
Poor	>50°	>20°	Pain/neurovascular lesion	0

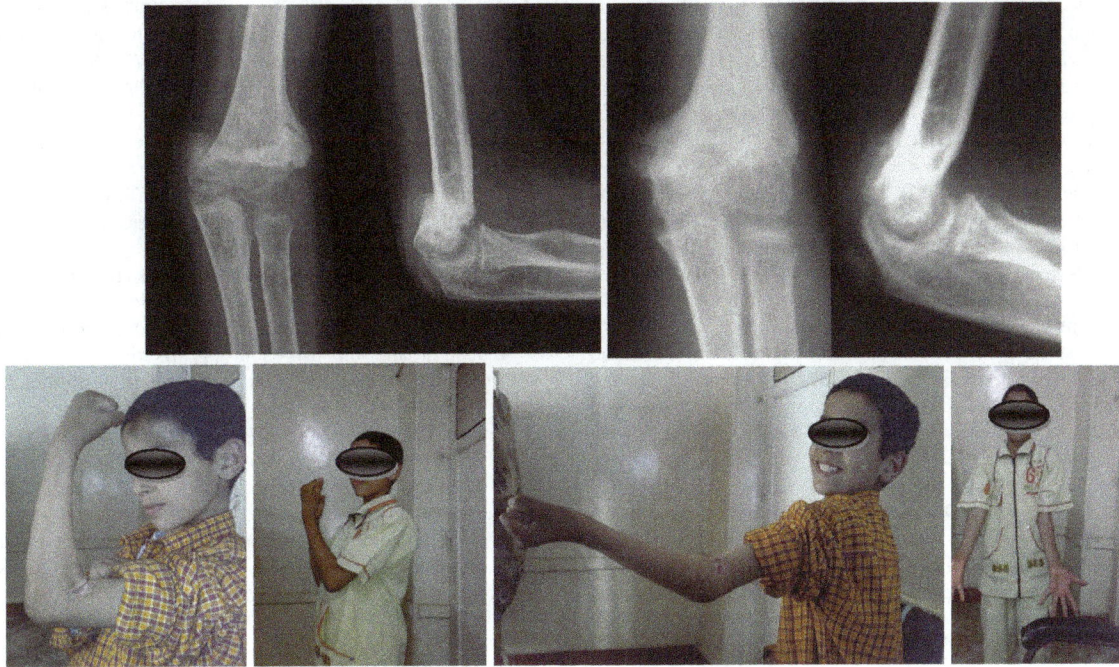

Fig. 10 The patient with iatrogenic re-fracture after complete union and remodeling with loss of more than 30° of motion, denoting a fair result according to the criteria given by Mark et al. Full finger and wrist functions denoting spontaneous recovery of the previously affected radial nerve (patient 1)

flexion–extension arc exceeding 100°, and maintenance of 90 % of elbow extension strength compared with that of the contralateral, normal elbow.

In comparison with the other studies, the current study is characterized by an older age group of patients, a longer time interval of neglected treatment and a wide variety of cases including flexion and extension types of supracondylar fractures and also lower humeral fractures.

In conclusion, patients with neglected supracondylar fractures of the humerus are those who presented for treatment after 14 days of injury and in such neglected cases—especially those with early appearance of callus—there is no place for trials of closed reduction and percutaneous pinning. Finally, we can conclude that triceps-sparing approach isan easy, simple and safe approach for exposure and internal fixationof neglected supracondylar and distal humeral fractures in childrenwith excellent functional outcome.

Conflict of interest None.

Ethical standards The procedure was performed in accordance with the ethical standards of the responsible committee on human experimentation (institutional and national) and with the Helsinki Declaration of 1975, as revised in 2000 and 2008.

Informed consent All patients' parents gave informed consent before inclusion in the study; the study was authorized by the institutional review board.

References

1. Ozkoc G, Gonc U, Kayaalp A, Teker K, Peker TT (2004) Displaced supracondylar humeral fractures in children: open reduction vs. closed reduction and pinning. Arch Orthop Trauma Surg 124(8):547–551

2. Pretell Mazzini J, Rodriguez Martin J, Andres-Esteban EM (2010) Surgical approaches for open reduction and pinning in severely displaced supracondylar humerus fractures in children: a systematic review. J Child Orthop 4(2):143–152

3. Abdullah Eren, Güven Melih, Erol Bülent, Çakar Murat (2008) Delayed surgical treatment of supracondylar humerus fractures in children using a medial approach. J Child Orthop 2(1):21–27

4. Kazimoglu C, Cetin M, Sener M, Agus H, Kalanderer O (2009) Operative management of type III extension supracondylar fractures in children. Int Orthop 33(4):1089–1094

5. Sadiq MZ, Syed T, Travlos J (2007) Management of grade III supracondylar fracture of the humerus by straight-arm lateral traction. Int Orthop 31(2):155–158

6. Oh CW, Park BC, Kim PT, Park IH, Kyung HS, Ihn JC (2003) Completely displaced supracondylar humerus fractures in children: results of open reduction versus closed reduction. J Orthop Sci. 8(2):137–141

7. Turhan E, Aksoy C, Ege A, Bayar A, Keser S, Alpaslan M (2008) Sagittal plane analysis of the open and closed methods in children with displaced supracondylar fractures of the humerus (a radiological study). Arch Orthop Trauma Surg 128(7):739–744

8. Aronson DC, Vollenhoven E, Meeuwis JD (1993) K-wire fixation of supracondylar humeral fractures in children: results of open reduction via a ventral approach in comparison with closed treatment. Injury 24(3):179–181

9. Barlas K, Baga T (2005) Medial approach for fixation of displaced supracondylar fractures of the humerus in children. Acta Orthop Belg 71(2):149–153

10. Ay S, Akinci M, Kamiloglu S, Ercetin O (2005) Open reduction of displaced pediatric supracondylar humeral fractures through the anterior cubital approach. J Pediatr Orthop 25:149–153

11. Rasool MN, Naidoo KS (1999) Supracondylar fractures: posterolateral type with brachialis muscle penetration and neurovascular injury. J Pediatr Orthop 19:518–522

12. Erpelding Jason M, Mailander Adam, High Robin, Mormino Matthew A, Fehringer Edward V (2012) Outcomes following distal humeral fracture fixation with an extensor mechanism-on approach. J Bone Joint Surg Am 94:548–553

13. Mark G, Innocenti M, Ruedi T, Yacchia GE (1985) Die supracondylare Humerusfraktur beim Kind. Helv Chir Acta 51:617–620

14. Turchin DC, Beaton DE, Richards RR (1998) Validity of observer-based aggregate scoring systems as descriptors of elbow pain, function, and disability. J Bone Joint Surg 80:154–162

15. Peters CL, Scott SM, Stevens PM (1995) Closed reduction and percutaneous pinning of displaced supracondylar humerus fractures in children: description of a new closed reduction technique for fractures with brachialis muscle entrapment. J Orthop Trauma 9:430–434

16. Tiwari A, Kanojia RK, Kapoor SK (2007) Surgical management for late presentation of supracondylar humeral fracture in children. J Orthop Surg (Hong Kong) 15:177–182

17. Brauer CA, Lee BM, Bae DS (2007) A systematic review of medial and lateral entry pinning versus lateral entry pinning for supracondylar fractures of the humerus. J Pediatr Orthop 27:181–186

18. Kumar R, Kiran EK, Malhotra R, Bhan S (2002) Surgical management of the severely displaced supracondylar fracture of the humerus in children. Injury 33:517–522

19. Lal GM, Bhan S (1991) Delayed open reduction for supracondylar fractures of the humerus. Int Orthop 15(3):189–191

20. Dehao Fu, Xiao Baojun, Yang Shuhua, Jin Li (2011) Open reduction and bioabsorbable pin fixation for late presenting irreducible supracondylar humeral fracture in children. Int Orthop 35(5):725–730

21. Fowles JV, Kassab MT (1974) Displaced supracondylar fractures of the elbow in children. A report on the fixation of extension and flexion fractures by two lateral percutaneous pins. J Bone Joint Surg Am 56:490–500

22. Lyons J, Ashley E, Hoffer MM (1998) Ulnar nerve palsies after percutaneous cross-pinning of supracondylar fractures in children's elbows. J Pediatr Orthop 18:43–45

18

Barbed suture vs conventional tenorrhaphy: biomechanical analysis in an animal model

A. Clemente · F. Bergamin · C. Surace ·
E. Lepore · N. Pugno

Abstract

Background The advantages of barbed suture for tendon repair could be to eliminate the need for a knot and to better distribute the load throughout the tendon so as to reduce the deformation at the repair site. The purpose of this study was to evaluate the breaking force and the repair site deformation of a new barbed tenorrhaphy technique in an animal model.

Materials and methods Sixty porcine flexor tendons were divided randomly into three groups and repaired with one of the following techniques: a new 4-strand barbed technique using 2/0 polypropylene Quill™ SRS or 2/0 polydioxanone Quill™ SRS and a modified Kessler technique using 3/0 prolene. All tendons underwent mechanical testing to assess the 2-mm gap formation force, the breaking force and the mode of failure. The percentage change in tendon cross-sectional area before and after repair was calculated.

Results The two-sample Student *t*-test demonstrated a significant increase in 2-mm gap formation force and in breaking force with barbed sutures, independently from suture material, when compared to traditional Kessler suture. Concerning the tendon profile, we registered less bunching at the repair site in the two barbed groups compared with the Kessler group.

Conclusions This study confirms the promising results achieved in previous ex vivo studies about the use of barbed suture in flexor tendon repair. In our animal model, tenorrhaphy with Quill™ SRS suture guarantees a breaking force of repair that exceeds the 40–50 N suggested as sufficient to initiate early active motion, and a smoother profile at the repair site.

Level of evidence Not applicable.

Keywords Barbed suture · Breaking force · Tenorrhaphy · Biomechanical testing

A. Clemente · F. Bergamin (✉)
Department of Hand, Plastic and Reconstructive Surgery, Maria Vittoria Hospital, Turin, Italy
e-mail: federicabergamin@yahoo.it

C. Surace
Laboratory of Bio-inspired Nanomechanics "Giuseppe Maria Pugno", Department of Structural, Building and Geotechnical Engineering, Politecnico di Torino, Turin, Italy

E. Lepore · N. Pugno
Laboratory of Bio-inspired and Graphene Nanomechanics, Department of Civil, Environmental and Mechanical Engineering, University of Trento, Via Mesiano 77, 38123 Trento, Italy

N. Pugno
Centre of Materials and Microsystems, Bruno Kessler Foundation, Via Santa Croce 77, 38122 Trento, Italy

N. Pugno
School of Engineering and Materials Science, Queen Mary University, Mile End Rd, London E1 4NS, UK

Introduction

An ideal tendon repair would ensure a sufficient breaking force with a minimal deformity in the tendon repair site to allow early passive and active motion so as to reduce tendon adhesions and improve the functional outcome. In a conventional tenorrhaphy, knots are the weak point of tendon repair, being operator dependent and causing decreased tendon apposition. Increased suture diameter and number of knots increases the force of repair but also the tendon cross-sectional area, causing an increased gliding resistance. To avoid the potential weakness from knots, and to improve the interaction between tendon tissue and suture materials, it is proposed that barbed sutures could be utilized.

In 1967, McKenzie described the first account for the use of an internal multiple barbed suture to repair flexor tendons in a canine model [1, 2]. Recently, with the improvement in biomaterial and US Food and Drug Administration approval of barbed nylon, polydioxanone and polypropylene sutures, a renascent interest in this kind of suture material was registered. Quill[TM] Self-Retaining System (SRS) (Angiotech, Vancouver, BC, Canada) is a barbed bidirectional suture, created using absorbable and non-absorbable materials, with barbs spiraling around the central core suture and armed with a surgical needle on each end. The barbs anchor tissues so Quill[TM] SRS does not require knots to approximate opposing edges of a wound.

Up until now, few studies concerning the breaking force[1] of tenorrhaphy with barbed sutures have been published, and all in cadaver or animal models. The purpose of this study was to evaluate the breaking force and repair site characteristics of a new 4-strand technique using Quill[TM] SRS, compared with the traditional modified Kessler technique in flexor tendon repair in a porcine model.

Materials and methods

Sixty tendons of similar size were obtained from the forelegs of adult pigs for slaughter. The pig model was chosen for the similarity in structure and strength to a human tendons [3]. Tendons were examined for abnormalities, such as synovitis and degeneration, and were rejected if an anomaly was present. Sheaths were excised and tendons were stored with refrigeration. During tendon harvest, preparation and repair (Fig. 1), desiccation was prevented with application of normal saline. Each tendon was transected at the midpoint and was measured by a single observer with a digital caliper to determine the pre-repair (A_{PR}) and post-repair (A_R) cross-sectional area. The cross-sectional area was calculated assuming an elliptic cross-sectional area, i.e., equal to πab, where a and b are equal one-half tendon height and width, respectively. The change between the post-repair and the pre-repair cross-sectional areas was determined as $(A_{PR} - A_R)/A_{PR}$ (%). A single surgeon harvested all tendons and performed all sutures.

The tendons were randomly assigned to three repair groups: 20 tendons sutured using 3/0 prolene with a 2-strand modified Kessler technique (group A) (Fig. 2); 20 using 2/0 polypropylene Quill[TM] SRS with a new 4-strand barbed technique (group B) (Fig. 3); 20 using 2/0 polydioxanone (PDO) Quill[TM] SRS with the same new 4-strand barbed technique (group C). No suture was performed in the epitenon.

The 2/0 Quill[TM] SRS barbed suture was chosen because it has a breaking force that most closely resembles that of 3/0 unbarbed suture [4], according to the manufacturer's data. After testing the new 4-strand barbed technique with 2/0 polypropylene Quill[TM] SRS, the same tenorrhaphy was performed with 2/0 PDO Quill[TM] SRS, a monofilament synthetic absorbable suture, to assess whether there was an improvement in breaking force with this suture material.

For knotless tendon repair, the following new technique was used (Fig. 3). The beginning is like a Kessler technique, but each needle enters the lateral wall of the proximal tendon stump perpendicular to the fibrils before turning 90 ° and exiting the stump. In the distal stump, each needle was advanced parallel to the direction of the fibrils for a distance of 0.5 cm before exiting the tendon surface. Next, each needle was used to make two transverse passes perpendicular to the direction of the tendon fibrils. Each needle was then reintroduced into the tendon and advanced parallel to the fibrils to traverse the injury site and enter the opposite end of the tendon for a distance of 0.5 cm before exiting the tendon surface. Again, two transverse passes were made to anchor the suture, and following the second pass, the excess suture and needle were cut off. This process resulted in a knotless repair with four strands crossing the injury site and four transverse passes at each end of the tenorrhaphy.

All biomechanical tensile tests were done in the Laboratory of Bio-inspired Nanomechanics "Giuseppe Maria Pugno" (Politecnico di Torino, Italy) with an air temperature of 22 ± 1 °C and 31 ± 2 % of relative humidity. Tendons were kept moist up until the test with normal saline.

The tensile tests were conducted using a testing machine (Insight 1 kN, MTS, Minnesota, USA), equipped with a 100-N cell load with pneumatic saw-tooth-shaped clamps (closure pressure of 275.6 kPa), which prevent tendon slippage during testing (Fig. 4). The clamps were brought to zero tension before starting mounting tendons, which were placed between clamps defining an initial length l_0 of 50 mm. Once tendons were in place, a preload of ~ 2 N was applied by slightly raising the actuator, leaving the tendons loose to properly extend between the clamps, without placing significant tension on the repair, in accordance with previously published papers [5, 6]. The specimens were pulled until they completely broke using a

---

[1] The articles cited in the literature improperly use the term "tensile strength", which is force per unit area, as they present the measured data in Newtons (the SI derived unit of force). Therefore, in this paper only the correct term of "breaking force" will be utilized.

Fig. 1 Tendons before and after the suture: repair site distortion with the modified Kessler technique (*above*), with the new 4-strand barbed technique with 2/0 polypropylene Quill™ SRS (*center*) and with the new 4-strand barbed technique with 2/0 PDO Quill™ SRS (*below*) in comparison with uninjured tendon (*on the left*)

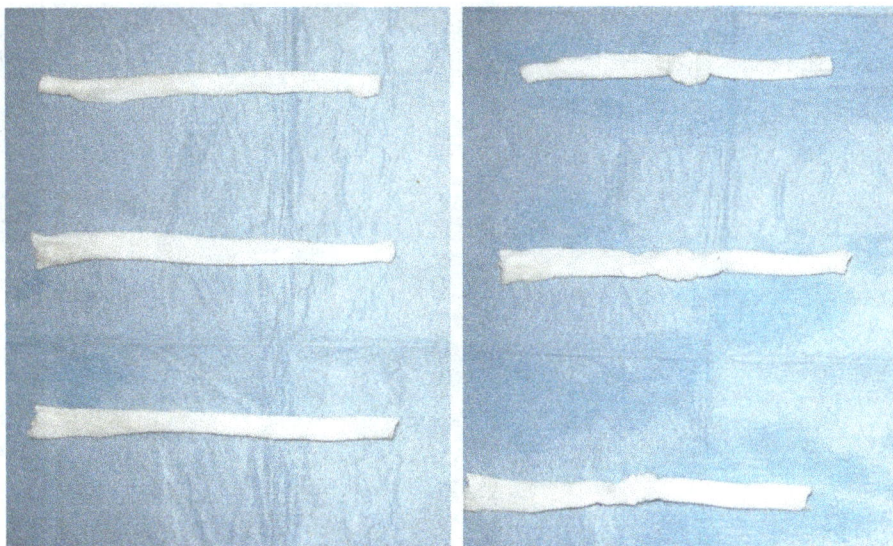

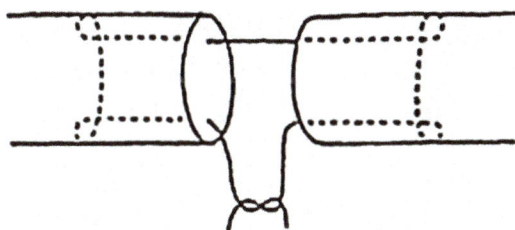

Fig. 2 The modified Kessler technique used in group A

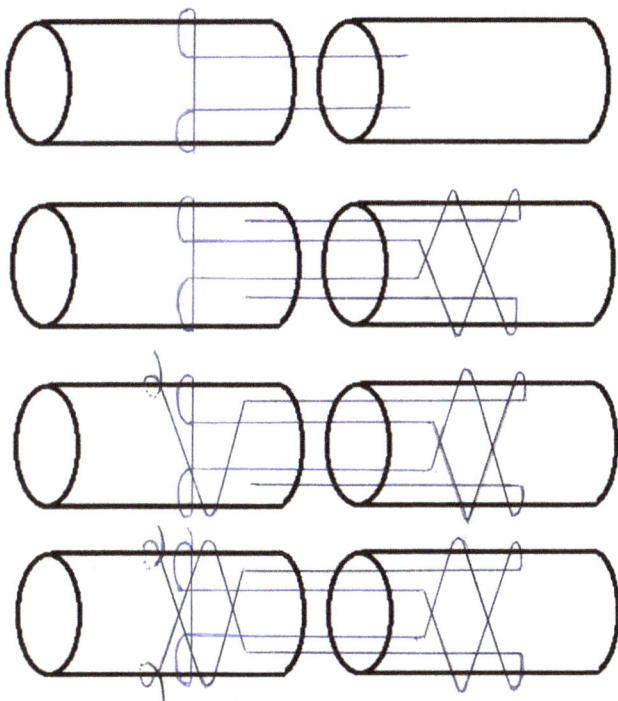

Fig. 3 The new 4-strand barbed technique used in groups B and C

displacement-controlled uniaxial tension at a constant rate of 20 mm/min, as in previous studies [7]. This preload and rate were selected because they best simulate forces acting on an immobilized tendon during active flexion.

In addition, tensile tests were performed for the suture materials, fixing the same initial length l_0 and the same constant rate of 20 mm/min, without the 2-N preload.

The computer program Test Works 4 (MTS, Minnesota, USA) recorded the experimental data of the applied tensile force and displacement. All tendons underwent mechanical testing to assess the 2-mm formation force, which was calculated using a bar scale placed near the repaired tendon and captured with a DCR SR55E SONY digital video camera. Linear traction continued until the suture materials were ruptured or tendons failed, and the breaking force was recorded immediately before failure.

A two-sample Student t-test was performed to determine whether there was a significant difference in load at 2-mm gap formation, maximum load or pre-repair areas among the three repair groups. Differences at the $P \leq 0.01$ level were considered significant.

Results

The force corresponding to 2-mm gap formation and to breaking of the suture, the mode of sample failure, the pre-repair (A_{PR}) and post-repair (A_R) cross-sectional areas and the changes (%) in tendon dimensions are listed in Table 1. Table 2 reports the mechanical data of the suture materials alone. All values are reported as mean $\pm$ SD.

The two-sample Student t-test demonstrated a significant increase in mean load at 2-mm gap formation with barbed sutures, independently from suture material, when

Fig. 4 Flexor tendon in tension on MTS with pneumatic saw-tooth-shaped clamps holding the tendon

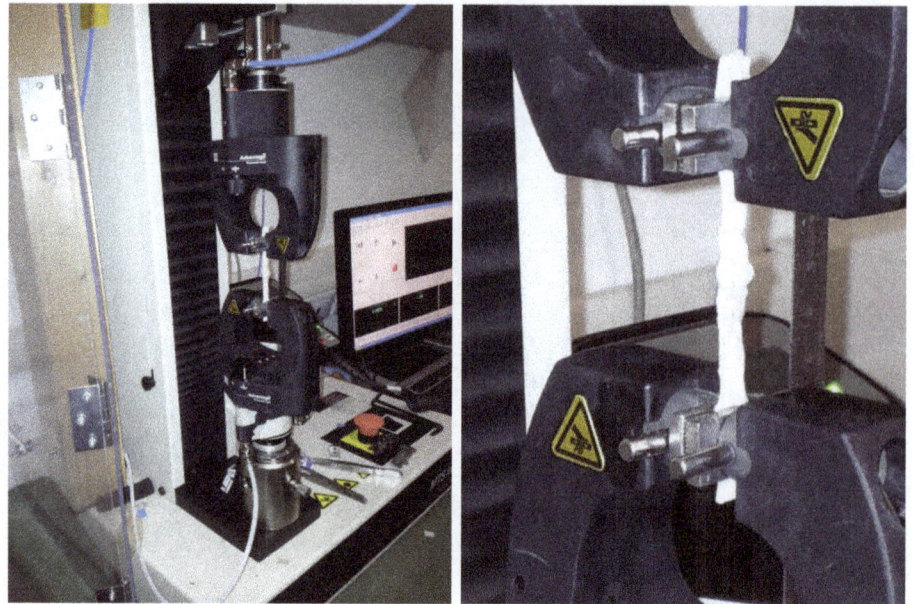

Table 1 Results of biomechanical tensile tests of tendon repairs including tensile force of 2-mm gap formation, the breaking force, the mode of sample failure, the pre-repair (A_{PR}) and post-repair (A_R) cross-sectional area and the changes (%) in tendon dimensions

Repair technique	Tensile force (N)		Failure mode (observed number)		Repair site cross-sectional area (mm^2)		
	2-mm gap formation	Breaking force	Suture breakage	Suture pull-out	Pre-repair (A_{PR})	Post-repair (A_R)	Change (%)
Group A	21.2 ± 5.9	28.2 ± 6.2	12	8	12.4 ± 3.1	24.7 ± 7.6	99.6
Group B	38.2 ± 9.3	50.3 ± 9.9	20	0	14.6 ± 2.8	25.7 ± 10.0	76.3
Group C	41.0 ± 11.4	61.5 ± 11.0	20	0	15.4 ± 2.3	25.0 ± 6.1	61.8

Group A: modified Kessler technique. Group B: 4-strand barbed technique with 2/0 polypropylene Quill^{TM} SRS. Group C: 4-strand barbed technique with 2/0 PDO Quill^{TM} SRS

Table 2 Results of biomechanical tensile tests of suture materials alone

Suture material	Tensile force (N) Breaking force
3/0 prolene	23.5 ± 0.9
2/0 polypropylene Quill^{TM} SRS	27.1 ± 1.2
2/0 PDO Quill^{TM} SRS	28.3 ± 1.0

Table 3 Results of the two-sample Student t-test applied to 2-mm gap formation load

Student t-test/2-mm gap formation load			
	Group A	Group B	Group C
Group A	//	6.914 ($P < 0.01$)	6.893 ($P < 0.01$)
Group B		//	0.853 ($P = 0.399$)
Group C			//

compared to a traditional Kessler suture. No statistically significant differences in mean load at 2-mm gap formation were registered between the two barbed groups. As regards load to failure, the two barbed groups demonstrated a significantly increased breaking force when compared to the Kessler group, and also the 4-strand technique with Quill^{TM} SRS PDO suture demonstrated significantly better resistance to failure relative to the 4-strand repair with Quill^{TM} SRS polypropylene suture (Tables 3, 4; Fig. 5).

Note that the differences between pre-repair areas are not significant, except between the barbed group with Quill^{TM} SRS PDO suture and the Kessler group where a significant difference emerges (Table 5). Nevertheless, this difference is irrelevant because we calculated the breaking force of the suture that is not affected by the area of the tendon. Indeed, in all tests the failure mode is due to the breakage of the suture or suture pull-out, but never due to tendon failure.

Table 4 Results of the two-sample Student *t*-test applied to breaking force

Student *t*-test/breaking force

	Group A	Group B	Group C
Group A	//	8.5 ($P < 0.01$)	11.759 ($P < 0.01$)
Group B		//	3.375 ($P < 0.01$)
Group C			//

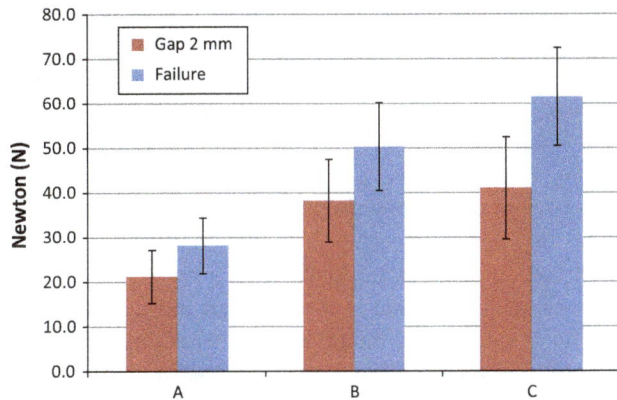

Fig. 5 Comparison of forces among tendon repair techniques (*A* Kessler suture, *B* barbed technique with 2/0 polypropylene Quill™ SRS and *C* barbed technique with 2/0 PDO Quill™ SRS): the average 2-mm gap formation force (*red bars*) and the breaking force (*blue bars*) are shown for each tendon repair technique

Table 5 Results of the two-sample Student *t*-test applied to pre-repair area

Student *t*-test/pre-repair area

	Group A	Group B	Group C
Group A	//	2.432 ($P = 0.025$)	3.981 ($P < 0.01$)
Group B		//	1.287 ($P = 0.205$)
Group C			//

Discussion

Initially, the breaking force of tendon repair depends on the biomechanics of tendon sutures. Immobilized tendon sutures lose 50 % of their initial strength within the first week due to tenomalacia at the suture-tendon junction [8]. Early passive and especially active motion rehabilitation programs have been shown to prevent the initial weakening at the repair site by improving tendon nutrition, healing and remodeling [9, 10]. Therefore, it is absolutely essential that the tendon repair is sufficiently strong to tolerate the forces generated during early active motion, which are of 40–50 N as described by Amadioet al. [11].

The breaking force of the repair can be improved by increasing the number of strands crossing the repair site, the suture caliber and the number of knots; however, in this way the tendon cross-sectional area is enlarged, causing increased gliding resistance [12].

Consequently, the ideal suture technique must be strong enough to allow early active motion with minimal deformity of the cross-sectional area at the repair site.

All conventional tenorrhaphy techniques require knots, but knots are potential weak points in tendon sutures. If a knot lies within the tendon, it may reduce vascularization, tendon apposition and intrinsic healing, causing extrinsic neovascularization and adhesion formation. Furthermore, bulky knots enlarge the tendon cross-sectional area, increasing gliding resistance during active flexion and therefore the risk of gapping or suture failure.

The advantages of barbed sutures are to eliminate the need for a knot and to better distribute the load throughout the tendon repaired due to a greater number of points for barb-tendon interaction along the length of the suture. In this way, the bunching at the repair site is reduced and the breaking force improved.

Previous studies hypothesized that a knotless flexor tendon repair using bidirectional barbed suture has a similar breaking force to a traditional knotted technique but with a smaller change in the repair site cross-sectional area. This was proven by McClellan et al. [7] who compared, in a porcine model, two conventional techniques, the 2-strand Kessler and the 4-strand Savage, with a 4-strand barbed tenorrhaphy. By testing the 2-mm gap formation force and the load to failure, they demonstrated that Savage and barbed techniques have equivalent breaking force, both significantly greater than the Kessler method. As regards tendon deformity, the repair site cross-sectional area of tendon repaired with the knotless technique was significantly smaller than that of tendons repaired with Kessler and Savage techniques. Parikh et al. [5] compared, in cadaver flexor tendons, 3-strand and 6-strand barbed suture techniques to a knotted 4-strand cruciate technique, demonstrating that the 3-strand barbed suture achieved a breaking force comparable to that of 4-strand cruciate repair, but with significantly less repair site bunching. In the 6-strand barbed suture technique an increased breaking force and significantly less repair site bunching have been recorded, compared with 4-strand cruciate repair. When trying to critically analyze the literature, in each study one finds that the tendon repair technique, number of strands, suture material and suture diameter between control and experimental groups change, making it difficult to compare the results. Another disadvantage of these studies lies in the lack of cyclical testing that models in vivo situations more realistically than linear tests alone. Recently, Zeplin et al. [13] compared a knotted with a knotless tendon repair technique, applying linear and cyclical loads, without detecting any difference in breaking force between the two groups in both situations.

In our study, we wanted to test a new 4-strand repair technique using Quill™ SRS suture. The control group was represented by a modified Kessler technique. Although it is not appropriate to compare a 4-strand with a 2-strand tenorrhaphy, the purpose was to test a new technique using barbed suture against a well-studied, widely accepted standard in flexor tendon repair. To maximize the purchase of the barb of the suture on the tendon fibrils, the repair was designed to traverse the tendon several times perpendicular to the direction of the collagen fibers.

As regards the suture material, after testing barbed suture using Quill™ SRS polypropylene 2/0, it was decided to try an absorbable material, Quill™ SRS polydioxanone 2/0, since, according to data provided by the manufacturer, it should have a higher suture breaking force, i.e., 1.77 kgf (17.36 N) versus 0.96 kgf (9.42 N). Furthermore, we did not want to leave a non-absorbable barbed material in the repaired tendon indefinitely. Before performing the tendon repair, the breaking force of the suture materials was measured and a higher load to failure compared to the declaration of the manufacturer was recorded. This data could be related to a safety factor utilized by the manufacturer. According to Quill™ SRS's manufacturer, the results of implantation studies in animals using PDO indicate that for sizes larger than 3/0, approximately 80 % of the original strength remains after 4 weeks of implantation. The absorption of PDO is declared be minimal until about 120 days and essentially complete within 180 days. However, additional in vivo studies are needed in order to understand better the biological behavior of this absorbable suture material, to determine whether it is absorbed prematurely or if it creates denser scarring.

In this study, a significant increase in mean load at 2-mm gap formation with barbed sutures was exhibited, independently of suture material, compared with a traditional Kessler suture. No statistically significant difference in mean load at 2-mm gap formation was registered between the two barbed groups. As regards load to failure, the two barbed groups demonstrated a significantly increased breaking force when compared to the Kessler group, and the 4-strand technique with Quill™ SRS PDO suture also had a significantly higher load to failure when compared with the 4-strand repair using Quill™ SRS polypropylene suture. In barbed tenorrhaphy using the Quill™ SRS suture, the breaking force of the repair exceeded the 40–50 N suggested by Amadio [11] as sufficient to initiate early active motion.

Concerning repair site profile, less bunching was recorded at the repair site with the barbed suture compared with the conventional modified Kessler technique. This result improves tendon gliding through the sheath, and avoids peripheral epitendinous suturing.

As regards the failure mode, it was observed that all barbed suture repairs failed by suture breakage, whereas unbarbed control repair failed in 40 % of cases by suture pull-out and in 60 % by suture breakage. This suggests that inadequate suture-tendon interaction was the limiting factor in achieving a high breaking force with the modified Kessler technique, whereas in barbed repair the native strength of the suture material, rather than slippage, was the weak point. By increasing the suture diameter or by applying barbs to materials with higher tensile strength, an improvement in repair site breaking force could be gained.

Despite the encouraging results of this study, it is acknowledged that a number of possible limitations and difficulties may exist with respect to the clinical application of this new barbed tenorrhaphy. Firstly, as this new technique was not performed in situ, it has not been possible to assess the ease of suturing in a clinical setting under the constraints of limited exposure, tendon retraction and tension, especially in zone II. Secondly, it has not been possible to assess in vivo factors such as tendon ischemia and healing after repair, edema, and adhesion formation of this new repair. Another critical aspect is that to maintain the integrity of the barbs, no direct handling of the suture is to be performed with fingers or instruments, so if there is a technical error during repair, the suture has to be cut and removed completely, since it is impossible to back up the suture to rethrow a stitch without damaging the barbs. Finally, our biomechanical testing used a linear load to failure, which may not reflect the physiologic conditions as well as cyclic loading models.

In conclusion, this study confirms the promising results achieved in previous studies concerning the use of barbed suture in flexor tendon repair. In our animal model, tenorrhaphy with Quill™ SRS suture guarantees a breaking force of repair that exceeds the 40–50 N suggested as sufficient to initiate early active motion, and a smoother profile of the repair site. Further in vivo testing is warranted to evaluate the clinical applicability of this new barbed suture tenorrhaphy, especially in zone II tendon flexor laceration, where a more aggressive rehabilitation plan is desired to reduce tendon adhesions and improve the functional outcome.

Acknowledgments NP is supported by the European Research Council (ERC StG Ideas 2011 BIHSNAM n. 279985 on "Bio-Inspired hierarchical super-nanomaterials", ERC PoC 2013-1 REP-LICA2 n. 619448 on "Large-area replication of biological anti-adhesive nanosurfaces", ERC PoC 2013-2 KNOTOUGH n. 632277 on "Super-tough knotted fibres"), by the European Commission under the Graphene Flagship (WP10 "Nanocomposites", n. 604391) and by the Provincia Autonoma di Trento ("Graphene Nanocomposites", n. S116/2012-242637 and reg. delib. n. 2266).

Conflict of interest None.

Ethical standards No animal was purposely killed for this study. All pigs were animals for slaughter. The tendons were provided by an official veterinarian and harvested after animal death in the slaughterhouse. The slaughter conforms to the European Convention for the Protection of Animals for Slaughter. All applicable international, national and institutional guidelines for the care and use of animals were followed.

References

1. McKenzie AR (1967) An experimental multiple barbed suture for the long flexor tendons of the palm and fingers. Preliminary report. J Bone Jt Surg Br 49(3):440–447
2. McKenzie AR (1967) Function after reconstruction of severed long flexor tendons of the hand. A review of 297 tendons. J Bone Jt Surg Br 49(3):424–439
3. Havulinna J et al (2011) Comparison of modified Kessler tendon suture at different levels in the human flexor digitorumprofundus tendon and porcine flexors and porcine extensors: an experimental biomechanical study. J Hand Surg Eur Vol 36(8):670–676
4. Rashid R, Sartori M, White LE et al (2007) Breaking strength of barbed polypropylene sutures: rater-blinded, controlled comparison with nonbarbed sutures of various calibers. Arch Dermatol 143(7):869–872
5. Parikh PM, Davison SP, Higgins JP (2009) Barbed suture tenorrhaphy: an ex vivo biomechanical analysis. Plast Reconstr Surg 124:1551–1558
6. Trocchia AM, Aho HN, Sobol G (2009) A re-exploration of the use of barbed suture in flexor tendon repairs. Orthopedics 32:731–735
7. McClellan WT, Schessler MJ, Ruch DS et al (2011) A knotless flexor tendon repair technique using a bidirectional barbed suture: an ex vivo comparison of three methods. Plast Reconstr Surg 128(4):322e–327e
8. McDowell CL, Marqueen TJ, Yager D et al (2002) Characterization of the tensile properties and histologic/biochemical changes in normal chicken tendon at the site of suture insertion. J Hand Surg 27A:605–614
9. Hitchcock TF, Light TR, Bunch WH et al (1987) The effect of immediate constrained digital motion on the strength of flexor tendon repairs in chickens. J Hand Surg 12A:590–595
10. Wada A, Kubota H, Miyanishi K et al (2001) Comparison of postoperative early active mobilization and immobilization in vivo utilizing four-strand flexor tendon repair. J Hand Surg 26B:301–306
11. Amadio P, An KN, Ejeskar A et al (2005) IFSSH flexor tendon committee report. J Hand Surg (Br.) 30:100–116
12. Momose T, Amadio PC, Zhao C, Zobitz ME et al (2000) The effect of knot location, suture material and suture size on the gliding resistance of flexor tendons. J Biomed Mater Res 53:806–811
13. Zeplin PH, Henle M, Zahn RK et al (2012) Tensile strength of flexor tendon repair using barbed suture material in a dynamic ex vivo model. J Hand Microsurg 4(1):16–20

19

Intramedullary nailing versus proximal plating in the management of closed extra-articular proximal tibial fracture: a randomized controlled trial

Ramesh Chand Meena · Umesh Kumar Meena · Gopal Lal Gupta · Nitesh Gahlot · Sahil Gaba

Abstract

Background Extra-articular proximal tibial fractures account for 5–11 % of all tibial shaft fractures. In recent years, closed reduction and minimally invasive plating and multidirectional locked intramedullary nailing have both become widely used treatment modalities for proximal and distal tibial metaphyseal fractures. This study was performed to compare plating and nailing options in proximal tibia extra-articular fractures.

Materials and methods This randomized prospective clinical study was conducted on 58 skeletally mature patients with a closed extra-articular fracture of the proximal tibia treated with minimally invasive proximal tibial plating (PTP) or intramedullary nailing (IMN) by trained surgeons at a tertiary trauma center.

Results Postoperative hospital stay ($p = 0.035$), time to full weight-bearing, and union time ($p = 0.004$) were significantly less in the IMN group than in the PTP group, but there was no clear advantage of either technique in terms of operative time ($p = 0.082$), infection rate ($p = 0.738$), range of motion of the knee ($p = 0.462$), or degrees of malunion and nonunion.

Conclusion Both implants have shown promising results in extra-articular proximal tibial fractures, and provide rigid fixation that prevents secondary fracture collapse.

Level of evidence Level 2, randomized controlled trial.

Keywords Intramedullary nailing (IMN) · Proximal tibial plate (PTP) · Proximal tibial extra-articular fractures · Prospective trial

R. C. Meena · U. K. Meena (✉) · G. L. Gupta · S. Gaba
Department of Orthopaedics, SMS Medical College and
Hospital, Jaipur 302004, India
e-mail: drumesh_meena@yahoo.co.in

R. C. Meena
e-mail: rc.meena@yahoo.com

G. L. Gupta
e-mail: drglg4u@gmail.com

S. Gaba
e-mail: drsahilgaba@gmail.com

N. Gahlot
Department of Orthopaedics, Postgraduate Institute of Medical
Education and Research, Chandigarh, India
e-mail: doc.nitesh@gmail.com

Introduction

Extra-articular proximal tibial fractures account for 5–11 % of all tibial shaft fractures [1, 9] and often result from high-velocity trauma. They lead to complex tissue injuries involving bone and surrounding soft tissues [1]. Conservative management of these fractures has often resulted in malunion, nonunion, rotational deformity, or stiffness of adjacent joints [2–4], so there has been a shift towards operative management of these fractures in recent times. However, the optimal method of surgically treating these fractures remains debatable. Options include intramedullary implant, half-pin external fixation, hybrid or thin-wire external fixation, plate fixation, or a combination of these techniques [5, 17]. In recent years, closed reduction with minimally invasive plating and locked intramedullary nailing have both become widely used treatment modalities for proximal and distal tibial metaphyseal fractures [6–8], despite the absence of any conclusive proof of the superiority of one modality over the other.

Due to the paucity of the relevant literature and the lack of conclusive evidence to guide the selection of treatment options in such cases, we designed this randomized controlled study (RCT) in order to compare the plating and nailing options in proximal tibia extra-articular fractures. We intended to compare these options in terms of operative time, duration of hospital stay, period of non-weight-bearing, degree of reduction, union rate, malunion rate, infection rate, and rates of other possible complications which could possibly affect decision-making in relation to such fracture patterns.

Materials and methods

This randomized prospective clinical study was conducted on 58 patients with extra-articular fracture of the proximal tibia (OTA 41-A2/A3) treated with minimally invasive proximal tibial plating (PTP) or intramedullary nailing (IMN) by trained surgeons at a tertiary trauma care center in the Department of Orthopedics, SMS Medical College and Hospital, Jaipur, between January 2009 and December 2012. After excluding 14 patients who were lost to follow-up, a total of 44 patients were included in the final outcome analysis. Ethical committee approval was obtained, and patients were recruited once written informed consent had been provided.

Skeletally mature patients with closed proximal tibial metadiaphyseal fractures were included in this study. The proximal tibia was defined as the region extending from the articular surface up to 1.5 times the medial to lateral width of the articular surface [6]. Patients with metadiaphyseal tibial fractures with an intra-articular extension, tibial shaft fractures, open fractures, pathological fractures, and patients with multiple musculoskeletal injuries to the same or opposite lower limb were excluded from the study.

Patient allocation to groups was randomized by computer prospectively through the use of sequentially numbered opaque envelopes. Envelopes were opened inside the operating theater by a nurse who was blind to the allocation. Group A patients were treated with IMN and group B patients received PTP.

The intramedullary nailing performed in group A was done by creating an entry point just medial to the lateral intercondylar eminence of the tibial plateau through a medial parapatellar approach. Temporary blocking screws, a reduction clamp, a reduction unicortical plate, or a universal fixator was used to achieve reduction and removed after fracture fixation, except for the reduction unicortical plate when used with a reamed intramedullary tibial nail. The intramedullary nail used had a proximal Herzog band and four multilevel, multiplanar, and multidirectional screws (Expert Tibial Nail, Synthes, Zuchwil, Switzerland) (Fig. 1).

Patients in group B were treated by minimally invasive PTP using curvilinear incision over the lateral aspect of the proximal tibia. Indirect reduction was achieved using axial traction and/or the application of a reduction clamp or distractor. Internal fixation was then achieved with a proximal tibial lateral locking compression plate (LCP). A minimum of three screws were used on both sides of the fracture, and plating was done using a minimally invasive technique (Fig. 2).

Postoperatively, patients in both groups were given intravenous third-generation cephalosporin antibiotics for 3 days. Ankle pumps and isometric quadriceps strengthening exercises were started on the first postoperative day, followed by active and assisted knee bending on the second postoperative day. Partial weight-bearing was allowed from the second postoperative day, depending upon the stability of the construct, whereas full weight-bearing was allowed only after complete clinical and radiological union.

All patients were followed up at 2 and 6 weeks, 3 and 6 months, and 1 year postoperatively. Both the immediate postoperative and the final follow-up radiographs were compared to assess the accuracy of reduction and final alignment. Measurements were performed for coronal (varus and valgus) and sagittal (procurvatum and recurvatum) plane deformities using the measuring technique described by Freedman and Johnson [9]. In AP view, varus/valgus deformity was evaluated by measuring the angle between the lines drawn perpendicular to the proximal and distal tibial articular surfaces. In lateral view, the procurvatum/recurvatum was measured similarly and 8° of posterior slope was subtracted. Malreduction was defined as a deformity of >5° in any plane. Rotational alignment, shortening, and knee ROM were assessed clinically [9, 10]. The fracture was considered united if three or more cortices were continuous on two radiographic views. Nonunion was defined as three consecutive months of X-rays that did not show progressive healing.

All data were entered into a pro forma. The statistical analysis was performed by an independent statistician using the Statistical Package for the Social Sciences (SPSS version 22.0; SPSS, Chicago, IL, USA). The chosen level of significance was $p < 0.05$. The two groups were compared with respect to age, sex, operating time, hospital stay, infection rate, fracture union time, angulation of the fracture, and the knee range of motion. The parameters were compared between the groups. A paired-sample t test was used for the interval data (age, operating time, length of hospital stay, fracture union time, postoperative angulation, and range of motion of the knee).

Results

Out of a total of 58 patients, 14 (6 in the IMN group, 8 in the plating group) were excluded from the study as they were absent for follow-up, meaning that 44 patients were

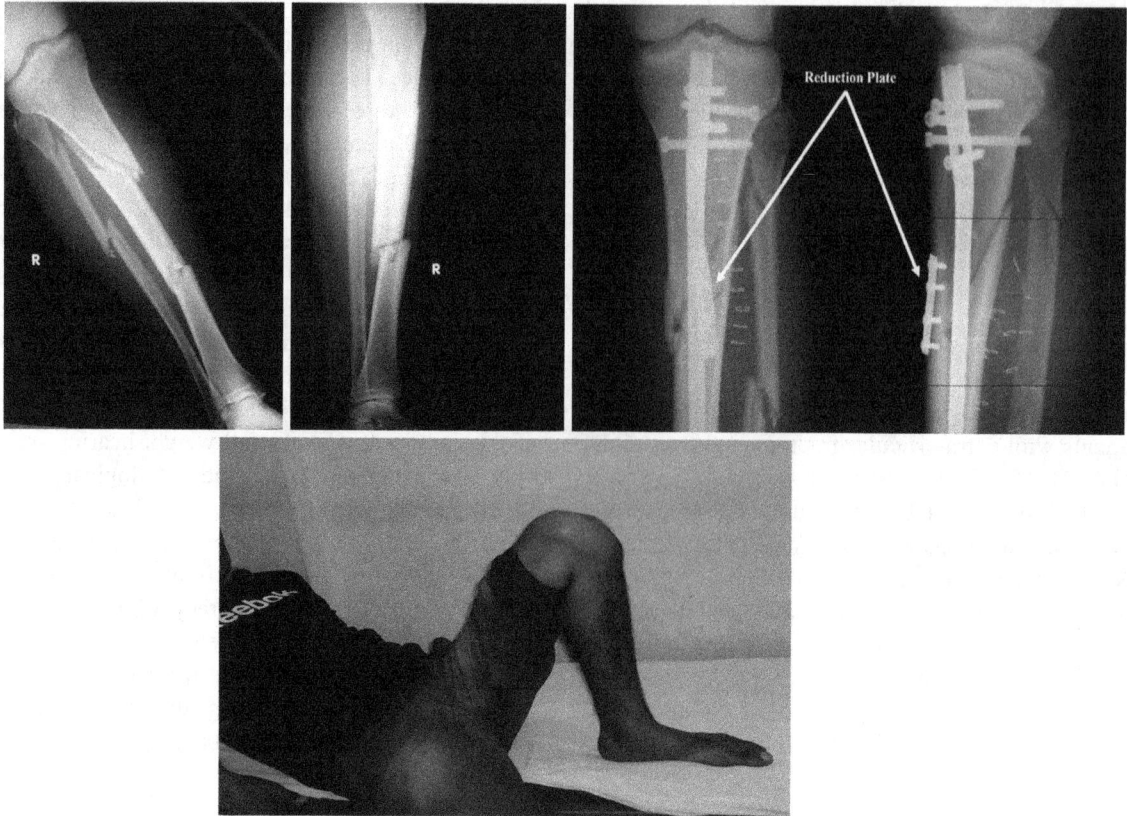

Fig. 1 Patient with a segmental tibial fracture treated with expert tibial nail, showing a good range of motion of the knee postoperatively

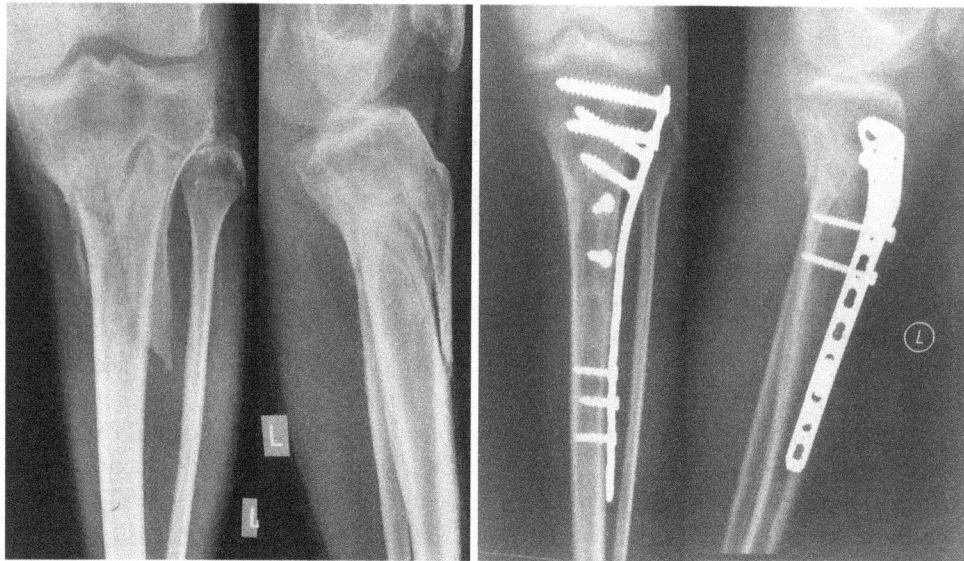

Fig. 2 Preoperative and postoperative radiographs of a patient treated with plating

included in the final outcome analysis. Preoperative characteristics including age, sex, classification, mode of injury, and time period from injury to operation were comparable in both groups (Table 1).

Postoperative hospital stay, time period to full weight-bearing, and union time were significantly less in the IMN group as compared to the PTP group (Table 1). Surgical site infections (SSIs) were seen in two patients in the PTP group, one of which was resolved with debridement while the other necessitated implant removal due to infection.

Delayed union occurred in two patients in the IMN group, for which dynamization was performed by

Table 1 Comparison of the demographic and postoperative data for both groups

	IMN group (group A)	PTP group (group B)	p value
Sex			
Male	14	18	0.961
Female	5	7	
Age	39 (18–65)	36 (19–62)	0.525
AO/OTA classification (OTA 41-A2/A3)	10/9	10/15	0.405
Operative time (h)	81.57 (60–110)	87.91 (60–120)	0.082
Hospital stay (days)	4.1 (2–8)	5.3 (3–10)	0.035
Union time (weeks) or time required before full weight-bearing (weeks)	18.26 (10–30)	22.84 (16–34)	0.004
Infection	0	2	0.738
Malalignment			
Coronal plane	2.77 (0–7)	2.08 (0–8)	0.296
Sagittal plane	2.57 (0–8)	2.19 (0–9)	0.415
Range of motion of knee	119.7 (90–150)	115.2 (80–150)	0.462
Delayed union/nonunion	2/1	0/1	0.849

removing the distal screw. One case in the nailing group presented nonunion, which ultimately required exchange nailing with bone grafting and fibular osteotomy. There was nonunion in one patient in the PTP group; bone grafting was done in that case, which eventually led to fracture healing.

The alignment of the tibia, as measured by an independent observer in the immediate postoperative and 1-year follow-up X-rays, did not show any significant difference between the groups, indicating that there was no secondary loss of reduction. The mean postoperative angulation in the coronal plane (varus/valgus) was 2.7° (range 0–7°, SD = 1.98) in the IMN group and 2.1° (range 0–8°, SD = 1.77) in the PTP group; both of these tended towards a varus inclination, but there was no statistically significant difference between the groups ($p = 0.296$). In the sagittal plane, the mean extent of postoperative procurvatum/recurvatum was 2.6° (range 0–8°, SD = 1.82) in the IMN group and 2.2° (range 0–9°, SD = 1.98) in the PTP group; both of these tended towards procurvatum, but there was no statistically significant difference between the groups ($p = 0.415$). >5° of malalignment was seen in four patients (21.1 %) in the IMN group (one patient had varus and three had anterior apex deformity) and in four patients (16 %) in the PTP group (two patients had varus and two patients had procurvatum). The average range of motion was 119.7° (range 90–150°, SD = 19.18) in group A and 115.2° (range 80–150°, SD = 17.28) in group B ($p = 0.462$). There were complaints of occasional anterior knee pain and discomfort upon kneeling on the floor from six patients (31.6 %) in group A and two patients (8.0 %) in group B ($p = 0.097$).

Discussion

Data allowing a comparison of tibial nail and minimally invasive plating for extra-articular proximal tibial fractures are scarce. The primary goal of this prospective study was to compare the results of tibial nailing and minimally invasive plating from various aspects.

In the present study, patients in the IMN group had a significantly shorter length of hospital stay compared with those in the PTP group ($p < 0.05$) because of the smaller incision made during closed nailing, meaning that IMN results in less of an economic burden and a lower cost of healthcare to society than PTP.

Although early weight-bearing is inherently associated with a load-sharing device such as an IMN, the literature does not accurately predict an accepted time at which full weight-bearing should be initiated with either procedure. Various studies have often stated that weight-bearing should be initiated when it can be tolerated by the patient [6]. In previous studies of extra-articular proximal tibial fractures treated with IMN, full weight-bearing was initiated at various times ranging from 0 to 16 weeks, depending on the fracture location, fracture pattern, and surgeon's preference [11, 19]. Similarly, in extra-articular proximal tibial fractures treated with PLP, time to full weight-bearing has ranged from 6 to 13 weeks for the same reasons [6, 8, 18]. In our study, the time required before full weight-bearing, which was done only after complete radiological union, was significantly less in the IMN group (18.26 weeks) as compared to the PTP group (22.84 weeks). Although these times are longer than those stated in previously published reports, we started full weight-bearing only after complete clinical and

Table 2 Comparison of data obtained in the present work with data presented in the literature

References	Infection		Union rate		Malunion	
	IMN group (%)	PTP group (%)	IMN group (%)	PTP group (%)	IMN group (%)	PTP group (%)
Bhandari et al. [17]	2.5	14	96.5	98	20	10
Lindvall et al. [6]	28	24	77	94	40.9	20.6
Beuhler et al. [12]	0		92.9		7.1	
Tornetta and Collons [15]	0		0		10	
Present study	5.3	8	94.7	96	21.1	16

radiological fracture union. That being said, we started passive and active assisted movements early—from day 2, progressing later to partial weight-bearing. Hence, we found no significant differences in range of motion of the knee between the groups.

Reported infection rates range from 0 to 8 % in nailing patients [5, 12, 17] and from 0 to 14 % in plating patients [17, 18, 20]. But, in the study by Lindvall et al. [6], the authors reported significantly higher infection rates: 28 % in the nailing group and 24 % in the plating group. The most probable reason for this is the higher proportion (42.8 %) of patients with open fractures in their study [6]. In the systemic review by Bhandari et al. [17], the infection rates were 2.5 % in the nailing group and 14 % in the plating group. The infection rates in our series were 5.3 % in the IMN group and 8 % in the PTP group ($p = 0.738$).

Malunion is a documented complication of the nailing of proximal tibia fractures and has been reported to occur in 3–100 % of cases in previous studies (Table 2) [9, 11, 17]. In our study, there was a malreduction/malunion rate of >5° in the IMN group (four patients, 21.1 %): varus malalignment in one patient and anterior apex deformity in three patients. Various techniques have been described for preventing malreduction, including the use of blocking screws [5, 6], unicortical plating [13], a universal distractor [14], nailing in the semiextended position [15], or the use of a nail with a more proximal Herzog bend [16]. In our study, we used blocking screws in three cases, reduction plating in one case, and a universal distractor in two cases. In the other cases, a reduction clamp was used to prevent proximal fragment extension while inserting the nail. A common technique employed in all of the nailing cases was to make a slightly higher entry point than that normally used for tibial nail insertion. This modification brought our insertion point more in line with the medullary canal of the tibia, hence reducing the extension of the proximal fragment. The plating group also had four cases of malunion (16 %), but the difference was not statistically significant. In a systemic review of 17 studies by Bhandari et al. [17], the authors reported a higher malunion rate in the nailing group (20 %) than in the plating group (10 %). Similarly,

Lindvall et al. [6] reported a higher malunion rate in the nailing group—apex anterior malreduction occurred in 36 % of the patients in the IMN group and 15 % of those in the locking plate group—although this difference was not statistically significant.

When union rates after the initial fixation were analyzed in our study, it was found that the union rate in the IMN group was 94.7 and that in the PTP group was 96 % ($p = 0.849$). The high union rates observed in our series are consistent with those stated in various published reports, which range from 91 to 100 % [6, 8, 11, 19]. Our results were, however, higher than seen in a study performed by Lindvell et al. [6], where the authors noted union rates of 77 % in the IMN group and 94 % in the PTP group. We believe that this difference in union rates arose because open fractures were excluded from our series, not because of the type of procedure performed. The locked nail technique demonstrated advantages in terms of the operation time, hospital stay, early full weight-bearing, and time required for bony union.

We concluded from our study that intramedullary nail is superior to minimally invasive plating in terms of brevity of hospital stay and speed of union along with early full weight-bearing, but there was no clear advantage of either technique in terms of operative time, infection rate, range of motion of the knee, and rates of malunion and nonunion. Both implants yielded promising results with extra-articular proximal tibial fractures and provided rigid fixation that prevented secondary fracture collapse.

Limitations of this study include the small number of patients, the involvement of multiple surgeons, the absence of long-term follow-up to evaluate the outcome of malalignment in terms of the development of osteoarthritis of the knee, and the use of both stainless steel and titanium implants, which may affect infection rates because titanium is more biocompatible than stainless steel, meaning that using titanium reduces the soft-tissue reaction and reduces the chance of infection.

Conflict of interest The authors declare that they have no conflict of interest related to the publication of this manuscript.

Ethical standards All of the patients provided informed consent prior to enrollment, ethical clearance was obtained from the institutional review board, and the study was performed in accordance with the ethical standards of the 1964 Declaration of Helsinki as revised in 2000.

References

1. Court-Brown CM, McBirnie J (1995) The epidemiology of tibial fractures. J Bone Jt Surg Br 77(3):417–421
2. DeCoster TA, Nepola JV, el-Khoury GY (1988) Cast brace treatment of proximal tibia fractures. A 10-year follow-up study. Clin Orthop Relat Res 231:196–204
3. Jensen DB, Rude C, Duus B, Bjerg-Nielsen A (1990) Tibial plateau fractures. A comparison of conservative and surgical treatment. J Bone Jt Surg Br 72(1):49–52
4. Milner SA, Davis TR, Muir KR, Greenwood DC, Doherty M (2002) Long-term outcome after tibial shaft fracture: is malunion important? J Bone Jt Surg Am 84-A(6):971–980
5. Nork SE, Barei DP, Schildhauer TA, Agel J, Holt SK, Schrick JL et al (2006) Intramedullary nailing of proximal quarter tibial fractures. J Orthop Trauma 20(8):523–528
6. Lindvall E, Sanders R, Dipasquale T, Herscovici D, Haidukewych G, Sagi C (2009) Intramedullary nailing versus percutaneous locked plating of extra-articular proximal tibial fractures: comparison of 56 cases. J Orthop Trauma 23:485–492
7. Hiesterman TG, Shafiq BX, Cole PA (2011) Intramedullary nailing of extra-articular proximal tibia fractures. J Am Acad Orthop Surg 19(11):690–700
8. Naik MA, Arora G, Tripathy SK, Sujir P, Rao SK (2013) Clinical and radiological outcome of percutaneous plating in extra-articular proximal tibia fractures: a prospective study. Injury 44(8):1081–1086
9. Freedman EL, Johnson EE (1995) Radiographic analysis of tibial fracture malalignment following intramedullary nailing. Clin Orthop Relat Res 315:25–33
10. Milner SA (1997) A more accurate method of measurement of angulation after fractures of the tibia. J Bone Jt Surg 79(6):972–974
11. Krettek C, Stephan C, Schandelmaier P et al (1999) The use of Poller screws as blocking screws in stabilizing tibial fractures treated with small diameter intramedullary nails. J Bone Jt Surg Br 81:963–968
12. Beuhler KC, Green J, Woll TS, Duwelius PJ (1997) A technique for intramedullary nailing of proximal third tibia fractures. J Orthop Trauma 11(3):218–223
13. Moed BR, Watson JT (1994) Intramedullary nailing of the tibia without a fracture table: the transfixation pin distractor technique. J Orthop Trauma 8(3):195–202
14. Archdeacon MT, Wyrick JD (2006) Reduction plating for provisional fracture fixation. J Orthop Trauma 20(3):206–211
15. Tornetta P, Collons E (1996) Semiextended position of intramedullary nailing of the proximal tibia. Clin Orthop Relat Res 328:185–189
16. Henley MB, Meier M, Tencer AF (1993) Influences of some design parameters on the biomechanics of the unreamed tibial intramedullary nail. J Orthop Trauma 7(4):311–319
17. Bhandari M, Audige L, Ellis T (2003) Operative treatment of extraarticular proximal tibial fractures. J Orthop Trauma 17(8):591–595
18. Cole PA, Zlowodzki M, Kregor PJ (2004) Treatment of proximal tibia fractures using the less invasive stabilization system: surgical experience and early clinical results in 77 fractures. J Orthop Trauma 18(8):528–535
19. Koval K, Clapper M, Brumback R et al (1991) Complications of reamed intramedullary nailing of the tibia. J Orthop Trauma 5(2):184–189
20. Schutz M, Kaab MJ, Haas N (2003) Stabilization of proximal tibia fractures with the LIS-System: early clinical experience in Berlin. Injury 34(Suppl 1):A30–A35
21. Uhthoff HK, Bardos DI, Liskova-Kiar M (1981) The advantages of titanium alloy over stainless steel plates for the internal fixation of fractures: an experimental study in dogs. J Bone Jt Surg Br 63-B(3):427–484

20

The effect of tranexamic acid on artificial joint materials: a biomechanical study (the bioTRANX study)

Sattar Alshryda · James M. Mason ·
Praveen Sarda · T. Lou · Martin Stanley ·
Junjie Wu · Anthony Unsworth

Abstract

Background Tranexamic acid (TXA) has been success-fully used to reduce bleeding in joint replacement. Recently local TXA has been advocated to reduce blood loss in total knee or hip replacement; however, this raised concerns about potential adverse effects of TXA upon the artificial joint replacement.

Materials and methods In this biomechanical study we compared the effects of TXA and saline upon the following biomechanical properties of artificial joint materials—(1) tensile properties (ultimate strength, stiffness and Young's modulus), (2) the wear rate using a multi-directional pin-on-plate machine, and (3) the surface topography of pins and plates before and after wear rate testing.

Results There were no significant differences in tensile strength, wear rates or surface topography of either ultra-high-molecular-weight polyethylene pins or cobalt chromium molybdenum metal plates between specimens soaked in TXA and specimens soaked in saline.

Conclusion Biomechanical testing shows that there are no biomechanical adverse affects on the properties of common artificial joint materials from using topical TXA.

Level of evidence V

Keywords Topical · Local · Tranexamic acid · Arthroplasty · Joint replacement · Blood loss · Blood transfusion · Wear rate · Surface topography · Biomechanical profile

S. Alshryda (✉) · T. Lou
Departments of Trauma and Orthopaedics, Central Manchester University Hospitals, Oxford Road,
Manchester M13 9WL, Lancashire, UK
e-mail: Sattar26@doctors.org.uk

T. Lou
e-mail: nurn1981@yahoo.co.uk

J. M. Mason
School of Medicine and Health, Wolfson Research Centre,
Queen Campus, Durham University,
Stockton on Tees TS17 6BH, UK
e-mail: j.m.mason@durham.ac.uk

P. Sarda
Departments of Trauma and Orthopaedics, Medway Maritime Hospital, Windmill Road, Gillingham, Kent ME7 5NY, UK
e-mail: praveensarda2003@yahoo.com

M. Stanley · J. Wu · A. Unsworth
Centre for Biomedical Engineering School of Engineering and Computing Sciences, Durham University, Durham DH1 3LE,
UK
e-mail: m.j.stanley@leeds.ac.uk

J. Wu
e-mail: junjie.wu@durham.ac.uk

A. Unsworth
e-mail: tony.unsworth@durham.ac.uk

Introduction

A major cause of artificial joint failure is the loosening that occurs as a consequence of wear and tear of the bearing surfaces. Even a well performing prosthetic joint releases billions of microscopic wear particles (debris) into the joint space. When an excessive amount of debris is generated it may stimulate a severe body reaction in the capsular tissues and bone leading to inflammation and osteolysis. The resulting loss of supporting bone may lead to loosening of the implants requiring difficult revision surgery.

Most artificial joints consist of two metal surfaces, commonly made of cobalt chromium molybdenum (Co–Cr–Mo) alloy and an insert, commonly made of ultra-high-molecular-weight polyethylene (UHMWPE). The mechanical properties of these two materials are influenced by several chemical and physical factors. Oxidation breaks down the molecular chains in UHMWPE resulting in increased brittleness and reduced resistance to crack propagation. Historically, there have been unfortunate consequences within artificial joints when unexpected and unwanted chemical or physical reactions led to severe wear and joint failure. One example arose from the storage of artificial implants in air-filled packets after sterilisation using gamma radiation. This mode of storage led to gradual oxidation of the UHMWPE and deterioration of its mechanical properties. This was partly overcome by storage within a vacuum-sealed packet. Another example was post-irradiation thermal treatment to reduce free radicals in the polyethylene. This could cause a partial reduction in crystallinity of the material that, in turn, reduced the resistance to crack propagation [1].

Intravenous tranexamic acid (TXA) has been shown to reduce blood loss and transfusion in joint replacement [2–16]; however, fear of systemic side-effects precludes its wide use in orthopaedic practice. Locally administered TXA has been advocated as a better alternative due its easier preparation and administration, higher concentration at the bleeding site and less systemic side-effects [17–21]. There is a legitimate concern that TXA might adversely affect the biomechanical properties of artificial implants, especially the wear rate which might lead to subsequent loosening and failure. A rigorous search of the published literature, contact with manufacturers and contact with the community publishing on the use of TXA uncovered no research to address this issue. Consequently, this is the first study to investigate the effect of local TXA upon artificial joint biomechanical properties and performance. The research is named the bioTRANX study.

Materials and methods

In this biomechanical study we investigated the effects of TXA on the following biomechanical properties of artificial joint materials as surrogates for long-term effects:

1. Tensile properties of the UHMWPE (ultimate strength, stiffness and Young's modulus).
2. The wear rate using a multi-directional pin-on-plate machine. Pins were made of UHMWPE and plates were made of Co–Cr–Mo.
3. The surface topography of pins and plates before and after wear rate testing:

   (a) Peak-valley ratio (PV): the distance between the highest peak and the deepest valley over the entire evaluation length (Fig. 1).
   (b) Root mean square roughness (rms): the standard deviation of the surface roughness measurements relative to mean plane of all the data.
   (c) Arithmetic mean roughness (R_a): the average roughness or deviation of all points from a plane (centre line) fitted to the test surface (Fig. 2).

All tested materials are made from identical materials used in the DePuy artificial knee joint replacement (P.F.C.® Sigma® Revision Knee System).

Tensile testing was conducted by gripping the ends of a standardised test specimen made of UHMWPE in a tensile testing machine (Fig. 3) and then applying a gradually increasing axial load until failure occurred. Several calculations to describe the biomechanical properties of the material were obtained. Stress is the force applied per unit cross-sectional area (N/m^2). Strain is the change in length divided by the original length. The stress obtained at the highest applied force is the ultimate tensile strength. The stiffness is the resistance of material to deformation while

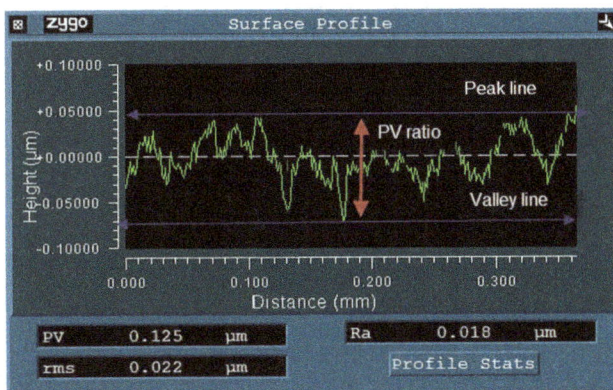

Fig. 1 Peak-valley ratio (PV): the distance between the highest peak and the deepest valley over the entire evaluation length

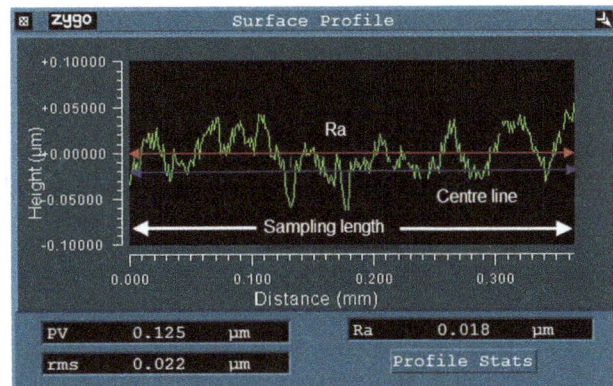

Fig. 2 Surface roughness average (R_a): the arithmetic mean roughness of all points from a plane (*centre line*) fitted to the test surface

Fig. 3 Tensile testing machine with a mounted specimen made of UHMWPE

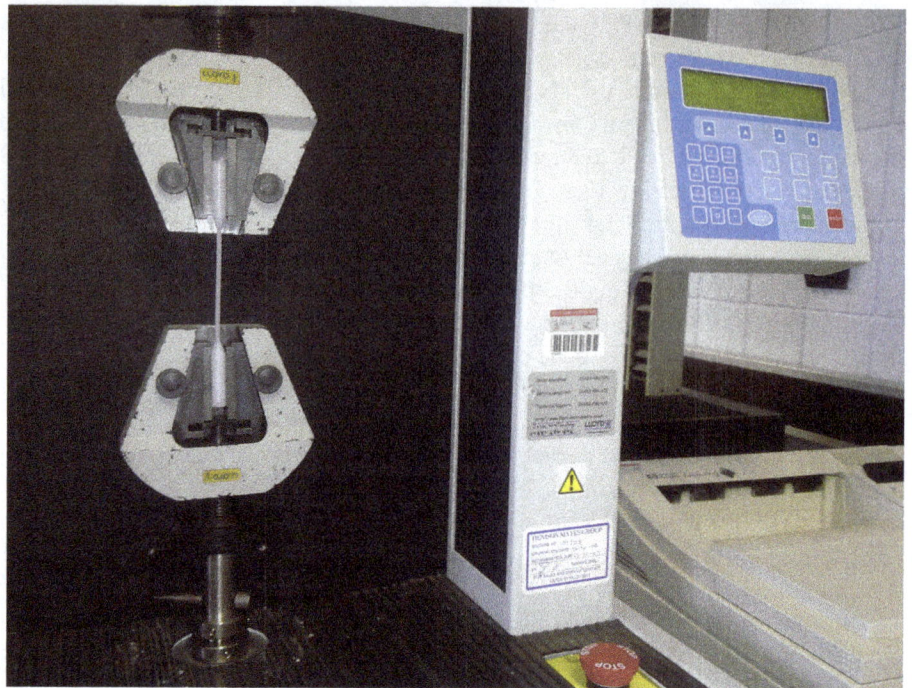

Young's modulus is found by dividing the stress by the strain over the linear portion of stress strain curve [22].

Fifteen dumbbell-shaped tensile specimens were made of UHMWPE—five were soaked in TXA solution (1 g/50 ml saline) for 48 h, five were soaked in 50 ml of saline and the other five were used to standardise the tensile testing machine. The duration of soaking of the tested material was based on the pharmacokinetics properties of TXA in the human body. TXA half-life time is 3.5 h and the human body needs 24 h to clear 90 % of administered TXA.

Wear rate testing was performed to assess the influence of TXA under accelerated body wear conditions. This test was performed using a multidirectional pin-on-plate machine (Fig. 4). It is a four-station machine applying both reciprocational and rotational motion. The reciprocation was applied by a sledge moving forward and backward over a 4 cm range at 60 cycles/min. The heated bed, lubricant tray, level sensor and plate holders were positioned on this sledge.

The plates were made of Co–Cr–Mo. Four plates were fitted to the tray and secured with three metal plates and screws. They were covered with lubricant and heated to 37° C (body temperature). The pins were made of UHMWPE. Each pin was numbered, notched and tightly fitted to the pin holders at the end of each motor. The rotational frequency was also set at 60 cycles/min (1 Hz).

The lubricant used in all tests was a 24.5 % concentration of bovine serum (protein content 15 g/l) and was prepared following a standardised protocol.

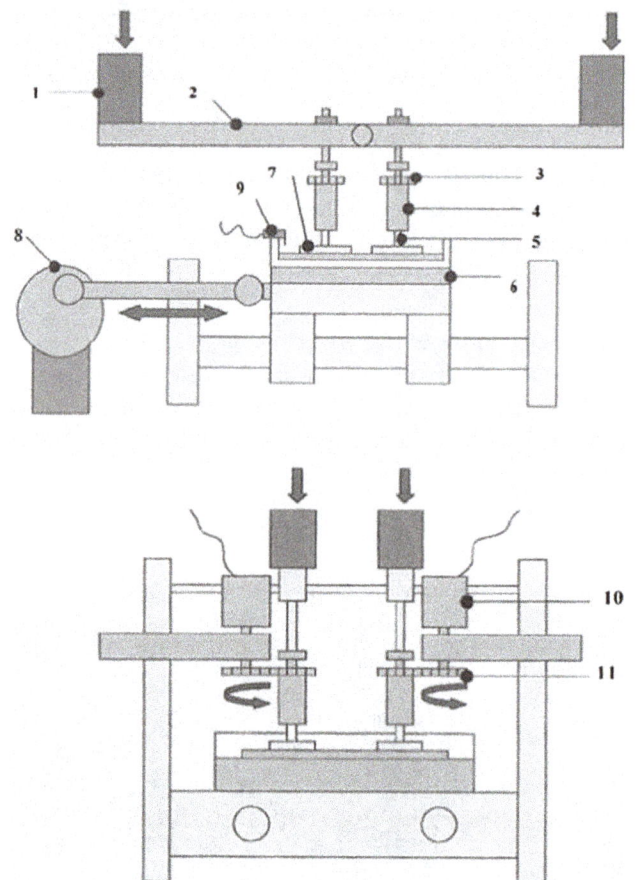

Fig. 4 Schematic diagram of the pin-on-plate machine. *1* weight to provide load, *2* lever arm, *3* gear, *4* pin holder, *5* UHMWPE pin, *6* heater bed, *7* Co–Cr–Mo plate, *8* motor to provide reciprocation, *9* level sensor, *10* motor, *11* gear. Reproduced with permission of SAGE Publications Ltd, London, UK

Fig. 5 Profilemeter view of surface topography of a Co–Cr–Mo plate

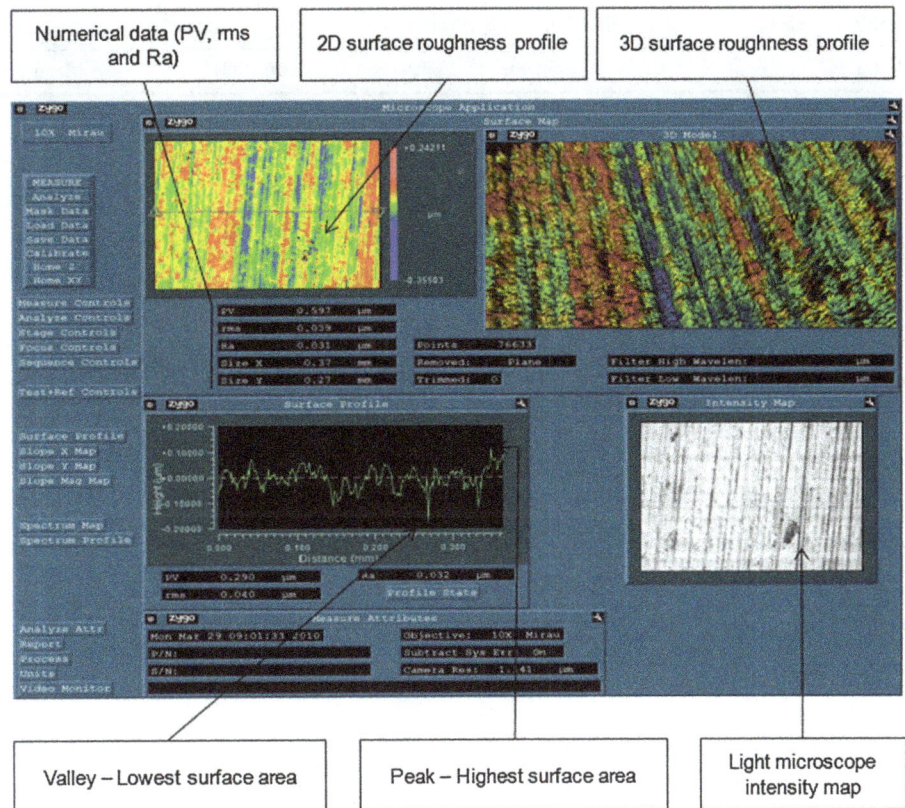

Numerical data (PV, rms and Ra)

2D surface roughness profile

3D surface roughness profile

Valley – Lowest surface area

Peak – Highest surface area

Light microscope intensity map

A lubricant level sensor was attached to the lubricant tray to allow the lubricant to be maintained at an almost constant level. Any lubricant loss was assumed to be evaporation of water so this was topped up from a reservoir of distilled water. The rotational motion was provided by four small motors. The four loaded pins were held in stainless steel holders and mounted so that each pin rested on the corresponding plate. A load of 40 N was applied to each station via a static mass and lever arm mechanism.

The wear was assessed gravimetrically (loss of weight) and volumetric loss was calculated by dividing the mass by the density. Twice a week (approximately every 0.25 million cycles), the machine was stopped to allow for gravimetric assessment and machine maintenance. The pins and plates were cleaned, dried and weighed following a standardised protocol.

Control specimens were used to take account of the absorption of lubricants by both the pins and plates during the test. The wear volumes were plotted against the sliding distance and the gradient of the line provided the wear rate. Wear rate was divided by the load to determine the wear factor, k (mm^3/Nm).

Surface topography measurements were performed using a Zygo NewView 100 non-contacting three-dimensional (3-D) profilemeter. Ten measurements were taken of the pins and plates before and after wear testing. Each measurement provided visual and numerical data of the surface profile of the specimens (Fig. 5). Visual data includes intensity map, 2- and 3-D profiles of surface roughness. This provided a quick scan of a wider area of the specimens to get an overall impression of the roughness of the surfaces. Numerical data included PV, rms and R_a.

Results

The tensile test showed that the stiffness, Young's modulus, load to fracture and stress at fracture values were not affected by immersion in TXA or saline for 48 h.

The two groups were comparable in term of stiffness, Young's modulus of elasticity, load at break and stress at break (Table 1). There were no statistically significant differences between saline- and TXA-immersed UHMWPE.

The stiffness, Young's modulus, load to fracture and stress at fracture of the soaked specimens (TXA and saline) were comparable to those of control specimens (non-soaked specimen) (ANOVA; $P = 0.79$, 0.79, 0.67 and 0.67, respectively).

The stress strain curves of the ten tensile specimens are shown in Fig. 6. The graph shows all specimens have an almost identical stress strain curve apart from control specimen number five which failed at a lower stress. However, this did not adversely affect the overall findings.

Table 1 Tensile test results of the UHMWPE specimens

Variable	Specimens	N	Mean (SD)	Mean difference	P value (95 % CI)
Stiffness (N/m)	Saline	5	81,588 (10,518)	1,964	0.740 (−15,146 to 11,218)
	TXA	5	83,552 (7,262)		
Young's modulus (MPa)	Saline	5	923 (119)	23	0.740 (−171 to 127)
	TXA	5	946 (82)		
Load at break (N)	Saline	5	330 (33)	12	0.523 (17 to −52)
	TXA	5	342 (20)		
Stress at break (MPa)	Saline	5	47 (5)	1	0.526 (2 to −7)
	TXA	5	48 (3)		

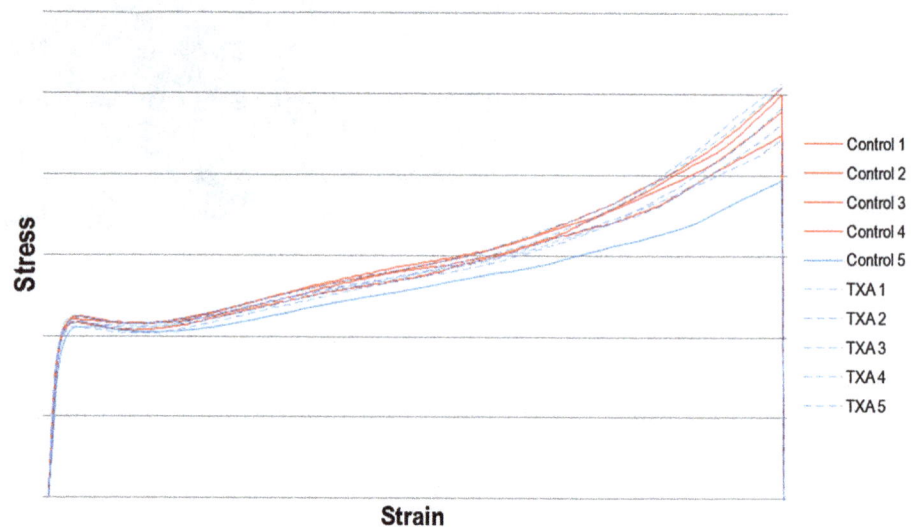

Fig. 6 Stress strain curves of tensile. Control specimen number 5 which failed at a lower stress is represented with a *blue solid line* (colour figure online)

It is not unusual to have a faulty specimen with a small scratch or defect that affects its tensile properties.

The wear test involved two multidirectional pin-on-plate machines each with four test stations, four control pins and four control plates which were soaked with saline, and four TXA-soaked pins and four-TXA soaked plates. Another two pins and two plates were used as controls to measure the weight changes caused by lubricant absorption. This was deducted from the test specimens at every gravimetric assessment.

Table 2 and Fig. 7 show the cumulative volume changes in the pins and plates in each group (placebo or TXA) as measured each time the machines were stopped. As expected, the main weight loss occurred in the UHMWPE pins rather than the Co–Cr–Mo plates as they are softer and prone to wear more rapidly than plates. Wear factors were calculated for all pins and plates using the following equation:

$$\text{Wear factor} = \text{Volume loss (mm}^3) / [\text{sliding distance (m)} \times \text{load (N)}]$$

There were no statistically significant differences between the mean wear factor when comparing either plates or pins which were soaked in saline or TXA as shown in Table 3.

The surface topography testing revealed no significant difference in the PV, rms and R_a of the plates and pins between the two groups before and after the pin-on-plate wear tests (see Table 4). Hence, the null hypothesis of no difference was supported.

Discussion

It may take many years to determine the effectiveness of new and innovative designs of artificial joint replacements since many journals refuse to publish new implants series or interventions with <10 years follow-up. Surgeons are cautious about introducing a new intervention without it being carefully studied and assessed. The history of artificial joint replacement supports this caution.

Table 2 Cumulative volume loss in mm³ in plates and pins

Distance (km)		Plates				Pins			
Test 1	Test 2	TXA test 1 plate	TXA test 2 plate	Placebo test 1 plate	Placebo test 2 plate	TXA test 1 pin	TXA test 2 pin	Placebo test 1 pin	Placebo test 2 pin
0	0	0.00000	0.00000	0.00000	0.00000	0.00000	0.00000	0.00000	0.00000
4	14.2	−0.12659	0.02191	−0.00913	0.13309	−0.14354	−0.87560	−0.46651	−0.71412
12.4	24.2	−0.19679	−0.00406	−0.00162	0.11503	−0.44677	−1.89833	−0.93122	−1.67405
30.5	34.8	−0.19517	−0.07608	−0.00446	0.16575	−1.05862	−2.73446	−1.13756	−2.70755
38.9	47.4	−0.18441	−0.07993	0.00426	0.15276	−1.84989	−3.74284	−1.90192	−3.99762
49.6	60.7	−0.18949	−0.04098	0.01603	0.14566	−2.76676	−5.03112	−3.31760	−4.91449
60.8	73.7	−0.19922	−0.01440	0.00751	0.13511	−3.86485	−6.43065	−4.53590	−6.34094
73.1	88.5	−0.19598	−0.01481	0.01298	0.14262	−5.21055	−8.03652	−5.83495	−7.95219
84.6	109.5	−0.22113	−0.02090	−0.01116	0.09170	−6.11306	−9.82719	−7.16450	−9.54908
100.9	130.6	−0.20308	−0.01075	−0.00122	0.14992	−7.75661	−10.77636	−8.57839	−10.65973
121.9	162.6	−0.21119	0.05336	0.00467	0.14161	−8.64477	−12.32661	−9.52037	−12.13821
149.2		−0.20308		0.00426		−10.81583		−11.57660	

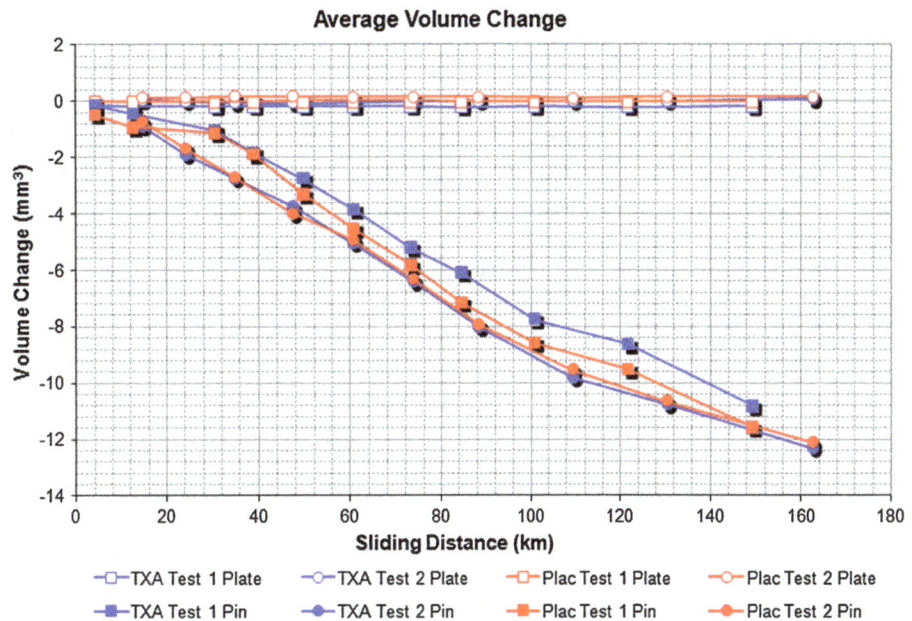

Fig. 7 Graph of volume losses of the pins and plates plotted against sliding distance

There has been a recent increase in the use of TXA to reduce bleeding and blood transfusion after joint replacement and, more recently, topical application has been advocated without proper safety profile assessment. In this study we investigated the effects of TXA on three important material properties. Tensile testing and surface topography were studied using gold standard methods. This showed there was no difference in the tensile properties and surface topography between the artificial implants that had been soaked in saline and those soaked with TXA.

There are several methods to assess the rate of wear. Clinical and radiological survival analysis of implanted joints is probably the most useful method; however, it takes an extremely long time as some implants can last >30 years. Furthermore, patients are often lost to follow-up during such a long period. Joint simulation is a reliable predictor but it is expensive with limited access. Multidirectional pin-on-plate machines are a reasonable alternative and several studies have confirmed that they are comparable to joint simulators [23–26].

Comparing results from eight stations, there was no significant difference in the wear factor between the two groups and findings were comparable with the wear factors reported in other studies [23, 27].

Table 3 The wear factors of plates and pins; parametric t test

	Groups	N	Mean[a]	SD[a]	Mean difference[a]	P value (95 % CI)
Plates wear factor	Placebo	4	0.00100	0.013515	0.0035	0.768 (−0.161 to 0.023)
	TXA	4	−0.00250	0.008583		
Pins wear factor	Placebo	4	2.15925	0.240433	0.046	0.677 (−0.319 to 0.411)
	TXA	4	2.11325	0.177184		

[a] $\times 10^{-9}$ mm^3/Nm

Table 4 Post wear surface topography findings

	Group	N	Mean	SD	Mean difference	P value (95 % CI)
Plates (PV)	Placebo	3	0.279	0.228	−0.0340	0.856 (−0.5 to 0.4)
	TXA	4	0.313	0.240		
Plates (rms)	Placebo	3	0.021	0.0075	−0.0115	0.141 (−0.0284 to 0.0054)
	TXA	4	0.0325	0.0092		
Plates (R_a)	Placebo	3	0.019	0.002	−0.007	0.187 (−0.02 to 0.005)
	TXA	4	0.026	0.007		
Pins (PV)	Placebo	4	3.504	1.780	−1.959	0.195 (−5.24 to 1.32)
	TXA	4	5.463	2.010		
Pins (rms)	Placebo	4	0.3167	0.199	−0.0715	0.612 (−0.542 to 0.3531)
	TXA	4	0.3882	0.2216		
Pins (R_a)	Placebo	4	0.247	0.119	0.043	0.616 (−0.16 to 0.24)
	TXA	4	0.203	0.113		

PV Peak-valley ratio (μm), *rms* root mean square roughness (μm), R_a surface roughness average (μm)

Authors acknowledge the fact that biomechanical studies do not always correlate well with the clinical outcomes; however, biomechanical tests are widely accepted as the best available predictors and surrogates for future outcomes. Public expectation is that materials used for health reasons need to be tested mechanically or in animal studies before human use. With increasing medical litigation against health care providers, waiting for clinical outcome studies which may take years may not be the option. This study supports the localised usage of TXA around artificial joints used in humans, while accepting the limitations of a laboratory-based study. Separately, members of the team are investigating the 5-year clinical and radiological outcomes of the first 157 patient who underwent total knee replacement using topical TXA in our centre and this will be reported separately.

In summary, laboratory biomechanical testing shows that there are no biomechanical adverse affects on common artificial joint materials exposed to topical TXA. Nonetheless, surgeons using topical TXA are strongly recommended to be vigilant and encouraged to report unexpected premature joint failures associated with topical use of TXA. The National Joint Registry should collect and analyse data on the use of topical TXA, to help inform on-going research into the safety profile of topical TXA in joint replacement.

Acknowledgments The research team would like to thank Dr Roy Harvey and Mr Pete Copley from DePuy International Ltd, Leeds, UK for their support in providing the tested specimens.

Conflict of interest The bioTRANX study was conducted in the Bioengineering Laboratory of the School of Engineering and Computing Sciences, Durham University, Durham, UK between October 2009 and April 2010. All testing materials were provided free of charge by DePuy International Ltd; however, they did not play any role in the investigation.

References

1. Fischgrund J (2009) Orthopaedic Knowledge Update, 9th edn. The American Academy of Orthopaedic Surgeons, Rosemont, p 840
2. Camarasa MA et al (2006) Efficacy of aminocaproic, tranexamic acids in the control of bleeding during total knee replacement: a randomized clinical trial. Br J Anaesth 96(5):576–582
3. Jansen AJ et al (1999) Use of tranexamic acid for an effective blood conservation strategy after total knee arthroplasty. Br J Anaesth 83(4):596–601
4. Sorin A et al (1999) Reduction of blood loss by tranexamic acid in total knee replacement. J Bone Joint Surg 81-B(Suppl.II):234–234
5. Veien M et al (2002) Tranexamic acid given intraoperatively reduces blood loss after total knee replacement: a randomized, controlled study. Acta Anaesthesiol Scand 46(10):1206–1211
6. Zhang F, Gao Z, Yu J (2007) Clinical comparative studies on effect of tranexamic acid on blood loss associated with total knee arthroplasty. Zhongguo Xiu Fu Chong Jian Wai Ke Za Zhi 21(12):1302–1304

7. Benoni G et al (1995) Does tranexamic acid reduce blood loss in knee arthroplasty? Am J Knee Surg 8(3):88–92

8. Benoni G, Fredin H (1996) Fibrinolytic inhibition with tranexamic acid reduces blood loss and blood transfusion after knee arthroplasty: a prospective, randomised, double-blind study of 86 patients. J Bone Joint Surg Br 78(3):434–440

9. Benoni G et al (2001) Blood conservation with tranexamic acid in total hip arthroplasty: a randomized, double-blind study in 40 primary operations. Acta Orthop Scand 72(5):442–448

10. Benoni G, Lethagen S, Fredin H (1997) The effect of tranexamic acid on local and plasma fibrinolysis during total knee arthroplasty. Thromb Res 85(3):195–206

11. Benoni G et al (2000) Tranexamic acid, given at the end of the operation, does not reduce postoperative blood loss in hip arthroplasty. Acta Orthop Scand 71(3):250–254

12. Molloy DO et al (2007) Comparison of topical fibrin spray and tranexamic acid on blood loss after total knee replacement: a prospective, randomised controlled trial. J Bone Joint Surg Br 89(3):306–309

13. Orpen NM et al (2006) Tranexamic acid reduces early post-operative blood loss after total knee arthroplasty: a prospective randomised controlled trial of 29 patients. Knee 13(2):106–110

14. Lozano M et al (2008) Effectiveness and safety of tranexamic acid administration during total knee arthroplasty. Vox Sang 95(1):39–44

15. Alshryda S et al (2011) Tranexamic acid in total knee replacement: a systematic review and meta-analysis. J Bone Joint Surg Br 93(12):1577–1585

16. Sukeik M et al (2011) Systematic review and meta-analysis of the use of tranexamic acid in total hip replacement. J Bone Joint Surg Br 93(1):39–46

17. Wong J et al (2010) Topical application of tranexamic acid reduces postoperative blood loss in total knee arthroplasty: a randomized, controlled trial. J Bone Joint Surg Am 92(15):2503–2513

18. Ishida K et al (2011) Intra-articular injection of tranexamic acid reduces not only blood loss but also knee joint swelling after total knee arthroplasty. Int Orthop 35(11):1639–1645

19. Alshryda S et al (2013) Topical (intra-articular) tranexamic acid reduces blood loss and transfusion rates following total hip replacement: a randomized controlled trial (TRANX-H). J Bone Joint Surg Am 95(21):1969–1974

20. Alshryda S et al (2013) Topical (intra-articular) tranexamic acid reduces blood loss and transfusion rates following total knee replacement: a randomized controlled trial (TRANX-K). J Bone Joint Surg Am 95(21):1961–1968

21. Panteli M et al (2013) Topical tranexamic acid in total knee replacement: a systematic review and meta-analysis. Knee 20(5):300–309

22. Ramachandran M (2007) Basic orthopaedic sciences. The Stanmore guide. Hodder Arnold, UK, p 304

23. Saikko V (1998) A multidirectional motion pin-on-disk wear test method for prosthetic joint materials. J Biomed Mater Res 41(1):58–64

24. Joyce TJ et al (2000) A multi-directional wear screening device and preliminary results of UHMWPE articulating against stainless steel. Biomed Mater Eng 10(3–4):241–249

25. Scholes SC, Unsworth A (2007) The wear properties of CFR-PEEK-OPTIMA articulating against ceramic assessed on a multidirectional pin-on-plate machine. Proc Inst Mech Eng H 221(3):281–289

26. Scholes SC, Unsworth A (2001) Pin-on-plate studies on the effect of rotation on the wear of metal-on-metal samples. J Mater Sci Mater Med 12(4):299–303

27. McKellop H et al (1978) Wear characteristics of UHMW polyethylene: a method for accurately measuring extremely low wear rates. J Biomed Mater Res 12(6):895–927

21

Patellar mobility can be reproducibly measured using ultrasound

**Takashi Kanamoto · Yoshinari Tanaka · Yasukazu Yonetani ·
Keisuke Kita · Hiroshi Amano · Masashi Kusano ·
Mie Fukamatsu · Shinji Hirabayashi · Shuji Horibe**

Abstract The present study was performed to examine
the reliability of ultrasound in evaluating patellar mobility
in the superior–inferior direction. Twelve healthy men
volunteered for the study. Patellar mobility in the superior–
inferior direction during isometric knee extension contraction with the knee immobilized in a semi-flexed knee
brace was measured using ultrasound. Both intra-observer
and inter-observer reliability were assessed by intra-class
correlation coefficients (ICCs). Bland–Altman analysis was
used for assessing agreement between measurements. ICC
values were excellent for both intra-observer and inter-
observer reliability at 0.97 and 0.93, respectively. In 95 %
of measurements, the same observer measured within
−0.55 to 0.61 mm, while different observers measured
within −0.82 to 0.85 mm. In conclusion, patellar mobility
in the superior–inferior direction during an isometric knee
extension exercise can be reproducibly measured using
ultrasound.
The level of evidence VI (basic study of a novel evaluation method).

Keywords Patellar mobility · Ultrasound ·
Rehabilitation · Isometric knee extension exercise ·
Reliability

Introduction

To prevent postoperative complications, it is important to
regain normal patellar mobility after knee surgeries such as
anterior cruciate ligament reconstruction and total knee
arthroplasty. Patellar immobility leads to decreased range
of motion, quadriceps inhibition, altered gait pattern, and
prolonged rehabilitation [1]. Thus, multidirectional mobilization of the patella and quadriceps muscle setting exercises are initiated in the early postoperative period to
improve patellar mobility and quadriceps function. Despite
the importance of this being generally accepted, a single
gold standard evaluation method of patellar mobility has
not been established [2–4].

With the recent development of high-resolution probes,
the use of musculoskeletal ultrasound has significantly
increased [5]. The superficial localization of the knee
extensor apparatus, including the patella and patellar tendon,
makes it suitable for ultrasound evaluation [6, 7]. The purpose of this report was to determine if ultrasonography can be
useful in evaluating patellar mobility in the superior–inferior
direction during an isometric knee extension exercise.

Materials and methods

Participants

Twelve healthy men with no signs of musculoskeletal
injury or disorder that would prevent their participation

T. Kanamoto (✉) · S. Hirabayashi
Department of Rehabilitation, Osaka Rosai Hospital,
1179-3 Nagasone-cho, Kita-ku, Sakai, Osaka 597-8025, Japan
e-mail: takanamoto2@gmail.com

Y. Tanaka · Y. Yonetani · K. Kita · H. Amano · M. Kusano ·
S. Horibe
Department of Orthopaedic Surgery, Osaka Rosai Hospital,
1179-3 Nagasone-cho, Kita-ku, Sakai, Osaka 597-8025, Japan

M. Fukamatsu
Department of Clinical Laboratory, Osaka Rosai Hospital,
1179-3 Nagasone-cho, Kita-ku, Sakai, Osaka 597-8025, Japan

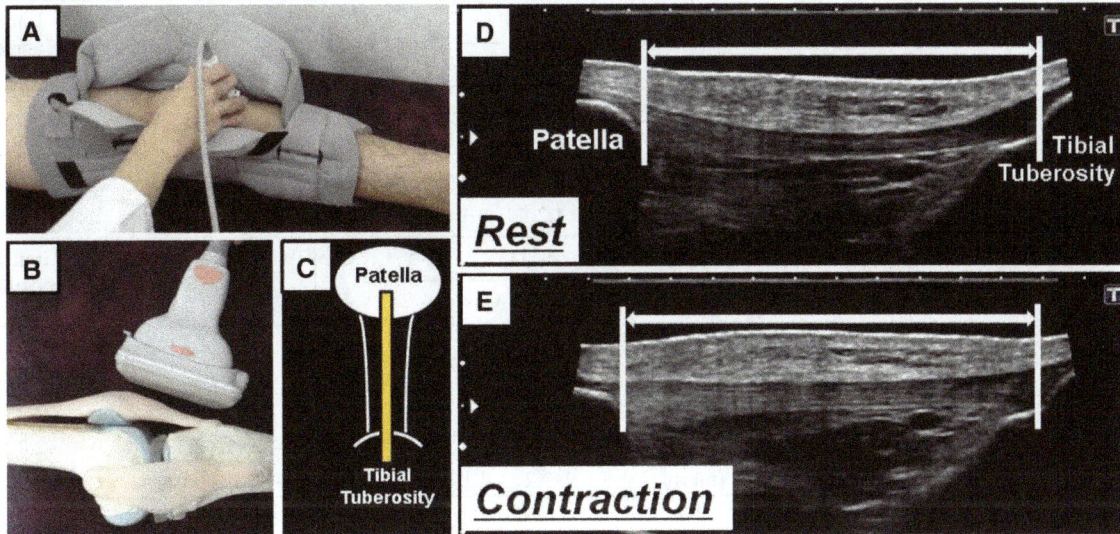

Fig. 1 Ultrasound examination of the patellar mobility in the superior–inferior direction during isometric knee extension exercise. **a** The participants were evaluated in a supine position with the knee immobilized with a semi-flexed brace. **b** An ultrasound probe was fitted onto the skin overlying the patellar tendon in the sagittal plane using water bag kit. **c** The probe was positioned so that the caudal pole of the patella and the tibia tuberosity were visible within the viewing field. **d**, **e** Ultrasound images of the patella, patellar tendon, and tibial tuberosity at rest and during isometric knee extension contraction. The patellar mobility in the superior–inferior direction was measured as the change in distance between manually marked points of the deep insertion to the caudal pole of the patella and tibia tuberosity

volunteered for the study. Mean (±SD) age, height, and weight were 31.2 ± 6.9 years, 175 ± 3.7 cm, and 67.8 ± 8.6 kg, respectively. Ultrasound examinations were performed by an orthopedic surgeon and an ultrasonographer experienced in musculoskeletal ultrasound measurements.

Procedure

Participants performed three trials of maximal knee extension contractions in the supine position with the knee immobilized by a semi-flexed knee brace (Fig. 1a). An 8.0 MHz, 58-mm ultrasound probe (Aplio^{TM} 300, Toshiba, Tokyo, Japan) was fitted onto the skin overlying the patellar tendon in the sagittal plane using a water bag kit (UAWB-022A, Toshiba). The probe was positioned so that the inferior pole of the patella and the tibial tuberosity were within the viewing field during isometric knee extension contraction (Fig. 1b–e).

All trials were performed on two different days and analyzed independently by two observers. Using recorded ultrasound images, the observer manually marked the points of the inferior pole of the patella and the tibial tuberosity frame by frame. The patellar mobility in the superior–inferior direction was defined as the change in distance between the two points during isometric knee extension contraction.

Statistical analysis

Continuous variables are expressed as mean ± SD. Both intra-observer and inter-observer reliability were assessed using intra-class correlation coefficients (ICC). Bland–Altman analysis was used to assess agreement between measurements. All statistical analyses were performed using SPSS (SPSS Inc., Chicago, IL, USA).

Results

The intra-observer reproducibility for patellar mobility was excellent, with an ICC (1, 3) of 0.97. In Bland–Altman plots, the mean difference between paired measurements by two observers was 0.03 mm. The corresponding 95 % limits of agreement were −0.55 to 0.61 mm (Table 1).

The inter-observer reproducibility for patellar mobility was also excellent, with an ICC (2, 3) of 0.93. In Bland–Altman plots, the mean difference between paired measurements by two observers was 0.02 mm. The corresponding 95 % limits of agreement were −0.82 to 0.85 mm (Table 1).

Discussion

The principal findings of the present study were that patellar mobility in the superior–inferior direction during

Table 1 .

Intra-observer	Mean ± SD		ICC (95 % CI)	Mean difference	Limits of agreement
	Day 1	Day 2			
Patella–tuberosity distance (mm)					
Rest	44.2 ± 5.3	44.4 ± 5.2	0.99 (0.96–1.00)	−0.22	−1.88 to 1.43
Contraction	47.3 ± 5.4	47.5 ± 4.7	0.98 (0.94–1.00)	−0.2	−2.1 to 1.8
Patellar mobility (mm)	3.1 ± 1.2	3.1 ± 1.2	0.97 (0.91–0.99)	0.03	−0.55 to 0.61

Interobserver	Mean ± SD		ICC (95 % CI)	Mean difference	Limits of agreement
	Observer 1	Observer 2			
Patella–tuberosity distance (mm)					
Rest	44.2 ± 5.3	44.0 ± 5.2	0.98 (0.93–0.99)	0.2	−2.2 to 2.5
Contraction	47.3 ± 5.4	47.1 ± 5.4	0.98 (0.94–0.99)	0.2	−2.0 to 2.3
Patellar mobility (mm)	3.1 ± 1.2	3.1 ± 0.9	0.93 (0.77–0.98)	0.02	−0.82 to 0.85

an isometric knee extension exercise could be reproducibly measured using ultrasound. ICC values were excellent for both intra-observer and inter-observer reliability at 0.97 and 0.93, respectively. In 95 % of measurements, the same observer measured within −0.55 to 0.61 mm, while different observers measured within −0.82 to 0.85 mm.

Ultrasound evaluation of the patellar tendon has been used extensively in recent years. There are several publications describing the ultrasound appearance of patellar tendinopathy and ultrasound measurements of mechanical properties of the patellar tendon [6, 7]. However, to our knowledge, this is the first report showing the utility of ultrasound in evaluating patellar mobility during a knee rehabilitation exercise.

Measurement of patellar tendon length with ultrasound using adjustable surface markers and calipers is highly accurate and has good inter-observer reliability [8]. Hansen et al. [6] performed patellar tendon measurements, keeping 90° of flexion with a custom made rigid cast to position an ultrasound probe, and showed high accuracy and reproducibility using measurements from two trials after discarding trials with the smallest and largest measurements. In a recent report, Schulze et al. [9] concluded that 5–6 trials are required for reliably measuring tendon elongation. In the present study, simple tools available in the clinical setting were used to perform the measurements, and an average of three trials showed sufficient reliability for clinical application.

Although abnormal patellar mobility potentially contributes to several knee disorders, such as anterior knee pain, patellofemoral pain, and arthrofibrosis, there is no strong evidence to support its importance, partially due to the lack of a standard measurement method [1, 3, 4, 10]. Considering the patient tolerability, low cost, and lower time commitment of our simple method, clinicians can easily evaluate patellar mobility before and after treatment. In addition to the conventional assessment of quadriceps

muscle strength, this method will help establish appropriate and effective treatment strategies [1]. Furthermore, objective evaluation of patellar mobility in the clinical context has the potential to provide clues to underlying causes of knee disorders as well as monitor treatment effects.

Limitations of the current study include the small sample size and the fact that the general condition of participants was not assessed. Although ICCs of intra-observer and inter-observer reproducibility were high, further study is required to clarify the utility of the present method for a large cohort. Another limitation is that we did not include measures of quadriceps muscle force. In the future, it would also be interesting to test the relationship between muscle force and patellar mobility.

In conclusion, patellar mobility in the superior–inferior direction during an isometric knee extension exercise can be reproducibly measured using ultrasound. Clinical application should provide useful information for treatment evaluation and planning in rehabilitation therapy.

Conflict of interest None.

Ethical standards We followed the Helsinki Declaration, and all experiments in this study were conducted in accordance with a protocol approved by the Ethical Committee of our hospital. Written informed consent was obtained from all participants.

References

1. van Grinsven S, van Cingel RE, Holla CJ, van Loon CJ (2010) Evidence-based rehabilitation following anterior cruciate ligament reconstruction. Knee Surg Sports Traumatol Arthrosc 18:1128–1144

2. Joshi RP, Heatley FW (2000) Measurement of coronal plane patellar mobility in normal subjects. Knee Surg Sports Traumatol Arthrosc 8:40–45

3. Ota S, Nakashima T, Morisaka A, Ida K, Kawamura M (2008) Comparison of patellar mobility in female adults with and without patellofemoral pain. J Orthop Sports Phys Ther 38:396–402

4. Sweitzer BA, Cook C, Steadman JR, Hawkins RJ, Wyland DJ (2010) The inter-rater reliability and diagnostic accuracy of patellar mobility tests in patients with anterior knee pain. Phys Sportsmed 38:90–96

5. Fullerton BD (2008) High-resolution ultrasound and magnetic resonance imaging to document tissue repair after prolotherapy: a report of 3 cases. Arch Phys Med Rehabil 89:377–385

6. Hansen P, Bojsen-Moller J, Aagaard P, Kjaer M, Magnusson SP (2006) Mechanical properties of the human patellar tendon in vivo. Clin Biomech (Bristol, Avon) 21:54–58

7. Hoksrud A, Ohberg L, Alfredson H, Bahr R (2008) Color Doppler ultrasound findings in patellar tendinopathy (jumper's knee). Am J Sports Med 36:1813–1820

8. Gellhorn AC, Morgenroth DC, Goldstein B (2012) A novel sonographic method of measuring patellar tendon length. Ultrasound Med Biol 38:719–726

9. Schulze F, Mersmann F, Bohm S, Arampatzis A (2012) A wide number of trials is required to achieve acceptable reliability for measurement patellar tendon elongation in vivo. Gait Posture 35:334–338

10. Millett PJ, Wickiewicz TL, Warren RF (2001) Motion loss after ligament injuries to the knee. Part II: prevention and treatment. Am J Sports Med 29:822–828

22

Avulsion of both posterior meniscal roots associated with acute rupture of the anterior cruciate ligament

Pier Paolo Mariani · Germano Iannella ·
Guglielmo Cerullo · Marco Giacobbe

Abstract A rare case of acute avulsion of both posterior meniscal roots concomitant with an acute anterior cruciate ligament (ACL) tear in a professional soccer player is described. While avulsion of the lateral meniscal root has been extensively reported in association with ACL injuries, medial root avulsion has never been reported in association with acute ACL. A review of the video documentation of the match accident revealed the exact mechanism of injury was a forceful external rotation of the standing limb.

Keywords Meniscus · Meniscal root · ACL · Knee

Introduction

Root tears are a subset of meniscal injuries, which have become increasingly recognized as a cause of pain and impaired mobility. The root serves as the anchor point for the menisci. Occurring on either the medial or lateral meniscus, root tears refer to a radial tear or avulsion at the posterior horn attachment to the bone. Both radial tear and posterior horn avulsion defunction the menisci as load-bearing structures, with increasing local contact pressure and premature onset of knee arthritis [9]. Because the medial and lateral menisci differ in anatomy and biomechanics, the pathogenesis of posterior root avulsions is also different. Tearing of the lateral posterior meniscal root is

P. P. Mariani (✉)
Università Roma 4-Foro Italico, Piazza L. de Bosis 5,
00136 Rome, Italy
e-mail: ppmariani@virgilio.it; ppmariani@iusm.it

G. Iannella · G. Cerullo · M. Giacobbe
Clinic "Villa Stuart", via Trionfale 5952, 00136 Rome, Italy

traumatic and always associated with anterior cruciate ligament (ACL) injury [1, 22], while the medial posterior root [2, 8, 10, 19] is prone to chronic degenerative meniscal disease.

To date, only one case [15] has been reported of radial tear of both roots detected two years after an ACL injury. The authors hypothesised a traumatic origin for avulsion of the lateral meniscus and a degenerative origin for the medial meniscus.

Here, we describe a rare case of avulsion of both posterior roots in association with an acute ACL tear in a professional soccer player. A review of the video documentation of the match accident revealed the exact mechanism of injury.

Case report

A 20-year-old professional soccer player reported sustaining a forceful rotatory left knee injury during an official match of the Italian Second Division. The dynamics of the accident could be clearly followed on the video recording of the match. While the player was standing with one foot fixed on the field and the contralateral limb elevated for shooting the ball, a player from the opponent team collided into the elevated limb, causing a forceful external rotation of the standing limb.

At presentation two days after the injury, physical examination revealed signs of acute anterior laxity and pain was elicited over both lateral and medial joint lines. Full flexion was painful and restricted by knee swelling. Manual knee laxity tests, including the Lachman test, anterior drawer test and pivot shift test, were positive, as was the McMurray test. Measurement using a KT-2000 arthrometer (MEDmetric Corporation, San Diego, CA, USA) demonstrated a 5-mm

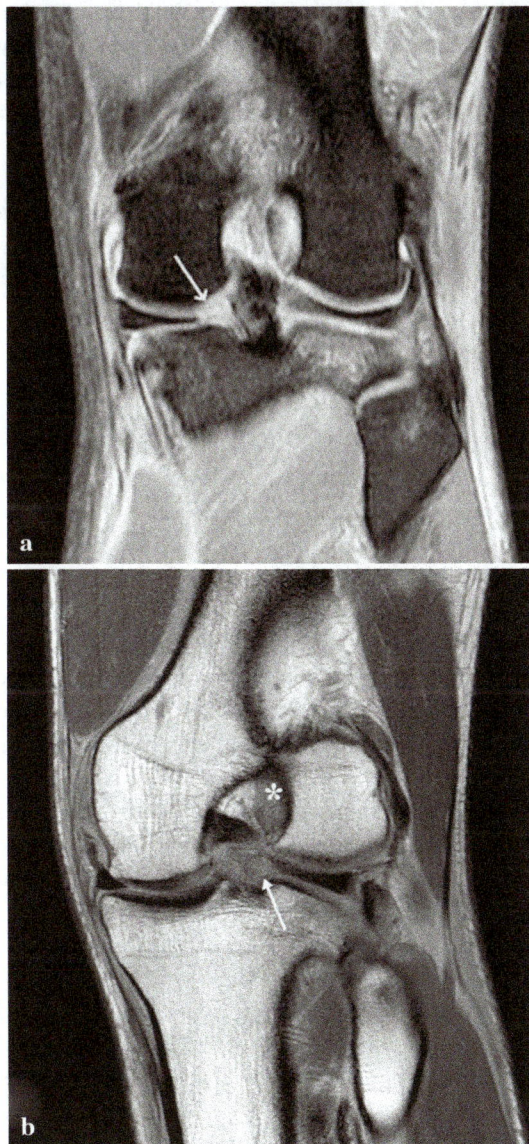

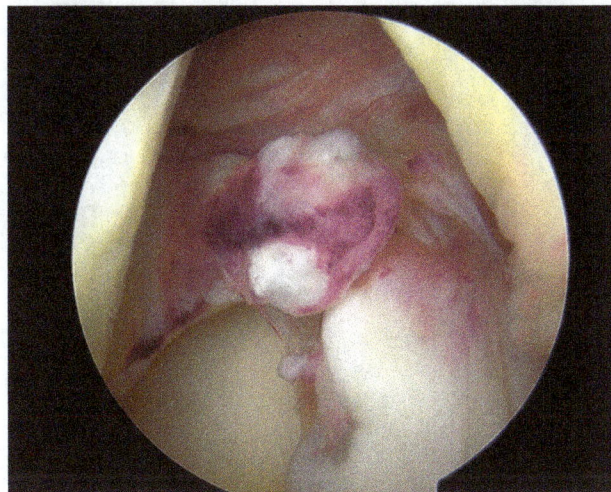

Fig. 2 Arthroscopic view of acute medial posterior root avulsion

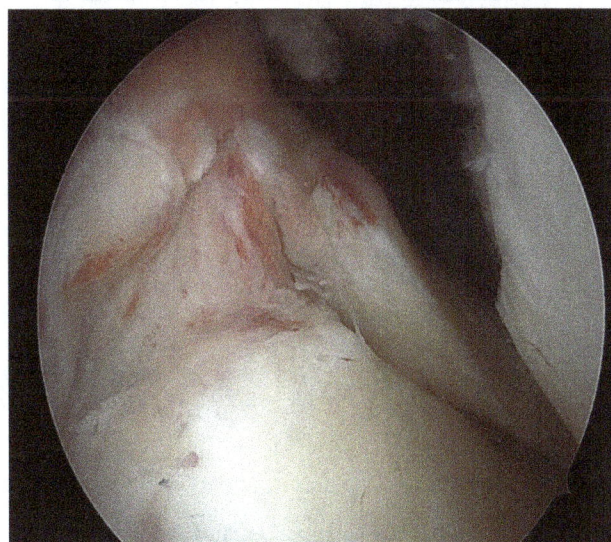

Fig. 1 a Preoperative coronal TSE-fat saturated MR image shows the ACL tear and an area of heterogeneous intrameniscal signal intensity of both meniscal roots with a void at the posterior attachment site of both menisci (*arrow*). b Preoperative coronal oblique 30° MR image. The *arrow* shows absence of tibial insertion of posterior lateral root. The *asterisk* shows hyperintensity signal at femoral ACL insertion

Fig. 3 Arthroscopic view of acute lateral posterior root avulsion

side-to-side difference. Preoperative radiographic evaluation was normal. Magnetic resonance imaging (MRI) disclosed acute rupture of the ACL and tears in the roots of the posterior horns of both lateral and medial menisci (Fig. 1). Arthroscopic evaluation under regional anesthesia revealed an acute tear of the ACL at its midsubstance. Avulsion of the posterior root of the lateral meniscus was present in addition to acute avulsion at the posterior root of the medial meniscus with posterior displacement (Figs. 2, 3). No other intraarticular lesions were detected.

Treatment consisted of arthroscopic pullout suturing of both menisci and ACL reconstruction with an autologous

bone-patellar tendon-bone graft. A transeptal approach was used for the medial meniscus root suture. The flat tip of an ACL guide (Arthrex, Naples, FL, USA) was introduced through the anterolateral portal at the footprint of the posterior root of the previously abraded medial meniscus. A tibial tunnel was made using a 2.9-mm guide pin from the anterolateral cortex of the proximal tibia to the footprint of the posterior root of the medial meniscus. Two nonabsorbable sutures were placed at the posterior root using a crescent-shaped suture hook. Both sutures ends were pulled out through the anterolateral cortex of the proximal tibia. The lateral meniscus was sutured in the same manner. The suture material for the lateral meniscus was pulled through the anteromedial cortex of the proximal tibia. The lateral and medial sutures were tied over two buttons after confirming sufficient reduction and tension.

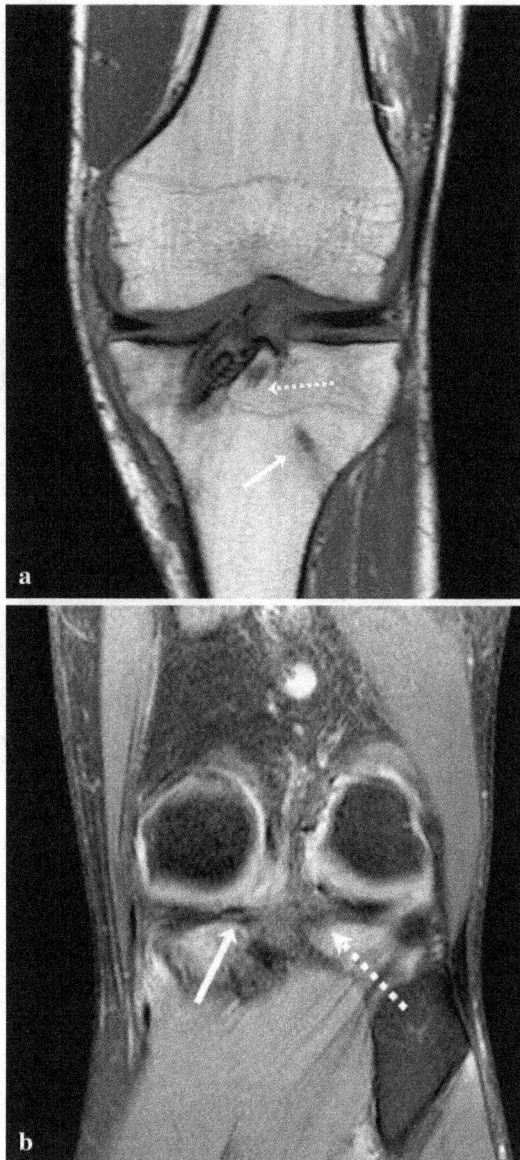

Fig. 4 At MRI follow-up at three months, the coronal T1-TSE view (**a**) shows the tibial tunnel for ACL reconstruction and the tunnels for the medial root (*white arrow*) and for the lateral root (*dashed arrow*). **b** The coronal TSE-fat saturated MR image shows both medial and lateral roots healed

Postoperatively, the knee was kept in full extension in a brace locked at 0° for four weeks. Passive motion was allowed after the first two weeks and active motion was restricted to 90° during the first four weeks. Partial weight bearing was permitted at four weeks postoperatively, followed by full weight bearing at six weeks. After six weeks closed-chain strengthening was begun, and full flexion exercises were allowed. During the second and the third month, strengthening exercises and hydrokinetic therapy were implemented. Running on a treadmill was started after two months and training on the field was permitted after four months. Six months postoperatively, the patient was able to return to play in an official match with full range of knee motion. At the last follow-up of one year, no meniscal signs and symptoms were present. Manual knee laxity tests, including the Lachman test, anterior drawer test and pivot shift test, were negative. The side-to-side difference was 0.4 mm, as measured by the KT-2000 manual maximal test. The postoperative MRI showed a good healing process of both roots (Fig. 4).

Discussion

The unusual finding in this case was avulsion of both posterior meniscal roots with a concomitant acute ACL tear. Medial posterior root avulsion usually results from chronic degenerative meniscal tears [2, 8, 10, 19] and is seldom associated with posterior cruciate ligament tears [14]. According to the radiological literature, the incidence of meniscal root tear is 8–9.8 % [3, 6, 20], whereas the orthopaedic literature reports a wider range between 6.7 % and 12.4 % [1, 9, 10]. This discrepancy stems from difficulties in radiographic diagnosis and in defining meniscal root tear. Two subcategories of meniscal root tear can be distinguished: root avulsion from the tibial plateau and meniscal posterior horn tear within 1 cm from the root. These tears are biomechanically similar because they can disrupt the circumferential fibers of the meniscus resulting in failure of the hoop strain mechanism [9, 11, 12]. Following rupture, the ability to resist extrusion under axial loading is definitely lost [4, 13].

In the only case described to date of a radial tear in both roots [15] concurrent with a chronic ACL tear, Lee et al. [15] postulated that the mechanism of injury was involvement of the posterior lateral root together with an ACL injury. The medial radial tear in the posterior root was caused by forceful mechanical stress secondary to instability. In the present case, avulsion of both meniscal roots was associated with an acute ACL tear. From a review of the video recording, the mechanism of injury was seen to be clearly due to forceful rotatory stress. As postulated by Park et al. [20], anterior tibial translation in an ACL injury may pull the lateral meniscus forward, stripping the meniscofemoral ligament away the meniscus attachment. The mechanism of medial meniscus root injury is more difficult to explain. Due to external rotation, for stress associated with compression axial load, the posterior horn is impinged by the femoral condyle. Markolf et al. [16] have shown that the anterior tibial force and the external tibial torque during knee loading produce relatively high posterior horn attachment forces, presumably by impinging the medial femoral condyle against the posterior meniscal rim.

In our patient, both meniscal roots were refixed with a transtibial technique. The sequelae of a medial root avulsion left in situ or misdiagnosed is functionally equivalent to total meniscectomy with meniscal extrusion and rapid progression to knee arthritis [17, 18]; however, there is no consensus on the treatment of lateral meniscal root tear. The fewer lateral meniscal tears in chronic versus acute ACL tears have led to conservative treatment of such lesions [5]. There are several reasons justifying this approach: concomitant ACL reconstruction creates blood clots and joint stability, increased blood supply to the posterior horn in comparison to the lateral meniscal pars intermedia, and absence of definitive clinical complaints when a lateral meniscus tear is left in situ. So, a radial or complex (radial and longitudinal) tear that occurs within 1 cm of the meniscal attachment may be more likely to heal spontaneously [7, 22]. Spontaneous healing after avulsion of the lateral root is less probable. The lateral meniscal root has two distinct insertions: one is anterior and attached to the posterior aspect of the tibial intercondylar eminence, and the other is posterior to and confluent with the meniscofemoral ligament. When root avulsion occurs, the latter insertion probably inhibits spontaneous healing because of continuous traction by the meniscofemoral ligament during knee movements. Recently, Schillamer et al. [21] demonstrated that posterior horn avulsion of the lateral meniscus causes peak tibiofemoral contact pressure to increase from 2.8 to 4.2 MPa, but that the peak pressure returns to normal after repair to bone via a transtibial tunnel.

In this rare case of tears in the roots of the posterior horns of both menisci, concomitant with an acute ACL tear, radiological and clinical outcome after surgery confirmed good healing. Both the lateral posterior horn and the medial posterior horn need to be considered when planning ACL reconstruction.

Conflict of interest None.

Ethical standards The patient provided his consent to the publication of this case report.

References

1. Ahn JH, Lee YS, Chang JY, Chang MJ, Eun SS, Kim SM (2009) Arthroscopic all inside repair of the lateral meniscus tear. Knee 16:77–80
2. Bin SI, Kim JM, Shin SJ (2004) Radial tears of the posterior horn of the medial meniscus. Arthroscopy 20:373–378
3. Brody JM, Lin HM, Hulstyn MJ, Tung GA (2006) Lateral meniscus root tear and meniscus extrusion with anterior cruciate ligament tear. Radiology 239:805–810
4. Choi C-J, Choi Y-J, Lee J-J, Choi C-H (2010) Magnetic resonance imaging evidence of meniscal extrusion in medial meniscus posterior root tear. Arthroscopy 26:1602–1606
5. Cipolla M, Scala A, Giannì E, Puddu G (1995) Different patterns of meniscal tears in acute anterior cruciate ligament (ACL) ruptures and in chronic ACL-deficient knees. Classification, staging and timing of treatment. Knee Surg Sports Traumatol Arthosc 3:130–134
6. De Smet AA, Blankenbaker DG, Kijowski R, Graf BK, Shinki K (2008) MR diagnosis of posterior root tears of the lateral meniscus using arthroscopy as the reference standard. Am J Radiol 192:480–486
7. Fitzgibbons RE, Shelbourne KD (1995) "Aggressive" nontreatment of lateral meniscal tears seen during anterior cruciate ligament reconstruction. Am J Sports Med 28:156–159
8. Habata T, Uematsu K, Hattori K, Takakura Y (2004) Clinical features of the posterior horn tear in the medial meniscus. Arch Orthop Trauma Surg 124:642–645
9. Han SB, Shetty GM, Lee DH, Chae DJ et al (2010) Unfavorable results of partial meniscectomy for complete posterior medial meniscus root tear with early osteoarthritis: a 5 to 8 year follow-up study. Arthroscopy 26:1326–1332
10. Hwang BY, Kim SL, Lee SW, Lee HE, Lee CK, Hunter DJ, Jung KA (2012) Risk factors for medial meniscus posterior root tear. Am J Sports Med. doi:10.1177/0363546512447792
11. Johannsen AM, Civitarese DM, Padalecki JR, Goldsmith MT, Wijdicks CA, LaPrade RF (2012) Qualitative and quantitative anatomic analysis of the posterior root attachments of the medial and lateral menisci. Am J Sports Med 40:2342–2347
12. Johnson DL, Swenson TM, Livesay GA, Fu FH, Harner CD (1995) Insertion-site anatomy of the human menisci: gross, arthroscopic, and topographical anatomy as a basis for meniscal transplantation. Arthroscopy 11:495–498
13. Jones RS, Keane GC, Learmonth DJ (1996) Direct measurement of hoop strains in the intact and torn human medial meniscus. Clin Biomech 11:295–300
14. Kim YJ, Kim JG, Chang SH, Shim JC, Kim JC, Lee MY (2010) Posterior root tear of the medial meniscus in multiple knee ligament injuries. Knee 17:324–328
15. Lee JH, Hwang BY, Lim YJ, Kim KH, Song JH (2009) Radial tears in the roots of the posterior horns of both the medial and lateral menisci combined with anterior cruciate ligament tear: a case report. Knee Surg Sport Traumatol Arthosc 17:1340–1343
16. Markolf KL, Jackson SR, McAllister DR (2012) Force measurements in the medial meniscus posterior horn attachment: effects on anterior cruciate removal. Am J Sports Med 40:332–338
17. Marzo JM, Gruske-De Perio J (2009) Effects of medial meniscus posterior avulsion and repair on tibiofemoral contact area and peak contact pressure with clinical implications. Am J Sports Med 37:124–129
18. Neogi DS, Kumar A, Rijal L, Yadav CS, Jaiman A, Nag HL (2013) Role of nonoperative treatment in managing degenerative tears of the medial meniscus posterior root. J Orthop Traumatol 14(3):193–199
19. Ozkoc G, Circi E, Gonc U, Irgit K, Pourbagher A, Tandogan R (2008) Radial tears in the root of the posterior horn of the medial meniscus. Knee Surg Sports Traumatol Arthosc 16:849–854
20. Park LS, Jacobson JA, Jamadar DA, Caoili E, Kalume M, Wojtys E (2007) Posterior horn lateral meniscus tear simulating meniscofemoral ligament attachment in the setting of ACL tear: MRI findings. Skelet Radiol 36:399–403
21. Schillamer CK, Werner FW, Scuderi MG, Cannizzaro JP (2012) Repair of lateral meniscus posterior horn detachment lesion. A biomechanical evaluation. Am J Sports Med 40:2604–2609
22. Shelbourne KD, Heinrich J (2004) The long term evaluation of lateral meniscus tears left in situ at the time of anterior cruciate ligament reconstruction. Arthroscopy 20:346–351

23

Asymptomatic peripheral vascular disease in total knee arthroplasty: preoperative prevalence and risk factors

Ill Ho Park · Su Chan Lee · Il Seok Park ·
Chang Hyun Nam · Hye Sun Ahn · Ha Young Park ·
Viralkumar Harilal Gondalia · Kwang Am Jung

Abstract

Background Although vascular disease is commonly accepted as a risk factor for wound complications and prosthetic joint infections, little is known about the preoperative prevalence of lower-extremity peripheral vascular disease in patients undergoing total knee arthroplasty (TKA). In this study, we investigated the prevalence of asymptomatic vascular disease and its risk factors.

Materials and methods A total of 1,000 knees of 692 patients who underwent primary TKA due to osteoarthritis were preoperatively evaluated by experienced musculoskeletal radiologists using Doppler ultrasonography of the lower extremity vessels. The mean age of the patients was 74.1 years (range 65–81). Risk factors for development of peripheral vascular disease were investigated.

Results Abnormal findings were identified in 38 knees of 32 patients (4.6 %); atherosclerotic changes in 31 knees of 25 patients (3.6 %), deep vein thrombosis (DVT) in two knees, and anomalous vessels in five knees. Three out of 31 knees with atherosclerotic changes showed severe luminal stenosis. Two knees were moderate and 26 knees showed mild changes according to our institutional criteria. Multivariate logistic regression analysis showed that age and diabetes mellitus were positively associated with vascular pathology.

Conclusion The prevalence of incidentally detected peripheral vascular disease was significant. Three of 31 knees had severe arterial stenosis and two knees had DVT. All patients with vascular pathologies had one or more risk factors related to vascular disease. Out of those patients, age was the most important risk factor. Understanding the prevalence of vascular pathology and related risk factors in TKA candidates may be important for successful TKA.

Level of Evidence Level III.

Keywords Vascular disease · TKA · DVT · Arterial complications

Introduction

Vascular complications after total knee arthroplasty (TKA) are rare but can be limb-threatening and sometimes life-threatening events. The incidence of arterial complications ranges from 0.03 % to 0.17 % [1, 2]. Limb-threatening complications include poor wound healing, deep infection and so on. The amputation rate is reported to be 25–43 % in patients with arterial complications after TKA [3, 4]. Although underlying vascular disease is commonly accepted as an identifiable risk factor for arterial insufficiency that can lead to wound complications and periprosthetic joint infection, little is known about the preoperative prevalence of lower extremity peripheral vascular disease in patients undergoing TKA. In this study, we investigated the prevalence of asymptomatic vascular disease and its risk factors in TKA candidates.

Materials and methods

Between January and May 2010, a total of 1,000 knees of 692 patients scheduled for primary TKA for the treatment of osteoarthritis were preoperatively evaluated with Doppler sonography of the lower extremity vessels. The

I. H. Park · S. C. Lee · I. S. Park · C. H. Nam ·
H. S. Ahn · H. Y. Park · V. H. Gondalia · K. A. Jung (✉)
Joint and Arthritis Research, Department of Orthopaedic
Surgery, Himchan Hospital, 20-8, Songpa-dong, Songpa-gu,
Seoul, Korea
e-mail: kwangamj@gmail.com

Table 1 Analysis demographic and baseline data

	Patient (knee)
Total number of patients	692 (1,000 knees)
Male:female	62:630
Mean age	74.1
Mean BMI (kg/m^2)	25.4
Doppler sonography	
Normal	660 (962 knees)
Abnormal	32 (38 knees) (4.6 %)
Atherosclerosis	25 (31 knees) (3.6 %)
Deep vein thrombosis	2 (2 knees) (0.3 %)
Anomaly of vessels	5 (5 knees) (0.7 %)

patients who had vascular-related symptoms, including intermittent pain, rest pain, or skin ulcers and had a previous history of percutaneous transluminal angioplasty (PTA) or bypass surgery, were excluded from this study. Doppler sonography was performed by experienced musculoskeletal radiologists with approximately ten years of clinical experience. The severity of peripheral vascular disease was graded as follows: mild—atherosclerotic plaque is present without luminal stenosis; moderate—luminal stenosis is present and multi-detector computed tomography (MDCT) is required; and severe—significant luminal stenosis identified with MDCT.

Risk factors for peripheral vascular disease were investigated in both groups. We reviewed demographic data including age, sex and body mass index (BMI). In addition, known risk factors including hypertension, diabetes mellitus, smoking, hyperlipidemia, and decreased renal function were investigated through the patients' medical records. Multivariate logistic regression analysis was performed to analyze the risk factors of preexisting vascular disease and statistical analyses of respective parameters were conducted using the SPSS (18.0 for Windows, Chicago, IL, USA) statistical software program.

Results

The mean age of the patients was 74.1 years (range 65–81), and the number of men and women were 62 and 630, respectively. The mean BMI of the patients was 25.4 kg/m^2 (Table 1). Abnormal Doppler sonography findings were identified in 38 knees of 32 patients (4.6 %): atherosclerotic changes in 31 knees of 25 patients (3.6 %), deep vein thrombosis (DVT) in two knees, and anomalous vessels in five knees. Six of the patients with atherosclerotic changes had bilateral involvement. Three out of 31 knees with atherosclerotic changes showed severe luminal stenosis associated with diffuse atherosclerotic and

calcified plaque on Doppler sonography, as well as abnormal waveform patterns on the spectral mode (Fig. 1). Two knees were moderate, and showed mild diffuse atherosclerotic plaque changes without significant stenosis, but with decreased peak flow velocity on spectral mode (Fig. 2). Twenty-six knees were mild according to our institutional criteria, and showed only multiple calcified atherosclerotic plaques without luminal stenosis and decreased peak flow velocity.

The most commonly affected vessels were the popliteal artery (64.5 %) and the common femoral artery (61.3 %). Anomalous vessels in five knees represented high origins of the anterior tibial artery.

Pertinent medical backgrounds in this study included diabetes (DM) (51 % of patients with peripheral vascular disease), hypertension (HTN) (87 %), hyperlipidemia (74 %), abnormal renal function (19 %), and smoking (0 %).

Multivariate logistic regression analysis showed that age (OR 5.26, 95 % CI 2.23–12.43) and diabetes mellitus (1.25, 95 % CI 1.15–1.37) were positively associated with vascular pathology. Two knees (one patient) out of 38 knees of incidence of DVT were septic arthritis occurring after primary TKA, and they had a both revision.

Discussion

Peripheral vascular disease is defined as decreased arterial perfusion to the lower extremities by any cause, and can be clinically identified by intermittent claudication or the absence of arterial pulses in the lower extremities. Although patients with subclinical status may be asymptomatic, the condition can become clinically significant through the worsening of thromboembolic lesions by a natural course or surgical events such as TKA. In particular, arterial complications following TKA can lead to delayed wound healing or skin necrosis, deep infections, and amputations of affected limbs. The development of septic conditions from periprosthetic joint infection in elderly patients can sometimes be life-threatening.

Many risk factors predisposing patients to arterial complications after TKA have been identified, including a history of arterial insufficiency, previous vascular surgery, absent or asymmetrical pedal pulses, preexisting atherosclerotic disease, presence of a popliteal aneurysm, and radiographic evidence of calcification of the distal superficial femoral artery or popliteal arteries [3–7].

In our study, the prevalence of peripheral vascular disease incidentally detected by Doppler sonography was 4.6 % (38 knees of 32 patients). Of these 38 knees, 31 knees showed arterial pathologies including atherosclerotic changes on Doppler sonography. Anomalous vessels

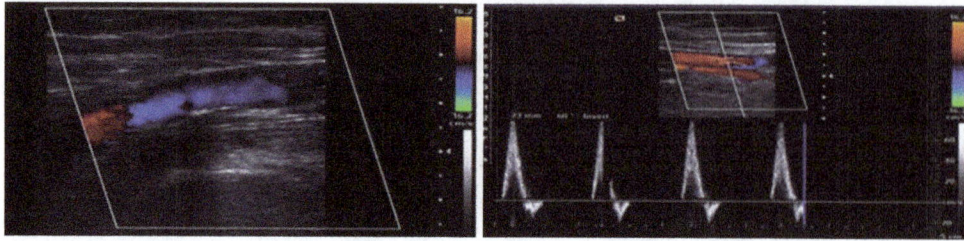

Fig. 1 Doppler sonography. Severe luminal stenosis associated with diffuse atherosclerotic and calcified plaque

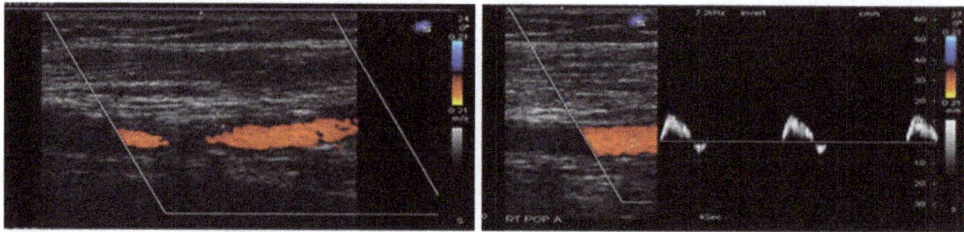

Fig. 2 Doppler sonography. Mild diffuse atherosclerotic plaque changes without significant stenosis, but with decreased peak flow velocity on spectral mode

(considered a normal variation) were present in five knees, and preoperative DVT was present in two knees. DeLaurentis et al. [5] previously demonstrated that only 24 (2 %) of 1,182 patients who underwent TKA in their series had an underlying peripheral vascular disease. The prevalence of peripheral vascular disease in population-based and clinical studies varies (5.1–38.9 % in diabetic patients, 2.6–12.2 % in nondiabetic patients) [8–11]. However, these previous studies uniformly concluded that the prevalence of vascular disease was higher in diabetic than nondiabetic patients, and that the incidence in patients with abnormal peripheral arterial findings increased with age [8–12].

Age, sex, diabetes, hyperlipidemia, hypertension, and smoking are significant risk factors for peripheral vascular disease of the lower extremities [15–17]. In our study, all of the patients with vascular pathologies had one or more of the risk factors mentioned above. Of these, age was the most important risk factor, followed by diabetes mellitus. Associated risk factors of not only peripheral vascular disease but also of sequent arterial complications should be assessed preoperatively to determine whether preoperative vascular consultation or immediate surgical revascularization is necessary. When a screening test such as Doppler sonography is highly suggestive of arterial insufficiency, the ankle-brachial index (ABI) should be determined. Because ABI represents the severity of ischemia, it is a useful method for the preoperative assessment of vascular patency. Proper consultation and interventions should be performed by vascular surgeons according to ABI values [1, 18].

In addition, the use of tourniquets and subsequent pressure on preexisting atheromatous plaques are associated with arterial ischemic complications after TKA [6, 13, 14]. The use of tourniquets during TKA is controversial. Most arterial complications after TKA are associated with tourniquet use, especially in previously pathological arteries [2, 4, 6, 19]. As a result, some authors have recommended that TKA should be performed without tourniquets in patients who are at risk [5, 6]. In addition, two prospective randomized studies suggested that TKA performed without tourniquets is safe [16, 18].

Orthopedic surgeons should understand mechanisms responsible for arterial complications after TKA and risk factors associated with arterial ischemia including preexisting vascular pathology. Careful preoperative assessment should be performed, particularly in elderly or diabetic patients, who are at especially high risk. If necessary, vascular consultations should be performed before TKA, and the use of tourniquets during TKA should be carefully considered to prevent arterial complications [20]. Although the preoperative prevalence of DVT is very rare, orthopedic surgeons should consider modifiable risk factors of DVT and prophylactic medication after TKA.

Although it remains to be determined whether incidentally detected vascular pathology is significantly related to clinical outcomes and periprosthetic joint infection, understanding the prevalence of vascular pathology and associated risk factors in TKA candidates is important for successful TKA.

Conflict of interest None.

Ethical standards (1) All the patients gave informed consent prior to being included in the study; and (2) the study was authorized by the local ethical committee and was performed in accordance with the ethical standards of the 1964 Declaration of Helsinki as revised in 2000.

References

1. Calligaro KD, DeLaurentis DA, Booth RE, Rothman RH, Savarese RP, Dougherty MJ (1994) Acute arterial thrombosis associated with total knee arthroplasty. J Vasc Surg 20(6):927–932. doi:10.1016/0741-5214(94)90229-1

2. Rand JA (1987) Vascular complications of total knee arthroplasty: report of three cases. J Arthroplasty 2(2):89–93. doi:10.1016/S0883-5403(87)80014-1

3. Holmberg A, Milbrink J, Bergqvist D (1996) Arterial complications after knee arthroplasty: four cases and a review of the literature. Acta Orthop Scand 67(1):75–78

4. Kumar SN, Chapman JA, Rawlins I (1998) Vascular injuries in total knee arthroplasty: a review of the problem with special reference to the possible effects of the tourniquet. J Arthroplasty 13(2):211–216. doi:10.1016/S0883-5403(98)90102-4

5. DeLaurentis DA, Levitsky KA, Booth RE, Rothman RH, Calligaro KD, Raviola CA, Savarese RP (1992) Arterial and ischemic aspects of total knee arthroplasty. Am J Surg 164(3):237–240. doi:10.1016/S0002-9610(05)81078-5

6. Hozack WJ, Cole PA, Gardner R, Corces A (1990) Popliteal aneurysm after total knee arthroplasty: case reports and review of the literature. J Arthroplasty 5(4):301–305. doi:10.1016/S0883-5403(08)80087-3

7. Klenerman L (1982) The tourniquet in operations on the knee: a review. J R Soc Med 75(1):31–32

8. Nilsson SE, Nilsson JE, Frostberg N, Emilsson T (1967) The Kristianstad survey II. Studies in a representative adult diabetic population with special reference to comparison with an adequate control group. Acta Med Scand Suppl 469:1–42

9. Melton LJ III, Macken KM, Palumbo PJ, Elveback LR (1980) Incidence and prevalence of clinical peripheral vascular disease in a population-based cohort of diabetic patients. Diabetes Care 3(6):650–654

10. Janka HU, Standl E, Mehnert H (1980) Peripheral vascular disease in diabetes mellitus and its relation to cardiovascular risk factors: screening with the Doppler ultrasonic technique. Diabetes Care 3(2):207–213

11. Bendick PJ, Glover JL, Keubler TW, Dilley RS (1983) Progression of atherosclerosis in diabetics. Surgery 93(6):834–838

12. Abbott RD, Brand FN, Kannel WB (1990) Epidemiology of some peripheral arterial findings in diabetic men and women: experiences from the Framingham study. Am J Med 88(4):376–381. doi:10.1016/0002-9343(90)90492-V

13. Jayasellan S, Stevenson TM, Pfitzner J (1981) Tourniquet failure and arterial calcification: case report and theoretical dangers. Anaesthesia 36(1):48–50. doi:10.1111/j.1365-2044.1981.tb08599.x

14. Parfenchuck T, Young T (1994) Intraoperative occlusion in total joint arthroplasty. J Arthroplasty 9(2):217–220. doi:10.1016/0883-5403(94)90071-X

15. Zimmermann BR, Palumbo PJ, O'Fallon WM, Osmundson PJ, Kazmier FJ (1981) A prospective study of peripheral occlusive arterial disease in diabetes. I. Clinical characteristics of the subjects. Mayo Clin Proc 56(4):217–222

16. Palumbo PJ, O'Fallon WM, Osmundson PJ, Zimmermann BR, Langworthy A, Kazmier F (1991) Progression of peripheral occlusive arterial disease in diabetes mellitus. Arch Intern Med 151(4):717–721. doi:10.1001/archinte.1991.00400040067015

17. Beach KW, Bedford GR, Bergelin RO, Martin DC, Vandenberghe N, Zaccardi M, Strandness DE (1988) Progression of lower-extremity arterial occlusive disease in type II diabetes mellitus. Diabetes Care 11(6):464–472

18. Smith DE, McGraw RW, Taylor DC, Masri BA (2001) Arterial complications and total knee arthroplasty. J Am Acad Orthop Surg 9(4):253–257

19. Schina MJ Jr, Atnip RG, Healy DA, Thiele BL (1994) Relative risks of limb revascularization and amputation in the modern era. Cardiovasc Surg 2(6):754–759

20. Butt U, Samuel R, Sahu A, Butt IS, Johnson DS, Turner PG (2010) Arterial injury in total knee arthroplasty. J Arthroplasty 25(8):1311–1318. doi:10.1016/j.arth.2010.05.018

24

Ossifying tendinitis of the rotator cuff after arthroscopic excision of calcium deposits: report of two cases and literature review

Giovanni Merolla · Arpit C. Dave · Paolo Paladini ·
Fabrizio Campi · Giuseppe Porcellini

Abstract Ossifying tendinitis (OT) is a type of heterotopic ossification, characterized by deposition of hydroxyapatite crystals in a histologic pattern of mature lamellar bone. It is usually associated with surgical intervention or trauma and is more commonly seen in Achilles or distal biceps tendons, and also in the gluteus maximus tendon. To our knowledge, there is no description of OT as a complication of calcifying tendinitis of the rotator cuff. In this report, we describe two cases in which the patients developed an OT of the supraspinatus after arthroscopic removal of calcium deposits. The related literature is reviewed.

Keywords Ossifying · Calcifying · Tendinitis ·
Shoulder · Arthroscopy

Introduction

Subacromial calcium deposits and calcifications in the tendons of the rotator cuff (RC), with histologic presence of chondrocytes along tenocytes, were identified as a cause of scapulo-humeral periarthritis in the early 1900s [1–3]. Later, the term calcifying tendinitis (CT) was coined, denoting an evolutionary process tending towards spontaneous healing [4]. Prevalence of CT was reported to be 2.7 % in asymptomatic individuals and it seems to be more common in females between their fourth and sixth decades, and sedentary workers [5]. Uhthoff and Sarkar [6] noted that CT evolves through a typical cycle in three distinct stages: pre-calcific, calcifying and post-calcific. The pre-calcific stage is characterized by metaplasia of tenocytes into chondrocytes that can be stimulated by multiple factors including hypoxia, microtrauma, disuse and hormonal action. The calcific stage can be divided into three phases: formation, resting and resorption; the process evolves from deposition of amorphous calcium phosphate followed by vascularisation to absorb the calcium deposits. The phase of resorption is associated with significant clinical pain experienced by the patient. The post-calcific stage marks collagenisation of the lesion by fibroblasts, thus ending the cycle of calcifying tendinitis.

Ossifying tendinitis (OT) is a type of heterotopic ossification (HO), characterized by deposition of hydroxyapatite crystals in a histologic pattern of mature lamellar bone [7, 8].

It is usually associated with surgical intervention or trauma [9] and is more commonly seen in the Achilles tendon [10] or following repair of ruptured distal biceps [11]. To our knowledge, there is no description of OT as a complication of calcifying tendinitis of the rotator cuff. In this report, we describe two cases in which patients developed an OT of the supraspinatus after arthroscopic removal of calcium deposits, and we review the literature.

G. Merolla (✉) · A. C. Dave · P. Paladini · F. Campi ·
G. Porcellini
Unit of Shoulder and Elbow Surgery, "D. Cervesi" Hospital,
AUSL della Romagna, Ambito Territoriale di Rimini, L.V
Beethowen 5, 47841 Cattolica, RN, Italy
e-mail: giovannimerolla@hotmail.com;
giovanni.merolla@auslrn.net

G. Merolla
Biomechanics Laboratory "Marco Simoncelli", D. Cervesi
Hospital, Cattolica, AUSL della Romagna,Ambito Territoriale di
Rimini, Cattolica, Italy

Case report

Case 1

In April 2005 the patient came to our outpatient office, complaining of severe pain and discomfort in the right

Fig. 1 Radiographic evaluation of case 1: **a** preoperative X-ray (November 2005) of the right shoulder showing a subacromial (S/A) calcification of 1.2 cm; **b** postoperative radiographs confirmed the complete excision of the calcium deposit; **c** preoperative X-ray performed before the 2nd operation (February 2011) highlighted recurrence of calcification as a dense area more than 1 cm in size in the S/A space; **d** last follow-up radiographic evaluation confirmed the absence of ossifying mass

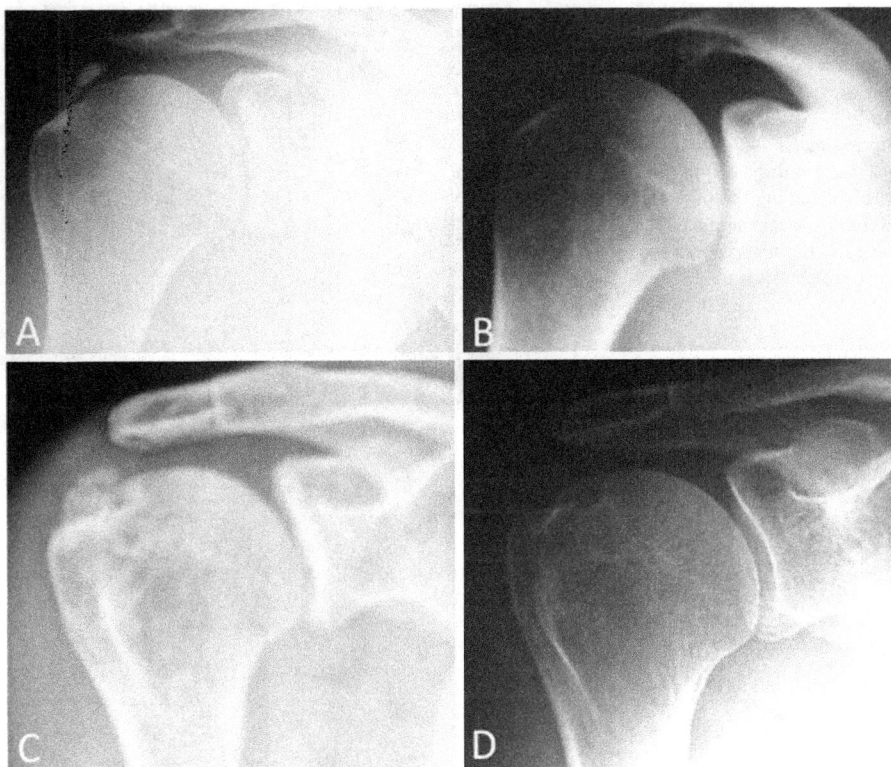

shoulder for 1 year. After radiological and ultrasound (US) examination, he was diagnosed with calcific tendinitis of the rotator cuff and he underwent two cycles of extracorporeal shock wave (ESW) therapy. At 1 year follow-up he had not had any improvement in pain and shoulder function and therefore was advised to undergo shoulder arthroscopy.

Preoperative shoulder examination showed the following range of motion (ROM): 160° in flexion and abduction, 80° in internal rotation(IR) and 90° in external rotation(ER). Impingement tests (Hawkins and cross-arm) and Empty Can Test were found positive. The Constant–Murley score (CS) was 67 points, and the Simple Shoulder Test (SST) had a 5/12 "yes" response. Laboratory exams showed normal values of peripheral blood counts, and X-ray showed a 1.2-cm calcification located on the bursal side of the supraspinatus tendon (Fig. 1a).

The patient underwent shoulder arthroscopy in November 2005. Intraoperatively we found a severe subacromial bursitis and a calcific deposit of 2 cm in the supraspinatus and in the superior portion of the infraspinatus. We performed a complete debridement up to the tendon edges devoid of calcific residuals and multiple needling in the surrounding tissue to ensure complete removal of the calcific deposit. The gap thus created was sutured with two side-to-side stitches and postoperative radiograms confirmed the complete excision of the calcific deposits (Fig. 1b). Postoperative rehabilitation included arm protection in a sling for 15 days, passive mobilization

in the scapular plane after 15 days, active exercises from the 5th week and strengthening exercises after 2 months. The patient was followed up in our unit at 45 days, 3, and 6 months, showing a satisfactory shoulder function, till November 2009 when he complained of pain in the right shoulder for 3 months. At this time he was prescribed a standard program of physiotherapy and stretching. X-ray showed a small focus of calcium deposit in the S/A space close enough to the greater tuberosity. We prescribed a cycle of ESW, but due to persistently increasing pain, he was advised for a second arthroscopic look. Before the second operation the pain was severe and the passive ROM was 45° in ER, 45° in IR, 140° in forward elevation (FE); the CS was 71 points and the SST had 7/12 "yes" responses. Laboratory investigations were normal. Preoperative X-ray performed on February 2011 confirmed the presence of a dense 1.5-cm area in the subacromial space that was suspected to be a recurrence of calcium deposit. The patient was operated upon in February 2011 (Fig. 1c) and, intraoperatively, dense hard calcific deposits were found over and into the substance of both supraspinatus and infraspinatus tendons (Fig. 2a–c). However, completed excision of the whole mass did not hamper the integrity of the tendons and so no cuff repair was planned. On histologic examination, the excised mass showed a widespread chondral and bony metaplasia with myxoid degenerative areas (Fig. 3a). Postoperative X-ray confirmed the excision of the mass. At 8 years follow-up examination he was

Fig. 2 Intraoperative findings of case 1 at the time of the second arthroscopy: **a** a dense and irregular area was found in the S/A space, above the supraspinatus and infraspinatus insertion; **b** the ossifying mass was isolated and prepared to be excised; **c** after the excision of the mass the tendon was found to be intact

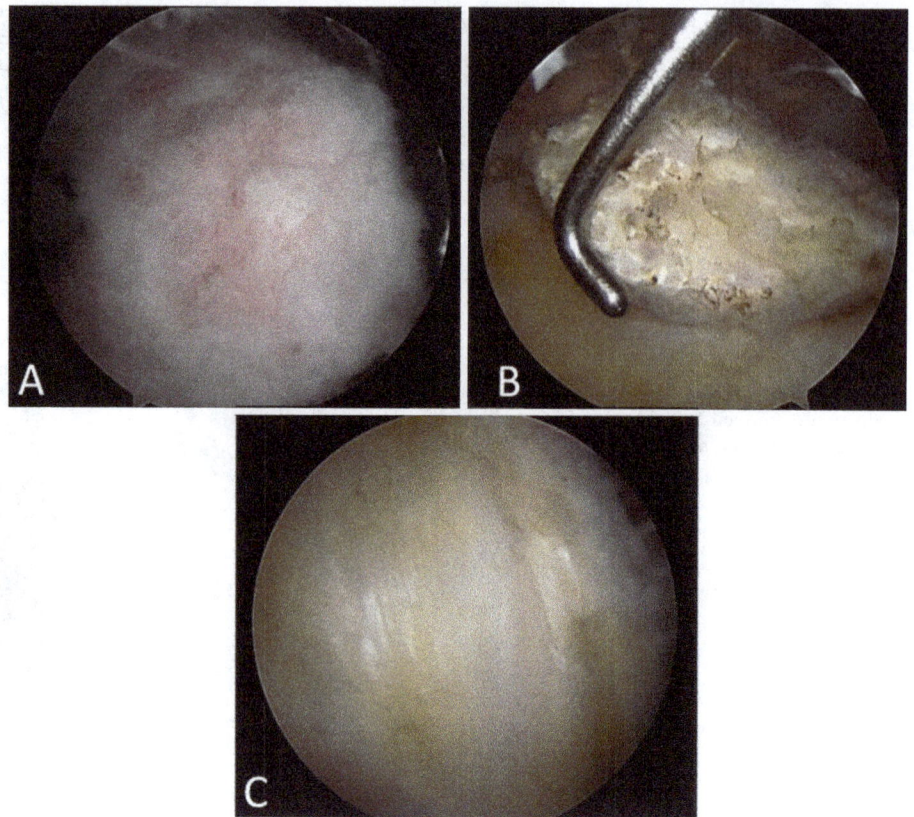

Fig. 3 Histologic examination of the mass excised (hematoxylin–eosin ×100): **a** case 1: tendinous tissue with areas of bone metaplasia, **b** case 2: bone and chondroid areas of metaplasia inside the tendinous tissues

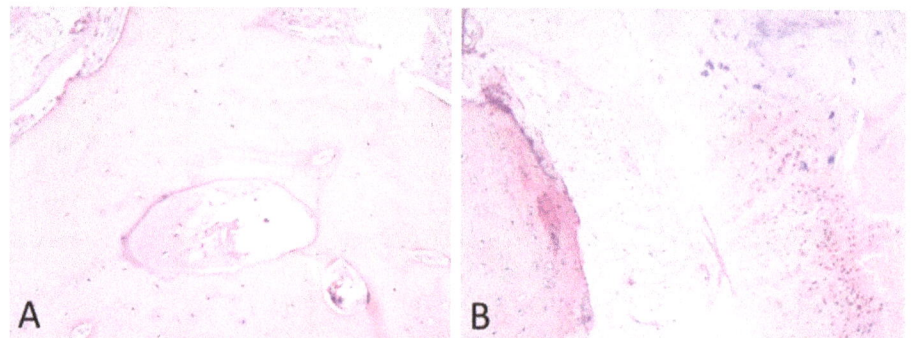

satisfied and pain free; the SST had 12/12 "yes" responses, the CS was 91 points and he had returned to previous work and sport activities. The supraspinatus tendon was anatomically intact and radiological examination confirmed the absence of any calcific or ossified mass (Fig. 1d).

Case 2

The patient was evaluated in our outpatient office in April 2005 for severe right shoulder pain and limitation in daily living activity. X-ray and US showed a calcific deposit of 1.5 cm in the supraspinatus tendon. He was given US-guided needling and bursal lavage, but there was no significant pain improvement. No signs of resorption were seen on the X-ray; therefore, in November 2005 he underwent shoulder arthroscopy. Preoperative ROM was 160° in FE, 70° in ER and 80° in IR. CS was 62 points and SST had 3 "yes" responses. Laboratory exams were normal for blood counts and preoperative X-ray confirmed subacromial calcification of the supraspinatus (Fig. 4a). In April 2006, he underwent arthroscopic removal of calcium deposits and 1 side-to-side suture of the supraspinatus tendon (Fig. 5a, b). Complete disappearance of calcification was noted on viewing the postoperative X-ray

Fig. 4 Radiographic evaluation of case 2: **a** preoperative X-ray (April 2006) of the right shoulder with a dense S/A calcification sized 1.5 cm; **b** postoperative radiographs showed the complete excision of the calcific deposit; **c** preoperative MRI (September 2007) before the second operation showed an area of high intensity (T1-weighted) at the supraspinatus insertion that was interpreted as recurrence of calcifying tendinitis with partial tendon tear; **d** MRI before the third operation showed high intensity in the area where the supraspinatus was fixed, but the tendon appeared healed

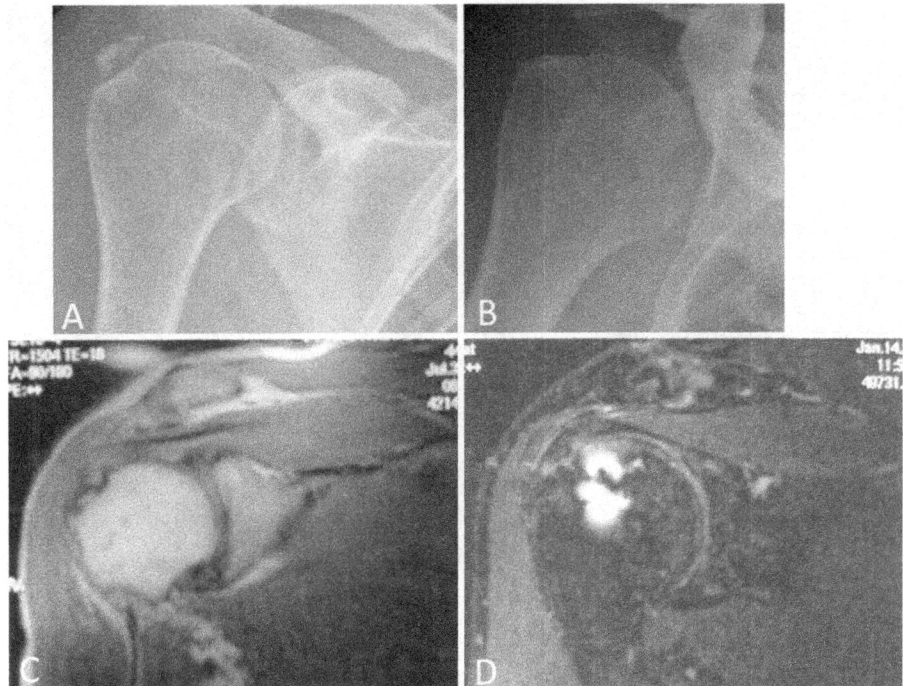

(Fig. 4b). A standard postoperative rehabilitation was prescribed as for case 1. At the follow-up examinations of 45 days, 3 and 6 months, 1 and 2 years he had a persistent pain with complete range of motion and good supraspinatus strength. In February 2007 he asked to be assessed and we found shoulder and cervical pain with loss of strength in abduction; at this time point US showed lamellar calcification in the subacromial space and he was prescribed shoulder X-rays, and cervical spine MRI. An addition, clinical evaluation by an expert rheumatologist excluded chronic inflammatory diseases and suggested electromyography investigations of the upper limbs that did not reveal alteration in the examined muscle groups. Cervical spine MRI showed no spinal nerve compression nor vertebral body discopathies. He was also assessed for parathyroid hormone, autoantibodies (ANA, ENA, anti ds-DNA, IMF), C-reactive protein (CRP) and eritrosedimentation rate (ASDAS-ESR) but all these laboratory exams were normal. X-rays showed recurrence of calcifications and therefore he underwent MRI that showed high signal intensity of the supraspinatus at its insertion which was considered to be a recurrence of CT with secondary tendon rupture (Fig. 4c). In October 2007 he had a second shoulder arthroscopy where we found a calcific deposit inside the supraspinatus that, when it was grasped with a forceps, appeared to have a consistency similar to bone tissue; the deposit was removed and the tendon was repaired with 1 anchor (Super-Revo HI-Fi, ConMed, Largo, Fl, USA) (Fig. 5c, d). Histologic examination showed chondral and myxoid tissues associated with bony metaplasia foci as found in case 1 (Fig. 3b).

After 1 year of moderate postoperative pain, the patient asked to be reassessed again due to severe disability during work and daily living activities Several attempts at conservative therapies (rehabilitation, laser therapy, NSAID, steroid injections) failed and he was therefore prescribed shoulder MRI that revealed slight changes in signal intensity (T1 weighted) of the supraspinatus insertion due to degenerative alterations of the tendon (Fig. 4d). A third arthroscopic approach in May 2009 showed a subacromial bursitis with fibrous adhesions and a complete tendon healing. We performed a S/A bursectomy, removal of adhesions and tendon stimulation with low radiofrequency (Fig. 5e, f).

The patient followed the standard postoperative program and he had slight pain for 3 years, especially during work activity. At the last FU examination in December 2013 (8 years) the CS was 87 and SST had 10/12 "yes" responses.

Discussion

CT of the shoulder is a widespread clinical condition with a significant impact on patient's quality of life. Although several treatments have been proposed, the best option to choose is still controversial [12–16]. Extracorporeal shock wave therapy (ESWT) has been described to be effective [13, 14], but a long-term follow-up study showed that about 20 % of the patients treated have required surgery [14]. US-guided needling, irrigation and aspiration may reduce pain and stimulate calcium resorption [15], while a

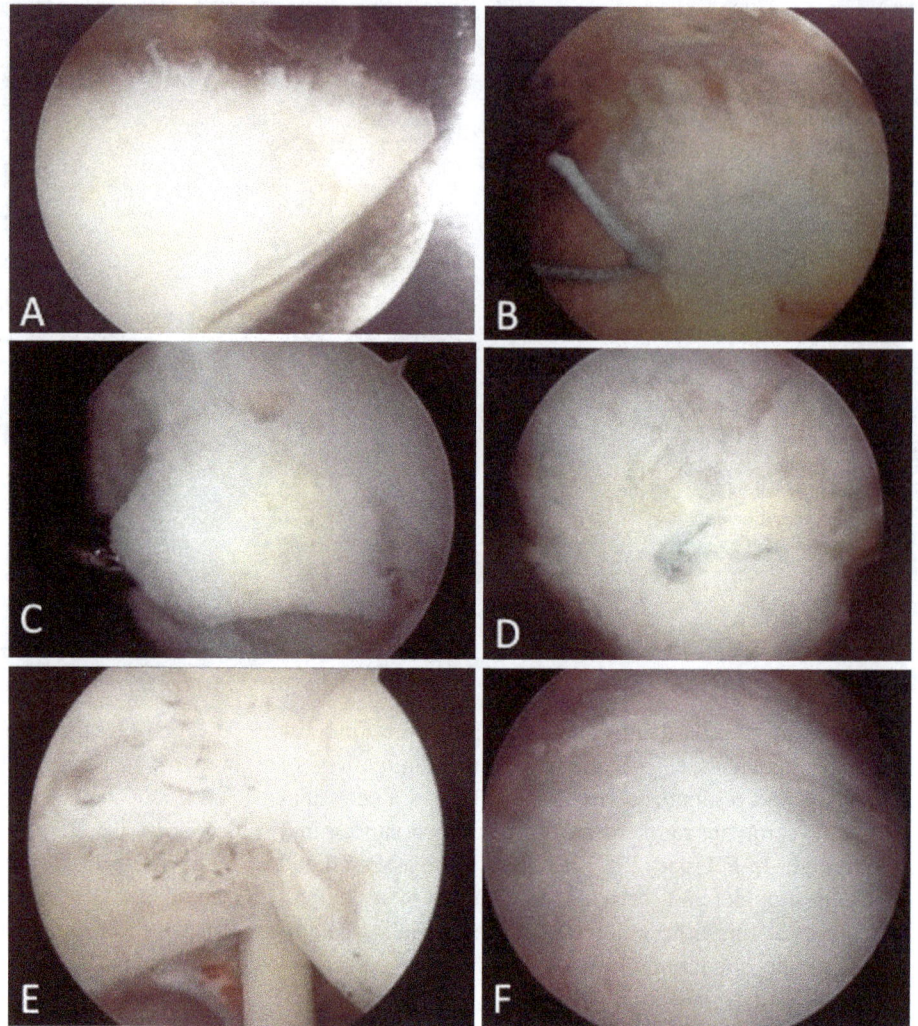

Fig. 5 Intraoperative findings in case 2: **a, b** first arthroscopy: the calcium deposit was identified, removed with a motorized shaver and the supraspinatus was repaired with 1 side-to-side suture; **c, d** an ossifying mass was isolated and removed, the tendon tear was repaired with a suture anchor (Super-Revo HI-Fi, ConMed, Largo, Fl, USA); the supraspinatus assessed from the articular (**e**) and bursal side (**f**) appeared completely healed

surgical approach is suggested in cases with persistent disabling symptoms for at least 6 months [16]. Some case-series studies reported good results with partial removal of the calcific deposits, so as to preserve the integrity of the tendon [17, 18]. However, in cases with arthroscopic removal of large and deep calcific deposits, it is recommended to repair the defect with side-to-side sutures or anchors [16, 18]. Recurrence is a known complication following surgical excision of calcific deposits of the shoulder with an incidence reported between 16 % and 18 % [19], but to our knowledge, there is no description of recurrence in the form of OT. Tendon involvement by HO was found in 26.7 % of patients after shoulder surgery and 80 % of these occurred after RC repair and acromioplasty, but the presence of ossifications seemed to be of minor clinical impact [7, 8, 20, 21].

In a case series of 892 patients treated with acromioplasty and distal clavicle resection, Berg et al. [22] reported 5 % with ectopic bone formation, including sites like S/A space, acromio-clavicular joint, coraco-acromial ligament and coraco-clavicular ligament: around 3.2 % of them were symptomatic.

HO of the deltoid muscle [23] and supraspinatus tendon [21] has also been described following open RC repair. The first was managed with resection of pathologic bone and soft tissue contracture by open interval release and manipulation followed by radiation therapy; in the second case the authors did not perform any additional surgery but they described the association with axillary nerve palsy and they highlighted that there were several risk factors present, including two operations within 2 months, smoking and chronic pulmonary disease. In fact, it has been postulated that hypoxia may drive metaplasia in bone-forming cells in patients who are chronic smokers and continue smoking in the peri-operative period and in patients suffering from chronic pulmonary diseases [22, 23].

The mechanism of origin of bone metaplasia in the RC tendon with calcium deposits is unknown, but some aspects of this phenomenon can be interpreted through the findings already known to us. The presence of resident progenitor cells with multi-differentiation potential in the human tendon [24] and local release of bone morphogenic proteins (BMP) which helps in differentiation of pluripotent mesenchymal cells into osteoblasts [25, 26] has been noted after acromioplasty and in cases with degenerated cuff tissue; these biologic changes may thus induce ectopic bone formation [22, 27]. Ectopic chondrogenesis and ossification have been reported in the patellar calcific tendinopathy rat model and to a lesser extent, in the traumatic patellar tendon injury model [28]. The authors detected BMP-2 protein in the chondrocyte-like cells and calcific deposits in both injury models but not in control samples, indicating that BMP-2 might be involved in the pathogenesis of ectopic chondrogenesis and ossification. HO is common after traumatic injuries requiring prolonged immobilization and rigorous passive physiotherapy [9] or can be associated with other specific rheumatic conditions [29]. An additional predisposing factor for HO is an altered balance within the autonomic nervous system, as seen in brain, spinal cord or peripheral nerve injury [30]. Finally, it can develop after minimally invasive surgery and arthroscopy, but the incidence is less common than after open shoulder surgery [31]. The dilution of osteoinductive marrow elements with irrigation fluid and also its continuous washout may be implicated in its formation [23]. We accurately investigated overall features of both our patients but we didn't find any of the supposed risk factors which are implicated in HO. Both patients were non-smokers with no history of any chronic neurological or internal diseases, and surgeries were performed arthroscopically without pre- or postoperative nerve involvement. The patients followed a protocol of physiotherapy as standardized for all our cases of CT arthroscopically managed. No significant anthropometric difference was found comparing the two patients, nor did they have a family history of inflammatory osteoarthritis, connectivitis or other rheumatic or metabolic disorders; both were employed with no potential habits (smoking, alcohol, drugs, dietary behaviour) or work-related risk factors.

In both cases the RC was involved with severe pain and functional impairment that required an arthroscopic second look to ascertain the origin and the characteristics of the mass.

During the surgical procedure of case 1 we found a formation of hard consistency above and partly within the supraspinatus tendon at the same site the first calcific deposit was removed from; in case 2 we found similar macroscopic characteristics of the ossification, with a tendency to infiltrate the tendon. The histologic features showed in both cases areas of chondrometaplasia and ossification that were diagnosed as a particular form of OT, without supposing such a kind of evolution before the intraoperative assessment.

The ossifications found above and within the substance of the tendon may be the result of a transformation of mesenchymal cells to bone-forming cells in response to the surgical excision of the calcium deposit and suturing of the tendon during the arthroscopic procedure.

Our preference for complete, meticulous excision of the mass might help avoid further recurrence of the ossifying mass. The long-term follow-up of the two cases described in this study showed no clinical or radiological recurrence of the deposits. Although the surgical approach may have been the trigger event inducing the chondrometaplasia, we have not enough data to support this speculative hypothesis, nor can we rule out that the ossification and cartilaginous metaplasia could be the natural evolution of the case. The surgical findings described in this study led us to consider with caution arthroscopic excision of calcium deposits and to be meticulous during the subacromial debridement of calcific foci to minimize the risk of recurrence. We do believe that the description of these two rare cases of OT will be useful to include this condition as a further complication of CT and also to consider the shoulder as an additional potential site of OT.

Conflict of interest   None.

Informed consent   Both patients provided informed consent to the publication of their clinical cases.

References

1. Painter CF (1907) Subdeltoid bursa. Bost Med Surg J 156:345–349
2. Codman EA (1909) Bursitis subacromialis, or periarthritis of the shoulder joint. Publications of the Mass Gen Hospital in Boston 2:521–591
3. Sandstrom C (1938) Peritendinitis calcarea: common disease of middle life: it's diagnosis, pathology and treatment. Am J Roentgenol 40:1–21
4. DeSeze S, Welfing J (1970) Calcifying tendinitis. Rheumatologie 22:45–50
5. Bosworth B (1941) Calcium deposits in the shoulder and subacromial bursitis: a survey of 12,122 shoulders. JAMA 116:2477–2482
6. Uhthoff HK, Sarkar K, Maynard JA (1976) Calcifying tendinits: a new concept of its pathogenesis. Clin Orthop Relat Res 118:164–168
7. Ozaki J, Kugai A, Tomita Y, Tamai S (1992) Tear of an ossified rotator cuff of the shoulder. A case report. Acta Orthop Scand 63:339–340
8. Erggelet C, Eggensperger G, Steinwachs M, Lahm A, Reichelt A (1999) Postoperative ossification of the shoulder. Incidence and clinical impact. Arch Orthop Trauma Surg 119:168–170

9. Ahmed SI, Burns TC, Landt C, Hayda R (2013) Heterotopic ossification in high-grade open fractures sustained in combat: risk factors and prevalence. J Orthop Trauma 27:162–169

10. Richards PJ, Braid JC, Carmont MR, Maffulli N (2008) Achilles tendon ossification: pathology, imaging and aetiology. Disabil Rehabil 30:1651–1665

11. Gallinet D, Dietsch E, Barbier-Brion B, Lerais JM, Obert L (2011) Suture anchor reinsertion of distal biceps rupture: clinical results and radiological assessment of tendon healing. Orthop Traumatol Surg Res 97:252–259

12. Krasny C, Enenkel M, Aigner N, Wlk M, Landsiedl F (2005) Ultrasound-guided needling combined with shock-wave therapy for the treatment of calcifying tendonitis of the shoulder. J Bone J Surg Br 87:501–517

13. Moretti B, Garofalo R, Genco S, Patella V, Mouhsine E (2005) Medium energy shock wave therapy in the treatment of rotator cuff calcifying tendonitis. Knee Surg Sports Traumatol Arthrosc 13:405–410

14. Daecke W, Kusnierczak D, Loew M (2002) Long-term effects of extracorporeal shockwave therapy in chronic calcific tendinitis of the shoulder. J Shoulder Elbow Surg 11:476–480

15. Sconfienza LM, Bandirali M, Serafini G, Lacelli F, Aliprandi A, Di Leo G et al (2012) Rotator cuff calcific tendinitis: does warm saline solution improve the short-term outcome of double-needle US-guided treatment? Radiology 262:560–566

16. Porcellini G, Paladini P, Campi F, Paganelli M (2004) Arthroscopic treatment of calcifying tendinitis of the shoulder: clinical and ultrasonographic follow-up findings at two to five years. J Shoulder Elbow Surg 13:503–508

17. Seil R, Litzenburger H, Kohn D, Rupp S (2006) Arthroscopic treatment of chronically painful calcifying tendinitis of the supraspinatus tendon. Arthroscopy 22:521–527

18. Yoo JC, Park WH, Koh KH, Kim SM (2010) Arthroscopic treatment of chronic calcific tendinitis with complete removal and rotator cuff tendon repair. Knee Surg Sports Traumatol Arthrosc 18:1694–1699

19. Wittenberg RH, Rubenthaler F, Wolk T et al (2001) Surgical or conservative treatment for chronic rotator cuff calcifying tendinitis — a matched pair analysis of 100 patients. Arch Orthop Trauma Surg 121:56–59

20. Matsumoto I, Ito Y, Tomo H, Nakao Y, Takaoka K (2005) Case reports: ossified mass of the rotator cuff tendon in the subacromial bursa. Clin Orthop Relat Res 437:247–250

21. Degreef I, Debeer P (2006) Heterotopic ossification of the supraspinatus tendon after rotator cuff repair: a case report. Clin Rheumatol 25:251–253

22. Berg EE, Ciullo JV (1995) Heterotopic ossification after acromioplasty and distal clavicle resection. J Shoulder Elbow Surg 4:188–193

23. Sanders BS, Wilcox RB 3rd, Higgins LD (2010) Heterotopic ossification of the deltoid muscle after arthroscopic rotator cuff repair. Am J Orthop (Belle Mead NJ) 39:e67–e71

24. Salingcarnboriboon R, Yoshitake H, Tsuji K, Obinata M, Amagasa T, Nifuji A, Noda M (2003) Establishment of tendon derived cell lines exhibiting pluripotent mesenchymal stem cell-like property. Exp Cell Res 287:289–300

25. Buring K (1975) On the origin of cells in heterotopic bone formation. Clin Orthop Relat Res 110:293–302

26. Craven PL, Urist MR (1971) Osteogenesis by radioisotope labelled cell populations in implants of bone matrix under influence of ionising radiation. Clin Orthop Relat Res 76:231–233

27. Neuwirth J, Fuhrmann RA, Veit A, Aurich M, Stonans I, Trommer T, Hortschansky P, Chubinskaya S, Mollenhauer JA (2006) Expression of bioactive bone morphogenetic proteins in the subacromial bursa of patients with chronic degeneration of the rotator cuff. Arthritis Res Ther 8:R92

28. Lui PP, Chan LS, Cheuk YC, Lee YW, Chan KM (2009) Expression of bone morphogenetic protein-2 in the chondrogenic and ossifying sites of calcific tendinopathy and traumatic tendon injury rat models. J Orthop Surg Res 21(4):27

29. Mader R, Buskila D, Verlaan JJ, Atzeni F, Olivieri I, Pappone N, Di Girolamo C et al (2013) Developing new classification criteria for diffuse idiopathic skeletal hyperostosis: back to square one. Rheumatology (Oxford) 52:326–330

30. Fuller DA, Mani US, Keenan MA (2013) Heterotopic ossification of the shoulder in patients with traumatic brain injury. J Shoulder Elbow Surg 22:52–56

31. Kircher J, Martinek V, Mittelmeier W (2007) Heterotopic ossification after minimally invasive rotator cuff repair. Arthroscopy 23:1359.e1–1359.e3

25

Pediatric medial epicondyle fractures with intra-articular elbow incarceration

Luigi Tarallo · Raffaele Mugnai · Francesco Fiacchi ·
Roberto Adani · Francesco Zambianchi ·
Fabio Catani

Abstract

Background Intra-articular incarceration of the epicondylar fragment occurs in 5–18 % of all cases of medial epicondyle fracture. It requires stable fixation to allow early motion, since elbow stiffness is the most common complication following medial epicondyle fracture. In this retrospective study, we report the clinical and functional outcomes and the complications that occurred following open reduction and screw fixation of medial epicondyle fractures with intra-articular fragment incarceration.

Methods Thirteen children who had a fracture of the medial epicondyle with incarceration of the fragment in the elbow joint (type III) were surgically treated in our university hospital between 1998 and 2012. There were eight male and five female patients. The mean age at the time of injury was 13 years (range 9–16). Operative treatment consisted of open reduction and internal fixation with one or two 4.0-mm cannulated screws under fluoroscopic control.

Results All of the patients were clinically reviewed at an average follow-up of 29 months. The overall range of motion limitation was about 5° for flexion–extension and 2° for pronation–supination. The score was excellent in all patients (mean 96.3). Complications occurred in four (31 %) children: two cases of symptomatic screw head prominence, irritation with partial lesion of the distal triceps myotendinous junction in one patient, and median nerve entrapment syndrome in one patient.

Conclusions In conclusion, open reduction and screw fixation yielded excellent clinical and functional outcomes for the treatment of medial epicondyle fractures with intra-articular fragment incarceration. However, particular attention is should be paid when treating these potentially serious injuries in order to minimize the risk of possible complications.

Level of evidence Therapeutic IV.

Keywords Medial epicondyle · Pediatric · Fractures · Incarceration · Outcome · Complications

Introduction

In the pediatric population, medial humeral epicondylar fractures account for nearly 12 % of all elbow fractures [1]. The medial epicondyle is the anatomic origin of the flexor carpi radialis, flexor carpi ulnaris, flexor digitorum superficialis, palmaris longus, part of the pronator teres, and the ulnar collateral ligament [2]. The major stabilizing ligamentous structure in the elbow is the anterior band of the ulnar collateral ligament; the posterior band only provides stability in flexion [3]. The fractured fragment is usually displaced distally due to traction forces exerted by its soft-tissue attachments [4].

There are three possible mechanisms of injury: a direct force applied to the medial epicondyle, an avulsive force from valgus or extension loading, and an association with elbow dislocation [5, 6].

Medial epicondyle fractures have been classified into four types depending on the extent of medial epicondyle displacement and the presence of a concomitant: a small

L. Tarallo (✉) · R. Mugnai · F. Fiacchi · F. Zambianchi ·
F. Catani
Department of Orthopaedic Surgery, University of Modena and
Reggio Emilia, Modena, Italy
e-mail: tarallo.luigi@policlinico.mo.it

R. Adani
Department of Hand Surgery, University Hospital of Verona,
Verona, Italy

degree of avulsion (type I); a non-entrapped avulsed fragment at the level of the joint (type II); a fragment incarcerated in the joint (type III); a fracture associated with elbow dislocation (type IV) [7].

Whereas previous studies have recommended open reduction and internal fixation when the epicondyle is displaced by >2–5 mm [8, 9], numerous studies have recently reported that nonsurgical treatment yields results that are similar to or better than those of surgical treatment [10, 11].

Current absolute indications for open reduction and internal fixation of medial epicondylar fractures include incarceration of the epicondylar fragment in the elbow joint, suspected entrapment and dysfunction of the ulnar nerve, marked instability, and open fracture [12]. Moreover, the surgical treatment must be taken into account in cases of high-energy trauma, elbow laxity or instability, and significant fracture displacement [11].

Intra-articular incarceration of the epicondylar fragment occurs in 5–18 % of cases [13] and requires stable fixation to allow early motion, since elbow stiffness is the most common complication following medial epicondyle fracture [14]. In the study reported in the present paper, we evaluated the clinical and functional outcomes and the complications that occurred following open reduction and fixation with screws of medial epicondyle fractures with intra-articular fragment incarceration.

Materials and methods

Thirteen children who had a fracture of the medial epicondyle with incarceration of the fragment in the elbow joint (type III) were surgically treated in our University Hospital between 1998 and 2012. All the fractures were closed and resulted from a fall on the outstretched hand. Four cases were associated with a posterolateral elbow dislocation.

There were eight male and five female patients. The dominant arm was involved in eight children. The age at the time of injury ranged from 9 to 16 years, with an average of 13 years.

Standard anteroposterior and lateral plain films of the injured elbow were obtained preoperatively for all patients.

The operations were performed under general anesthesia with the patient in the supine position and the injured elbow on an arm board. Operative treatment consisted of open reduction and internal fixation with a 4.0-mm cannulated screw under fluoroscopic control. When the epicondylar fragment was large enough, a second screw was used to provide rotational stability. The screws were placed up the medial column of the elbow, avoiding the olecranon fossa. The medial epicondyle was exposed using a medial

longitudinal incision. The ulnar nerve was routinely identified and protected but not transposed (case 1, see Fig. 1a–c). Postoperatively, patients were immobilized with a cast at 90° flexion and with the forearm in neutral rotation for 2 weeks. Patients were then placed in a posterior splint and encouraged to remove the splint to perform gentle passive and active range-of-motion exercises 3–5 times per day. The splint was removed after pain-free palpation of the medial epicondyle, usually at 1 month after surgery.

It is our routine practice to clinically evaluate all patients at 2 weeks and perform both clinical and radiological evaluations at 1 and 3 months. Moreover, we organized an additional clinical follow-up in September 2013.

The postoperative clinical evaluation was performed by one of the authors and included analysis of passive and active range of motion (ROM), functional results based on the Mayo Elbow Performance Score (MEPS) [15], pain levels during activities of daily life evaluated with a 10 cm Visual Analogue Scale (VAS) [16], elbow stability, and early or late complications. Flexion–extension of the elbows and pronation–supination of the forearm were measured by a goniometer. The uninjured elbows served as controls.

We decided to use the MEPS as it can be completed quickly, it assesses elbow function and pain via questions and elbow condition via objectively measured clinical data, and all of its items are applicable to pediatric subjects. The total MEPS score ranges from 5 to 100 points, with higher scores indicating better function. If the total score is between 90 and 100 points, it can be considered excellent; between 75 and 89 points, good; between 60 and 74 points, fair; less than 60 points, poor [15]. The stability of the elbow was evaluated with a manual valgus stress test at 15° of flexion.

Possible early or late complications were assessed and recorded at each follow-up evaluation.

Results

All of the patients were clinically reviewed an average follow-up of 29 months. X-rays showed solid union in all patients. At the final examination, all of the children presented an excellent range of motion. The overall ROM limitation was about 5° for flexion–extension and 2° for pronation–supination. The MEPS score was excellent in all children (mean 96.3, range 90–100).

Complications occurred in four (31 %) patients. There were three cases of screw removal due in two cases to symptomatic screw head prominence and in one case to irritation with partial lesion of the distal triceps myotendinous junction caused by the protrusion of the screw tip

(a)

(c)

(b)

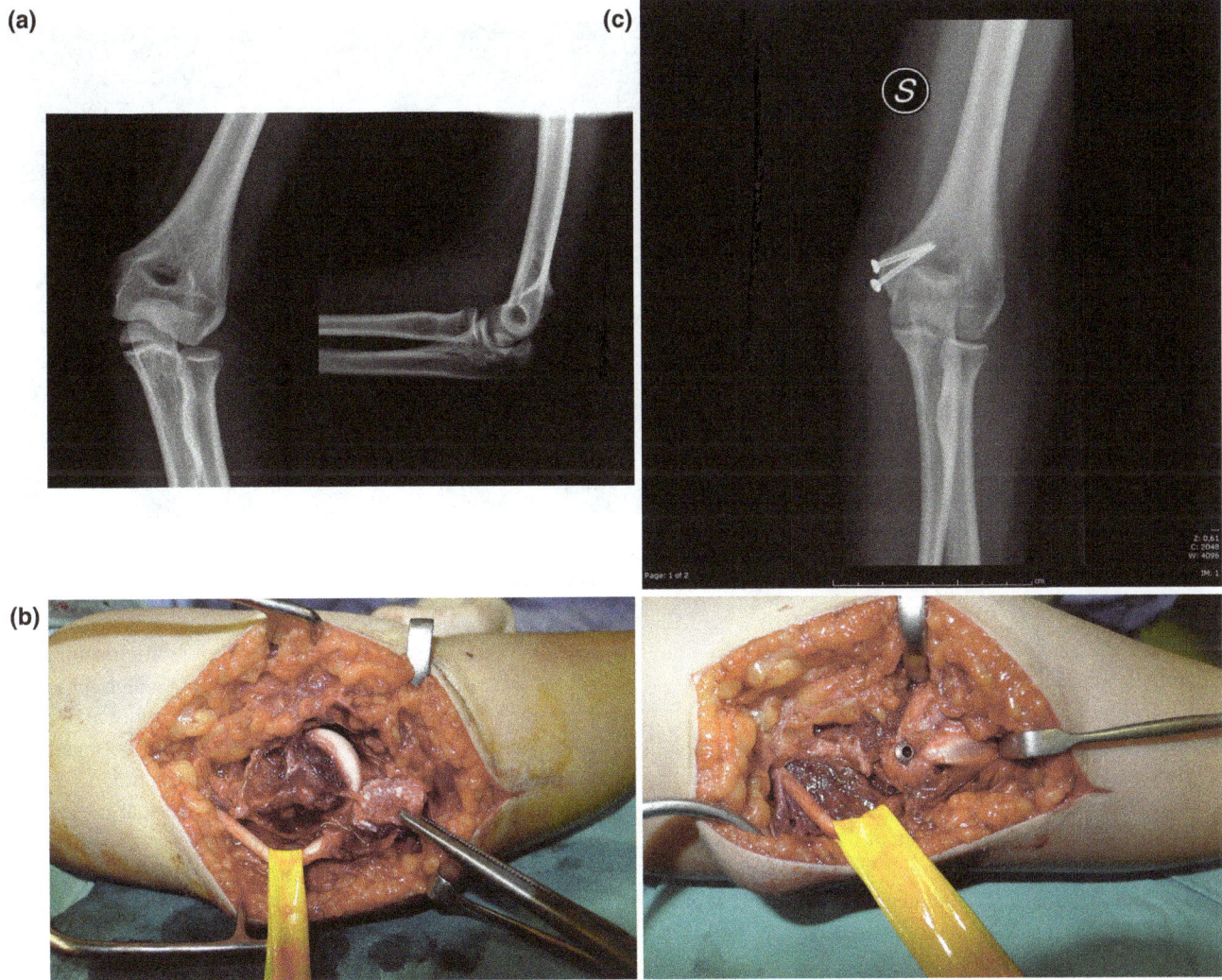

Fig. 1 Case 1. **a** X-ray showing medial epicondyle fracture with intra-articular fragment incarceration. **b** Intraoperative view of ulnar nerve identification and protection followed by open reduction and internal fixation with two cannulated screws. **c** X-ray at 3 months, showing complete healing of the fracture

posteriorly, causing impingement of the triceps tendon during elbow flexion–extension. The latter case was completely asymptomatic for the first 4 months after surgery, but the patient complained of pain during elbow flexion–extension after resuming sporting activity (swimming). The clinical examination revealed the presence of a painful swelling at the distal third of the humerus. The lateral X-ray projection showed that one screw was oriented posteriorly with the screw tip protruding slightly from the bone surface, and echography demonstrated a partial lesion of the myotendinous junction over the protruding screw tip (case 2, see Fig. 2a, b). After screw removal and splint immobilization for 2 weeks, complete recovery and pain relief were reported. Moreover, we observed persistent median nerve symptoms (anterior interosseous nerve syndrome with weakness of the flexor pollicis longus and flexor digitorum profundus muscles associated with pain centered over the

antecubital fossa and extending distally into the proximal forearm) after surgery in one case associated with posterolateral elbow dislocation. In this case, the median nerve was entrapped within the joint by the fragment and the medial collateral ligament after the trauma. The median nerve was not explored during surgery and remained entrapped within the joint (case 3, see Fig. 3a). The patient underwent a second surgery consisting of osteotomy of the previously fractured fragment, median nerve release (case 3, see Fig. 3b), and new fixation with one cannulated screw, leading to relief from symptoms within 2 months. No other neurological complications were observed. Pain during activities of daily life was absent in all patients at the final clinical evaluation, except in the patient who was re-operated on for median nerve entrapment.

No patient had elbow instability or valgus deformity. All patients resumed their sporting activities at a mean

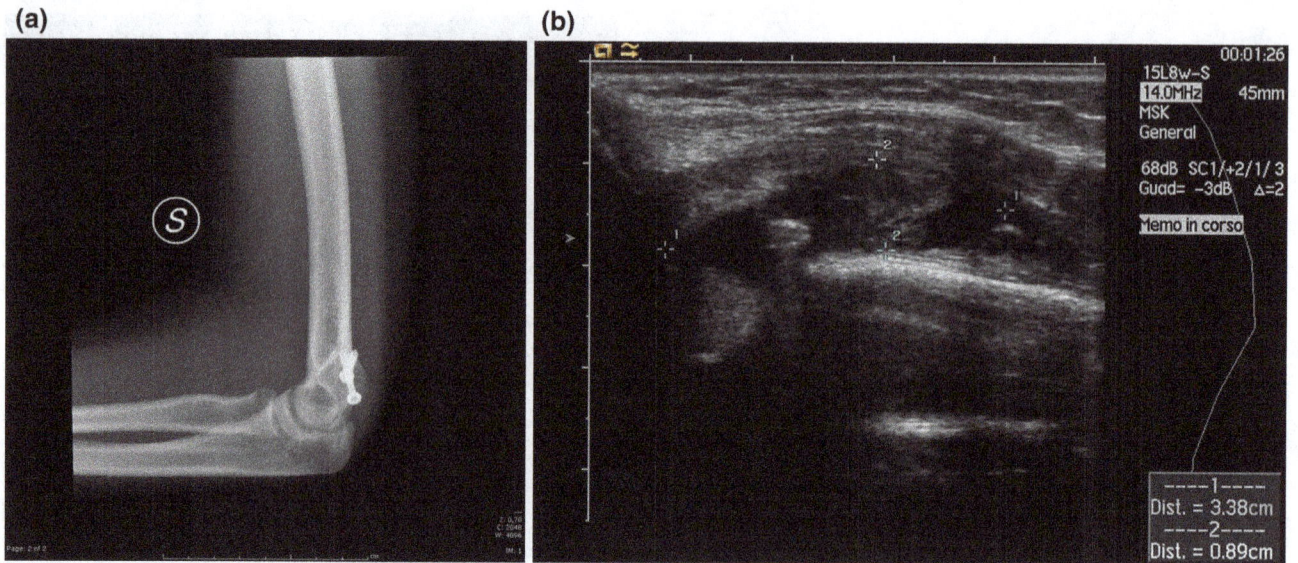

Fig. 2 Case 2. **a** X-ray showing a screw tip slightly protruding posteriorly from the bone surface. **b** Ultrasound examination showing the presence of a hematoma with a partial lesion of the myotendinous junction of the triceps over the protruding screw tip

4 months after surgery, and all patients returned to their previous level of activity (Table 1).

Discussion

Many authors agree that fractures of the medial epicondyle with incarceration of the fragment in the elbow joint (type III) should be surgically treated [12, 17–20]. Multiple methods of surgical treatment have been reported: fragment excision and sutures [10, 21], closed reduction and percutaneous Kirshner wires [22], open reduction and Kirshner wires [10, 23–25], open reduction and sutures [6, 9, 26], open reduction and smooth pins [9, 27], and open reduction and screws [11, 25, 28]. The goals of operative fixation are to maximize the possibility of early return to full function and high-level activity and to minimize late deformity and the likelihood of stiffness (as with prolonged cast immobilization). Therefore, the fracture fixation method employed must be secure enough to allow for early elbow mobilization [29]. Lee et al. stated that operative treatment with suture fixation is unstable and requires supplementary immobilization with a splint; K-wire fixation provides improved stability over sutures, but supplementary splint immobilization is also required [25]. Furthermore, if motion is attempted with Kirshner wire fixation, the wires tend to bind the skin and inhibit early ROM [29].

Moreover, Kamath et al. suggested in their systematic review that the use of Kirshner wires or smooth pins for fixation could not achieve adequate compression, leading in some cases to bony nonunion [30]. However, a potential drawback of screw fixation is the symptomatic prominence of the screw head over the epicondyle, which produces irritation that sometimes requires the removal of the hardware [9, 31]. Another factor that should be taken into account in the choice of the surgical technique is the patient's age. In fact, it has been suggested that the ratio of elbow growth to width has the same biomechanical importance as longitudinal growth in terms of muscle balance and stability [32]. Therefore, in very young patients, K-wire fixation should be preferred, since screws should be routinely removed to avoid growth anomalies [28, 33].

In the present research, open reduction and internal fixation with one or two cannulated screws provided stable fixation, leading to a 100 % rate of bony union and resulting in excellent functional and clinical outcomes in all patients, with early resumption of sporting activities. Our functional results are in line with those reported by Lee et al., who obtained good to excellent results at a mean follow-up of 27.2 months when evaluations were performed based on the Elbow Assessment Score of the Japanese Orthopedical Association in all surgically treated patients. In particular, the mean score was 97.1 points in patients who received screw fixation, 96.3 for those who received Kirshner wire fixation, 94.5 points after tension-band wire fixation, and 93.5 following interosseous suture [25]. When the ROM evaluations were considered, we calculated a mean loss of about 5° for flexion–extension and 2° for pronation–supination. Several studies in the literature evaluated the ROM in patients who had been surgically treated for medial epicondyle fractures. However, different methods of fixation were evaluated at the

(a)

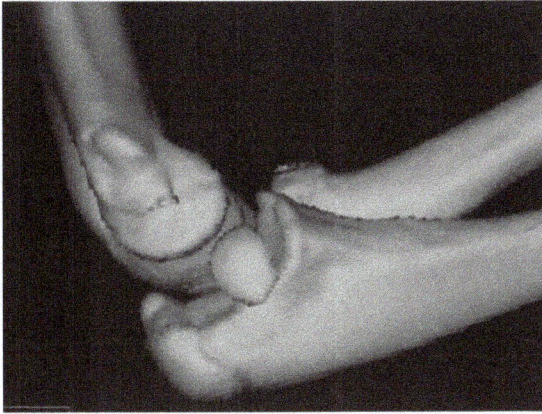
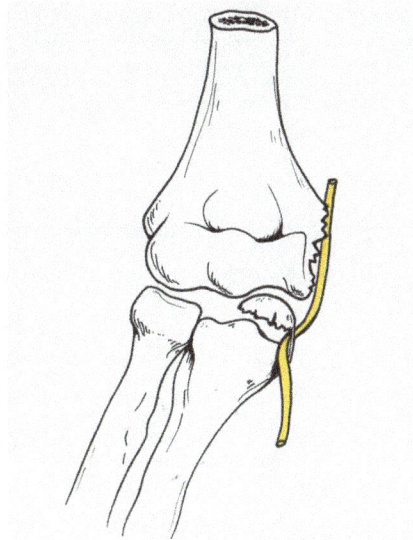

(b)

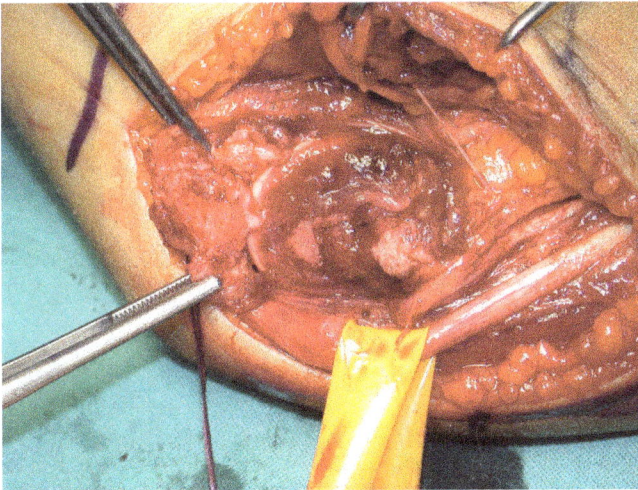
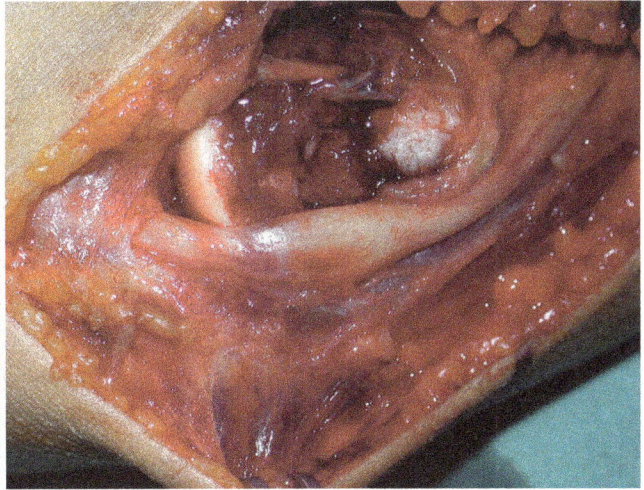

Fig. 3 Case 3. **a** Preoperative CT study with reconstruction showing the median nerve entrapped within the joint by the fragment and the medial collateral ligament after the trauma. **b** Intraoperative view showing median nerve release after osteotomy of the previously fractured fragment, with the presence of swelling at the site of compression

same time in these studies, and different fracture types were often included. In particular, Pimpalnerkar et al. found a mean loss of extension of 6.4° (range 0–15) and a mean loss of supination of 2.5° (range 0°–10°) in patients with type IV fractures treated with either Kirshner wires or screws [23]. Duun et al. reported that seven of their 33 surgically treated patients lost extension (5°–25°), one lost supination (10°), and two lost flexion (5°) [9]. Louahem et al. retrospectively evaluated 139 patients who were surgically treated with Kirshner wires in 129 cases and compressive screws in 10 cases, and reported normal elbow ROM at a mean follow-up of 3.9 years in 133 patients. The six remaining (three with a type III and three with a type IV fracture) had extension deficits of <20°. The final clinical result was excellent in 130 patients and good in nine [24].

Complications, including hardware removal, were documented in four (31 %) children. Painful screw head prominence was reported in two subjects, and irritation with partial lesion of the distal triceps myotendinous junction caused by the protrusion of the screw tip posteriorly was reported in one subject. This case suggests that particular attention must be paid when inserting the screw, as it must be placed up the medial column of the elbow, avoiding the olecranon fossa, and any eventual screw tip protrusion must be checked for by monitoring different fluoroscopic projections.

Moreover, we reported a case in which the median nerve was not explored during surgery; it remained entrapped within the joint, with consequent median nerve entrapment syndrome observed. Therefore, it is important to perform neurolysis of the nerve in addition to surgical exploration, particularly in the most complex fractures—especially those associated with elbow dislocation.

In conclusion, open reduction and screw fixation proved excellent clinical and functional outcomes for the treatment

Table 1 Patient details, clinical outcome at the latest follow-up, and complications

Range of motion (°)

Patient	Age	F.U. (months)	Δ Flexion	Δ Extension	Δ Pronation	Δ Supination	Pain during activities (VAS)	MEPS	Time until sporting activities were resumed (months)	Complications
1	10	27	0	0	0	0	0	100	3	
2	13	33	3	5	0	0	0	100	3	
3[a]	11	28	0	2	0	2	0	100	4	
4[a]	13	37	5	0	0	0	2	92	8	Median nerve intra-articular entrapment
5	9	25	0	0	3	3	0	92	2	
6	12	18	3	10	2	5	0	90	6	Pain (screw removal)
7	14	27	2	0	0	0	0	98	3	
8	16	29	7	5	2	2	0	93	2	
9[a]	15	35	0	3	0	5	0	94	6	
10	13	33	5	0	0	0	0	100	2	
11	15	31	0	0	0	0	0	98	2	Partial lesion of the distal triceps myotendinous junction (screw removal)
12[a]	10	22	2	7	0	0	0	95	3	
13	14	26	0	0	0	0	0	100	4	Pain (screw removal)

[a] Cases associated with posterolateral elbow dislocation

of medial epicondyle fractures with intra-articular fragment incarceration. However, particular attention must be paid when treating these potentially serious injuries in order to minimize the risk of possible complications.

Conflict of interest None.

Ethical standards (1) The patients and their parents provided informed consent prior to being included in the study. (2) The study was authorized by the local ethical committee and was performed in accordance with the ethical standards of the 1964 Declaration of Helsinki as revised in 2000.

References

1. Wilkins KE (1991) Fractures involving the medial epicondylar apophysis. In: Rockwood CA Jr, Wilkins KE, King RE (eds) Fractures in children, 3rd edn. JB Lippincott, Philadelphia, pp 509–828
2. Silberstein MJ, Brodeur AE, Graviss ER et al (1981) Some vagaries of the medial epicondyle. J Bone Joint Surg Am 63:524–528
3. Schwab GH, Bennett JB, Woods GW et al (1980) Biomechanics of elbow instability: the role of the medial collateral ligament. Clin Orthop Relat Res 146:42–52
4. Blount WP (1955) Fractures in children. Williams and Wilkins, Baltimore, pp 26–42
5. Smith FM (1950) Medial epicondyle injuries. JAMA 142:396–402
6. Fowles JV, Slimane N, Kassab MT (1990) Elbow dislocation with avulsion of the medial humeral epicondyle. J Bone Joint Surg Br 72:102–104
7. Papavasiliou VA, Crawford AH (1982) Fracture-separation of the medial epicondylar epiphysis of the elbow joint. Clin Orthop Relat Res 171:172–174
8. Hines RF, Herndon WA, Evans JP (1987) Operative treatment of medial epicondyle fractures in children. Clin Orthop Relat Res 223:170–174
9. Duun PS, Ravn P, Hansen LB et al (1994) Osteosynthesis of medial humeral epicondyle fractures in children. 8-year follow-up of 33 cases. Acta Orthop Scand 65:439–441
10. Farsetti P, Potenza V, Caterini R et al (2001) Long-term results of treatment of fractures of the medial humeral epicondyle in children. J Bone Joint Surg Am 83:1299–1305
11. Lawrence JT, Patel NM, Macknin J et al (2013) Return to competitive sports after medial epicondyle fractures in adolescent athletes: results of operative and nonoperative treatment. Am J Sports Med 41:1152–1157
12. Patel NM, Ganley TJ (2012) Medial epicondyle fractures of the humerus: how to evaluate and when to operate. J Pediatr Orthop 32:S10–S13
13. Chambers HG, Wilkins KE (1996) Fractures involving the medial condylar apophysis. In: Rockwood CA Jr, Wilkins KE, Beaty JH (eds) Fractures in children, 4th edn. Lippincott-Raven, Philadelphia, pp 801–819
14. Ireland ML, Andrews JR (1988) Shoulder and elbow injuries in the young athlete. Clin Sports Med 7:473–494

15. Morrey BF, An KN, Chao EYS (1993) Functional evaluation of the elbow. In: Morrey BF (ed) The elbow and its disorders, 2nd edn. WB Saunders, Philadelphia, pp 86–89

16. Carlsson AM (1983) Assessment of chronic pain. I. Aspects of the reliability and validity of the visual analogue scale. Pain 16:87–101

17. Bede WB, Lefebvre AR, Rosman MA (1975) Fractures of the medial humeral epicondyle in children. Can J Surg 18:137–142

18. Cain EL Jr, Dugas JR, Wolf RS et al (2003) Elbow injuries in throwing athletes: a current concepts review. Am J Sports Med 31:621–635

19. Case SL, Hennrikus WL (1997) Surgical treatment of displaced medial epicondyle fractures in adolescent athletes. Am J Sports Med 25:682–686

20. Gottschalk HP, Eisner E, Hosalkar HS (2012) Medial epicondyle fractures in the pediatric population. J Am Acad Orthop Surg 20:223–232

21. Gilchrist AD, McKee MD (2002) Valgus instability of the elbow due to medial epicondyle nonunion: treatment by fragment excision and ligament repair—a report of 5 cases. J Shoulder Elbow Surg 11:493–497

22. Hines RF, Herndon WA, Evans JP (1987) Operative treatment of medial epicondyle fractures in children. Clin Orthop Relat Res 223:170–174

23. Pimpalnerkar AL, Balasubramaniam G, Young SK et al (1998) Type four fracture of the medial epicondyle: a true indication for surgical intervention. Injury 29:751–756

24. Louahem DM, Bourelle S, Buscayret F et al (2010) Displaced medial epicondyle fractures of the humerus: surgical treatment and results. A report of 139 cases. Arch Orthop Trauma Surg 130:649–655

25. Lee HH, Shen HC, Chang JH et al (2005) Operative treatment of displaced medial epicondyle fractures in children and adolescents. J Shoulder Elbow Surg 14:178–185

26. Wilson NI, Ingram R, Rymaszewski L et al (1988) Treatment of fractures of the medial epicondyle of the humerus. Injury 19:342–344

27. Skak SV, Grossmann E, Wagn P (1994) Deformity after internal fixation of fracture separation of the medial epicondyle of the humerus. J Bone Joint Surg Br 76:297–302

28. Kamath AF, Cody SR, Hosalkar HS (2009) Open reduction of medial epicondyle fractures: operative tips for technical ease. J Child Orthop 3:331–336

29. Wilkins KE (1991) Fractures of the medial epicondyle in children. Instr Course Lect 40:3–10

30. Kamath AF, Baldwin K, Horneff J et al (2009) Operative versus non-operative management of pediatric medial epicondyle fractures: a systematic review. J Child Orthop 3:345–357

31. Partio EK, Hirvensalo E, Böstman O et al (1996) A prospective controlled trial of the fracture of the humeral medial epicondyle—how to treat? Ann Chir Gynaecol 85:67–71

32. Waters PM (2006) The upper limb. In: Morrissy RT, Weinstein SL (eds) Lovell and Winter's pediatric orthopaedics, 6th edn. Lippincott Williams & Wilkins, Philadelphia, pp 921–986

33. Haxhija EQ, Mayr JM, Grechenig W et al (2006) Treatment of medial epicondylar apophyseal avulsion injury in children. Oper Orthop Traumatol 18:120–134

26

Suture-related pseudoinfection after total hip arthroplasty

Luca Pierannunzii · Andrea Fossali ·
Orazio De Lucia · Arturo Guarino

Abstract Absorbable sutures are widely used for wound closure after total hip replacement. Here we present two cases of suture-related foreign-body reaction that perfectly mimicked a periprosthetic joint infection, with sterile abscess formation and physical and laboratory signs of inflammation acutely presenting 7–8 weeks after surgery, at the time of suture absorption. Both recurred with analogous timing after irrigation and debridement, likely due to re-using the same suture material. Multiple negative microbiological samples and positive histological samples showing a foreign-body reaction are the fundamental steps towards the diagnosis of a suture-related pseudoinfection (SRPI). Only three other cases have been reported to date, but the recurrence, together with the self-healing course after relapse, represents a completely novel feature and possibly the strongest demonstration of the supposed aetiopathogenesis. The knowledge of this possible complication leads to some clinical implications: all potential periprosthetic joint infections should routinely undergo not only microbiological but also histological sampling; caution should be used when recommending prosthesis exchange for potential infections occurring in the time range of suture absorption; lastly, if SRPI is suspected, a suture with low propensity to induce foreign-body reactions should be chosen after irrigation and debridement and the volume of absorbable material left in the wound should be as small as possible.

L. Pierannunzii (✉) · A. Fossali · O. De Lucia · A. Guarino
Gaetano Pini Orthopaedic Institute, P.zza Cardinal Ferrari, 1,
20122 Milan, Italy
e-mail: lmcpierannunzii@hotmail.com

Introduction

Infection is probably the most dangerous and feared complication after total hip arthroplasty (THA). Since timely treatment is mandatory to increase the chance of success, careful patient monitoring and prompt irrigation and debridement of possibly infected wounds are essential [1].

Absorbable sutures are widely used for wound closure after THA, and Vicryl Plus® (Ethicon, Johnson & Johnson) combines the features of a well known absorbable suture (Vicryl®) with a broad-spectrum antibacterial agent (Triclosan).

A few cases of adverse reactions to Vicryl®/Vicryl Plus® have reported to date [2] in contrast with the worldwide circulation of these products in most fields of surgery; however, interestingly, three cases were described as mimicking infection after THA [3].

The present paper aims to present another two cases, whose clinical history, histopathological and laboratory findings are so distinctive (and consistent with previous reports) as to define a novel, exceptional THA complication, the suture-related pseudoinfection (SRPI).

Case report

Case #1

A 63-year-old woman with displaced femoral neck fracture of the left hip underwent cementless ceramic-on-ceramic THA through straight lateral approach. The patient had no relevant risk factors for infection (immunocompetent, non-diabetic with normal body mass index and no history of recent infections) except light smoking (less than 10 cigarettes per day), and surgery was completed within 80 min.

Antibiotic prophylaxis was obtained with a short intravenous course of cefazolin (2 g before operation, followed by 1 g 6–14–22 h later). The trochanteric digastrics tendon split and the fascial incision were sutured with Vycril Plus® #2, while subcutaneous tissue was sutured with Vycril Plus® #2 and #0 in the deep layer and Vycril Plus® #2/0 in the superficial layer. Staples were used for skin closure. Two deep suction drains were maintained for 48 h and removed at first dressing change. The post-operative course was uneventful: body temperature normalized (below 37 °C) 2 days after surgery, the wound was dry with no signs of inflammation or hematoma, C-reactive protein (CRP) levels halved every 2 days, and the hip was mobile and pain-free. The patient was therefore discharged home 8 days after surgery. On the 14th postoperative day skin staples were removed and on the fifth week the patient was seen in the outpatient clinic; X-rays and clinical examination were extremely satisfactory, and she was allowed to abandon her crutches and to resume ordinary life activities.

In the ninth week from index surgery the patient, previously pain-free, started to complain of tenderness, warmth and redness of the skin around the scar. She was examined immediately after symptom onset and a minimal seropurulent discharge was noticed from a small sinus, which was carefully dilated with a sterile swab, allowing the exudate to drain and microbiological samples to be collected (with negative results). Blood tests detected mildly elevated CRP (1.4 mg/dL) and erythrocyte sedimentation rate (ESR) (60 mm/h), but no elevation of white blood cell (WBC) count. Ultrasonographic (US) examination of the hip demonstrated an abscess in the deep layer of the hypodermis, with several sinus tracts towards the surface. The presence of local signs (warmth, redness, swelling, tenderness and fluid discharge), US signs (abscess) and laboratory signs (elevated CRP) of surgical site infection convinced us to schedule immediate irrigation and debridement (ID) within 1 week from complication onset.

The debridement was performed through the pre-existing scar, with excision of multiple sinus tracts. A massive abscess, with purulent grey-yellowish content, was retrieved in the deep subcutaneous tissue, extending along the whole incision. After culture and histological sampling, the cavity was debrided and irrigated with diluted iodopovidone and saline solution. The fascia, apparently intact, was then incised and the pertrochanteric space was inspected. Since no signs of infection were retrieved below the fascia, surgical gowns, gloves and instruments were replaced before splitting the digastrics tendon and opening the periprosthetic capsule; within the joint just a few milliliters of clear fluid were found. Thorough irrigation was performed after microbiological sampling. Since the infection seemed not to have spread below the fascia, and

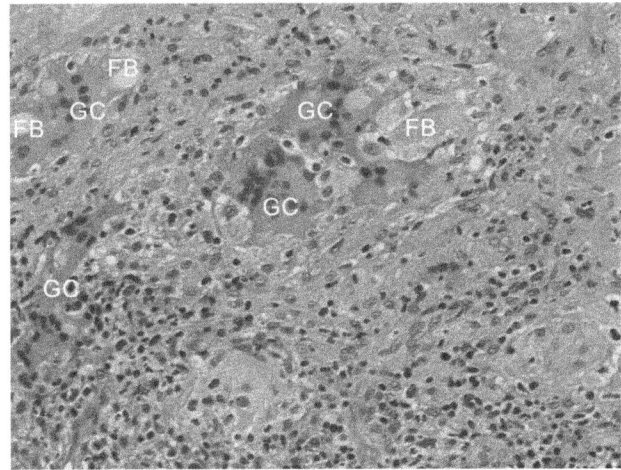

Fig. 1 Foreign-body reaction in the superficial hypodermis. *GC* giant cell, *FB* foreign body (haematoxylin and eosin, original magnification 200×)

given the risk of ceramic rupture associated with head and liner exchange, no attempt was made to remove them. The wound was closed in a standard fashion, but employing as few sutures as possible so as not to leave an excessive amount of foreign material in a potentially infected surgical site, and two suction drains (whose tips were sent to the microbiology laboratory for further cultures) were placed. During the procedure, immediately after culture sampling, an empirical course of antibiotics was started (teicoplanin 800 mg and levofloxacin 1 g i.v.) and was confirmed postoperatively (teicoplanin 600 mg q.d. and levofloxacin 500 mg b.i.d.).

On the first postoperative day the patient was already pain-free, her body temperature normalized and the wound healed regularly. CRP stayed within the range throughout the hospitalization, after normalizing with sinus drainage 3 days before surgery. No cultures were positive, but given the strong suspicion of infection and the absence of adverse reactions to antibiotics, the patient was discharged home 7 days after ID with an oral 4-week therapy (cotrimoxazole 800 mg/160 mg b.i.d. and levofloxacin 500 mg q.d.).

The histological examination of the collected material demonstrated a giant-cell foreign-body reaction, where some amorphous birefringent material was clearly visible (Fig. 1).

Even though the patient was asymptomatic, she was followed up monthly with physical examinations and blood tests (Fig. 2), and 8 weeks after ID another mild CRP elevation (1.6 mg/dL) was noticed without reasonable causes, except minimal scar inflammation and extrusion of suture material. The wound was treated with iodopovidone solution and daily dressing change and healed in a week after complete extrusion of the foreign material. CRP normalized and no further complications have occurred for over 20 months.

Fig. 2 C-reactive protein kinetics of patient #1. Weeks are calculated from the index surgery (THA). The *two grey vertical lines* represent the procedures (THA and ID), while the *grey horizontal line* represents the highest value of the normal CRP range (1 mg/dL)

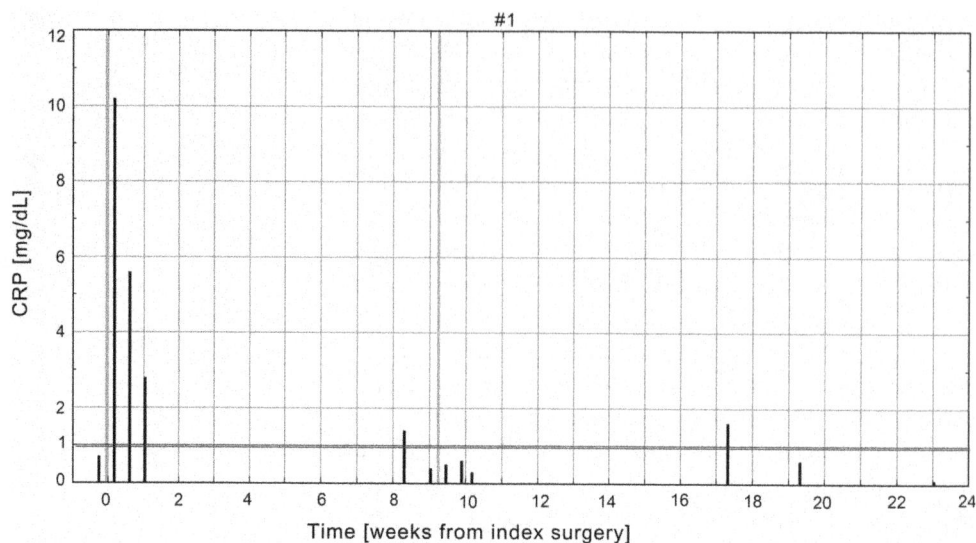

Case #2

A 64-year-old woman affected by bilateral hip osteoarthritis underwent cementless ceramic-on-ceramic right hip THA through straight lateral approach. She had no relevant risk factors for infection, surgery was uncomplicated and lasted about 70 min. The same antibiotic prophylaxis, surgical technique and suture materials were employed as in case #1. The post-operative course was similarly uneventful: body temperature never exceeded 37 °C, the wound was dry with no signs of inflammation or hematoma, CRP fell within the normal range in 12 days, and the hip was mobile and pain-free. The patient was therefore discharged to the rehabilitation facility as soon as an inpatient rehab bed was available, 8 days after surgery. On the 15th postoperative day skin staples were removed, she returned home and on the fifth week the patient was seen in the outpatient clinic with excellent functional recovery and X-rays. She was allowed to abandon her crutches and to resume ordinary life activities.

In the eighth week after THA, almost as in case #1, the patient, previously pain-free, started complaining of tenderness, warmth and redness of the scar, with mild elevation of body temperature (37.5 °C). Ambulation became painful as well as lying on the operated side. She was seen 3 days after symptom onset and no drainage was noticed from the scar, but it was extremely painful on palpation. Blood tests detected mildly elevated CRP (1.5 mg/dL) and ESR (50 mm/h), but no WBC count elevation. Ultrasonographic examination of the hip demonstrated a bulky pertrochanteric abscess, with several sinus tracts perforating the fascia towards the surface. No joint effusion was clearly documented. The presence of local signs (warmth, redness, swelling and tenderness), US signs (abscess) and laboratory

signs (elevated CRP) of surgical site infection persuaded us to schedule prompt reoperation for ID.

The debridement was performed through the pre-existing scar and a massive abscess, with purulent grey-yellowish material, was retrieved in the deep hypodermis. Several fistulae perforated the fascia and allowed the exudates to spread in the pertrochanteric space. After culture and histological sampling, the cavity was debrided and irrigated with diluted iodopovidone and saline solution. The fascia was then incised, trans-fascial fistulae excised and the pertrochanteric space debrided and irrigated similarly. Since the abductor mechanism seemed to be intact and the preoperative US examination did not show joint space effusion, surgical gowns, gloves and instruments were replaced before splitting the digastrics tendon and opening the joint capsule; the same healthy periprosthetic environment was found as in case #1. The procedure was completed as previously described, with microbiological sampling, careful joint irrigation but without head/liner exchange, and administering the same intravenous empirical antibiotic therapy.

On the first postoperative day the patient was already pain-free, with body temperature normalized. CRP normalized on the second day and the wound healed regularly. No cultures (either intraoperative or postoperative on drainage tube tips) were positive, but given the strong suspicion of infection and the absence of adverse reactions to antibiotics, the patient was discharged home 13 days after ID with an oral 4-week therapy (amoxicillin 1 g t.i.d. and levofloxacin 500 mg q.d.).

Histological examination of the material collected showed the same pattern of foreign-body reaction: a mixed inflammatory cell infiltrate, with multinucleated giant cells and amorphous birefringent material (Fig. 3).

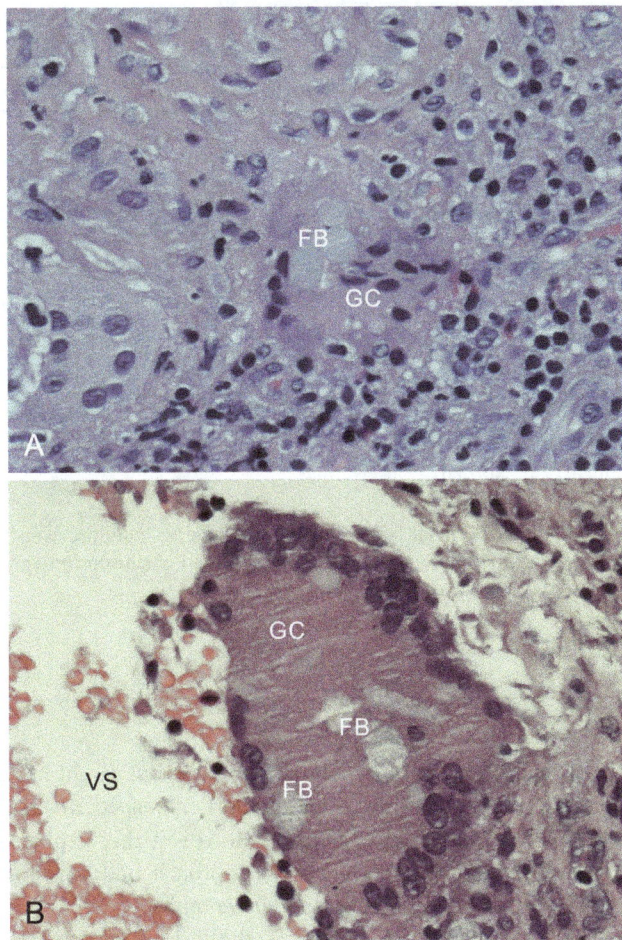

Fig. 3 Foreign-body reaction in the superficial (**a**) and deep (**b**) hypodermis. *GC* giant cell, *FB* foreign body, *VS* vascular space (haematoxylin and eosin, original magnification 400×)

During the postoperative clinical and laboratory follow-up (Fig. 4), the patient demonstrated an elevated CRP (1.3 mg/dL) 5 weeks after reoperation, associated with suture material extrusion. Frequent wound care allowed complete recovery and renormalization of CRP within 2 weeks, without any further recurrence.

Fourteen months after right hip THA, the patient, satisfied with the previous joint replacement despite the complication, requested left hip THA as originally planned. In order to minimize the risk of foreign-body reaction, a different suture material with no colouring or antibacterial agents was selected (undyed Polysorb™), and the closure was performed using as few and as thin sutures as possible. From the sixth to the ninth postoperative week the patient complained about suture material extrusion through the scar and mild local tenderness, but no blood test abnormalities, ultrasonographically detectable abscess or significant functional impairment occurred. This complication resolved with appropriate wound care. Two years after the first joint replacement and 10 months after the second one, the patient is extremely satisfied with her bilateral THA.

Discussion

The two cases presented demonstrate that an adverse reaction to an absorbable suture after total hip replacement might determine a clinical condition that cannot be reliably differentiated from a surgical site infection.

Both cases were standard, uncomplicated procedures performed on low-risk patients, had an uneventful early postoperative course with no complaints up to the 8th–9th postoperative week. They then developed local, systemic, US and laboratory signs of surgical site infection. Although no positive cultures were available, ID could not have been questioned or delayed, given the high probability of infection and the negative prognostic impact of the elapsed time [1, 4, 5]. Because of this latter concern, joint aspiration was not attempted and both hips were quickly

Fig. 4 C-reactive protein kinetics of patient #2. Weeks are calculated from the index surgery (THA). The *two grey vertical lines* represent the procedures (THA and ID), while the *grey horizontal line* represents the highest value of the normal CRP range (1 mg/dL)

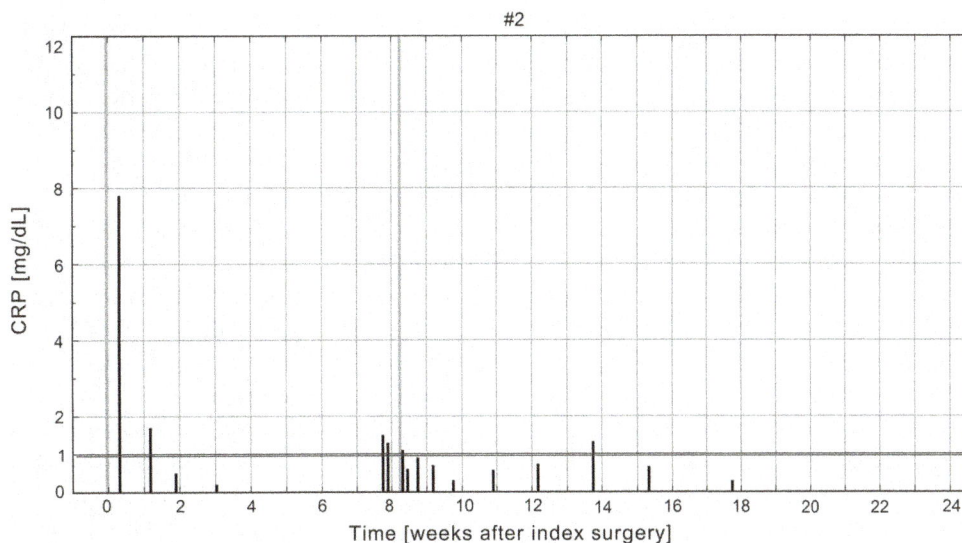

Table 1 Synoptic table summarizing the main clinical information from the three cases reported by Sayegh et al. [3] (I, II and III) and the two cases presented here (IV and V)

	I	II	III	IV (#1)	V (#2)
Suture material	Vicryl®	Vicryl®	Vicryl®	Vicryl Plus®	Vicryl Plus®
Presentation time (weeks after surgery)	8	9	6	8	7
Local inflammation	+	+	+	+	+
Draining sinus	+	+	–	+	–
Body temperature (°C)	37.9	37	39	<37	37.5
CRP	Elevated	Elevated	Elevated	Elevated	Elevated
WBC	Normal with eosinophilia	Normal with eosinophilia	Normal with eosinophilia	Normal	Normal
Abscess location	Extensive (from subcutaneous to intracapsular)	Extensive (from subcutaneous to intracapsular)	Extensive (from subcutaneous to intracapsular)	Superficial (prefascial)	Superficial and intermediate (pre- and subfascial, with no extension through the glutei muscles)
Recurrence	Not mentioned	Not mentioned	Not mentioned	Yes (8 weeks later)	Yes (5 weeks later)

reoperated. The patients had a mild recurrence 8 and 5 weeks, respectively, after ID, likely because the same suture material was used as in the primary surgery, but in a smaller amount. However, knowledge of the histological diagnosis, awareness of having reused the suture material that elicited the first foreign-body reaction, and the similar presentation and timing suggested that we provide simple wound care, without any surgical or antibiotic treatment, and the relapses self-healed without any consequences.

To the best of our knowledge, only three other cases of adverse reaction to suture material mimicking a periprosthetic joint infection have been reported to date, by Sayegh and coworkers [3] (Table 1). Those three patients received the same resorbable suture as in our series, but without antibacterial agent (Vicryl® instead of Vicryl Plus®). Interestingly, the timing is almost identical: 8 and 7 weeks after index sugery in our series (with recurrences 8 and 5 weeks after ID, respectively); 6, 8 and 9 weeks after index surgery in Sayegh et al.'s series (with no mention of possible relapses). On the other hand, the eosinophilia described by Sayegh et al. was not confirmed in our two patients, who showed a normal total WBC count, with minor elevation of neutrophil percentage but normal neutrophil count. Eosinophils were within the normal range for percentage and for count. While the three previously described patients had an extensive involvement of all the layers from the hypodermis to the intracapsular space, our two patients had a relatively superficial involvement, with no penetration of the glutei muscle cuff. We believe that this might depend on capsular repair, which we never

performed after a straight lateral approach, but might have been performed by Sayegh and coworkers, especially if a posterolateral approach was used. However, this explanation is conjectural, since surgical approach and capsular repair are not mentioned by the above authors.

The two cases presented are the first suture-related pseudoinfections whose recurrence after absorbable suture material re-implantation is documented. Similar timing but different extents between first episode and recurrence confirm the hypothetical aetiopathogenesis, since the same material was used but in different amounts.

All the reported five patients had the wound closed with coated Vicryl®, a synthetic suture material made of Polyglactin 910, which is a copolymer obtained from 90 % glycolide and 10 % L-lactide. Its resorption is completed by hydrolysis within 56–70 days from implantation (which corresponds perfectly to the latency of the psuedoinfection). It is used worldwide in most surgical fields, and recently became available associated with an antibacterial agent, triclosan (Vicryl Plus®). Few adverse reactions have been reported to date: Holzheimer described inflammation and occasional sinus discharge in 12 patients after subcutaneous suture with Vicryl® or Vicryl Plus® and skin closure with Dermabond® glue in patients operated for hernia, varicose veins and soft tissue tumors [2]. The complication occurred 3–8 weeks after the index procedure, and only in two patients was an infection demonstrated.

Local inflammation after wound healing is likely underreported, since suture extrusion is a common and benign complication of surgical wounds, often overlooked by patients and general practitioners. Drake and coworkers [6] clearly demonstrated that this phenomenon depends both on the material (Vicryl is more prone to extrusion than Polysorb) and on the volume (the more knots, the higher the risk). On the other hand, some cases of foreign-body reactions to suture material might have been classified as surgical site infection with false-negative cultures, since histological samples are not routinely collected by all surgeons. It is well known that preoperative culture sensitivity is only fair (0.70 from joint aspiration in infected THA according to Qu et al. [7], and possibly lower from sinus discharge swabs), and even intraoperative culture sensitivity is suboptimal (0.94 according to Spangehl et al. [8]). Dealing with a supposed periprosthetic joint infection with no positive cultures is thus not an exceptional experience for orthopaedic surgeons.

However, in the presented cases several elements make occult infection extremely unlikely: multiple cultures (preoperative swabs, three intraoperative samples and postoperative cultures on drain tips) were negative without any preoperative antibiotic administration, the histological examination found a mixed inflammatory infiltrate with lymphomonocytes prevailing over neutrophils, and the relapses self-healed after complete suture absorption or extrusion.

Remarkably, in our patient #2, who received a subsequent contralateral THA sutured with undyed Polysorb^{TM}, made of Lactomer (another glycolide/lactide copolymer) coated with a mixture of a caprolactone/glycolide copolymer and calcium stearoyl lactylate, the absorption phase was not uneventful, although the reaction was milder than after the first surgery. The role of the suture material therefore seems to be important, but likely less important than the patient's aptitude to foreign-body reaction.

In conclusion, the five cases described to date allow us to define a somewhat novel complication of total hip replacement, the suture-related pseudoinfection (SRPI). SRPI is characterized by local and systemic signs of inflammation occurring 6–9 weeks after THA, when sutures are absorbed. A sterile abscess is usually located in the subcutaneous tissue, with possible superficial seropurulent drainage and deep extension through the fascia. The phenomenon cannot be reliably differentiated from a postoperative infection at the time of its presentation, and only the negative result of all the microbiological samples, the benign course and the histological examination allow the differential diagnosis, which is always ex post. Thus, even though this complication might possibly self-heal after complete absorption of the foreign material, we strongly advice against nonsurgical management, which would surely worsen the prognosis of a true, more common postoperative infection.

The awareness of this exceptional phenomenon leads to some clinical considerations. First, the principle that only early periprosthetic joint infections are eligible for simple irrigation and debridement should not be overemphasized. If strict exclusion criteria were applied [4, 9–12], some of the reported five patients might have been candidates for two-stage revision arthroplasty, since more than 6 weeks had elapsed from implantation and no microbiological diagnosis was available. The acute onset and the short interval from onset to treatment, rather than from implantation to onset, should be considered a relevant positive factor in favour of a prosthesis-sparing surgery. Second, histological specimens should always be collected when potential periprosthetic joint infections are debrided. Third, the smallest possible volume of suture material should be left in every wound, especially in the subcutaneous tissue, where little tensile strength is required and foreign-body reactions seem to be more devastating due to extensive fat necrosis. In our routine surgical practice, deep subcutaneous suture after THA is now obtained with #0 suture only (instead of using two or three #2 stitches), and the number of knots has been reduced from four to three. Fourth, if a SRPI is suspected, closing the wound after ID with a suture material with low propensity to induce foreign-body reaction might lower the chance and the severity of possible recurrences.

Acknowledgments The authors thank Antonia Parafioriti, MD, and Elisabetta Ammiraglio, MD, from the Gaetano Pini Orthopaedic Institute Pathology Service for the histopathological investigations.

Conflict of interest The authors certify there is no actual or potential conflict of interest in relation to this article.

Ethical standards The patients provided informed consent to the publication of their case reports.

References

1. Crockarell JR, Hansen AD, Osmon DR, Morrey BF (1988) Treatment of infection with debridement and retention of the components following hip arthroplasty. J Bone Joint Surg Am 80(9):1306–1313
2. Holzheimer RG (2005) Adverse events of sutures: possible interactions of biomaterials? Eur J Med Res 10(12):521–526
3. Sayegh S, Bernard L, Stern R, Pache JC, Szalay I, Hoffmeyer P (2003) Suture granuloma mimicking infection following total hip arthroplasty. A report of three cases. J Bone Joint Surg Am 85(10):2006–2009

4. Marculescu CE, Berbari EF, Hanssen AD et al (2006) Outcome of prosthetic joint infections treated with debridement and retention of components. Clin Infect Dis 42:471–478

5. Tattevin P, Cremieux AC, Pottier P, Huten D, Carbon C (1999) Prosthetic joint infection: when can prosthesis salvage be considered? Clin Infect Dis 29:292–295

6. Drake DB, Rodeheaver PF, Edlich RF, Rodeheaver GT (2004) Experimental studies in swine for measurement of suture extrusion. J Long Term Eff Med Implants 14(3):251–259

7. Qu X, Zhai Z, Wu C, Jin F, Li H, Wang L et al (2013) Preoperative aspiration culture for preoperative diagnosis of infection in total hip or knee arthroplasty. J Clin Microbiol 51(11):3830–3834

8. Spangehl MJ, Masri BA, O'Connell JX, Duncan CP (1999) Prospective analysis of preoperative and intraoperative investigations for the diagnosis of infection at the sites of two hundred and two revision total hip arthroplasties. J Bone Joint Surg Am 81(5):672–683

9. Tsukayama DT, Estrada R, Gustilo RB (1996) Infection after total hip arthroplasty. A study of the treatment of one hundred and six infections. J Bone Joint Surg Am 78:512–523

10. Hartman MB, Fehring TK, Jordan L, Noton HJ (1991) Periprosthetic knee sepsis. The role of irrigation and debridement. Clin Orthop Relat Res 273:113–118

11. Burger RR, Basch T, Hopson CN (1991) Implant salvage in infected total knee arthroplasty. Clin Orthop Relat Res 273:105–112

12. Silva M, Tharani R, Schmalzried TP (2002) Results of direct exchange or debridement of the infected total knee arthroplasty. Clin Orthop Relat Res 404:125–131

27

Primary lipoma arborescens of the knee may involve the development of early osteoarthritis if prompt synovectomy is not performed

Luis Natera · Pablo E. Gelber · Juan I. Erquicia · Juan Carlos Monllau

Abstract

Background Primary lipoma arborescens (LA) is a rare, benign intra-articular hyperplastic tumor that has been associated with osteoarthritis (OA). The aim of this study was to determine whether prompt synovectomy could avoid progressive joint degeneration in cases of primary LA of the knee.

Materials and methods A review of currently available literature about the disease was carried out. The clinical, histological and radiological records of a series of nine knees with primary LA diagnosed and treated between 2002 and 2012 were retrospectively reviewed. Eight of the knees had histological confirmation of LA and none had evidence of condropathy on the initial magnetic resonance image or degenerative changes at the initial radiographic examination.

Results At the final follow-up no evidence of OA was found in the three knees that underwent synovectomy when symptoms did not last more than 1 year. The five knees in which synovectomy was delayed developed progressive joint degeneration.

Conclusion In this series, primary LA of the knee involved the development of early osteoarthritis when prompt synovectomy was not performed. Timely synovectomy is strongly recommended, if not mandatory. *Level of evidence* IV.

Keywords Lipoma · Arborescens · Knee · Osteoarthritis · Synovectomy

L. Natera (✉) · P. E. Gelber · J. C. Monllau
Hospital de la Santa Creu i Sant Pau, Universitat Autònoma de Barcelona, C/Sant Antoni Maria Claret 167, 08025 Barcelona, Spain
e-mail: lnatera@santpau.cat

P. E. Gelber · J. I. Erquicia · J. C. Monllau
Hospital Universitari Quirón Dexeus, Universitat Autònoma de Barcelona, C/Sabino Arana, 5-19, 08028 Barcelona, Spain

Introduction

Primary lipoma arborescens (LA) is a rare, benign intra-articular hyperplastic tumor characterized by villous, polypoidal, and lipomatous proliferation of the synovium [1, 2]. Although some cases have been reported in the glenohumeral joint, the subdeltoid bursa, the elbow, the wrist, the hip and the ankle [3–6], nearly all the cases involve the suprapatellar pouch of the knee [7]. It is considered a primary benign tumor of unknown etiology [8]. Histology shows a hyperplastic process characterized by a diffuse replacement of the subsynovial tissue with mature fat cells [9]. This leads to prominent villous polypoidal proliferation of the synovium. Patients usually present with a chronic or recurrent painless swelling of the knee joint [2]. However, patients look for medical attention at different stages of the disease and in some cases, they may be referred by other specialists after unsuccessful conservative treatment and after having been misdiagnosed. This has a clear impact on their prognosis as the progression of the disease frequently leads to osteoarthritis (OA) over a short period of time. Although it is usually postulated that most cases of primary LA of the knee have similar presenting clinical characteristics [10], different clinical situations with different prognoses are presented in this series of nine cases (Table 1). The aim of this study was to determine if

Table 1 Details of seven patients with lipoma arborescens of the knee

Case	1	2	3	4	5	6	7
Age	39	53	53	37	34	57	40
Gender	Woman	Woman	Woman	Man	Man	Man	Woman
Additional conditions/ situations	None	None	None	Marathon runner	-Lymphoma B	-High blood pressure -Dyslipidemia -Obesity -Smoking -Alcoholism	None
Trigger or particular debut	None	None	None	After a twist playing soccer	None	Sudden, oppressive and atraumatic left knee pain with a large effusion	None
Prior to surgery	12 months	37 months	30 months	4 months	11 months in the right knee	23 months	10 months
Prior to surgery Physical symptoms and Findings	Recurrent effusions and discomfort	Recurrent effusions, swelling and a large palpable supra-patellar mass	Recurrent effusions and anterior knee pain	Soft tissue palpable mass above the superior aspect of the patella and anterior knee pain	Recurrent effusions, pain and swelling in both knees	Oppressive left knee pain.	Pain, swelling and recurrent effusions
Laterality	Right	Right	Right	Left	Bilateral	Bilateral	Left
Treatment	AS	OS	2 AS. PFA*. 1 AS after PFA	AS	AS in both knees	OS in the left knee, no treatment in the right knee	AS
Results	Pain free. No effusions	Pain free. No effusions	Still pain. Still effusions	Pain free. No effusions	Asymptomatic in both knees	The symptoms of the left knee subsided almost completely. Still pain in the right knee	Pain free. No effusions
Surgical Findings	Bright yellow villi in the whole suprapatellar pouch	Large, pedicled and encapsulated tumor	Synovitic villi in the whole knee	Synovitic villi in the suprapatellar pouch	Synovitic villi at the suprapatellar pouch of both knees	An elongated diffuse synovial proliferation in the whole knee	Synovitic villi in the whole knee
Follow up	14 months	22 months	25 months	12 months	27 months in the right knee	29 months	44 months
Evidence of osteoarthritis	No	Yes	Yes	No	Yes, in the right knee	Yes, in both knees	No

AS arthroscopic synovectomy

OS open synovectomy

* PFA patellofemoral arthroplasty

prompt synovectomy could avoid progressive joint degeneration in cases of primary LA of the knee.

Materials and methods

We retrospectively reviewed the clinical, histological and radiological records of patients diagnosed with primary LA of the knee and treated by two senior surgeons in three institutions between 2002 and 2012. We asked in the Pathology Departments of these three institutions for histological records coded as "lipoma arborescens". We excluded cases involving other joints different to the knee, patients older than 60 years old, and cases where the initial magnetic resonance image (MRI) diagnosis of LA was accompanied by condropathy. The final population consisted of seven patients. Two of the patients had bilateral LA, so the total number of cases was nine. There were four men and three women with a mean age of 44.7 (34–57) years old. All of the patients had an MRI, which showed in all cases an exophytic mass in continuity with the synovium with villous-like projections invading the suprapatellar pouch with a fat signal intensity (Fig. 1) and no evidence of condropathy. Initial radiographs showed no evidence of degenerative changes in any of the cases. The establishment of the diagnosis of osteoarthritis was made by means of the observation in the X-ray of joint sclerosis, joint space narrowing and/or osteophytes. The diagnosis of secondary OA was established by means of the observation via X-rays of degenerative changes that were not present at the initial radiological examination. The main symptoms in all patients consisted of increasing and progressive discomfort, pain, swelling and recurrent effusions. The magnitude of the symptoms was not graded. We quantified the pain and the effusions in a dichotomic manner: present or absent. One of the patients had history of lymphoma-B and other of hyperuricemia. One of them said that the initial symptom was a sudden oppressive atraumatic knee pain with a large effusion, and another related the onset of symptoms due to a traumatic episode. The remaining patients did not relate the onset of symptoms to a particular situation. In eight of the nine knees, resection of the tumor was performed: six arthroscopic and two open. The two patients with bilateral LA underwent arthroscopic synovectomy: one of them in both knees and the other only in the left one, because, despite our recommendations, he rejected surgical treatment due to personal reasons. The timing of the synovectomy was agreed by the patient and the surgeon; and it was mostly related to the magnitude of the initial discomfort. The synovial tissue excised in the eight cases was afterwards sent for histological examination. The mean duration of the symptoms from debut until surgery was 19.13 months (4–37). The findings from the

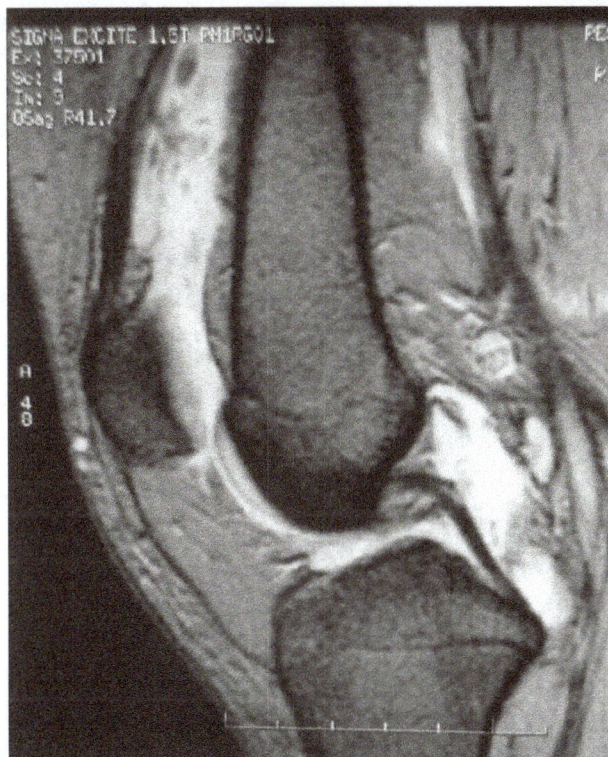

Fig. 1 Sagittal reconstruction of the MRI showing villous-like projections invading the suprapatellar pouch with a fat signal intensity on T2

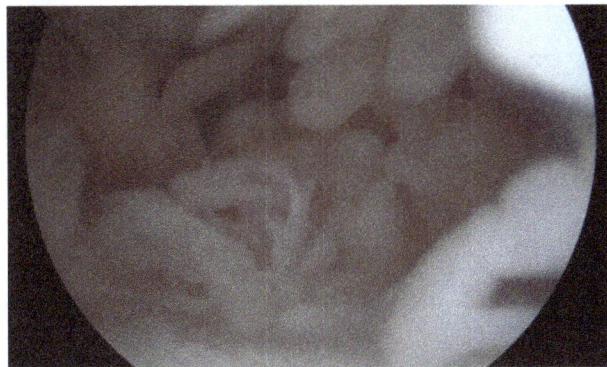

Fig. 2 An arthroscopic view from the anterolateral portal of a villous synovitic mass in the suprapatellar pouch

six knees that underwent arthroscopic surgery consisted of a marked villous proliferation of the synovial membrane and bright yellow and slightly firm villi on the whole suprapatellar pouch (Fig. 2). The histologic evaluation confirmed the diagnosis in all cases (Fig. 3). In one patient the excision could not be done arthroscopically because of the size, consistency and location of the tumor. A 60 × 45 mm mass was firmly attached to the anterior aspect of the joint capsule at the level of the fat pad, so a longitudinal anteromedial parapatellar arthrotomy had to be performed for a complete resection of the mass. The

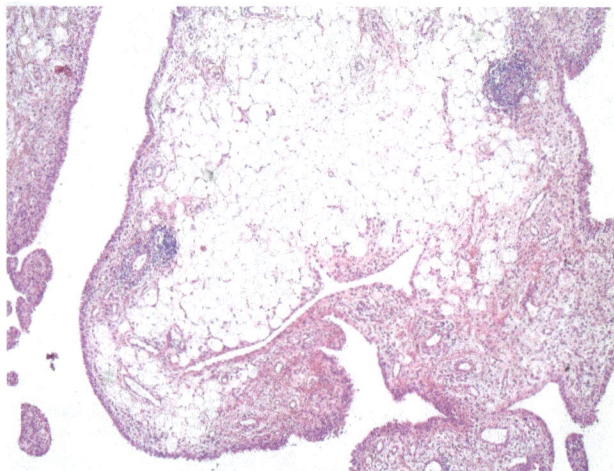

Fig. 3 Histological view of a hyperplastic process characterized by a diffuse replacement of the subsynovial tissue with mature fat cells, causing villous expansion of the synovium. Inflammatory cells are observed around capillaries (haematoxylin and eosin ×30)

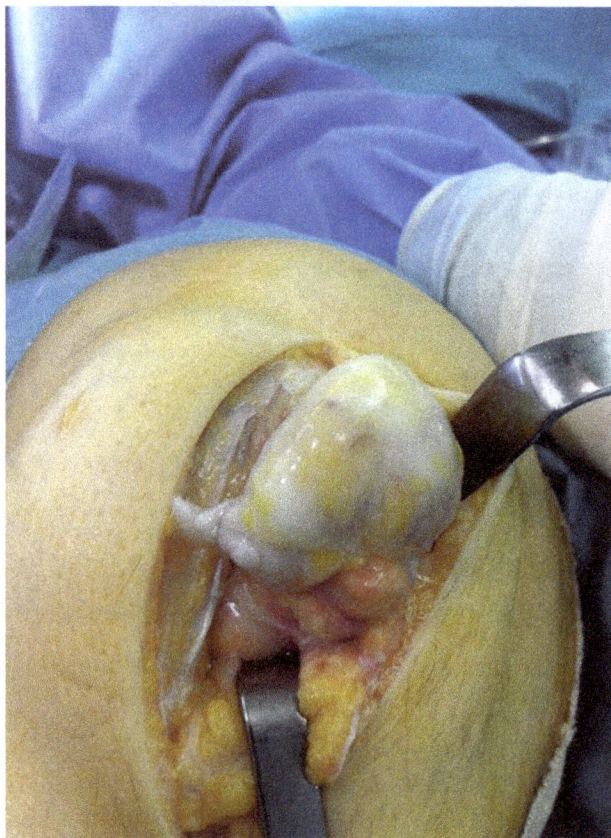

Fig. 4 Large encapsulated tumor attached with a pedicle to the anterior aspect of the joint capsule at the level of the fat pad, seen during an anteromedial parapatellar arthrotomy

tumor was pedicled and encapsulated, as shown in Fig. 4. In another patient who underwent an arthroscopic synovectomy with no evidence of osteoarthritic changes, due to

persistent and recurrent effusions, 15 months later another MRI revealed a remaining soft tissue mass in the suprapatellar pouch, but with concomitant patellofemoral degenerative changes at that moment. A second arthroscopic procedure was then performed. A pediculated synovial tumor with concomitant exposed subchondral bone in both the patella and femoral trochlea were found. A second synovectomy was performed. Eight months later the patient was still complaining of disabilities in daily life activities that was attributed to patellofemoral OA. A patellofemoral arthroplasty was then performed. Although the symptoms subsided for 6 months, recurrent effusions started again. A third arthroscopic surgery was subsequently performed. A diffuse synovitic proliferation with concomitant advanced degenerative changes in the medial tibiofemoral compartment were seen (Fig. 5). The mean follow-up from synovectomy until the last visit was 23 months (11–44). We arbitrarily established the threshold between prompt and delayed synovectomy at 1 year. We expose in detail the patterns of presentation and clinical conditions of this series of patients with primary LA (Table 1), in which we looked for a possible relationship between the time of synovectomy and the development of OA.

Results

Synovectomy was performed in 88.89 % (8/9) of the knees. At the latest follow-up, 12.5 % (1/8) of the knees in which synovectomy was performed were pain and swelling free. Of the operated knees, 12.5 % (1/8) had recurrent effusions despite synovectomy. One of the patients with bilateral LA rejected synovectomy in the right knee, so it remained symptomatic. Of the knees that underwent synovectomy, 62.5 % (5/8) developed OA. One of the patients with bilateral LA, whose initial MRIs showed no evidence of condropathy in either knee, eventually developed OA in the knee that was not surgically treated. Of the operated knees, 37.5 % (3/8) underwent synovectomy in the first year after the onset of symptoms and 62.5 % (5/8) after the first year. All (3/3) of the knees that had undergone synovectomy when symptoms did not last more than 1 year showed no evidence of OA. All (5/5) of the knees in which synovectomy was delayed more than 1 year after clinical debut developed progressive joint degeneration.

Discussion

This series of seven patients and nine knees diagnosed with primary LA with a variety of presentations of the same disease showed different prognosis conditions. The two

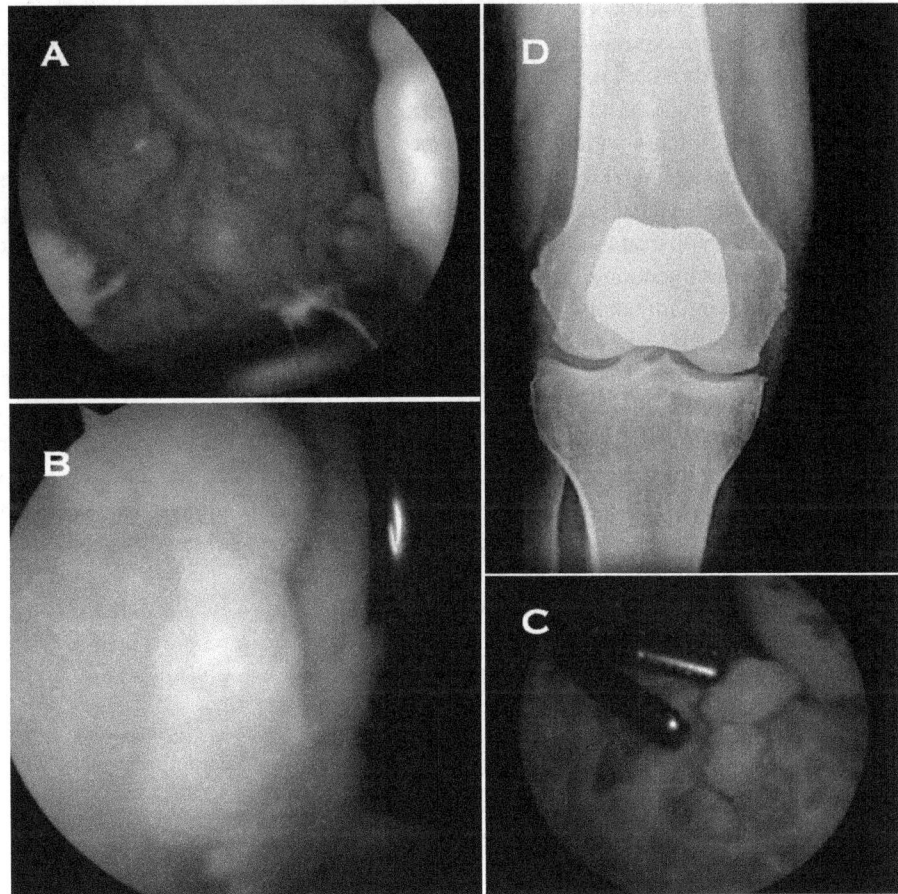

Fig. 5 a, b, c Arthroscopic view of a right knee with a patellofemoral arthroplasty, subchondral bone exposure in the femoral condyle and diffuse synovitic proliferation. **d** AP view of patellofemoral arthroplasty

most common complications were recurrence and development of secondary degenerative changes. The fact that the three cases where synovectomy was promptly performed did not develop degenerative changes, makes us conclude that timely excision of the tumor is strongly recommended, if not mandatory.

LA was first described in detail in 1957 [11]. It is an uncommon, benign intra-articular lesion of unknown etiology in which there is diffuse replacement of the sub-synovial tissue by mature fat cells along with prominent villous transformation of the synovium. Although the knee is the joint most commonly involved, it has been described in other locations [3–6]. It most commonly affects people in the fourth and fifth decade of life [12]. Once considered more frequent in the male population, it is currently considered to be equally distributed in both genders [13]. The majority of cases are monoarticular [7]. In fact, there have been only a few cases of bilateral LA described in the literature [2, 11, 14–17], as were cases five and six of this series. A few reports have described polyarticular involvement [6, 17].

Almost all reports on primary LA of the knee have been single-case reports. Two short series previously published had six [18] and eight cases [19], respectively. A recent publication describes a group of 39 cases of secondary LA, as the consequence of chronic reactive changes in patients with OA [20]. In their series, only three of the cases had no evidence of OA. All of the patients in our series had an initial MRI with evidence of LA and no evidence of condropathy, as well as an initial radiographic examination without evidence of OA. We believe that primary and secondary LA should be considered as different entities.

Patients with LA usually have long-standing, slowly progressive swelling of the involved knee, which may be associated with effusion, decreased range of motion and pain. However, two patients in this series had started with a sudden onset of pain and effusion. A soft, painless, boggy swelling in the suprapatellar pouch can frequently be palpated. Due to the fact that the tumor is painless, patients usually seek medical evaluation after several years of mechanical symptoms, as was the case in some of the patients in this series. The laboratory tests are usually unremarkable and negative for HLA B27 and rheumatoid factor [8]. The joint aspirate is negative for crystals and cultures of the fluid are sterile [21].

Plain radiographs are generally normal during the first stages of the disease [16], but a soft-tissue density in the suprapatellar pouch can be observed if it is meticulously evaluated. In more advanced stages, subchondral bone erosions suggesting synovial invasion, cyst formation or secondary osteoarthritic changes can be seen.

The MRI is considered the gold standard for the diagnosis of LA [16]. It has a pathognomonic aspect consisting of an intra-articular synovial mass with frond-like architecture and a high signal intensity which is suppressed using fat-selective presaturation [16]. There is lack of enhancement after injection of gadolinium, which helps to exclude synovial inflammatory or neoplastic processes, and there are no magnetic susceptibility effects due to hemosiderin or calcification. MRI also allows for the correct evaluation of the size and extension of the tumor, accurate preoperative planning, evaluation of the state of the cartilage and effective follow-up while avoiding the need for synovial biopsy [22]. These findings in the MRI should be correlated with the histology that should be performed after resection, to confirm the diagnosis, and then medical professionals should be aware of recurrences that could have a clear influence on prognosis.

Macroscopically, LA has a frond-like appearance with numerous broad-based polypoid or thin papillary villi composed of fatty yellow tissue [7]. Histologically, the villi are composed of mature adipose tissue, and enlarged or congested hyperemic capillaries may be present [7]. The overlying synovial membrane may contain mononuclear chronic inflammatory cells and the synovial cells may seem to be enlarged and reactive with abundant eosinophilic cytoplasm.

An association between LA and OA has been postulated [14, 23], but the causal relationship between these two entities has not been fully clarified. It has been suggested that the long-standing synovial thickening effusions caused by repeated mechanical injury to the proliferated villi eventually lead to OA [2]. Subchondral cysts and bone erosions can also be observed in some patients [9], as were seen in case six of this report.

The severity of the degenerative changes might have some relationship with the duration of symptoms. Conversely, LA has been suggested to be secondary to OA in elderly patients [23]. Authors have classified this as a secondary type, which is much more common than primary cases. This secondary LA is thought to be a lipomatosis secondary to chronic irritation [24]. The same mechanism could be observed in cases of meniscal injuries, trauma and chronic synovitis. However, this is not an actual neoplasm, so it should not be considered as LA. Although the patient in case four related the onset of symptoms to a traumatic episode, due to the results of the MRI and histology compatible with LA, the traumatic injury was considered only a coincidence.

The recommended treatment for symptomatic LA is open or arthroscopic synovectomy [9, 20]. The election of one technique over the other mainly relies on the size of the tumor and on the personal experience and preferences of the surgeon. Those few previous reports that had performed the synovectomy arthroscopically reported favorable outcomes at 1 year [9] and 2 years [21, 25]. In this series, synovectomy was performed in 8 of the 9 knees. Recurrence of LA after surgical treatment is considered very rare [25]. In this scenario, the patient in case three, with several recurrences and who had undergone three arthroscopic synovectomies and a patellofemoral arthroplasty, is a very atypical case. In fact, despite the four surgical procedures, she is still symptomatic.

This retrospective case series of a low number of patients is, however, one of the largest series ever reported on primary LA. These patients were seen at different stages of the disease and treated with different surgical techniques. This heterogeneity might be a logical consequence of the different clinical expressions and the evolution of the disease observed among these patients.

We conclude that progressive joint degeneration could be prevented or at least delayed, if prompt synovectomy is performed.

Acknowledgments We want to thank Eric Goode for his help in correcting the manuscript.

Conflict of interest None.

Ethical standards The patients gave their informed consent prior to being included in the study. The study was authorized by the local ethical committee and performed in accordance with the ethical standards of the 1964 Declaration of Helsinki as revised in 2000.

References

1. Weitzman G (1965) Lipoma arborescens of the knee: report of a case. J Bone Jt Surg [Am] 47-A:1030–1033
2. Hallel T, Lew S, Saba K, Bansal M (1988) Villous lipomatous proliferation of the synovial membrane (lipoma arborescens). J Bone Jt Surg [Am] 70-A:264–270
3. Teusink M, El-Khoury G, Buckwalter J (2010) Lipoma arborescens of the subdeltoid bursa: a case report. Iowa Orthop J 30:177–178
4. Hubscher O, Costanza E, Eisner B (1990) Chronic monoarthritis due to lipoma arborescens. J Rheumatol 17:861–862
5. Noel E, Tebib J, Dumontet C, Colson F, Carret J, Vauzelle J, Bouvier M (1987) Synovial lipoma arborescens of the hip. Clin Rheumatol 6:92–96
6. Siva C, Brasington R, Totty W, Sotelo A, Atkinson J (2002) Synovial lipomatosis (lipoma arborescens) affecting multiple joints in a patient with congenital short bowel syndrome. J Rheumatol 29:1088–1092
7. Sailhan F, Hautefort P, Coulomb A, Mary P, Damsin J (2011) Bilateral lipoma arborescens of the knee: a case report. J Bone Jt Surg Am 93:195–198

8. Azzouz D, Tekaya R, Hamdi W, Montacer Kchir M (2008) Lipoma arborescens of the knee. J Clin Rheumatol 14(6):370–372

9. Kim RS, Song JS, Park SW, Kim L, Park SR, Jung JH, Park W (2004) Lipoma arborescens of the knee. Arthroscopy 20:e95–e99

10. Finotti LT, Araújo DB, Vituli LF, Giorgi RD, Chahade WH (2011) Synovial lipoma arborescens. Acta Reumatol Port 36(2):171–175

11. Arzimanoglu A (1957) Bilateral arborescent lipoma of the knee. J Bone Jt Surg Am 39:976–979

12. Mestiri M, Kooli M, Charfi F (1996) Lipoma arborescens of the knee: contribution of X-ray computed tomography. A propos of a new case. Rev Chir Orthop Rep Appar Mot 82:340–343

13. Ensafdaran A, Vosoughi AR, Khozai A, Torabi A, Ensafdaran MR (2010) Lipoma arborescens of the knee: report of a case with full range of motion. Middle East J Cancer 1(1):51–54

14. Al-Ismail K, Torreggiani WC, Al-Sheikh F, Keogh C, Munk PL (2002) Bilateral lipoma arborescens associated with early osteo-arthritis. Eur Radiol 12:2799–2802

15. Cil A, Atay OA, Aydingöz U, Tetik O, Gedikoğlu G, Doral MN (2002) Bilateral lipoma arborescens of the knee in a child: a case report. Knee Surg Sports Traumatol Arthrosc 2005(13):463–467

16. Soler T, Rodríguez E, Bargiela A, Da Riba M (1998) Lipoma arborescens of the knee: MR characteristics in 13 joints. J Comput Assist Tomogr 22:605–609

17. Pandey T, Alkhulaifi Y (2006) Bilateral lipoma arborescens of the subdeltoid bursa. Australas Radiol 50:487–489

18. Kloen P, Keel SB, Chandler HP (1998) Lipoma arborescens of the knee. J Bone Jt Surg Br 80:298–301

19. Ryu KN, Jaovisidha S, Schweitzer M, Motta AO, Resnick D (1996) MR imaging of lipoma arborescens of the knee joint. AJR Am J Roentgenol 167:1229–1232

20. Howe BM, Wenger DE (2013) Lipoma arborescens: comparison of typical and atypical disease presentations. Clin Radiol 68(12):1220–1226. doi:10.1016/j.crad.2013.07.002

21. Sola JB, Wright RW (1998) Arthroscopic treatment for lipoma arborescens of the knee: a case report. J Bone Jt Surg Am 80(1):99–103

22. Lovane A, Sorrentino F, Pace L (2005) MR findings in lipoma arborescens of the knee: our experience. Radiol Med (Torino) 109:540–546

23. Xiao J, Xu Y, Wang J, Feng J, Shi Z (2011) Bilateral knee lipoma arborescens combined with osteoarthritis in elderly patients. J Int Med Res 39(4):1563–1569

24. Yan CH, Wong JW, Yip DK (2008) Bilateral knee lipoma arborescens: a case report. J Orthop Surg 16(1):107–110

25. Franco M, Puch JM, Carayon MJ, Bortolotti D, Albano L, Lallemand A (2004) Lipoma arborescens of the knee: report of a case managed by arthroscopic synovectomy. Jt Bone Spine 71:73–75

28

Low-grade periprosthetic knee infection: diagnosis and management

Michele Vasso · Alfredo Schiavone Panni

Abstract Diagnosis and management of low-grade periprosthetic knee infection are still controversial and debatable. The diagnosis of low-grade infection after total knee arthroplasty is often complex, as clinical symptomatology and diagnostic studies are highly conflicting and knees often exhibit well-fixed components. Although the criterion standard for staged reimplantation is interim placement of an antibiotic-loaded spacer, less-invasive surgical procedures have been advocated for managing infections caused by low-virulence bacteria. Debridement with polyethylene exchange and single-stage reimplantation could offer advantages, such as fewer surgeries, reduced potential for intraoperative complications, and lower direct social costs. The aim of this narrative review was to analyze the literature to evaluate the effectiveness of different surgical procedures in managing low-grade periprosthetic knee infections. Additionally, the most reliable investigations for diagnosing total knee infection caused by low-virulence bacteria were reviewed.
Level of evidence Level V.

Keywords Total knee arthroplasty · Low-grade infection · Diagnosis · Debridement · Reimplantation

Introduction

Infection continues to be a rare but devastating complication of total knee arthroplasty (TKA), occurring in 1–3 % of cases [1–5]. Despite the low incidence, infection is associated with patient morbidity, increased healthcare costs, and recurrence

M. Vasso (✉) · A. Schiavone Panni
Department of Medicine and Science for Health, University of Molise, Via Francesco De Sanctis, Campobasso, Italy
e-mail: vassomichele@gmail.com

and is also challenging to control [6]. TKA infections are often attributable to staphylococci and streptococci, whereas aerobic gram-negative bacteria cause 10–20 % of all infections and anaerobic bacteria are responsible for another 10 % [7]. Methicillin-sensitive staphylococci, streptococci, and anaerobic cocci are commonly considered as low-virulence bacteria causing low-grade periprosthetic infections; methicillin-resistant staphylococci, enterococci, and gram-negative organisms are certainly considered bacteria of high virulence due to their intrinsic resistance to antimicrobial agents and antibiotics [8]. The diagnosis of a TKA infection, itself very challenging, becomes highly complex in the presence of low-virulence organisms, as clinical features and diagnostic tests may be conflicting. Common clinical signs of infection are often absent, and a gold standard for preoperative diagnosis does not exist.

Whereas two-stage reimplantation is considered worldwide to be the most successful procedure in treating TKA infections, regardless of the etiology of the infecting organism(s) (and timing of infection) [2, 4, 6, 9–12], treatment of a low-grade prosthetic knee infection remains controversial and debatable. Less-invasive and more viable surgical procedures have been advocated for managing low-grade TKA infections (especially if early): debridement with insert exchange and single-stage reimplantation has the advantage of less surgery, ability to maintain motion and soft-tissue health, and lower costs. Furthermore, these procedures mean that the patient is never without prosthetic components, clearly improving comfort [1, 12–14]. Regardless of the virulence of the infecting organisms, debridement and component retention results in inconsistent infection control rates of 16–80 % [15], whereas single-stage revision, in which new, sterile components are implanted and secured with antibiotic-loaded bone cement, presents a large variability in successful infection control of

73–100 % [6, 15]. However, few data exist about the success rates of these different treatments strategies in TKA infections caused by low-virulence bacteria. Therefore, the purpose of this review was to analyze the literature to determine the most effective surgical treatment for managing low-grade periprosthetic knee infection. We also reviewed the most reliable investigations for diagnosing TKA infection caused by low-virulence bacteria.

Diagnosing low-grade periprosthetic knee infection

Diagnosing low-grade infection after TKA is often highly complex, as clinical symptomatology and diagnostic studies may be conflicting. Moreover, patients often present with well-fixed components, even in in acute infections. We believe the diagnostic process should be developed using the following steps.

History and clinical features

Early postoperative low-grade TKA infections generally present only with moderate knee pain and stiffness and/or difficult and delayed rehabilitation; persistent fever, severe pain, local warmth, erythema, and swelling are often absent. Hematogenous low-grade infection is quite rare and characterized by a sudden and unexpected deterioration in a previously well-functioning joint. There may also be a history of acute illness followed by sudden deterioration in knee function, with fever and chills [14, 16]. Chronic low-grade TKA infections do not show evident onset. Classic presentation with pain, fever, and local signs such as sinus tract, redness, and swelling is uncommon. More frequently, patients claim only moderate pain and stiffness, which exist since knee replacement [14, 16].

Radiographs

Standard X-rays are not very useful in the diagnosis of low-grade infection after TKA, particularly in acute infections in which X-rays are always normal. Radiographs showing periosteal new bone formation, scattered foci of osteolysis, and subchondral bone resorption are highly suggestive of infection but typically may be late findings. Periprosthetic radiolucency may be unrelated to a septic process, and serial radiographs help rule out other conditions, such as wear, osteolysis, or fracture [16].

Laboratory findings

Peripheral white blood cell (WBC) count is frequently normal in low-grade TKA infections and affords little diagnostic help [17]. Erythrocyte sedimentation rate (ESR) and C-reactive protein (CRP) remain the most useful laboratory investigation, even though their sensitivity may be diminished [19]. An ESR >30 mm/h or CRP >10 mg/L should be considered abnormal [7, 18]. Due to this lower sensitivity, serum interleukin-6 (IL-6) could represent a more reliable marker of periprosthetic low-grade infection [17, 19]. With a threshold of <10 pg/ml, serum IL-6 test shows sensitivity, specificity, positive predictive value (PPV), negative predictive value (NPV), and accuracy of 1.0, 0.95, 0.89, 1.0, and 97 %, respectively, thus being a more accurate marker than ESR and CRP [17, 19]. Due to its excellent sensitivity, IL-6 could be an optimal tool for diagnosing low-grade TKA infection [16, 19].

Radionucleotide scanning

Technetium-99 bisphosphonate scan in conjunction with indium-111-labeled leukocyte scan can contribute to the diagnosis of low-grade TKA infection. Technetium scan is quite reliable in detecting bone-remodelling changes around prosthetic components; however, when positive, it cannot distinguish between aseptic loosening and infection [22]. It has a low NPV in low-grade infections: a normal scan suggests that loosening is not the likely cause of pain, but it does not rule out the possibility of infection [16]. Leukocyte scan is more sensitive but has low specificity. Combining a leukocyte with a technetium scan improves the accuracy for detecting low-grade infection [16]. In particular, if uptake on leukocyte scan is more intense than on technetium scan, it is probable that the TKA is infected. Isotope scanning may present false-positive results: within the first postoperative year, increased scan activity may be present around 85–90 % of tibial and 60–65 % of femoral components in asymptomatic knees [23].

Aspiration

In the setting of a low-grade infection, knee aspiration could present poor sensitivity due to the low bacterial load. Antibiotic therapy must be suspended at least 2 weeks before aspiration to avoid further false-negative results [18]. The aspirate should be sent for aerobic, anaerobic, and fungal cultures. If the first aspirate is negative, then at least two additional aspirations should be performed [23]. Specimens obtained from the joint must be separated into two or three samples: if all samples are positive for the same organism, the aspiration is considered positive; if only one sample is positive or presents an unexpected positive result, aspiration must be repeated given the high suspicion of contamination [24]. Synovial-fluid WBC count and differential are two helpful parameters: cutoff values for optimal accuracy iare >1,100 cells/mm^3 for fluid leukocyte count and >64 % for neutrophil differential [25].

Molecular tests

The detection of bacterial DNA or RNA in synovial fluid using polymerase chain reaction (PCR) studies could be helpful in low-grade TKA infections in which bacterial load is low. PCR amplifies strains of bacterial (deoxy) RNA and can detect nonviable bacteria that do not grow on culture as well as bacteria lysed by ultrasonication, providing results within 12–13 h. Results of PCR are unaffected by the administration of antibiotics [16]. However, molecular techniques cannot distinguish between live or dead organisms, generating false-positive results (low specificity) and therefore being of little clinical utility [26].

Intraoperative histopathology

Gram staining of intraoperative specimens obtained from the joint capsule or periprosthetic membrane has been reported as being of little help in diagnosing low-grade TKA infection [27]. Intraoperative frozen section for identifying neutrophils in periprosthetic tissue is used to help intraoperative decision making. The exact histologic criteria used for diagnosing infection are not uniform. However, five to ten polymorphonuclear leukocytes per high power field ($\times 400$) (PMNs/HPF) in at least five fields is considered consistent with infection [7, 16]. This method is highly dependent on the tissue selected and interpretation by the pathologist. The poor sensitivity of this technique in low-grade infection is probably due to the low inflammatory response caused by coagulase-negative staphylococci, the organisms most commonly infecting TKA [7].

Sonication

At the time of prosthesis removal, sonication could improve sensitivity of microbiological investigations that, as mentioned above, is significantly diminished in low-grade infections [28]. Sonication uses ultrasound (US) energy to mechanically disrupt biofilm on removed implants following revision surgery. This increases the number of bacteria isolated on culture, or molecular techniques enabling detection of bacteria that would have been missed by conventional tissue culture [28]. Improvement in sensitivity is particularly notable in TKA infected by low-virulence organisms and in patients on antibiotics within 2 weeks prior to surgery [21].

Surgical management of low-grade periprosthetic knee infection

The goal of treatment is infection eradication and maintenance of a pain-free and functional joint. Different treatment options have been advocated: suppressive antibiotic therapy, irrigation and debridement, single-stage reimplantation, two-stage reimplantation, salvage procedures, and above-knee amputation. Whereas two-stage exchange is considered the best approach regardless of the infecting organism virulence and timing of infection [2, 4, 6, 9–12], optimal management of low-grade TKA infection remains controversial, as open debridement with insert exchange and single-stage reimplantation have been proposed as valid surgical alternatives with the least impact. Suppressive antibiotic therapy has been reserved for patients medically unable to undergo surgery, with limited success rates in low-grade infection [11, 16]. Salvage procedures, such as resection arthroplasty or arthrodesis, and amputation have never been necessary in TKA infected by sensitive bacteria [14]. Therefore, open debridement and single- and two-stage reimplantation are the only procedures reviewed in this paper.

Irrigation and debridement

In the setting of a low-grade TKA infection, debridement with component retention, and local and systemic antibiotic application could be indicated in healthy patients affected by acute (early postoperative and hematogenous) gram-positive infection with a stable and well-functioning prosthesis and good soft tissue envelope with no fistula [8, 28]. When attempting component retention, thorough debridement and rapid antibiotic treatment prior to the accumulation of biofilm are paramount for a successful outcome [16, 29, 30]. Contraindications are chronic infection, implant loosening, poor soft tissue envelope, and patients with other arthroplasties or a defective heart valve [16, 28]. Polyethylene exchange is always preferred, as it allows complete synovectomy and better debridement of the posterior synovium, and eliminates biofilm formation on the polyethylene [29, 31]. One reason for the failure of arthroscopic debridement is likely due to the inability to eliminate biofilm at the polyethylene–prosthesis interface and debride the posterior aspect of the knee [28, 29]. Intraoperative cultures are performed on synovial fluid and membrane, infected tissues, and polyethylene–implant interface. Organism-specific intravenous antibiotic application is initiated for 4–6 weeks, followed by protracted oral antibiotic administration.

Single-stage reimplantation

Low-grade infection after TKA has been considered to be potentially susceptible to a single-stage revision due to the low virulence of the infecting bacteria [5, 32, 33]. Factors associated with successful single-stage reimplantation include pathogen identification before revision, infections caused by gram-positive bacteria, absence of sinus tract, and use of antibiotic-loaded bone cement for new component fixation [34]. Single-stage reimplantation involves explantation of all components and cement, thorough debridement, copious irrigation, and reimplantation of new and appropriate prosthetic components with antibiotic-impregnated cement, followed by 6–12 weeks of systemic antibiotic therapy. Then, oral antibiotic therapy should be considered for 3–6 additional months based on recommendations [32]. In low-grade infection, single-stage revision may be advantageous, decreasing recovery time and costs and avoiding some of the problems of two-stage procedures, such as stiffness and arthrofibrosis resulting from a period with a spacer in situ. Furthermore, debridement and a single-stage strategy allows the patient to retain their prosthetic components [13].

Two-stage reimplantation

Two-stage reimplantation is actually considered state of the art for treating both acute and chronic TKA infections, with reported success rates of 88–96 % regardless the etiology of the infecting organism [2, 4, 6, 9–12]. During the first stage, removal of all components and cement, complete synovectomy, and debridement of all necrotic and infected tissue are performed. Multiple specimens are obtained from deep synovial biopsies and sent for aerobic, anaerobic, and fungal cultures. Resected bone ends and joint space are thoroughly irrigated with pulsatile lavage. Successively, an antibiotic-impregnated cement spacer is positioned into the joint [6, 12, 35, 36]. In low-grade infection, 2 g of vancomycin for a 40-g pack of bone cement could be sufficient [18, 37], as the majority of preformed spacers contain gentamicin. The choice of antibiotic should depend upon the antibiogram: in fact, even though virulence is low, antibiotic susceptibility might be low also [38]. Between stages, targeted intravenously and orally administered antibiotics are generally used for 6–12 weeks on the basis of recommendations of an infectious disease consultant [1, 10].

Decision for second-stage reimplantation is made after a minimum 2-week antibiotic-free interval, when clinical signs of infection have subsided and ESR and CRP levels have steadily trended toward to normal [18, 37]. In low-grade infection, laboratory markers may also normalize in patients with persistent infection, so that knee aspiration before reimplantation should be performed in patients with suspected persistent infection [18, 20, 39]. The second stage includes explantation of the cement spacer, removal of all cement fragments, thorough debridement of the joint and intramedullary canals, copious irrigation, and placement of the appropriate new prosthetic components fixed with vancomycin-impregnated bone cement [18, 40, 41].

After reimplantation, patients receive antibiotics intravenously until intraoperative cultures return to normal.

Results

In the setting of low-grade TKA infections, irrigation and debridement has shown unsatisfactory success rates, ranging on average from 16 % to 70 % [8, 14]. In acute (early postoperative or hematogenous) infections, primary open debridement is reported as successful in 56 % of patients infected by low-virulence organisms, such as *Staphylococcus epidermidis* or *Streptococcal* species, but only in 8 % of patients infected by *S. aureus* [42]. Assessing 247 knees, Buller et al. [31] reported an overall 45 % failure rate of debridement; higher failure rates were found in infections by resistant organisms and in patients with symptoms ≥ 21 days. A 34 % failure rate was also reported in low-grade infections. Barberan et al. [43] reported an overall debridement failure rate of 35 % in low-grade infections, which ranged from 17 % in patients with symptom duration <1 month to 69 % in patients with symptoms duration >6 weeks. Better results were reported when considering only early postoperative (and not hematogenous) infections: Kim et al. [44] reported that 27 of 32 knees (84 %) were treated successfully with perioperative debridement.

Certainly, debridement is reportedly unsuccessful for treating chronic low-grade infections, with a final failure rate of 100 % [8, 29, 45]. The most compelling evidence to discourage the use of debridement in low-grade infections is the 34 % failure rate of two-stage reimplantation after failed irrigation and debridement [8]. Fehring et al. [8] suggested limiting its use to early postoperative infections, in which the date of inoculation is well defined and perioperative debridement should improve infection control because intervention may occur before the establishment of drug-resistant biofilm on the implant or before osteomyelitis becomes entrenched in periprosthetic bone.

Reports related to single-stage revision are generally sparse and of poor quality [5]. Single-stage reimplantation has been successful in highly selected cases or small series, with an average success rate of 81 % [5, 12, 15]. In low-grade infections, reinfection rates are reported ranging from 5 % to 11, although in studies with small case series and short follow-ups [5, 11, 13, 34]. Silva et al. [34] reported a success rate of 89 % and found that factors associated with success are absence of sinus formation, gram-positive infection, use of antibiotic-impregnated bone cement in reimplantation, and 12 weeks of antibiotic therapy. Baker et al. [13] reported no significant differences between single- and two-stage revision in terms of postoperative knee score, general health perception, or satisfaction in patients with low-grade TKA infection. They concluded that single-stage treatment may be functionally superior in cases in which infection is successfully eradicated but be may be prone to higher rates of reinfection, which are associated with poorer outcomes. Singer et al. [5] reported that single-stage revision achieved a control rate of 95 % in low-grade TKA infections in which patients with methicillin-resistant *S. aureus* (MRSA), methicillin-resistant *S. epidermidis* (MRSE), or unknown microorganisms were excluded from the study. Higher rates of recurrent infection appeared to be associated with long-term chronic infections of hinged prostheses. Given the very limited number of reliable studies assessing the efficacy of single-stage reimplantation in eradicating low-grade infection following TKA, further investigations are warranted [12].

The success rates of two-stage reimplantation in eradicating infection and restoring function are almost constantly reported to be >90 %, regardless of the etiology of infecting organisms and the timing of infection [2, 4, 6, 9–12], so that this procedure is now considered the most reliable treatment option for infected TKA. Additionally, two-stage reimplantation is reported to be even more successful when used in low-grade TKA infections [2, 4, 9, 39, 46–48]. Volin et al. [48] reported a 94.6 % success rate in methicillin-sensitive *S. aureus* infections. Salgado et al. [47] reported a 17 % failure rate for treated MRSA infections, whereas no failures were noted among infections caused by methicillin-sensitive *S. aureus*. Cordero-Ampuero et al. [9] reported that infection was eradicated in 22 of 25 (88 %) patients infected by methicillin-resistant staphylococci and in 14 of 14 (100 %) infected by methicillin-sensitive staphylococci.

Conclusions

The diagnosis of a TKA infection, which in itself is highly challenging, may be extremely complex in the presence of low-virulence organisms. Clinical features are often conflicting, whereas classic presentation of pain, fever, and local signs such as sinus tract, redness, and swelling is uncommon. ESR and CRP levels remain the first-line investigation, even though the sensitivity of their results is often diminished in low-grade infections. In these cases, IL-6 levels should support ESR and CRP evaluation to significantly increase the sensitivity of the laboratory findings. Technetium and leukocyte scanning should both be used, and prosthesis sonication may help detect bacteria missed by conventional tissue culture. In patients with an acute postoperative low-grade infection, the strategy of irrigation and debridement with insert exchange persists given the emotional investment in dealing with this

complication by both patient and surgeon. Therefore, an attempt to "save the implant" through open debridement appears well intentioned despite a high reported failure rate. In the event of failed debridement or of chronic infections, resection of all components is necessitated. A single-stage exchange has the potential to decrease the number of surgeries and, subsequently, costs. However, infection eradication rates of direct exchange show this method is less safe and predictable than the two-stage revision. This suggests that two-stage reimplantation, with placement of an intrastage antibiotic-loaded spacer, should represent the gold standard for managing low-grade infections.

Conflict of interest   The authors declare that they have no conflict of interest.

References

1. Johnson AJ, Sayeed SA, Naziri Q, Khanuja HS, Mont MA (2012) Minimizing dynamic knee spacer complications in infected revision arthroplasty. Clin Orthop Relat Res 470:220–227
2. Kurd MF, Ghanem E, Steinbrecher J, Parvizi J (2010) Two-stage exchange knee arthroplasty: does resistance of the infecting organism influence the outcome? Clin Orthop Relat Res 468:2060–2066
3. Laudermilch DJ, Fedorka CJ, Heyl A, Rao N, McGough RL (2010) Outcomes of revision total knee arthroplasty after methicillin-resistant *Staphylococcus aureus* infection. Clin Orthop Relat Res 468:2067–2073
4. Siddiqui MM, Lo NN, Ab Rahman S, Chin PL, Chia SL, Yeo SJ (2013) Two-year outcome of early deep MRSA infections after primary total knee arthroplasty: a joint registry review. J Arthroplast 28:44–48
5. Singer J, Merz A, Frommelt L, Fink B (2012) High rate of infection control with one-stage revision of septic knee prostheses excluding MRSA and MRSE. Clin Orthop Relat Res 470:1461–1471
6. Jaekel DJ, Day JS, Klein GR, Levine H, Parvizi J, Kurtz SM (2012) Do dynamic cement-on-cement knee spacers provide better function and activity during two-stage exchange? Clin Orthop Relat Res 470:2599–2604
7. Bori G, Soriano A, Garcia S, Mallofrè C, Riba J, Mensa J (2007) Usefulness of histological analysis for predicting the presence of microorganisms at the time of reimplantation after hip resection arthroplasty for the treatment of infection. J Bone Joint Surg Am A 89:1232–1237
8. Fehring TK, Odum SM, Berend KR, Jiranek WA, Parvizi J, Bozic KJ, Della Valle CJ, Gioe TJ (2013) Failure of irrigation and débridement for early postoperative periprosthetic infection. Clin Orthop Relat Res 471:250–257
9. Cordero-Ampuero J, Esteban J, Garcia-Rey E (2010) Results after late polymicrobial, gram-negative, and methicillin-resistant infections in knee arthroplasty. Clin Orthop Relat Res 468:1229–1236

10. Kalore NV, Maheshwari A, Sharma A, Cheng E, Gioe TJ (2012) Is there a preferred articulating spacer technique for infected knee arthroplasty? A preliminary study. Clin Orthop Relat Res 470:228–235

11. Masters JP, Smith NA, Foguet P, Reed M, Parsons H, Sprowson AP (2013) A systematic review of the evidence for single stage and two stage revision of infected knee replacement. BMC Musculoskelet Disord 14:222

12. Romanò CL, Gala L, Logoluso N, Romanò D, Drago L (2012) Two-stage revision of septic knee prosthesis with articulating knee spacers yields better infection eradication rate than one-stage or two-stage revision with static spacers. Knee Surg Sports Traumatol Arthrosc 20:2445–2453

13. Baker P, Petheram TG, Kurtz S, Konttinen YT, Gregg P, Deehan D (2013) Patient reported outcome measures after revision of the infected TKR: comparison of single versus two-stage revision. Knee Surg Sports Traumatol Arthrosc 21:2713–2720

14. Chun KC, Kim KM, Chun CH (2013) Infection following total knee arthroplasty. Knee Surg Relat Res 25:93–99

15. Parvizi J, Zmistowski B, Adeli B (2010) Periprosthetic joint infection: treatment options. Orthopedics 33:659

16. Kalore NV, Gioe TJ, Singh JA (2011) Diagnosis and management of infected total knee arthroplasty. Open Orthop J 5:86–91

17. Berbari E, Mabry T, Tsaras G, Spangehl M, Erwin PJ, Murad MH, Steckelberg J, Osmon D (2010) Inflammatory blood laboratory levels as markers of prosthetic joint infection: a systematic review and meta-analysis. J Bone Joint Surg Am 92:2102–2109

18. Kusuma SK, Ward J, Jacofsky M, Sporer SM, Della Valle CJ (2011) What is the role of serological testing between stages of two-stage reconstruction of the infected prosthetic knee? Clin Orthop Relat Res 469:1002–1008

19. Garvin KL, Konigsberg BS (2012) Infection following total knee arthroplasty: prevention and management. Instr Course Lect 61:411–419

20. Ghanem E, Azzam K, Seeley M, Joshi A, Parvizi J (2009) Staged revision for knee arthroplasty infection: what is the role of serologic tests before reimplantation? Clin Orthop Relat Res 467:1699–1705

21. Savarino L, Tigani D, Baldini N, Bochicchio V, Giunti A (2009) Pre-operative diagnosis of infection in total knee arthroplasty: an algorithm. Knee Surg Sports Traumatol Arthrosc 17:667–675

22. Love C, Marwin SE, Palestro CJ (2009) Nuclear medicine and the infected joint replacement. Semin Nucl Med 39:66–78

23. Tsukayama DT, Goldberg VM, Kyle R (2003) Diagnosis and management of infection after total knee arthroplasty. J Bone Joint Surg Am 85A(Suppl 1):S75–S80

24. Neut D, Van Horn JR, Van Kooten TG, Van Der Mei HC, Busscher HJ (2003) Detection of biomaterial-associated infections in orthopaedic joint implants. Clin Orthop Relat Res 413:261–268

25. Ghanem E, Parvizi J, Burnett RS, Sharkey PF, Keshavarzi N, Aggarwal A, Barrack RL (2008) Cell count and differential of aspirated fluid in the diagnosis of infection at the site of total knee arthroplasty. J Bone Joint Surg Am 90:1637–1643

26. Bergin PF, Doppelt JD, Hamilton WG, Mirick GE, Jones AE, Sritulanondha S, Helm JM, Tuan RS (2010) Detection of periprosthetic infections with use of ribosomal RNA-based polymerase chain reaction. J Bone Joint Surg Am 92:654–663

27. Portillo ME, Salvadó M, Trampuz A, Plasencia V, Rodriguez-Villasante M, Sorli L, Puig L, Horcajada JP (2013) Sonication versus vortexing of implants for diagnosis of prosthetic joint infection. J Clin Microbiol 51:591–594

28. Choi HR, von Knoch F, Zurakowski D, Nelson SB, Malchau H (2011) Can implant retention be recommended for treatment of infected TKA? Clin Orthop Relat Res 469:961–969

29. Gardner J, Gioe TJ, Tatman P (2011) Can this prosthesis be saved?: implant salvage attempts in infected primary TKA. Clin Orthop Relat Res 469:970–976

30. Kuiper JW, Vos SJ, Saouti R, Vergroesen DA, Graat HC, Debets-Ossenkopp YJ, Peters EJ, Nolte PA (2013) Prosthetic joint-associated infections treated with DAIR (debridement, antibiotics, irrigation, and retention): analysis of risk factors and local antibiotic carriers in 91 patients. Acta Orthop 84:380–386

31. Buller LT, Sabry FY, Easton RW, Klika AK, Barsoum WK (2012) The preoperative prediction of success following irrigation and debridement with polyethylene exchange for hip and knee prosthetic joint infections. J Arthroplast 27:857–864

32. Gulhane S, Vanhegan IS, Haddad FS (2012) Single stage revision: regaining momentum. J Bone Joint Surg Br 94(11 Suppl A):120–122

33. Whiteside LA, Peppers M, Nayfeh TA, Roy ME (2011) Methicillin-resistant *Staphylococcus aureus* in TKA treated with revision and direct intra-articular antibiotic infusion. Clin Orthop Relat Res 469:26–33

34. Silva M, Tharani R, Schmalzried TP (2002) Results of direct exchange or debridement of the infected total knee arthroplasty. Clin Orthop Relat Res 404:125–131

35. Nettrour JF, Polikandriotis JA, Bernasek TL, Gustke KA, Lyons ST (2013) Articulating spacers for the treatment of infected total knee arthroplasty: effect of antibiotic combinations and concentrations. Orthopedics 36:19–24

36. Silvestre A, Almeida F, Renovell P, Morante E, López R (2013) Revision of infected total knee arthroplasty: two-stage reimplantation using an antibiotic-impregnated static spacer. Clin Orthop Surg 5:180–187

37. Hsu YC, Cheng HC, Ng TP, Chiu KY (2007) Antibiotic-loaded cement articulating spacer for 2-stage reimplantation in infected total knee arthroplasty: a simple and economic method. J Arthroplast 22:1060–1066

38. Martínez JL, Baquero F (2002) Interactions among strategies associated with bacterial infection: pathogenicity, epidemicity, and antibiotic resistance. Clin Microbiol Rev 15:647–679

39. Mittal Y, Fehring TK, Hanssen A, Marculescu C, Odum SM, Osmon D (2007) Two-stage reimplantation for periprosthetic knee infection involving resistant organisms. J Bone Joint Surg Am 89A:1227–1231

40. Panni AS, Vasso M, Cerciello S (2013) Modular augmentation in revision total knee arthroplasty. Knee Surg Sports Traumatol Arthrosc 21:2837–2843

41. Vasso M, Beaufils P, Schiavone Panni A (2013) Constraint choice in revision knee arthroplasty. Int Orthop 37:1279–1284

42. Deirmengian C, Greenbaum J, Stern J, Braffamn M, Lotke PA, Booth RE Jr, Lonner JH (2003) Open debridement of acute gram-positive infections after total knee arthroplasty. Clin Orthop Relat Res 416:129–134

43. Barberan J, Aguilar L, Carroquino G, Gimenez MJ, Sanchez B, Martinez D, Prieto J (2006) Conservative treatment of staphylococcal prosthetic joint infections in elderly patients. Am J Med 119:993.e7–10

44. Kim YH, Choi Y, Kim JS (2011) Treatment based on the type of infected TKA improves infection control. Clin Orthop Relat Res 469:977–984

45. Azzam KA, Seeley M, Ghanem E, Austin MS, Purtill JJ, Parvizi J (2010) Irrigation and debridement in the management of prosthetic joint infection: traditional indications revisited. J Arthroplast 25:1022–1027

46. Mortazavi SM, Vegari D, Ho A, Zmistowski B, Parvizi J (2011) Two-stage exchange arthroplasty for infected total knee arthroplasty: predictors of failure. Clin Orthop Relat Res 469:3049–3054

47. Salgado CD, Dash S, Cantey JR, Marculescu CE (2007) Higher risk of failure of methicillin-resistant *Staphylococcus aureus* prosthetic joint infections. Clin Orthop Relat Res 461:48–53

48. Volin S, Hinrichs S, Garvin K (2004) Two-stage reimplantation of total joint infections: a comparison of resistant and nonresistant organisms. Clin Orthop Relat Res 427:94–100

29

Assessment of functional treatment versus plaster of Paris in the treatment of grade 1 and 2 lateral ankle sprains

Muhammad Naeem · Muhammad Kazim Rahimnajjad ·
Nasir Ali Rahimnajjad · Zaki Idrees ·
Ghazanfar Ali Shah · Ghulam Abbas

Abstract

Background Despite the common occurrence of ankle sprains, no treatment is considered to be the gold standard for the management of such sprains. We assessed functional treatment versus plaster of Paris (POP) for the treatment of lateral ankle sprains, with pain and function employed as the outcome measures.

Materials and methods 126 Patients were eligible for inclusion. They were assigned to either the functional treatment Tubigrip (TG) group or the POP group after applying block randomization. Characteristics such as age, dominant ankle, and gender were assessed at baseline. Pain and functional assessments were done using the visual analog scale (VAS) and the Karlsson score (KS) at baseline (at the start of the study) and during the 2nd and 6th weeks, respectively. Data on other subjective parameters, such as the number of painkillers used, the number of days taken off work, and the number of sleepless nights, were requested from the patients at the end of the study. SPSS version 16 was used for analysis, and $p < 0.05$ was taken to indicate significance.

Results 60 Patients completed the trial in each group. The mean ages were 28.77 ± 6.72 in the TG group and 29.83 ± 6.30 in the POP group ($p = 0.034$). There was a slight female predominance. Right and left ankles were equally involved in the TG group, while left ankles were mainly involved in the POP group. Mean differences in VAS and KS between the two groups were statistically significant at the end of the study. The mean number of painkillers used by the patients in the TG group was higher than the number used in the POP group ($p < 0.001$). The mean number of days taken off work was 4.18 ± 1.73 days in the TG group, and 6.25 ± 2.73 days in the POP group ($p < 0.001$). The mean number of sleepless nights was higher in the POP group.

Conclusion The results of our study indicate that functional treatment provides better functional support and pain reduction than a below-knee POP cast.

Level of evidence Level I.

Keywords Ankle injury · Visual analog scale · Plaster of Paris

M. Naeem and M. K. Rahimnajjad contributed equally to this work.

ClinicalTrials.gov Identifier: NCT01499966.

M. Naeem (✉) · M. K. Rahimnajjad · N. A. Rahimnajjad ·
Z. Idrees · G. A. Shah · G. Abbas
B-8, Akbar Apartments, Bleak House Road, Civil Lines,
Cantt. Karachi, Karachi 74200, Pakistan
e-mail: dowgrad2012@gmail.com

Introduction

The recent emphasis of health professionals on physical fitness has resulted in decreases in morbidity and mortality but a rise in sports-related injuries [1, 2]. Ankle injuries, particularly ankle sprains, are the most common sports-related injuries, and are currently the reason for 3–5 % of all ER visits in the UK, and 10 % of them in the USA [3]. The mechanism of injury in a lateral ankle sprain may include inversion of the plantarflexed foot [2–4]. Crichton proposed the grading of these injuries based on ankle sprain severity [2].

The shibboleth RICE (rest, ice, compression, and elevation) is still used despite a lack of evidence for the benefit of compression. Conventional treatment includes early mobilization with weight bearing with or without the use of external support. External supports include tape, a brace, or elastic bandages, which are preferred to plaster of Paris (POP) because they gave better functional outcomes in previous studies [5]. A meta-analysis by Kerkhoffs and colleagues [6] showed no significant difference in the functional outcomes of cast immobilization and functional treatment. Contrary to the results obtained by Kerkhoffs, another study [7] provided evidence from a controlled clinical trial that a below-knee POP cast can increase the rate of healing of the sprained ankle, and they showed that cast immobilization was superior to other treatments during the first three months, but that with other functional treatments were equally effective after 9 months. Although no ankle sprain treatment is currently considered the gold standard, one survey found that functional treatment is being used by nearly 70 % of all doctors [8]. Studies also advocate that surgical management is a good option for sprains that result in instability, but this has not been shown to be superior over other treatments [9, 10].

Quality of life is another significant concern among these patients: while treatment may result in the resolution of symptoms, late manifestations in the form of recurrent sprains, pain, swelling, and instability may affect 30–50 % of such patients [2]. We hypothesized that functional treatment provides better resolution of pain and functionality than a below-knee POP cast; therefore, bearing in mind the treatment strategies currently being practiced, we assessed functional treatment versus POP for the treatment of lateral ankle sprains of grade 1 or 2, employing functionality and pain reduction as the outcomes of the study.

Materials and methods

This study was performed at the Department of Emergency and Trauma in a tertiary care teaching hospital from January 2011 until July 2011. During this period, 200 patients were enrolled after meeting the following inclusion criteria: grade 1 or 2 lateral ankle sprain (according to the Crichton classification, ankle sprains are grouped into three grades: I stretched ligaments (not torn), with a stable joint and a negative anterior drawer test; II partially torn ligament with a lax joint and a partially positive anterior drawer test; III complete ligament rupture with an unstable joint and a positive anterior drawer test [2]); <40 years of age for both sexes; presentation within 48 h of injury. Emergency radiographs were taken of both anteroposterior and lateral views to rule out any fractures. Only patients >18 years were included. Patients aged <18 years; those who presented >48 h after the injury; those with fractures, multiple injuries, any neurological or musculoskeletal illness, or any comorbidity associated with long-term disability; and non-local residents were excluded from the study. All patients gave their informed consent prior to

inclusion in the study. Only 126 patients agreed to participate in the study. After obtaining informed consent, the patients were randomized such that each patient was allocated to either a functional treatment (group A) or treatment with a plaster of Paris cast (group B). None of the patients opted for a particular treatment on their own; they were all assigned to the groups by the investigators using the block randomization technique. The standardized treatment based on the RICE (rest, ice, compression, and elevation) protocol was given to all patients. Either "TG" (denoting the functional treatment) or "POP" (for plaster of Paris) was written on each of 126 sheets of white paper which were placed in envelopes. The patients were allowed to pick the envelope of their choice. The authors were blinded until the opening of the envelopes by the patients. Each patient's usage of analgesia (in the form of paracetamol) was specifically noted. The patients in the TG group received the functional treatment and the patients in the POP group were given a below-knee plaster cast. Patients were followed up at 2 weeks and again at 6 weeks. The Karlsson score was noted at the time of presentation, as well as at 2 and 6 weeks. Pain was scored on the visual analog scale (VAS) at the time of presentation and again at 2 and 6 weeks. The CONSORT diagram for patient participation in the trial is shown in Fig. 1.

All information was gathered using a structured questionnaire in which characteristics such as age, dominant ankle, and gender were assessed at baseline. Pain and functional assessments were done using the visual analog scale and Karlsson score, respectively, at baseline and in the 2nd and 6th weeks. Data on other subjective parameters such as the number of painkillers used, the number of days taken off work, and the number of sleepless nights were requested from the patients at the end of the study. All data were analyzed using the Statistical Package for Social Sciences software (SPSS), version 16.0. Student's t test and chi square were used to assess the p value. $p < 0.05$ was taken to indicate significance. By setting Cohen's d to 0.5, the probability value to 0.05, and the sample size to 120, the power (calculated after the completion of the trial) of the study was found to be 85.93 % for a one-tailed hypothesis.

Results

Among the 120 patients who completed the study, 60 were assigned to the functional treatment group, and the other 60 to the POP group. The mean ± SD age of the patients in the TG group was 28.77 ± 6.72 years, and that of the patients in the POP group was 29.83 ± 6.30 years. The difference between the two groups was statistically significant ($p = 0.034$). Right and left ankles were equally

Fig. 1 CONSORT diagram

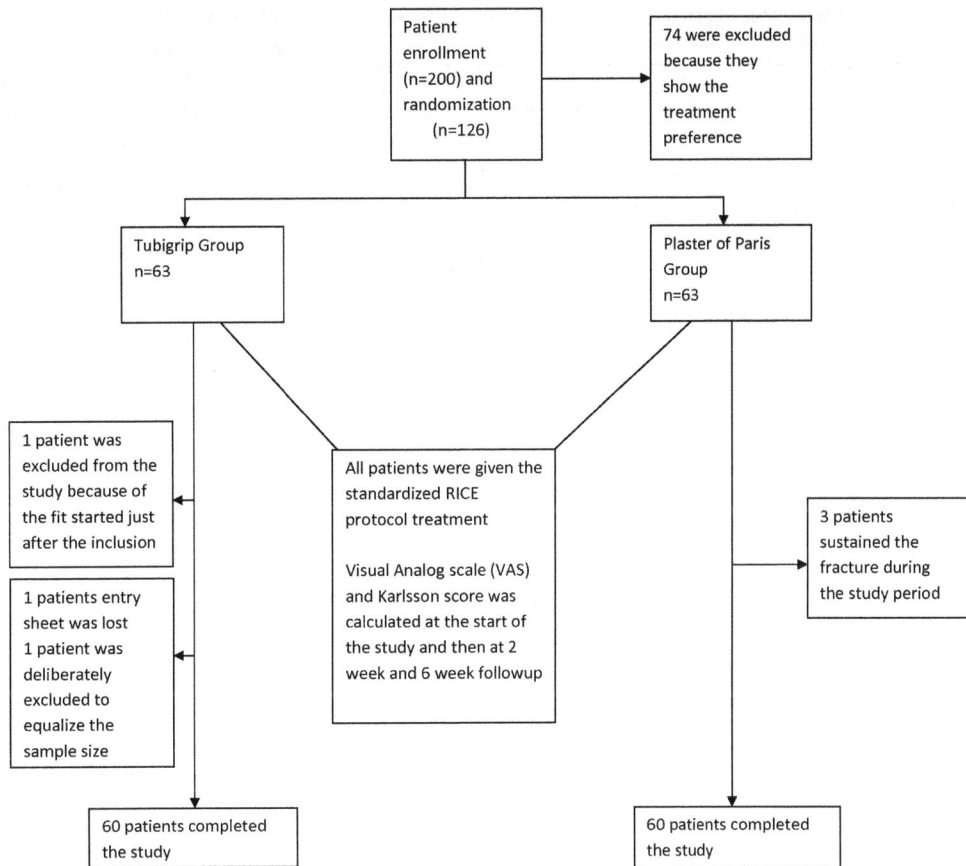

affected in the TG group (i.e., there were 30 right and 30 left ankles that were affected), while the dominant ankle involved was the left one in 39 patients in the POP group and the right one in 21 patients ($p < 0.001$). There was a slight female predominance in both groups (i.e., 35 in the TG group and 42 in the POP group), while the remaining patients were male; the significance level of this female predominance was $p < 0.001$.

The mean visual analog scale score at presentation was 8.40 ± 0.92 in the TG group and 8.27 ± 0.94 in the POP group. This difference in the scores of the groups was statistically nonsignificant ($p = 0.434$). The mean visual analog scale score at 2 weeks was 6.15 ± 0.75 in the TG group and 6.28 ± 0.11 in the POP group. This difference in the scores of the groups was statistically nonsignificant ($p = 0.376$). The mean visual analog scale score at 6 weeks was 3.88 ± 0.85 in the TG group and 4.97 ± 0.82 in the POP group. This difference in the scores of the groups was statistically significant ($p < 0.001$). The mean Karlsson score at presentation was 21.17 ± 6.31 in the TG group and 23.67 ± 5.24 in the POP group; this difference in the scores of the groups had a statistical significance of $p = 0.020$. The mean Karlsson score at 2 weeks was 52.03 ± 6.47 in the TG group and 52.37 ± 5.33 in the POP group. This difference in the scores of the groups was

Table 1 Pretreatment characteristics, visual analog scale scores, and Karlsson scores of the patients

Variable	TG	POP	p value
Age (years)	28.77 ± 6.72	29.83 ± 6.30	0.034*
Ankle			
Right	30	21	<0.001*
Left	30	39	
Sex			
Male	25	18	<0.001*
Female	35	42	
VAS at presentation	8.40 ± 0.92	8.27 ± 0.94	0.434
Karlsson score at presentation	21.17 ± 6.31	23.67 ± 5.24	0.571

VAS visual analog scale for pain, *TG* Tubigrip, *POP* plaster of Paris
* Denotes a statistically significant difference between the groups

statistically nonsignificant ($p = 0.759$). The mean Karlsson score at 6 weeks was 76.25 ± 10.67 in the TG group and 70.10 ± 6.35 in the POP group; the difference in the scores of the groups had a statistical significance of $p < 0.001$.

The mean number of painkillers used by the patients in the TG group was 6 ± 2.85, and it was 8 ± 2.58 in the POP group. The difference in the scores of the groups was statistically significant ($p < 0.001$). The mean number of

Table 2 Post-treatment characteristics, visual analog scale scores, and Karlsson scores of the patients

Variable	TG	POP	p value
VAS at 2 weeks	6.15 ± 0.75	6.28 ± 0.11	0.376
VAS at 6 weeks	3.88 ± 0.85	4.97 ± 0.82	<0.001*
Karlsson score at 2 weeks	52.03 ± 6.47	52.37 ± 5.33	0.759
Karlsson score at 6 weeks	76.25 ± 10.67	70.10 ± 6.35	<0.001*
Number of painkillers	6 ± 2.85	8 ± 2.58	<0.001*
Number of days taken off work	4.18 ± 1.73	6.25 ± 2.73	<0.001*
Number of sleepless nights	3.57 ± 1.56	5.45 ± 1.88	<0.001*

VAS visual analog scale for pain, *TG* Tubigrip, *POP* plaster of Paris

* Denotes a statistically significant difference between the groups

days taken off from work was 4.18 ± 1.73 days in the TG group and 6.25 ± 2.73 days in the POP group ($p < 0.001$). The mean number of sleepless nights was 3.57 ± 1.56 days in the TG group and 5.45 ± 1.88 days in the POP group. The difference in the scores of the groups had a significant p value of <0.001. All of these results are presented in tabulated form in Tables 1 and 2.

Discussion

The results of our study indicate that the functional treatment is a better treatment than a POP cast for lateral ankle sprains. We found that functional treatment provides better support in terms of pain reduction and provides more functional stability than a POP cast. Although many previous studies have compared one of the available treatments with another, none of them have provided sufficient evidence for the superiority of a particular treatment protocol, which may be the result of the use of poor study and assessment techniques. Cast immobilization, surgical repair, and functional treatments are considered the treatment options in the scientific literature [11, 12]. Cast immobilization utilizing a below-knee plaster cast is a double-edged sword, as it can help to speed up healing but can also result in functional impairment through muscle wasting (although evidence for such effects is lacking). A study by Lamb et al. [7] supports the usage of below-knee plaster cast immobilization. They found that functionality was improved at the 3-month interval when such a cast was used, but that all treatments (Aircast brace, Bledsoe boot, or 10-day below-knee cast and double-layer tubular compression bandage) were equally effective at the 9-month interval [7, 9, 10].

In our study, female patients were more affected. An epidemiological study from the United States [13] found that more sprains occurred between the ages of 10 and 19 years, while the mean affected age was higher in our study. The same study found that, among males, those between 15 and 24 years old were most commonly affected; among females, those >30 years old were most affected. Hosea and colleagues [14] found in their prospective study that grade 1 injuries were more prevalent among females, but the difference between the sexes was not statistically significant for grade 2 and 3 injuries. Both ankles were equally affected in the TG group, while left ankles were more likely to be affected in the POP group. Many studies have found that limb dominance does not manifest itself in ankle injuries, while one study found that limb dominance does indeed play a role in the injury mechanism [15].

The mean visual analog scale score was slightly higher in the TG group at the start of the study, while it was lower in the 2nd and 6th weeks. The difference between groups was statistically significant in the 6th week, showing that functional treatment is superior to POP in terms of pain reduction in patients with lateral ankle sprains. A prospective trial showed that patients treated with functional elastic wraps rather than cast immobilization experienced less pain in the third week (57 versus 87 %, $p = 0.02$) [16]. A meta-analysis showed that functional treatments provide better outcomes than immobilization when mild to moderate injuries were considered, but immobilization can speed up recovery from severe sprains [17].

The mean number of painkillers used by patients in the POP group was significantly higher than the mean number used by patients in the functional treatment group. One previous study found paracetamol to be just as effective as more potent NSAIDs at reducing pain [18]; considering the significant side effects of NSAIDs, paracetamol is therefore the better option. In our opinion, patients in the POP group may be more aware of their injuries, which was why more painkillers were consumed by that group. Hertel [19] found that painkillers along with the application of cold can reduce further injury caused by free radicals. These treatments can alleviate the pain and inflammation, but tissue repair requires a further period of 3 weeks. During this period, type III collagen replaces the type I collagen, increasing ligament strength, and the application of stress can aid proper fiber alignment. Other studies have also advocated proper muscular training after the injury [20, 21]. Since POP does not offer significant weight bearing, we believe that it may not aid proper healing.

As far as ankle rehabilitation is concerned, several studies have provided evidence that rehabilitation should improve the proprioception of the joints, thus reducing the rate of re-injury [22–24]. We found that the Karlsson scores were higher in the POP group at the start of the study, but they were significantly lower at the 6th week in the POP group when compared with the TG group. This might be because cast immobilization decreases functionality due to muscle wasting, although it contrasts with the findings of Lamb and colleagues [7], who advocated the use of a plaster cast due the resulting improved functional outcomes.

Our study found that the patients in the TG group required significantly fewer days off from work as compared to those in the POP group. Eiff and colleagues [16] also found that patients who underwent functional treatment returned to work earlier than those treated with cast immobilization (54 versus 13 %, $p < 0.001$). This indicates that ankle stability is not improved by immobilization. The management of acute sprains should consist of pain and swelling control along with range-of-motion exercises, including neuromuscular and strengthening exercises. Functionality is improved by early mobilization, and this leads to an earlier return to activities of daily life [25]. Many previous prospective studies have found that functional treatment is better at helping patients to maintain their mobility, which can strengthen the ankle joint and thus prevent further sprains [26–28]. Kerkhoffs and colleagues [29] found using an meta-analysis that functional treatment is superior to cast immobilization when treating sprains, but they further added that many of the trials reported so far were either of low quality or had high levels of bias.

Based on our results, and in the light of previous studies, we advocate that functional treatment provides better functional outcomes and pain reduction than POP. Given that its single-center setting is one of the main limitations of this study, a multi-center trial comparing the three treatment arms (functional treatment, plaster of Paris, and surgery) for all kinds of ankle sprains is needed. The other main limitation is the small observation period of this study, because we did not follow the patients beyond 6 weeks after the injury, which would have helped us to assess the long-term benefits of the treatments. At the end of the study, the patients were asked about their number of days off work, the number of painkillers they had used, and the number of sleepless nights they had endured, which may have a recall bias component. Finally, this was an unblinded study, which may also have influenced the outcomes.

Acknowledgments We are grateful to all of the participants in this study, as well as the paramedical staff of the Department of Orthopaedics, Liaquat National Hospital; without their help, this study could not have been conducted.

Conflict of interest The authors declare that they have no conflict of interest related to the publication of this manuscript.

Ethical standards The study was authorized by the local ethical committee and was performed in accordance with the ethical standards of the 1964 Declaration of Helsinki as revised in 2000. All of the enrolled patients provided their informed consent.

References

1. Fong DTP, Chan YY, Mok KM, Yung PSH, Chan KM (2009) Understanding acute ankle ligamentous sprain injury in sports. Sports Med Arthrosc Rehabil Ther Technol 1:14
2. Lamb SE, Nakash RA, Withers EJ, clark M, Marsh JL, Wilson S et al (2005) Clinical and cost effectiveness of mechanical support for severe ankle sprains: design of a randomised controlled trial in the emergency department. BMC Musculoskelet Disord 6:1
3. Wedmore IS, Charette J (2000) Emergency department evaluation and treatment of ankle and foot injuries. Emerg Med Clin North Am 18:85–113
4. Wolfe MW, Uhl TL, Mattacola CG, McCluskey LC (2001) Management of ankle sprains. Am Fam Physician 63:93–104
5. Ellen K, Van de Port I, Frank B, van Dijk Niek (2011) A systematic review on the treatment of acute ankle sprain: brace versus other functional treatment types. Sports Med 41:185–197
6. Kerkhoffs GMMJ, Rowe BH, Assendelft WJJ, Kelly KD, Struijs PAA, Niek van Dijk C (2001) Immobilisation for acute ankle sprain—a systematic review. Arch Orthop Trauma Surg 121:462–471
7. Lamb SE, Marsh JL, Hutton JL, Nakash R, Cooke MW, CAST Group (2009) Mechanical supports for acute, severe ankle sprain: a pragmatic, multicentre, randomised controlled trial. Lancet 373:575–581
8. Cooke MW, Lamb SE, Marsh J, Dale J (2003) A survey of current consultant practice of treatment of severe ankle sprains in emergency departments in the United Kingdom. Emerg Med J 20:505–507
9. Klenerman L (1998) The management of sprained ankle. Br J Bone Jt Surg 80:11–12
10. Povacz P, Salzburg M, Unger F et al (1998) A randomized, prospective study of operative and non-operative treatment of injuries of the fibular collateral ligaments of the ankle. J Bone Jt Surg 80:345–351
11. Boyce SH, Quigley MA, Campbell S (2005) Management of ankle sprains: a randomized controlled trial of the treatment of inversion injuries using an elastic support bandage or an air cast ankle brace. Br J Sports Med 39:91–96
12. Ogilvie-Harris DJ, Gilbart M (1995) Treatment modalities for soft tissue injuries of the ankle: a critical review. Clin J Sport Med 5:175–186
13. Waterman BR, Owens BD, Davey S, Zacchilli MA, Balmont PJ (2010) The epidemiology of ankle sprains in the United States. J Bone Jt Surg Am 92:2279–2284
14. Hosea TM, Carey CC, Harrer MF (2000) The gender issue: epidemiology of ankle injuries in athletes who participate in basketball. Clin Orthop 372:45–49
15. Beynnon BD, Murphy DF, Alosa DM (2000) Predictive factors for lateral ankle sprains: a literature review. J Athl Train 37:376–380
16. Eiff MP, Smith AT, Smith GE (1994) Early mobilization versus immobilization in the treatment of lateral ankle sprains. Am J Sports Med 22:83–88

17. Seah R, Mani-Babu S (2011) Managing ankle sprains in primary care: what is best practice? A systematic review of the last 10 years of evidence. Br Med Bull 97:105–135

18. Lyrtzis C, Papadopoulos C, Natsis K, Noussios G (2011) The effect of diclofenac sodium and paracetamol on active and passive range of motion after sprains. J Hum Sport Exerc 6:40–48

19. Hertel J (1997) The role of nonsteroidal anti-inflammatory drugs in the treatment of acute soft tissue injuries. J Athl Train 32:350–358

20. Bleakley C, McDonough Suzanne M, MacAuley Domhnall C (2008) Some conservative strategies are effective when added to controlled mobilisation with external support after acute ankle sprain: a systematic review. Aust J Physiother 54:7–20

21. Ashton-Miller JA, Ottaviani RA, Hutchinson C, Wojtys EM (1996) What best protects the inverted weight-bearing ankle against further inversion. Am J Sports Med 24:800–809

22. Uh BS, Beynnon BD, Helie BV, Alosa DM, Renstrom PA (2000) The benefit of a single-leg strength training program for the muscles around the untrained ankle. Am J Sports Med 28:568–573

23. Eils E, Rosenbaum D (2001) A multi-station proprioceptive exercise program in patients with ankle instability. Med Sci Sports Exerc 33:1991–1998

24. Matsusaka N, Yokoyama S, Tsurusaki T, Inokuchi S, Okita M (2001) Effect of ankle disk training combined with tactile stimulation to the leg and foot on functional instability of the ankle. Am J Sports Med 29:25–30

25. Denegar CR, Miller SJ III (2002) Can chronic ankle instability be prevented? Rethinking management of lateral ankle sprains. J Athl Train 37:430–435

26. McKay GD, Goldie PA, Payne WR, Oakes BW (2001) Ankle injuries in basketball: injury rate and risk factors. Br J Sports Med 35:103–108

27. Surve I, Schwellnus MP, Noakes T, Lombard C (1994) A fivefold reduction in the incidence of recurrent ankle sprains in soccer players using the sport-stirrup orthosis. Am J Sports Med 22:601–606

28. Sitler MR, Ryan J, Wheeler B et al (1994) The efficacy of a semirigid ankle stabilizer to reduce acute ankle injuries in basketball: a randomized clinical study at West Point. Am J Sports Med 22:454–461

29. Kerkhoffs GMMJ, Rowe BH, Assendelft WJJ, Kelly KD, Struijs PAA, van Dijk CN (2002) Immobilisation and functional treatment for acute lateral ankle ligament injuries in adults. Cochrane Database Syst Rev 3:CD003762

30

Carpometacarpal dislocation of the thumb associated with fracture of the trapezium

Ozkan Kose · Mert Keskinbora · Ferhat Guler

Abstract Carpometacarpal dislocation (CMC) of the thumb associated with fracture of trapezium is an extremely rare injury, with only 12 cases that sustained similar injuries reported in the literature. In this article, another patient with this rare injury was reported, and all previously published cases were extensively reviewed. The presented case and all previously published cases had a longitudinally oriented trapezium fracture, which is naturally unstable and almost always associated with dislocation of the CMC joint. In contrast to previous descriptions, we believe that CMC joint dislocation and trapezium fracture are not two distinct pathologies that occur simultaneously by chance but share cause and consequence.

Keywords CMC dislocation · Trapezium fracture · Trapeziometacarpal fracture–dislocation

Introduction

Pure carpometacarpal (CMC) dislocations of the thumb are rare injuries that account for <1 % of all hand injuries [1]. However, these injuries frequently occur in conjunction with avulsion of the metacarpal base due to thick and strong volar ligamentous attachments, the so-called Bennett's fracture–dislocation [1–4]. On the other hand, CMC

O. Kose (✉) · F. Guler
Department of Orthopaedics and Traumatology, Antalya Education and Research Hospital, Kultur mah. 3025 sk. Durukent Sit. F Blok Daire 22, Kepez, Antalya, Turkey
e-mail: drozkankose@hotmail.com

M. Keskinbora
Faculty of Medicine, Department of Orthoapedics and Traumatology, Medipol University, Istanbul, Turkey

dislocation of the thumb associated with fracture of trapezium is an extremely rare injury. To the best of our knowledge, only a few cases of the combination of such injuries are reported in English literature (Table 1) [5–15]. The purpose of this report is to describe a patient with CMC dislocation of the thumb associated with fracture of trapezium and to discuss anatomy, mechanism of injury, treatment options, and outcomes in light of current literature.

Case report

A 26-year-old electrician was involved in a motorcycle accident and brought to our emergency department. He complained of pain, swelling, and functional impairment of his left thumb. On physical examination, there was edema and tenderness over the thenar area (Fig. 1). Dorsoradial subcutaneous prominence was palpated at the base of right thumb. Thumb movements were restricted and painful in all directions. Neurovascular examination was normal. Anteroposterior and oblique hand radiographs revealed CMC dislocation of the thumb associated with trapezium fracture (Fig. 2).

With the patient under conscious sedation, closed reduction was achieved by applying distraction to the thumb, followed by volarly directed pressure over the base of the thumb metacarpal. During reduction, a palpable click was felt, and the dorsoradial bony prominence disappeared. The thumb was immobilized in a plaster cast, and postreduction radiographs confirmed concentric relocation of the joint and the fracture without a significant step in the articular surface (Fig. 3). Immobilization continued for 6 weeks, and the patient was referred for physiotherapy. After cast removal, passive and active range of motion (ROM) exercises were started immediately and encouraged.

Table 1 Previously published cases in the English literature of carpometacarpal (CMC) dislocation of the thumb associated with trapezium fracture

References	Sex	Age (years)	Mechanism of injury	Trapezium fracture classification	Treatment	Follow-up (months)	Result
Tolat and Jones [7]	Male	14	Fall onto an outstretched hand (skateboard)	IIa	Closed reduction splinting 6 weeks	2	Excellent without instability, full ROM
Mody and Dias [14]	Male	24	Motorbike accident	IIa	Open reduction and K-wire fixation; ligament reconstruction	6	Excellent
Kukreti and Harrington [13]	Not reported	26	Sport injury (rugby tackling)	IIa	Closed reduction and K-wire fixation	12	Slight pain, minimal loss of CMC flexion of CMC
Garavaglia et al. [11]	Female	20	Fall while holding the handle of a bucket	IIa	Open reduction and screw fixation	12	Excellent
Garneti and Tuson [9]	Male	24	Sport injury (rugby tackling)	IV	Open reduction and internal fixation with a minifragment 2.7-mm lag compression screw	12	Excellent
	Male	18	Sport injury (rugby)	IV	Open reduction and internal fixation with a single 2.7-mm lag screw	9	Excellent
Afshar and Mirzatoloei [6]	Male	30	Motorbike accident	IIa	Closed reduction and K-wire fixation	Not reported	No pain and instability, full ROM
Parker et al. [10]	Male	12	Fall onto an outstretched hand (rollerblade)	IIa	Closed reduction, spanning external fixation	36	Excellent
Morizaki and Miura [15]	Male	31	Fall onto flexed thumb	IIa	Open reduction and internal fixation using suture anchor and K-wire fixation	12	Excellent
Chamseddine et al. [5]	Male	23	Road accident	IV	Open reduction and K-wire fixation	9	Excellent
Ramoutar et al. [12]	Male	27	Fall onto an outstretched hand (football)	IIa	Closed reduction and K-wire fixation	6	Excellent
Mumtaz and Drabu [8]	Male	14	Direct trauma due to hammer hit (open injury)	IV	Irrigation, debridement, and K-wire fixation	12	Gross impairment in opposition and abduction
This case	Male	32	Motorbike accident	IIa	Closed reduction and splinting for 6 weeks	6	Excellent

ROM range of motion

To strengthen thumb grip and pinch, the patient was advised to clench a sponge ball as many times as possible. At the final follow-up 6 months after initial injury, the patient had gained full ROM in the CMC joint, without pain or instability. Final hand radiographs displayed a congruent CMC joint and trapezium fracture union (Fig. 4).

Discussion

Although the thumb CMC joint has wide ROM, which goes from extension through abduction to flexion, it is a highly stable joint. Integrity between mobility and stability is essential for performing an effective key pinch and grasp [5]. Thumb CMC joint stability is provided by several structures, including the joint capsule, dorsal and volar ligaments, tendons transpassing the joint, and the saddle-shaped trapeziometacarpal (TMP) joint configuration [3, 4]. Four main ligamentous structures are accepted to be the primary source of static stability: anterior oblique ligament (AOL), intermetacarpal ligament, radial collateral ligament (RCL), and palmar oblique ligament [3]. Several biomechanical and cadaver studies investigating the contribution of these ligaments to thumb stability and preventing

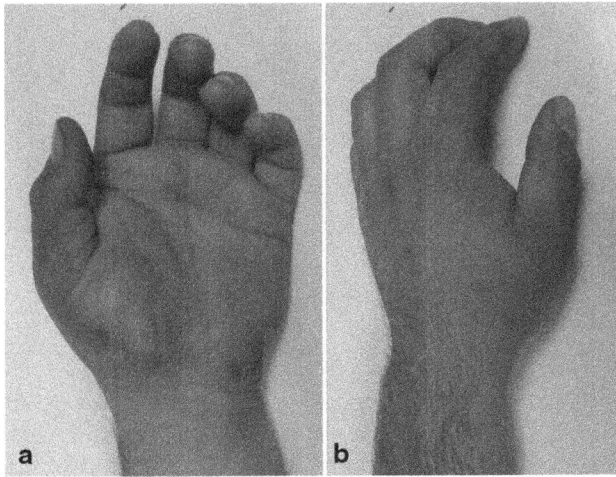

Fig. 1 Volar (a) and dorsal (b) appearance at presentation

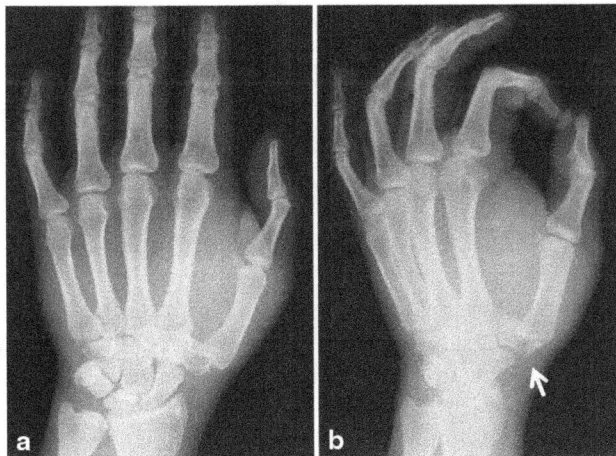

Fig. 3 Postreduction radiograph of the carpometacarpal (CMC) joint showing adequate reduction and a congruent joint

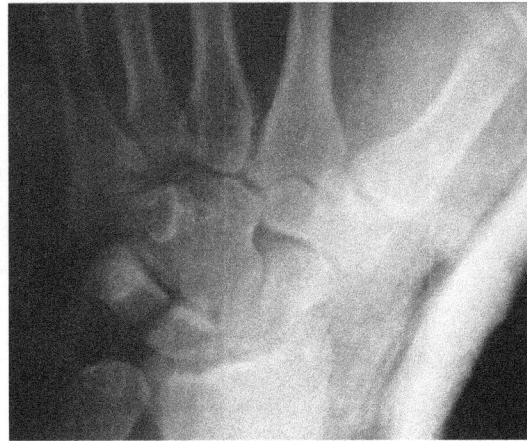

Fig. 2 Anteroposterior (a) and oblique (b) radiographs. *White arrow* trapezium fracture

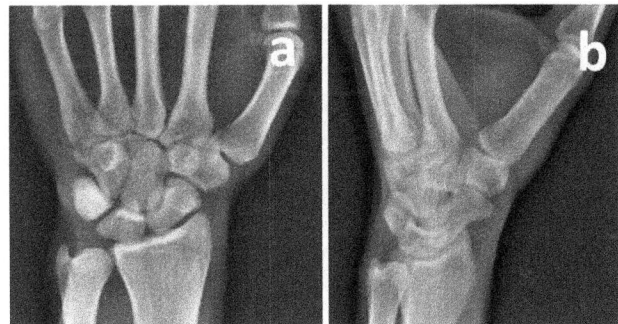

Fig. 4 Final hand radiographs 6 months after injury

dorsoradial dislocation of the TMP joint showed that RCL is the primary restraint against dorsal dislocation [1–4].

Two different mechanism of injury have been proposed for CMC dislocation and associated fractures of the trapezium [1, 2, 16]. According to the first mechanism of injury, CMC dislocation of the thumb occurs from axial loading on a flexed thumb metacarpal, which drives the metacarpal base dorsally over the trapezium and ruptures the RCL. TCL rupture results in dorsal dislocation, which may be a pure dislocation without any accompanying fracture [2]. In pure CMC dislocations, the AOL is also torn or stripped subperiosteally. During this injury, if AOL avulses a piece of bone fragment from the base of the first metacarpal, Bennett's fracture–dislocation occurs [6]. In some instances, a vertical split fracture of the trapezium may occur, with the pullout effect of the intact RCL and axial loading of the metacarpal base on the trapezium. In

the second proposed mechanism of injury, a commissural shearing produced by the impact of an object against the first web space causes CMC joint dislocation. This type of injury may happen with a fall while grasping an object, or if the individual is thrown forward while holding the handlebar of a motorcycle. Varying impact angles result pure CMC dislocation, Bennett's fracture–dislocation, or a trapezium fracture. If the vector of the force passes toward the trapezium, a trapezium fracture will occur [16]. Our patient was involved in a motorcycle accident and was thus more likely to be injured by commissural shearing forces produced by one of the handlebars during the collision. Other than these mechanisms of injuries, direct trauma (hit by a heavy hammer), fall onto an outstretched hand, and sporting injuries, have been reported in published cases [7–10].

Trapezium fractures are rare injuries and comprise about 3 % of all carpal bone fractures [16]. In 1988, Walker et al. classified trapezium fractures into five different fracture patterns in a series of ten cases (Fig. 5). Most reported cases with a combination of thumb CMC dislocation and trapezium fracture presented as types IIa, IIb, or IV

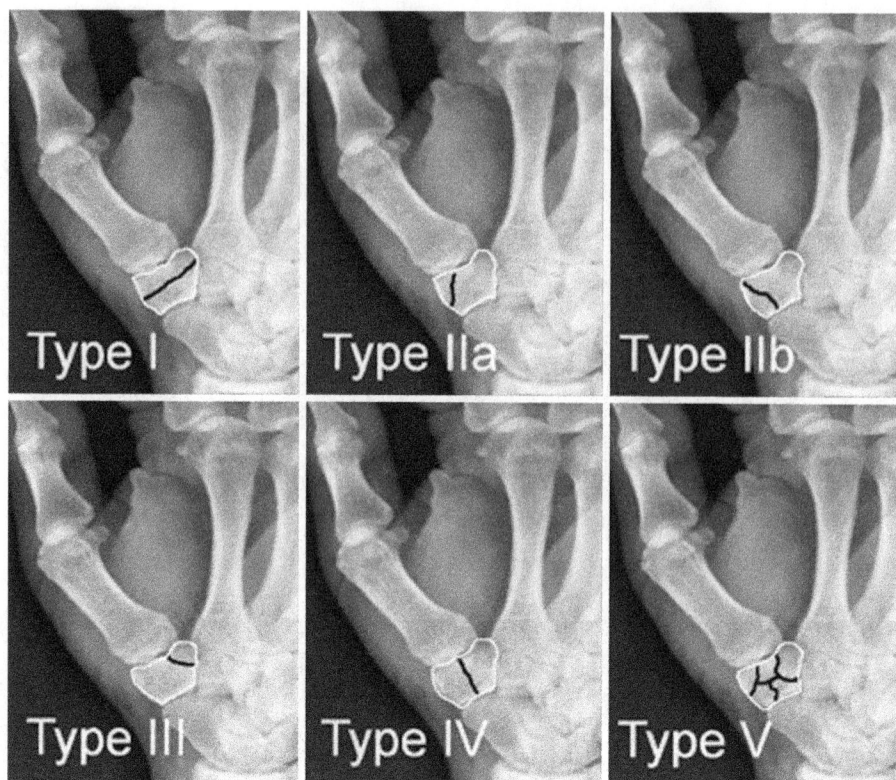

Fig. 5 Classification of trapezium fractures by Walker et al. [16]. *Black lines* show the fracture

(longitudinally oriented trapezium fractures). Similarly, in the series presented by Walker et al., types IIb and IV were simultaneous thumb CMC dislocations. Therefore, it appears that types IIa, IIb, and IV fractures are almost always accompany by thumb CMC dislocation. Garavaglia et al. [11] described this injury as transtrapezium carpometacarpal dislocation of the thumb, which seems to be the appropriate nomenclature for this specific injury.

Isolated nondisplaced trapezium fractures may be missed on direct radiographs due to overlapping adjacent bones, particularly on anteroposterior hand radiographs. In addition to meticulous physical examination and standard anteroposterior and oblique hand X-rays; a true anteroposterior view of the CMC joint of the thumb (Robert's view) with full pronation of the thumb is an effective imaging technique by which to visualize these fractures. In case of suspicion, CT imaging can be utilized for further detailed demonstration [12]. However, CMC dislocation associated with a trapezium fracture is usually evident, and there are only two cases which were initially missed the emergency department [11, 13]. Dorsoradial shift of the metacarpal, positive stress views and comparison with contralateral normal hand will be useful in confirming the subtle dislocations of the CMC joint. With an obvious dislocation of the thumb, attention must be paid for associated injuries including Bennett's fracture-dislocation or trapezium fracture.

Several treatment methods are reported in the literature, ranging from closed reduction and cast immobilization to open reduction and ligamentous reconstruction, as summarized in Table 1. Usually, the dislocation can be reduced easily by thumb traction and abduction while gently pushing the metacarpal base medially [7, 13]. Nevertheless, the major factor affecting treatment outcome is reduction adequacy and maintenance. In this combination of injury, the RCL remains intact; therefore, if the joint is stable and reduction quality is good after closed manipulation, a thumb spica cast may be chosen [7]. Thumb extension and slight pronation in the cast allows approximation of the stripped AOL and may enable ligamentous healing while contributing the joint stability [10]. If conservative treatment is preferred, the patient should be checked for any radiological signs of reduction loss, particularly during the first 2 weeks after the injury. Serial radiographic follow-up is advocated to monitor the reduction quality achieved at initial reduction. Tolat et al. reported excellent outcome after conservative treatment in a skeletally immature patient (14 years old) [7]. Although, our patient was an adult, conservative treatment yielded an excellent outcome. However, closed reduction and percutaneous pin fixation seems to be a more appropriate treatment method, as it is both minimally invasive and safe against loss of reduction during follow-up. We believe that extensive surgery, such as ligamentous reconstruction using tendon grafts, is overtreatment, because trapezium union and AOL healing provide adequate joint stability [6, 17].

As the follow-up period for reported cases is short (mean 11.1 months, range 2–36 months), it is difficult to comment on long-term consequences and prognosis, particularly the development of posttraumatic osteoarthritis. Theoretically, inadequate TMP joint reduction or trapezium malunion that leads to incongruency of the articular surface leads to osteoarthritis and loss of thumb function in the long term [16]. However, all reported cases expect one, a severe crush injury, resulted in good and excellent outcomes.

In conclusion thumb CMC dislocation associated with trapezium fracture is a rare injury, with few reported cases to date. Probable mechanism of injury is either axial loading on a flexed thumb or commissural shearing forces acting on the first web space. Radiographic evaluation of these patients should be done carefully to prevent missed diagnosis. Closed reduction and percutaneous K-wire fixation is sufficient to obtain a stable joint and promote proper ligamentous and bony healing. Although long-term follow-up is not available, prognosis is excellent in the short term.

Conflict of interest None.

Ethical standards The patient gave informed consent for publication of his medical records prior being included into this case study.

References

1. Bosmans B, Verhofstad MH, Gosens T (2008) Traumatic thumb carpometacarpal joint dislocations. J Hand Surg Am 33(3):438–441
2. Fotiadis E, Svarnas T, Lyrtzis C, Papadopoulos A, Akritopoulos P, Chalidis B (2010) Isolated thumb carpometacarpal joint dislocation: a case report and review of the literature. J Orthop Surg Res 5:16. doi:10.1186/1749-799X-5-16
3. Van Brenk BRR, Mackay MB, Boynton EL (1998) A biomechanical assessment of ligaments preventing dorsoradial subluxation of the trapeziometacarpal joint. J Hand Surg Am 23(4):607–611
4. Pagalidis T, Kuczynski K, Lamb DW (1981) Ligamentous stability of the base of the thumb. Hand 13:29–36
5. Chamseddine A, Hamdan H, Zein H, Obeid B, Tabsh I (2009) Fracture of trapezium with trapeziometacarpal subluxation. Eur J Orthop Surg Traumatol 19:499–503
6. Afshar A, Mirzatoloei F (2006) Carpometacarpal joint dislocation of the thumb associated with the fracture of the trapezium. Arch Iran Med 9(3):282–283
7. Tolat AR, Jones MW (1990) Carpometacarpal dislocation of the thumb associated with fracture of the trapezium. Injury 21(6):411–412
8. Mumtaz MU, Drabu NA (2009) Open complete dislocation of trapezium with a vertically split fracture: a case report. Cases J 2:9092
9. Garneti N, Tuson CE (2004) Sagittally split fracture of trapezium associated with subluxated carpo-metacarpal joint of thumb. Injury 35:1172–1175
10. Parker WL, Czerwinski M, Lee C (2008) First carpal-metacarpal joint dislocation and trapezial fracture treated with external fixation in an adolescent. Ann Plast Surg 61(5):506–510
11. Garavaglia G, Bianchi S, Santa DD, Fusetti C (2004) Transtrapezium carpo-metacarpal dislocation of the thumb. Arch Orthop Trauma Surg 124(1):67–68
12. Ramoutar DN, Katevu C, Titchener AG, Patel A (2009) Trapezium fracture—a common technique to fix a rare injury: a case report. Cases J 2:8304
13. Kukreti S, Harrington P (2004) Carpometacarpal joint dislocation of the thumb associated with fracture of the trapezium: a case report. Eur J Orthop Surg Traumatol 14(1):38–39
14. Mody BS, Dias JJ (1993) Carpometacarpal dislocation of the thumb associated with fracture of the trapezium. J Hand Surg Br 18(2):197–199
15. Morizaki Y, Miura T (2009) Unusual pattern of dislocation of the trapeziometacarpal joint with avulsion fracture of the trapezium: case report. Hand Surg 14(2–3):149–152
16. Walker JL, Greene TL, Lunseth PA (1998) Fractures of the body of the trapezium. J Orthop Trauma 2(1):22–28
17. El Ibrahimi A, Amar F, Chbani B, Daoudi A, Elmrini A, Boutayeb F (2009) Dislocation of the carpometacarpal joint of the thumb associated with trapezium and Bennett's fractures. Hand (N Y) 4(2):191–193

31

Influence of coincident distal radius fracture in patients with hip fracture: single-centre series and meta-analysis

C. E. Uzoigwe · M. Venkatesan · N. Johnson ·
K. Lee · S. Magaji · L. Cutler

Abstract

Background Hip and wrist fractures are the most common orthopaedic injuries. Combined hip and distal radius fractures are an important clinical and public health problem, since mobilisation and rehabilitation is challenging and likely to be prolonged in this setting. Few studies have explored the influence of an associated wrist fracture in patients with hip fracture. We present the largest series of patients with concomitant hip and wrist fractures. We perform the first meta-analysis of the literature on patients with concurrent hip and wrist fractures.
Material and methods In this single-centre retrospective study we compared 88 consecutive patients with simultaneous hip and wrist fractures with 772 consecutive patients who suffered isolated hip fractures.
Results Patients with the combined fracture were of a similar age compared to those with isolated hip fracture. There were a significantly higher proportion of women in the cohort with both hip and wrist fractures (female:male ratio of 9:1 versus 4:1 $p < 0.0001$). The combination fracture group had a greater length of hospitalisation (18 vs 13 days $p < 0.0001$). The survivorship of both groups was not significantly different even after adjustment for age and gender. Meta-analysis of the literature showed female preponderance, increased length of stay but no significant difference in survival in patients with concomitant hip and wrist fractures.
Conclusion The combination fracture occurs much more commonly in women and patients require a greater length of hospitalisation. The patients who sustained simultaneous hip and wrist fractures experienced no statistically significant difference in survivorship when compared to those who suffer isolated hip fractures. This is not withstanding the presence of two fractures. This difference in mortality did not reach statistical significance.
Level of evidence Level III (retrospective comparative study).

Keywords Concomitant fracture · Hip · Wrist · Distal radius · Fracture · Mortality · Outcome

Introduction

In England and Wales, the National Institute for Health and Clinical Excellence guidance on the management of patients with hip fractures reflects the ascendancy this injury has achieved in recent years over other injuries [1]. The hip fracture is arguably the most clinically significant fracture treated by the orthopaedic surgeon, given the high mortality associated with the injury. The wrist fracture is one of the most common fractures treated by the orthopaedic community. Few studies have explored the outcome of wrist fractures associated with neck of femur fractures. The purpose of the study is to compare the mortality of patients who sustain simultaneous hip and distal radius fractures to those who suffer isolated hip fractures.

Materials and methods

Clinical study

We identified all patients presenting to our unit with concomitant hip and wrist fractures between July 2004 and

C. E. Uzoigwe · M. Venkatesan (✉) · N. Johnson · K. Lee ·
S. Magaji · L. Cutler
Department of Trauma and Orthopaedics, University Hospitals
of Leicester, Infirmary Square, Leicester LE1 5WW, UK
e-mail: muraliv@doctors.org.uk

April 2011. We recorded the length of stay and date of mortality. We collected and compared similar data on patients presenting to our institution with isolated hip fracture between January 2010 and December 2010. Demographic data and information relating to the injury was collected, including the laterality of fracture for both groups. Our analysis looked retrospectively at outcomes for a large cohort of patients treated.

Normality testing was performed with the Shapiro–Wilk test. Normally distributed data was compared with the two-sample t-test. Non-parametric data underwent analysis with the Mann–Whitney U test. Nominal data was compared using Fisher's exact test. The 95 % confidence interval for proportions was calculated using standard methods. Cox's proportional hazards ratio was used to determine the effect of concomitant wrist fracture in patients with hip fracture while adjusting for age and gender.

Meta-analysis

A PubMed search was performed to conduct the meta-analysis. Search terms were the MeSH term (neck of femur fracture) in combination with "wrist", "upper limb" or "distal radius". An iterative process was then used with the papers identified and their references. Meta-analysis was performed by pooling numerical data. When values were heterogeneous, in particular when combining data regarding early mortality, where some studies looked at in-hospital mortality and others recorded 30-day mortality, the random effects model was used.

Results

Clinical study

Of the 5,164 patients presenting to our unit with hip fracture between July 2004 and April 2011, we identified 88 patients with concomitant hip and distal radius fractures. The injuries were ipsilateral in 91 % (80) and contralateral in only 9 % (8). There were 9 men and 79 (89 %) women. The mean age was 79 years (range 26–99). Most (16 %) of the patients with combined hip fractures presented in 2010.

The control group thus consisted of all the patients presenting to our unit from January 2010 to December 2010. Seven hundred and seventy-two patients with isolated hip fractures were identified presenting to our unit in the relevant time frame (January 2010–December 2010). There were 532 (69 %) women and 240 men. The mean age was 80 years (range 22–105). There was a statistically significant difference in gender distribution between the isolated hip fracture and combination hip and wrist fracture

Table 1 Comparison of patients with isolated fracture and combination hip and wrist fractures

	Isolated hip fracture	Hip and wrist fracture	p value
Age	80	79	0.45
Female:male ratio	9:1	4:1	<0.0001
30-day mortality (%)	9.6	9.1	0.33
90-day mortality	18	16	0.66
1-year mortality (%)	31	25	0.33
Median length of stay	13	18	<0.001

Table 2 Cox regression analysis for patients with hip fracture examining the effect of age, gender and concurrent wrist fracture

Covariate	Risk ratio	Lower 95 % CI	Upper 95 % CI	p value
Age	1.05	1.04	1.06	<0.0001
Gender	0.54	0.42	0.68	<0.0001
Concomitant wrist fracture	0.86	0.57	1.28	0.45

CI confidence interval

cohorts (Table 1). There was a female preponderance in both groups. This was much more marked in the cohort with concomitant wrist fractures ($p < 0.0001$). The 30-day and 1-year mortality was not significantly different for the combined fracture group compared to the isolated fracture group. Those with concurrent fractures had a longer in-hospital stay compared to those with isolated hip fractures (median 18 vs 13 days $p < 0.0001$) (Table 1).

Cox's proportional hazard analysis, adjusting for gender and age, showed that the presence of a concomitant wrist fracture did not significantly affect mortality ($p = 0.45$) (Table 2). Age and gender were strong predictors of survivorship. Female sex and youth were associated with improved survivorship. The risk ratio of 1.05 for age means that for every year increase in age, the odds of death at any given time increase by a factor of 1.05. Similarly, as far as gender is concerned, the odds of death for women at any given time is 0.54 that for men. The survivorship curves for patients with isolated hip fracture and the combination hip and wrist fracture had a similar profile (Figs. 1, 2).

There was no statistical significance between the groups in the method of fixation of hip fractures of the two groups (Table 3).

Meta-analysis

Four studies matched the search criteria (Mulhall et al. [2], Shabat et al. [3], Tow et al. [4], Robinson et al. [5]). Two percent (95 % CI 1.7–2.4) of patients with hip fracture suffered a concurrent wrist fracture. Pooling our

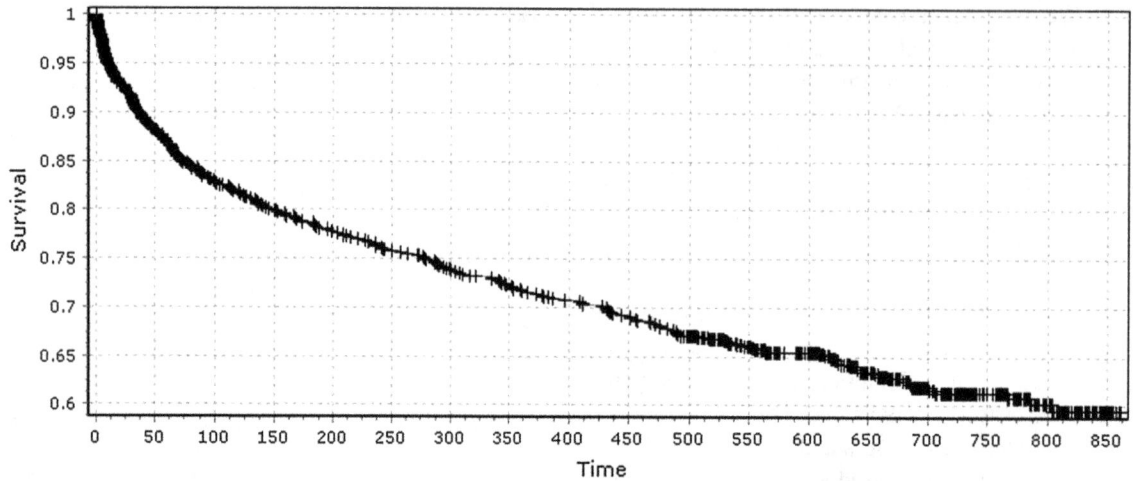

Fig. 1 Survivorship curve of patients with isolated hip fracture

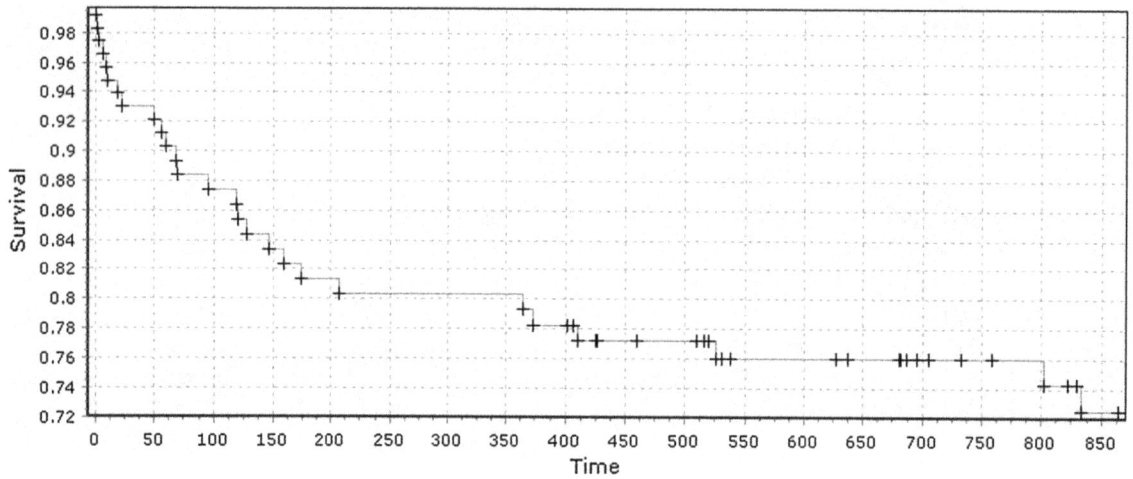

Fig. 2 Survivorship curve of patients with combined hip and wrist fracture

Table 3 Methods of fixation of hip fracture in patients with isolated hip fracture and combined hip and wrist fracture

	Isolated hip fracture	Hip and wrist fracture
Hemiarthroplasty	350 (45 %)	41 (47 %)
Nail	99 (13 %)	15 (17 %)
Dynamic screw	276 (36 %)	28 (32 %)
Cannulated screw	19 (2 %)	1 (1 %)

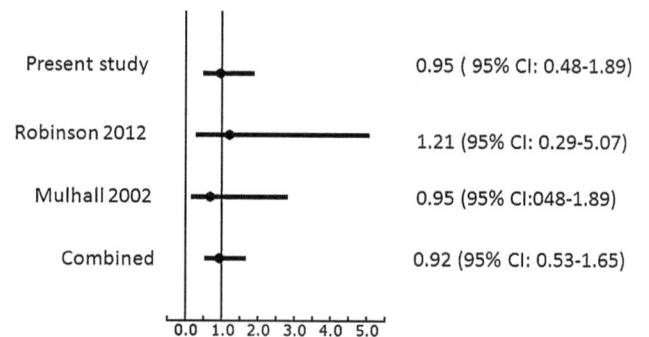

Fig. 3 Forest plot of studies exploring the effect of concomitant wrist fracture on early mortality in patients with hip fracture. Early mortality refers to in-hospital or 30-day mortality

data with that of Robinson et al., the presence of a wrist fracture did not adversely affect risk of death at 1 year. Performing a random effects meta-analysis, given the slightly different time frames, of the three studies (Robinson et al. [5], Mulhall et al. [2]), we found that the presence of a wrist fracture with hip fracture resulted in no difference in survivorship in the short term (namely 30-day or in-hospital mortality). This is confirmed in the forest plot (Fig. 3).

Discussion

Wrist and hip fractures are two of the most common and clinically significant fractures treated by the orthopaedic

Table 4 Meta-analysis of studies exploring effect of coincident hip fracture in patients with hip and wrist fracture

Study	Number of patients	Prevalence of hip fracture with wrist fracture	Mean age isolated hip vs combined fracture	Female: male isolated hip vs combined fracture	30-day mortality isolated hip vs combined fracture	1-year mortality isolated hip vs combined fracture	Length of stay isolated hip vs combined fracture (median)	Adjusted mortality ratio isolated hip vs combined fracture
Mulhall et al. [2]	28	3.7 %	77 vs 84*	3:1 vs 8:1*	10.3 vs 5.6 % (in-hospital mortality)*		15.6 vs 20.4 (mean)	
Tow et al. [4]	33	2.6 %	78 vs 79	2:1 vs 6:1			17 vs 23	
Robinson et al. [5]	34	1.8 %	82 vs 83	4:1 vs 7:1	6.4 vs 7.7 %	28 vs 19 %	13 vs 17.5	
Shabat et al. [3]	46			7:1 (no data of isolated hip fracture)			13 (no data of isolated hip fracture)	
This study	88	1.7 %	80 vs 79	4:1 vs 9:1	9.6 vs 9.1 %	30.6 vs 25 %	13 vs 18	0.86 (95 % CI 0.57–1.28)
Meta-analysis	229	2.0 (95 % CI 1.7–2.4)	79.8 vs 80.5	3:1 vs 7:1 (p < 0.0001)	Relative risk 0.93 (95 % CI 0.53–1.65)	29 vs 24 % (p = 0.2) relative risk 0.81 (95 % CI 0.58–1.13)		

* For all patients with hip and upper limb fractures

surgeon. When they occur in combination they pose a peculiar challenge. Expeditious surgery is mandated in hip fracture patients as it is thought to improve survivorship [6]. In England and Wales, the Department of Health provides financial incentives, in the form of the Best Practice Tariff, to National Health Service Trusts where patient care meets a minimum standard [7]. Surgery within 36 h is one criterion to be satisfied if trusts are to enjoy the Tariff. Functionality and independence are dependent upon hip and wrist function. No previous studies have examined the effect of concomitant wrist fractures in hip fracture patients, correcting for potential confounders.

In the present study the combination and singular fracture cohorts were recruited from different time frames. This was necessary to include sufficient numbers of patients with hip and distal radius fractures. This may potentially impact upon our findings. Over the periods in question (2004–2011 for hip/wrist and 2010 for hip fracture) operative fixation remained the mainstay of treatment for hip fractures. In particular, there was no significant difference in the method of fracture fixation for the two cohorts (Table 3).

Those with combination hip and wrist fractures did not have a significantly different 30-day, 90-day and 1-year mortality compared to those with isolated hip fractures. There was a considerably higher proportion of women in the combination fracture group (89 vs 69 %, respectively p < 0.0001). Correcting for both age and gender with Cox's proportional hazard regression analysis, we found that the presence of an associated wrist fracture did not significantly impact upon mortality in patients with hip fractures.

A review of the literature, involving smaller studies, suggests equally interesting findings (Table 4). In 2002 Mulhall [2] performed an analysis of all patients presenting to his institution with simultaneous hip and upper limb fractures. He found that wrist fractures were the most common upper limb fracture associated with hip fractures. He also observed a significant female preponderance when compared to patients with isolated hip fractures. The combination fracture cohort had a longer in-hospital stay and lower in-hospital mortality.

Tow et al. [4] performed a matched case–control study. In this they compared 33 patients with coincident hip and wrist fractures with 33 patients suffering from isolated hip fractures. The comparators were matched for age and gender. They observed a similar female predilection. Tow et al. interestingly observed that the combination fracture group were slightly more osteoporotic than those in the isolated hip fracture group, but the difference was not statistically significant.

Robinson and co-workers, in 2012, analysed the features of patients with concomitant hip and upper limb fractures. Similar to Mulhall they observed distal radius fractures to be the most common associated injury [5]. Consistent with our study and preceding works, Robinson noted that there was a high female:male ratio and longer length of hospital stay, in instances of hip and concomitant wrist fracture.

Pooling the available data from the literature, we observed that 2 % (95 % CI 1.7–2.4) of patients with hip fracture suffered a concurrent wrist fracture. The narrow confidence interval suggests the accuracy of the value. Both cohorts had a similar age. All previous studies found a much higher proportion of female patients in the group with combined wrist and hip fracture. We considered whether the similar survivorship observed in patients with simultaneous hip and wrist fractures, in spite of the presence of two fractures, was due to the female preponderance acting as a confounder. Male patients have a much higher mortality following hip fracture compared with women. The most recent meta-analysis, involving in excess of 64,000 patients, indicates that male sex engenders a 1.7-fold increase in mortality compared to female patients [8]. We thus decided to adjust mortality for gender and age. In this present study, using Cox's proportional hazard analysis adjusted for age and gender, there remained a non-significant difference in survivorship in patients with hip and wrist fractures compared to those with isolated wrist fractures. No adjustment was made for potential differences in co-morbidities between the two cohorts. However, both samples were sufficiently large to be representative and correction was made for the pre-eminent difference, namely gender. Further, differences in the mortality between male and female hip fracture patients are not related to co-morbid status [9].

A minority of patients with hip fractures sustain concomitant wrist fractures. However, given the incidence of hip fractures, this number is not negligible. This is the largest study exploring the outcome of concomitant hip and wrist fractures. This is the first meta-analysis of studies examining the natural history of patients with synchronous hip and wrist fractures. The combination fracture occurs much more commonly in women and patients require a greater length of hospitalisation. The patients who sustained simultaneous hip and wrist fractures suffered no significant difference in survivorship when compared to those who suffer isolated hip fractures. It is tempting to assume that the combination fracture is indicative of a frailer patient and poses a greater risk to life. However, our findings and the meta-analysis suggest that the combination hip and wrist fracture does not portend increased mortality compared to patients with isolated hip fractures.

Acknowledgments   No external funding was received for this study.

Conflict of interest   None.

Ethical standards   Patients gave informed consent for the use of their data anonymously for auditing or research purposes to improve healthcare and service provision. The study was permitted by the local institutional review board and was performed in accordance with the ethical standards of the 1964 Declaration of Helsinki as revised in 2000.

References

1. http://guidance.nice.org.uk/CG124/Guidance/pdf/English
2. Mulhall KJ, Ahmed A, Khan Y, Masterson E (2002) Simultaneous hip and upper limb fracture in the elderly: incidence, features and management considerations. Injury 33:29–31
3. Shabat S, Gepstein R, Mann G, Stern A, Nyska M (2003) Simultaneous distal radius and hip fractures in elderly patients—implications to rehabilitation. Disabil Rehabil 25:823–826
4. Tow BP, Chua BS, Fook-Chong S, Howe TS (2009) Concurrent fractures of the hip and wrist: a matched analysis of elderly patients. Injury 40:385–387
5. Robinson PM, Harrison T, Cook A, Parker MJ (2012) Orthopaedic injuries associated with hip fractures in those aged over 60 years: a study of patterns of injury and outcomes for 1,971 patients. Injury 43(7):1131–1134
6. Simonov N, Defraud JPG, Sprague S, Goat GHZ, Schematic E, DeBeers J, Bandar M (2010) Effect of early surgery after hip fracture on mortality and complications: systematic review and meta-analysis. Can Med Assoc J 182:1609–1616
7. http://www.dh.gov.uk/en/Publicationsandstatistics/Publications/PublicationsPolicyAndGuidance/DH_112284 No authors listed last accessed 25/06/2013
8. Hu F, Jiang C, Shen J, Tang P, Wang Y (2012) Preoperative predictors for mortality following hip fracture surgery: a systematic review and meta-analysis. Injury 43:676–685
9. Kannegaard PN, van der Mark S, Eiken P, Abrahamsen B (2010) Excess mortality in men compared with women following a hip fracture. National analysis of comedications, comorbidity and survival. Age Ageing 39:203–209

32

Bone metastases of unknown origin: epidemiology and principles of management

Andrea Piccioli · Giulio Maccauro ·
Maria Silvia Spinelli · Roberto Biagini ·
Barbara Rossi

Abstract   Metastases are the most common malignancies involving bone; breast, prostate, lung and thyroid are the main sites of primary cancer. However, up to 30 % of patients present with bone metastases of unknown origin, where the site of the primary neoplasm cannot be identified at the time of diagnosis despite a thorough history, physical examination, appropriate laboratory testing and modern imaging technology (CT, MRI, PET). Sometimes only extensive histopathological investigations on bone specimens from biopsy can suggest the primary malignancy. At other times, a bone lesion can have such a highly undifferentiated histological appearance that a precise pathological classification on routine hematoxylin–eosin-stained section is not possible. The authors reviewed the relevant literature in an attempt to investigate the epidemiology of the histological primaries finally identified in patients with bone metastases from occult cancer, and a strategy of management and treatment of bone metastases from occult carcinomas is suggested. Lung, liver, pancreas and gastrointestinal tract are common sites for primary occult tumors. Adenocarcinoma is the main histological type, accounting for 70 % of all cases, while undifferentiated cancer accounts for 20 %. Over the past 30 years, lung cancer is the main causative occult primary for bone metastases and has a poor prognosis with an average survival of 4–8 months. Most relevant literature focuses on the need for standardized diagnostic workup, as surgery for bone lesions should be aggressive only when they are solitary and/or the occult primaries have a good prognosis; in these cases, identification of the primary tumor may be important and warrants special diagnostic efforts. However, in most cases, the primary site remains unknown, even after autopsy. Thus, orthopedic surgery has a mainly palliative role in preventing or stabilizing pathological fractures, relieving pain and facilitating the care of the patient in an attempt to provide the most appropriate therapy for the primary tumor as soon as possible.

Level of evidence   5

Keywords   Bone metastases · Unknown origin · Carcinoma

A. Piccioli
Oncologic Center, "Palazzo Baleani", Teaching Hospital
Policlinico Umberto I, Rome, Italy

G. Maccauro · M. S. Spinelli
Department of Geriatrics, Orthopedics and Neurosciences,
Agostino Gemelli University Hospital, School of Medicine,
Catholic University of the SacredHeart, Rome, Italy

R. Biagini · B. Rossi (✉)
Unit of Oncological Orthopaedics, Regina Elena National
Cancer Institute, Rome, Italy
e-mail: barbararossi82@yahoo.it

Introduction

Metastases are the most common type of malignant tumor involving bone; the skeleton is the third most frequent site for metastatic carcinoma after the lung and liver. Any malignant tumor may metastasize to bone: the most common malignancies are breast in women and prostate in men but secondary lesions from lung cancer have risen in both sexes in the last two decades [1–4]. Skeletal lesions can be the first manifestation of malignancy in 25–30 % of cases [4–6]. In recent years, imaging studies have improved, the use of chest and abdominal computed tomography (CT) is increasing and diagnostic endoscopic techniques have advanced; new tumor markers have been identified, guided percutaneous bone biopsy has gained widespread acceptance, immunohistochemistry and even chromosomal analysis have been developed for studying histological specimens so that the primary malignancy is most often identified at an early stage [1, 4, 5, 7, 8]. However, among patients with bone metastases, 22.6–30 % have no evidence of the primary tumor at presentation [2, 8–12]. In fact, unknown primary malignancy is not a well-defined disease entity. On the one hand, it can be considered as a variety of different malignant and metastatic tumors with an occult source at initial presentation. Thus, the initial medical histories, physical examinations and routine laboratory tests fail to detect the site of the primary neoplasm as it is too small and dormant or it has disappeared [13]. In these cases, the histological findings such as immunohistochemical and other morphological parameters from the bone biopsy can be diagnostic. On the other hand, a bone lesion can have such a highly undifferentiated histological appearance that a precise pathological classification on routine hematoxylin–eosin-stained section is not possible [11, 14, 15].

As a consequence, screening and early diagnosis are impossible by definition. The lack of a detectable primary neoplasm delays staging, treatment is challenging, and prognosis and outcome can be uncertain. In any case, even when the primary cancer is unknown, the patient should always be referred as soon as possible to an oncologist after the diagnosis of bone metastasis has been confirmed at biopsy.

Epidemiology

Metastasis of unknown primary origin is reported to occur in 3–4 % of all cancer patients and 10–15 % of them present with skeletal localizations [2, 13, 16, 17]. The bone is the third most common site of metastatic cancer of unknown primary origin, after the lymph nodes and the lung [12, 17]. Lung, liver, pancreas and gastrointestinal tract are common sites of primary occult tumors. Adenocarcinoma is the main histological type, accounting for 70 % of all cases, while undifferentiated cancer accounts for 15 % and squamous cell carcinomas 10 % [12, 13]. Occult carcinomas are clinically different from their respective manifest forms: with regard to skeletal involvement, the incidence of bone metastases from pulmonary carcinoma is much lower if the primary is occult (4 %) than if it is known (30–50 %); similarly, bone lesions from occult prostate cancer are three times less common than from a known primary, whereas they are four times more common in cases of occult pancreatic primary [12]. Some unknown primary tumors are treatable, like lymphoma, extragonal germ cell neoplasms and ovarian cancer, but the majority of cases have a short fatal clinical course with very scarce possibilities of employing effective chemotherapy [12, 16, 18].

We reviewed the relevant literature in an attempt to investigate the epidemiology of the histological primaries finally identified in patients with bone metastases from occult cancer (Table 1). Since from the end of the 1980s, lung carcinoma was suggested to be the most commonly causative histotype of metastatic bone disease from occult primaries [2, 5, 11, 19–21]. Rougraff et al. [19] described a retrospective analysis of diagnostic workups in 40 patients: lung cancers accounted for 63 % of the identified primaries. Nottebaert et al. [2] found lung carcinomas to be responsible for 52 % of 51 cases of bone lesions from unknown origin, while they accounted for only 7 % of bone metastases with a diagnosed primary. Moreover, patients with skeletal metastases from occult carcinomas showed a high incidence of spinal metastases, cord compression and pathological fractures and a significantly shorter survival compared to bone lesions secondary to known primaries. Over 10 years later, Shih et al. [11] reported similar demographic data (incidence 30 %, male sex and lung prevalence), intractable pain as the predominant symptom, lytic appearance at radiography and poor prognosis. From an analysis of the Swedish Cancer Registry from 1993 to 2008, Hemminki et al. [13] found that patients with metastases from unknown origin diagnosed in the bone mostly died of lung cancer. Vandecandelarae et al. [1] investigated epidemiological changes from the middle of the last century to recent times: a marked increase in lung cancer was noted in all these patients over the last 40 years, especially among women as an obvious demographic effect of smoking; occult breast and prostate cancer reduced their incidence thanks to advances in diagnosis and treatment at an early stage [1]. Among patients admitted in recent years for bone metastases, different authors surprisingly reported an increased incidence of unidentified primaries despite the improvements in diagnostic examinations, new tumor markers, immunohistochemical methods and guided percutaneous biopsy techniques over a 30-year period [1, 5, 22]. Vandecandelarae et al. [1] compared two series of patients with bone metastases from the same rheumatology department, one extending from 1958 to 1967 and the other from 1989 to 1996. Investigations looking for a primary were negative in 9/34 (27 %) patients in the early series and 36/95 (38 %) patients in the recent series. However, these data may reflect the less effective diagnostic and treatment options available in rheumatological institutes, whereas specialized cancer centers now offer many sophisticated diagnostic procedures and valuable therapeutic protocols that can even be performed on an outpatient basis.

Thus, detection of bone metastases from occult primaries should raise the suspicion that the lungs are the tissue of origin and the suspicion should be stronger in relatively young patients (60–65 years) [1, 13]. After pulmonary origin, bone metastases from undiagnosed renal clear cell carcinomas have increased to 12 %, more than

Table 1 Review of the literature on case distribution and primaries identified in bone metastases of unknown origin

Authors	BMUO at diagnosis	Identified PC	Main PC	PC in order of frequency	Occult PC
Simon and Karluk [14]	12	6	Kidney 3 (50 %)	Kidney (3), lung (2), others (1)	6 (50 %)
Simon and Bartucci [31]	46	20	Lung 7 (35 %)	Lung (7), kidney (6), breast = prostate (2), ovarian = thyroid = liver (1)	26 (56 %)
Nottebaert et al. [2]	51	33	Lung 17 (51 %)	Lung (17), others (16)	18 (35 %)
Shih et al. [11]	52	28	Lung 9 (32 %)	Lung (9), liver (8), kidney (5), prostate (3), thyroid (2), rectum (1)	24 (46 %)
Rougraff et al. [19]	40	34	Lung 23 (67 %)	Lung (23), kidney (4), breast = colon = liver = bladder (1), others (3)	6 (15 %)
Jacobsen et al. [20]	29	24	Lung 11 (46 %)	Lung (11), prostate (3), breast = lymphomas (2), kidney = ovary = pancreas = stomach = small intestine carcinoid = retroperitoneal rhabdomyosarcoma (1)	5 (17 %)
Katagiri et al. [5]	64	59	Lung 23 (39 %)	Lung (23), prostate (11), breast = liver (5), others (15)	5 (8 %)
Vandecandelaere et al. [1]	129	84	Lung 36 (43 %)	Lung (36), prostate (17), kidney (15), breast (9), stomach (2), bladder = colon = testis = pancreas = liver (1)	45 (35 %)
Destombe et al. [24]	107	94	Lung 37 (39 %)	Lung (37), prostate (26), breast (20), bladder (11)	13 (12 %)
Iizuka et al. [25]	27	26	Myeloma 7 (27 %)	Myeloma (7), lymphoma (3), lung (6), prostate (4), kidney = thyroid = liver = pancreas = stomach = esophagus (1)	1 (4 %)
Hemminki et al. [13]	501	256	Lung 128 (50 %)	Lung (128), urinary (29), prostate (16), breast (14), colon (12), pancreas = gastrointestinal (10), liver (9), biliary system (4), stomach (3), mediastinum (2), ovarian (1), others (18)	203 (40 %)

BMUO bone metastases of unknown origin, *PC* primary carcinoma

prostate at 10 %, whereas occult thyroid carcinomas are extremely rare (3 %) [1].

As the spine is the most common site of bone metastases, it is also reported to be the most common site of lesions of unknown origin, followed by the pelvis and long bones; lung and thyroid carcinomas should be strongly suspected at this location [21, 23]. However, spinal malignancy of unknown origin is often derived not only from solid tumors, but also from hematological tumors [1, 21, 24, 25]. In the series reported by Iizuka et al. [25], myeloma was the most common etiology (22 %), followed by lung carcinoma, prostate carcinoma and lymphoma. Serological evaluation for monoclonal gammopathy was very useful in revealing the diagnosis of myeloma in all affected patients.

Acrometastases are extremely unusual (<0.1 %), especially as the first presentation of occult carcinoma, but strongly suggest bronchogenic or gastrointestinal cancer [3, 26, 27].

Strategy of diagnosis and treatment

In patients affected by bone metastases of unknown origin, one of the most important prognostic and treatment-conditioning factors is the histological type, and therefore biopsy is mandatory in an attempt to detect the primary cancer [6, 28, 29]. Biopsy should be performed in the most accessible osseous or concomitant visceral lesion [19, 20, 24] and should include histochemistry, immunohistology and electron microscopy; thus, the surgeon should obtain sufficient material to enable study with special stains, estrogen receptor activity, and hormonal and tumor markers [30]. Bone biopsy is a key component of the diagnostic strategy and histological confirmation is particularly valuable in patients who have a solitary bone metastasis or unusual radiological features suggesting a myeloma or a sarcoma rather than a carcinoma. Although histological studies rarely identify the exact nature of the primary, they often provide important diagnostic clues: highly suggestive histological patterns may be found in small-cell lung cancer, clear-cell renal cancer, or well-differentiated thyroid carcinoma. Immunohistochemistry helps to determine the nature of the primary, most notably when differentiation is minimal. However, Rougraff et al. [19] reported that biopsy alone was unable to identify the primary site of the malignant tumor in 60 % of cases.

Whole-body bone scintigraphy or positron emission tomography (PET)-CT scan, plain radiographs of painful bones and chest–abdominal–pelvic CT are always recommended when occult carcinoma presents with skeletal location regardless of gender. In men, prostate-specific antigen (PSA) levels should be investigated first. In women, mammography is indicated when appropriate immunohistochemistry confirms breast origin; if the mammogram is non-diagnostic and there is histopathological evidence of breast cancer, breast ultrasound and/or magnetic resonance imaging (MRI) should be suggested [31]. Serum protein electrophoresis should be performed as an initial routine study in patients with incidental spinal metastasis [25]. With regard to skeletal findings, the radiographic appearance of the bone lesions is a valuable clue for suggesting the primary; bone CT and MRI are generally used as complementary techniques to confirm the presence of the metastases and to characterize them [3, 6, 12, 18]. Osteolytic lesions typically result from myeloma, renal cell cancer, gastrointestinal tract cancer and melanoma. Osteoblastic metastases can occur from prostate cancer and bronchial carcinoid. The mixed type of metastasis may be seen with breast, lung and cervical cancer. Other morphological features can aid in assessing the source of malignant neoplasms: for example, an expansive and septated metastasis would strongly suggest primary renal cell cancer or thyroid cancer, while intralesional calcifications would suggest a mucinous tumor [3]. Highly hemorrhagic lesions are mostly related to hypernephroma, thyroid cancer and hepatocellular carcinoma [6]. Serum/urine immunofixation and osteomedullary biopsy are advised in the presence of lytic lesions; PSA and thyroglobulin levels are mostly recommended for osteoblastic metastases [12, 18]. Lung tumors can be detected by modern imaging techniques, including PET-CT scan or high resolution spiral CT. However, the sensitivity is low for tumors smaller than 1 cm [13].

On the basis of histology and/or organ-specific clinical symptoms, further diagnostic workup includes abdominal and pelvic ultrasound, bronchoscopy, gastric and intestinal endoscopy, intravenous urography, laparotomy and further site-specific tumor markers. Due to the overall poor prognosis, too many tests to identify the primary at all costs may be inappropriate. If these investigations fail to reveal the primary site, it is unlikely that it will be identified with further extensive diagnostic procedures, but is then mostly established at autopsy [2, 17, 30–32].

The mean survival of these patients has not changed in the last 30 years, ranging from 3 to 12 months from diagnosis [2, 11, 16, 20, 31]. In general, unfavorable prognostic factors for occult primary tumors are male gender, pathological diagnosis of adenocarcinoma and involvement of multiple organs, besides bone dissemination [12, 31]. In terms of histology of primary cancer, lung adversely influenced survival rate, whereas breast and myeloma are favorable [4, 6, 16, 28, 29]. The lung is reported to be the most common site of occult primary tumor with a poor prognosis

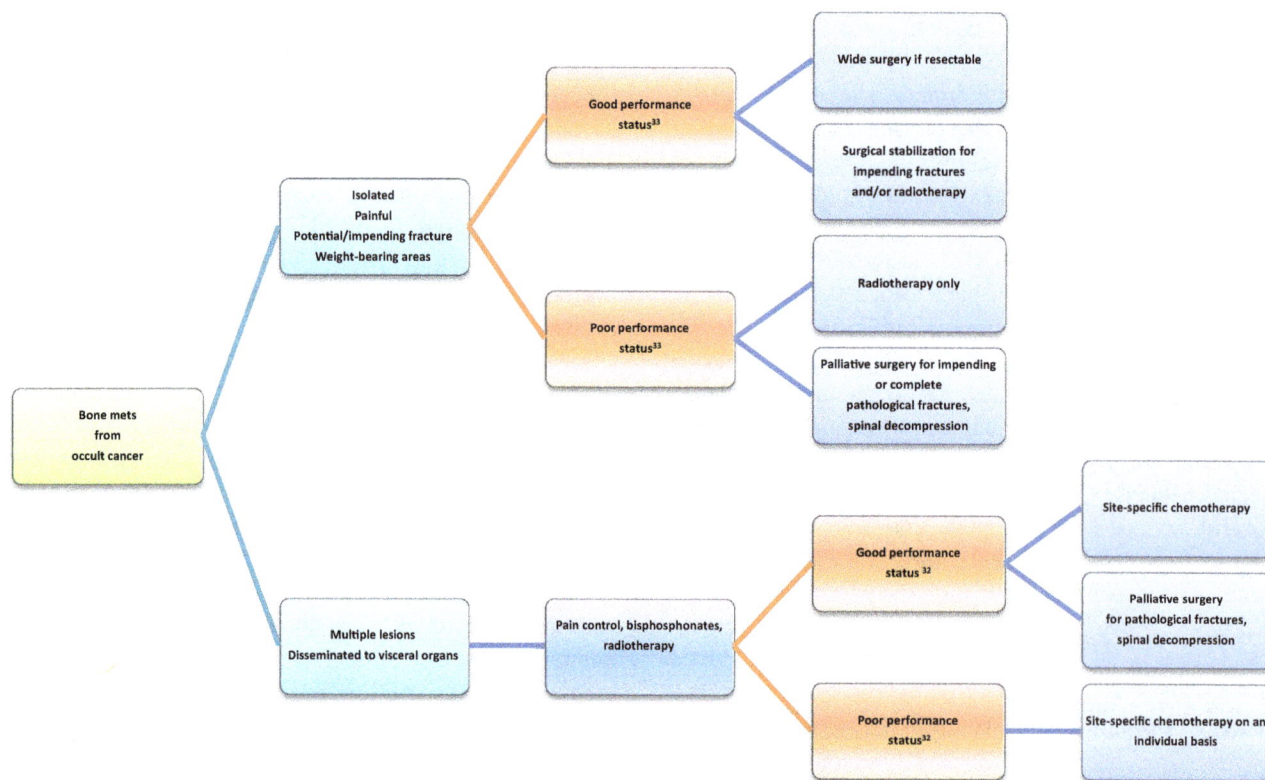

Fig. 1 Schematic indications for treatment of patients with bone metastases from occult primary tumor

of only 3 months, whereas breast and prostate cancer survival is relatively favorable at 15 and 23 months, respectively [12, 13, 16, 18, 29, 31, 32]. Patients with a favorable prognosis include men with blastic bone metastases from occult adenocarcinoma and elevated PSA and patients with a single, small and potentially resectable tumor [12, 18, 31].

Probably because of the rarity of occult cancer series and the short survival of bone metastatic patients in general, most of the literature on bone metastases from occult cancer focuses more on the need for a standardized diagnostic flowchart to detect the primary early rather than on a consensus about clinical management when the primary remains undiagnosed [1, 2, 5, 17, 19–21, 25, 32]. Multidisciplinary treatment should attempt to provide local and systemic tumor control in any case; as unknown origin is correlated with a short life expectancy, chemo-radiotherapy and surgery usually have only a palliative role [6, 29]. However, some integrated treatment protocols are potentially curative in a minority of favorable primary diagnoses [12, 18]. In according with current recommendations and guidelines [6, 12, 16, 18, 31, 33], we suggest a flowchart of therapeutic strategy: this approach depends on histological features, patients' performance status and survival estimation (Fig. 1). The foremost aims of surgery are to preserve the function of the affected bone, to prevent or stabilize pathological fractures, and to relieve pain and facilitate care of the patient while keeping hospitalization as short as possible. Obviously, anatomical site, multiple lesions, visceral involvement and performance status influence surgical options for bone metastases from occult cancer similarly to those of known origin; however, it is especially for bone metastases from unknown primaries that the principle of the more effective and feasible surgical procedures with the lowest rate of complications should be maintained [6, 28, 29, 33]. In the near future, further research on staging examinations, immunohistochemistry, hormone receptor staining and tumor markers may aid in understanding occult tumor characteristics and lead to the most appropriate therapies on an individual basis.

In conclusion, the epidemiology from analysis of the recent literature justifies firstly considering the lungs as the most probable site of primary carcinoma at the onset of bone metastases of undetected origin. The main goal of histology is to identify those primaries for which curative treatment may be available. Efforts should be made to identify the primary and to provide radical treatment in patients who have only one bone metastasis.

Conflict of interest None.

References

1. Vandecandelaere M, Flipo RM, Cortet B, Catanzariti L, Duquesnoy B, Delcambre B (2004) Bone metastases revealing primary tumors. Comparison of two series separated by 30 years. Jt Bone Spine 71(3):224–229
2. Nottebaert M, Exner GU, von Hochstetter AR, Schreiber A (1989) Metastatic bone disease from occult carcinoma: a profile. Int Orthop 13(2):119–123
3. Cooke KS, Kirpekar M, Abiri MM, Shreefter C (1997) US case of the day. Skeletal metastasis from poorly differentiated carcinoma of unknown origin. Radiographics 17(2):542–544
4. Piccioli A (2014) Breast cancer bone metastases: an orthopedic emergency. J Orthopaed Traumatol 15(2):143–144
5. Katagiri H, Takahashi M, Inagaki J, Sugiura H, Ito S, Iwata H (1999) Determining the site of the primary cancer in patients with skeletal metastasis of unknown origin: a retrospective study. Cancer 86(3):533–537
6. Piccioli A, Capanna R (2008) Il trattamento delle metastasi ossee. Linee Guida S.I.O.T
7. Wedin R, Bauer HC, Skoog L, Söderlund V, Tani E (2000) Cytological diagnosis of skeletal lesions. Fine-needle aspiration biopsy in 110 tumours. J Bone Jt Surg Br 82(5):673–678
8. Xu DL, Zhang XT, Wang GH, Li FB, Hu JY (2005) Clinical features of pathologically confirmed metastatic bone tumors—a report of 390 cases. Ai Zheng 24(11):1404
9. Conroy T, Platini C, Troufleau P, Dartois D, Lupors IE, Malissard L et al (1993) Presentation clinique et facteurspronostics au diagnostic de metastases osseuses. A propos de d'uneserie de 578 observations. Bull Cancer 80:S16e22
10. Papagelopoulos P, Savvidou O, Galanis E et al (2009) Advances and challenges in diagnosis and management of skeletal metastases. Orthopedics 29(7):609–620
11. Shih LY, Chen TH, Lo WH (1992) Skeletal metastasis from occult carcinoma. J Surg Oncol 51(2):109–113
12. Airoldi G (2012) Cancer of unknown primary origin: utility and futility in clinical practice. Ital J Med 6:315–326
13. Hemminki K, Riihimäki M, Sundquist K, Hemminki A (2013) Site-specific survival rates for cancer of unknown primary according to location of metastases. Int J Cancer 133(1):182–189
14. Simon MA, Karluk MB (1982) Skeletal metastases of unknown origin. Diagnostic strategy for orthopedic surgeons. Clin Orthop Relat Res 166:96–103
15. Bitran JD, Ultmann JE (1992) Malignancies of undetermined primary origin. Dis Mon 38(4):213–260
16. Schwartz H.S. (2008) Metastatic bone disease: diagnosis, evaluation and treatment. In: AAOS 2008, 75 h Annual Meeting Instructional Course Lecture Handout, pp 19–22 (Course n 386)
17. Le Chevalier T, Cvitkovic E, Caille P, Harvey J, Contesso G, Spielmann M, Rouesse J (1988) Early metastatic cancer of unknown primary origin at presentation. A clinical study of 302 consecutive autopsied patients. Arch Intern Med 148(9):2035–2039
18. Pavlidis N, Briasoulis E, Hainsworth J, Greco FA (2003) Diagnostic and therapeutic management of cancer of an unknown primary. Eur J Cancer 39(14):1990–2005
19. Rougraff BT, Kneisl JS, Simon MA (1993) Skeletal metastases of unknown origin. A prospective study of a diagnostic strategy. J Bone Jt Surg Am 75(9):1276–1281
20. Jacobsen S, Stephensen SL, Paaske BP, Lie PG, Lausten GS (1997) Skeletal metastases of unknown origin: a retrospective analysis of 29 cases. Acta Orthop Belg 63(1):15–22
21. Ugras N, Yalcinkaya U, Akesen B, Kanat O (2014) Solitary bone metastases of unknown origin. Acta Orthop Belg 80(1):139–143

22. Maillefert JF, Tebib J, Huguenin MC, Chauffert B, Pascaud F, Peere T et al (1993) Les metastases osseuses révélatrices: recherche du cancer primitif. Sem Hôp Paris 69:372–378

23. Khan MN, Sharfuzzaman A, Mostafa MG (2014) Spinal cord compression as initial presentation of metastatic occult follicular thyroid carcinoma. J Neurosci Rural Pract 5(2):155–159

24. Destombe C, Botton E, Le Gal G, Roudaut A, Jousse-Joulin S, Devauchelle-Pensec V, Saraux A (2007) Investigations for bone metastasis from an unknown primary. Jt Bone Spine 74(1):85–89 Epub 2006 Nov 30

25. Iizuka Y, Iizuka H, Tsutsumi S, Nakagawa Y, Nakajima T, Sorimachi Y, Ara T, Nishinome M, Seki T, Takagishi K (2009) Diagnosis of a previously unidentified primary site in patients with spinal metastasis: diagnostic usefulness of laboratory analysis, CT scanning and CT-guided biopsy. Eur Spine J 18(10):1431–1435

26. Wijayaratna R, Ng JW (2013) Metatarsal metastasis as the presenting feature of occult colorectal carcinoma. BMJ Case Rep

27. van Veenendaal LM, de Klerk G, van der Velde D (2014) A painful finger as first sign of a malignancy. Geriatr Orthop Surg Rehabil 5(1):18–20

28. Piccioli A, Rossi B, Scaramuzzo L, Spinelli MS, Yang Z, Maccauro G (2014) Intramedullary nailing for treatment of pathologic femoral fractures due to metastases. Injury 45(2):412–417

29. Forsberg JA, Eberhardt J, Boland PJ, Wedin R, Healey JH (2011) Estimating survival in patients with operable skeletal metastases: an application of a bayesian belief network. PLoS One 6(5):e19956

30. Perchalski JE, Hall KL, Dewar MA (1992) Metastasis of unknown origin. Prim Care 19(4):747–757

31. Ettinger DS, Handorf CR, Agulnik M, Bowles DW, Cates JM, Cristea M, Dotan E, Eaton KD, Fidias PM, Gierada D, Gilcrease GW, Godby K, Iyer R, Lenzi R, Phay J, Rashid A, Saltz L, Schwab RB, Shulman LN, Smerage JB, Stevenson MM, Varadhachary GR, Zager JS, Zhen WK, Bergman MA, Freedman-Cass DA (2014) Occult primary, version 3.2014. NCCN guidelines. J Natl Compr Cancer Netw 12(7):969–974

32. Simon MA, Bartucci EJ (1986) The search for the primary tumor in patients with skeletal metastases of unknown origin. Cancer 58(5):1088–1095

33. Oken MM, Creech RH, Tormey DC, Horton J, Davis TE, McFadden ET, Carbone PP (1982) Toxicity and response criteria of the Eastern Cooperative Oncology Group. Am J Clin Oncol 5:649–655

33

Biomechanical analysis of acromioclavicular joint dislocation repair using coracoclavicular suspension devices in two different configurations

Ferran Abat · Juan Sarasquete · Luis Gerardo Natera · Ángel Calvo · Manuel Pérez-España · Néstor Zurita · Jesús Ferrer · Juan Carlos del Real · Eva Paz-Jimenez · Francisco Forriol

Abstract

Background The best treatment option for some acromioclavicular (AC) joint dislocations is controversial. For this reason, the aim of this study was to evaluate the vertical biomechanical behavior of two techniques for the anatomic repair of coracoclavicular (CC) ligaments after an AC injury.

Materials and methods Eighteen human cadaveric shoulders in which repair using a coracoclavicular suspension device was initiated after injury to the acromioclavicular joint were included in the study. Three groups were formed; group I ($n = 6$): control; group II ($n = 6$): repair with a double tunnel in the clavicle and in the coracoid (with two CC suspension devices); group III ($n = 6$): repair in a "V" configuration with two tunnels in the clavicle and one in the coracoid (with one CC suspension device). The biomechanical study was performed with a universal testing machine (Electro Puls 3000, Instron, Boulder, MA, USA), with the clamping jaws set in a vertical position. The force required for acromioclavicular reconstruction system failure was analyzed for each cadaveric piece.

Results Group I reached a maximum force to failure of 635.59 N (mean 444.0 N). The corresponding force was 939.37 N (mean 495.6 N) for group II and 533.11 N (mean 343.9 N) for group III. A comparison of the three groups did not find any significant difference despite the loss of resistance presented by group III.

Conclusion Anatomic repair of coracoclavicular ligaments with a double system (double tunnel in the clavicle and in the coracoid) permits vertical translation that is more like that of the acromioclavicular joint. Acromioclavicular repair in a "V" configuration does not seem to be biomechanically sufficient.

Keywords Acromioclavicular dislocation · Joint · Anatomic repair · Biomechanics

F. Abat (✉)
Department of Sports Orthopaedics, ReSport Clinic, Barcelona, Spain
e-mail: ferranabat@gmail.com

F. Abat · J. Sarasquete · L. G. Natera
Department of Traumatology and Orthopaedic Surgery, Hospital de la Santa Creu i Sant Pau, Universitat Autónoma de Barcelona, Sant Quintí, 89, Barcelona 08026, Spain

Á. Calvo · N. Zurita
Hospital IMED Elche, Alicante, Spain

M. Pérez-España · J. Ferrer
Shoulder and Elbow Pathology Unit Shoulder of Madrid, Madrid, Spain

J. C. del Real · E. Paz-Jimenez
Engineering School (ICAI), University of Comillas, Madrid, Spain

F. Forriol
Universidad San Pablo CEU, Madrid, Spain

Introduction

Acromioclavicular (AC) dislocations usually present as the result of a fall that produces trauma to the lateral aspect of the shoulder. It brings about a variable separation of the acromioclavicular joint depending on the degree of damage to the capsule, the acromioclavicular ligaments, as well as the coracoclavicular (CC) ligaments. Rockwood classified them into grades I–VI depending on the severity of the injury and the degree of displacement [1]. Grade I–II injuries are treated conservatively, without surgery, leading to satisfactory results and a return to sporting activity in most cases [2]. The treatment of grade III injuries is controversial. However, surgical treatment is recommended for high-grade lesions IV–VI [3]. Despite their clinical impact, there is still no consensus for the surgical treatment of Rockwood high-grade lesions [4, 5].

From a biomechanical point of view, the importance of the acromioclavicular and coracoclavicular ligaments for maintaining the vertical and horizontal stability of the acromioclavicular joint has been shown [6]. There are many techniques that can be applied to the repair of the AC and CC ligaments in the literature [7, 8]. It is currently popular to perform these repairs in an anatomic way [5, 9].

To replace CC ligaments, some authors advocate using tendons (autograft or allograft) [10], while others perform repairs with synthetic devices [11, 12] which allow for the reduction of the AC joint, with the expectation that these devices might act as scaffolding while the injured ligaments heal.

Synthetic CC suspension devices placed arthroscopically permit the reduction of AC dislocations during the biological healing of the CC ligaments. Among the options for repairs with synthetic devices is anatomic reconstruction with a double tunnel in the clavicle as well as in the coracoid [5]. This technique allows the conoid and trapezoid ligaments to be emulated, and has shown biomechanical advantages [12], but there is also an increased risk of fracture of the clavicle during the construction of two tunnels and an increase in technical difficulty [5]. On the other hand, the isometric approach seeks to restore the anatomy of the conoid and trapezoid ligaments by using a single anchoring stitch in the coracoid at the midway point of the insertion of both ligaments.

The aim of the study reported in this paper was to evaluate the vertical biomechanical behavior of two techniques for the anatomic repair of coracoclavicular ligaments that can be used for the surgical treatment of acromioclavicular dislocations using synthetic CC suspension devices. The hypothesis was that anatomic CC repair with a double tunnel in both the coracoid and clavicle is the repair that comes closest to restoring the natural stability of the AC joint.

Materials and methods

Eighteen human cadaveric shoulders (9 men, 9 women) from individuals aged 41–63 years (mean 58) were used. All specimens studied were free of systemic diseases or previous acromioclavicular injury. The pieces were stored at −20 °C and subsequently prepared prior to study. Shoulders were sectioned and soft tissue was removed, leaving the bone and ligament structure. The scapula bound

to the clavicle with the intact coracoclavicular ligaments and acromioclavicular joint were obtained. In all cases, the ZipTight-type synthetic coracoclavicular suspension device was used (Biomet, Warsaw, IN, USA).

Three groups were formed: group I ($n = 6$), the control group; group II ($n = 6$), repair with a double tunnel in both the clavicle and coracoid (with two CC suspension devices); group III ($n = 6$), repair in a "V" configuration with two tunnels in the clavicle and one in the coracoid (with one CC suspension device).

Reconstruction techniques

For reconstruction with double tunnels in the coracoid (group II), anatomic repair of the CC, conoid, and trapezoid ligaments was performed (Fig. 1). This was done with two tunnels in the clavicle and another two tunnels at the base of the coracoid at the anatomic positions of the ligaments (4.5 cm from the acromial end of the clavicle for the conoid ligament tunnel and 2.5 cm for the trapezoid) [1, 5, 9, 12]. An individualized anatomic ligament repair of each ligament was performed.

In the reconstruction with a single tunnel in the coracoid (group III) for isometric repair of the CC ligaments in a "V" configuration (Fig. 2), two tunnels were created in the clavicle at the usual insertion of the conoid and trapezoid ligaments and one was made at the base of the coracoid (at the midpoint of the insertion of both ligaments). The CC suspension device was put in place with the titanium component locked into the base of the coracoid, passing

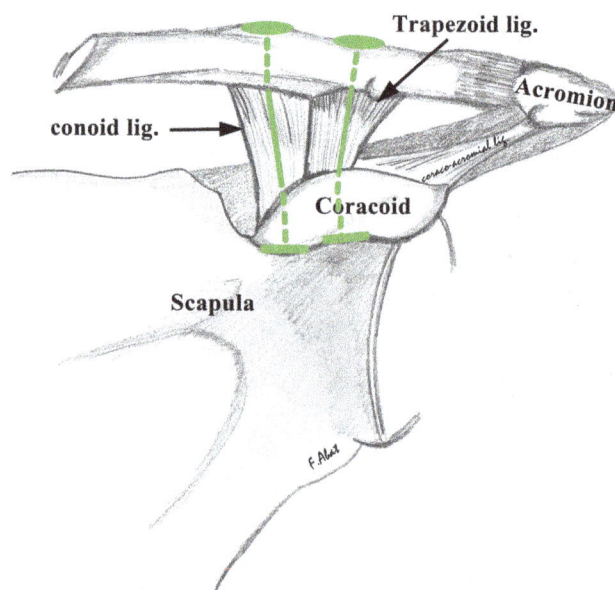

Fig. 1 Scheme for anatomic repair of the conoid and trapezoid ligaments with two CC suspension devices. Layout with a double tunnel in both the clavicle and coracoid

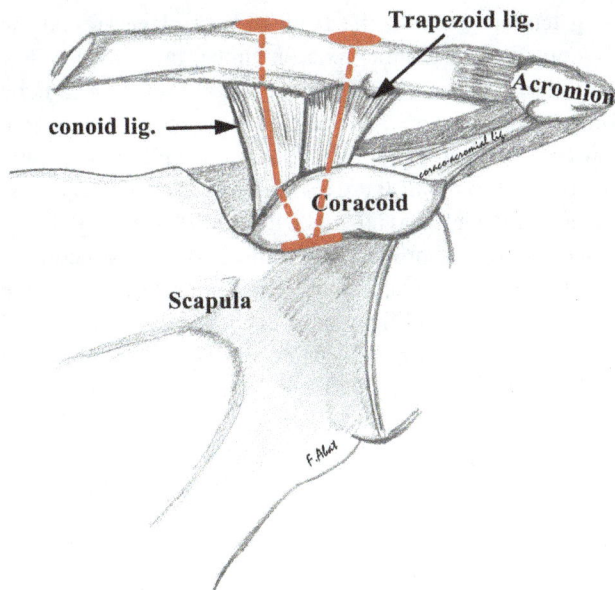

Fig. 2 Scheme for anatomic repair of the coracoclavicular ligaments in a "V" configuration. Note the arrangement of a single CC suspension device with two tunnels in the clavicle and one in the coracoid

through the tunnel inversely. Each loop of the device was then passed through the corresponding tunnel in the clavicle so as to obtain a repair of the CC ligaments with a single implant in a "V" configuration.

Biomechanical study protocol

The studied cadaveric pieces were placed in a universal testing machine (Electro Puls 3000, Instron, Boulder, MA, USA) with the clamping jaws vertical. The base of the scapula was fixed to the clamp by a compression system using two plates with screw tips to ensure proper fixation. By means of brackets, a bar contacting the upper edge of the scapula was fitted to prevent vertical movement.

To analyze the vertical behavior of the CC suspension systems, two rings were placed in the clavicle (one outside and one inside the fixations), which were connected by two chains to the vertical movement clamp. The chains allowed the traction system to be placed at the same distance. The traction test was performed at a speed of 15 mm/min. Pretensioning was performed at 15 N before the displacement of the bar of the testing machine was initiated. The test was stopped when the tensile force dropped by 60 % of the maximum applied force (Fmax 60 %) or when mobility of the part or implant failure was observed. In each test, the maximum breaking force (in N) was obtained. Group I (control) was tested first, thereby obtaining the reference values for a healthy shoulder. Groups II and III were tested later.

Statistical analysis

Mean values were calculated along with their standard deviations. Comparison was performed with an analysis of variance using the Tukey post-hoc test. SPSS (v.21.0) software was used. The level of significance was the usual 5 % ($\alpha = 0.05$, bilateral).

Results

The results obtained with the vertical traction biomechanical test to evaluate the maximum breaking force are shown in Table 1.

In group I and the control group ($n = 6$), the CC ligaments tore in all specimens upon reaching a maximum of 635.59 N and a minimum of 245.85 N. In group II (two tunnels and two fixations), two of the pieces were torn by the scapular fixation, so they were discarded. In the remaining four, the maximum force achieved was 939.37 N and the minimum was 278.75 N. In group III (two fixations and a single coracoid tunnel), the maximum value was 533.11 N and the minimum value was 210.30 N.

Upon performing a cluster analysis (Table 2), group I showed an average peak force of 444.0 N (SD 160.16) and group II averaged 495.6 N (SD 300.83). Group III had an average of 343.9 N (SD 111.46). A comparison of the three groups did not show any significant differences (ANOVA, $p = 0.446$), although the clear decline in resistance in group III is worth noting. Furthermore, no subsequent peer comparison indicated a significant difference from the overall value (Tukey post-hoc test, group I vs II, $p = 0.906$, group I vs III, $p = 0.638$, and group II vs III, $p = 0.448$).

Discussion

The main finding of this study was that the anatomic repair of the CC ligament with a double system (double tunnel in both the clavicle and coracoid) is biomechanically more

Table 1 Maximum breaking force in the vertical traction biomechanical test for each cadaveric piece

	Group I Control	Group II	Group III
1	534.44	412.43	374.12
2	529.94	351.99	274.10
3	245.85	278.75	533.11
4	253.49	939.37	371.50
5	464.81	*	300.05
6	635.59	*	210.30

Values expressed in Newtons (N)

Table 2 Mean values of maximum force according to study groups

Group	Average	SD	CV (%)	n
I	444.0	160.16	36.1	6
II	495.6	300.83	60.7	4
III	343.9	111.46	32.4	6
Total	419.4	186.73	44.5	16

Values expressed in Newtons (N)

like the AC joint than the AC repair with a single CC system in a "V" configuration is. Moreover, AC repair with a single CC system in a "V" configuration does not appear to be biomechanically sufficient, as it shows a clear tendency to offer less resistance. These findings confirm the hypothesis of the present study. We believe that compliance with these anatomical and biomechanical objectives allows for fewer recurrent subluxations and less residual pain, leading to a better clinical outcome.

A large number of AC dislocation repair techniques have been described, but there is still controversy over what the standard technique should be. Generally, repair focuses on reinforcing the CC ligaments with non-absorbable sutures, screws, pins, plates, or other methods of internal fixation [13–15]. Repairs with tendon grafts or fixation devices are based on the Weaver–Dunn technique and its variations [16, 17]. Initially, these coracoclavicular suspension devices were described for tibiofibular syndesmosis repair, but they have since been used in AC joint reconstruction too [18, 19]. Authors such as Salzmann [5] and Walz [12] argue that the placement of two CC suspension systems as replacements for the conoid and trapezoid ligaments is required to achieve proper primary stability. The precise anatomy of these two CC ligaments has already been described: the length of each ligament should be about 10 mm, giving a distance of 10–15 mm between the clavicle and coracoid [1, 5, 9, 12]. In agreement with a study by Breslow [20], the AC capsule and its ligaments work together to maintain horizontal stability, while the CC ligaments limit vertical displacement. Dimakopoulos et al. [21] were the first to provide clinical data on double-bundle repair for acute AC dislocations. The Mazzoca group [3, 7] described the open clamp technique with a semitendinosus tendon which, despite using an anatomic collarbone implementation, only uses a single point of traction on the coracoid. Lafosse et al. [22] reported a modified Weaver–Dunn technique performed arthroscopically, while Choi et al. [23] described procedures that use suture fixations to repair acute dislocations of the AC complex, with two sutures placed in the anatomic position to provide primary stability of the AC and CC ligaments. Recently, Tomlinson [24] and Baumgarten [25] described the anatomic repair of the CC complex

using tendon grafts in the form of a cerclage around the coracoid with anatomic fixation under the clavicle. Rehbein et al. [26] reported a transosseous suture technique with a cerclage in the AC and CC in an anatomic position.

Morrison et al. [15] suggest that a simple loop around the coracoid to repair the CC ligaments can cause the final position of the left clavicle to be displaced anteriorly. In the present study, we proposed that the best reconstruction is performed in the anatomical arrangement emulating the conoid and trapezoid ligaments. To achieve this, we tested two configurations, one of which was a "V" that emulated the fixation in the collarbone but with one tunnel placed at the isometric point of the coracoid, and the other a configuration with a double tunnel in the clavicle and a double tunnel in the coracoid that used two coracoclavicular suspension devices.

Chernchujit et al. [4] reported CC ligament tension results of 578 N, whereas they reached a value of 767 N with a double FiberWire® suture. Furthermore, Walz et al. [12] achieved a tension of 982 N using two coracoclavicular suspension systems (TightRope®). Wellmann et al. [27] reported a value of 663 N for a repair performed with polydioxanone (PDS), similar to the value recently reported by Martetschläger et al. [28]. Our study showed mean values for intact ligaments of 444.0 N (maximum 635.59 N), while the mean value for anatomic repairs involving double tunnels in the coracoid was 495.51 N (maximum 939.37 N). Although our study yielded lower values in terms of the average tension obtained with the repair compared to other reference works such as Motamedi et al. [29] and Wellmann et al. [27], the results reported here are very similar to those obtained in specimens with an intact acromioclavicular joint.

The main limitation of this study is that it is a cadaveric biomechanical study, so it inherently differed from the normal clinical situation. Nonetheless, this is a rigorous, well-controlled, and reproducible work. Another weakness is that we did not test the failure of the repair in combined craniocaudal, anterior–posterior, and rotational traction. The average age (58 years) of the donors of the cadaveric parts used is, however, comparable to those presented in previous studies, and is substantially higher than the normal average age at presentation of acromioclavicular dislocations (20 years). Since it has been shown that the mechanical qualities of the ligaments and bones deteriorate over the years, better results would be expected in younger individuals. One other weakness is that two specimens were lost from group II.

The results obtained in this study indicate that repair with a synthetic double CC suspension device with double tunneling in the coracoid as well as the clavicle gives vertical traction biomechanical results that resemble those of the native AC joint.

Acknowledgments We are grateful to E. Goode for his help in editing the manuscript.

Conflict of interest The authors declare that they have no conflict of interest related to the publication of this manuscript.

Ethical standards This is a cadaver study for which all ethical considerations and the international guidelines for cadaveric studies were followed.

References

1. Rockwood CJ, Williams G, Young D (1998) Disorders of the acromioclavicular joint. In: Rockwood CJ, Matsen FA III (eds) The shoulder, 2nd edn. WB Saunders, Philadelphia, pp 483–553
2. Jari R, Costic RS, Rodosky MW, Debski RE (2004) Biomechanical function of surgical procedures for acromioclavicular joint dislocations. Arthroscopy 20(3):237–245
3. Mazzocca AD, Santangelo SA, Johnson ST, Rios CG, Dumonski ML, Arciero RA (2006) A biomechanical evaluation of an anatomical coracoclavicular ligament reconstruction. Am J Sports Med 34(2):236–246
4. Chernchujit B, Tischer T, Imhoff AB (2006) Arthroscopic reconstruction of the acromioclavicular joint disruption: surgical technique and preliminary results. Arch Orthop Trauma Surg 126(9):575–581
5. Salzmann GM, Walz L, Buchmann S, Glabgly P, Venjakob A, Imhoff AB (2010) Arthroscopically assisted 2-bundle anatomical reduction of acute acromioclavicular joint separations. Am J Sports Med 38(6):1179–1187
6. Fukuda K, Craig EV, An KN, Cofield RH, Chao EY (1986) Biomechanical study of the ligamentous system of the acromioclavicular joint. J Bone Joint Surg Am 68(3):434–440
7. Mazzocca AD, Arciero RA, Bicos J (2007) Evaluation and treatment of acromioclavicular joint injuries. Am J Sports Med 35(2):316–329
8. Smith TO, Chester R, Pearse EO, Hing CB (2011) Operative versus non-operative management following Rockwood grade III acromioclavicular separation: a meta-analysis of the current evidence base. J Orthop Traumatol 12(1):19–27
9. Costic RS, Labriola JE, Rodosky MW, Debski RE (2004) Biomechanical rationale for development of anatomical reconstructions of coracoclavicular ligaments after complete acromioclavicular joint dislocations. Am J Sports Med 32(8):1929–1936
10. Lee SJ, Nicholas SJ, Akizuki KH, McHugh MP, Kremenic IJ, Ben-Avi S (2003) Reconstruction of the coracoclavicular ligaments with tendon grafts: a comparative biomechanical study. Am J Sports Med 31(5):648–655
11. Tischer T, Imhoff AB (2009) Minimally invasive coracoclavicular stabilization with suture anchors for acute acromioclavicular dislocation. Am J Sports Med 37(3):e5
12. Walz L, Salzmann GM, Fabbro T, Eichhorn S, Imhoff AB (2008) The anatomic reconstruction of acromioclavicular joint dislocations using 2 TightRope devices: a biomechanical study. Am J Sports Med 36(12):2398–2406
13. DeBerardino TM, Pensak MJ, Ferreira J, Mazzocca AD (2010) Arthroscopic stabilization of acromioclavicular joint dislocation using the AC graftrope system. J Shoulder Elbow Surg 19(2 Suppl):47–52
14. Mlasowsky B, Brenner P, Düben W, Heymann H (1988) Repair of complete acromioclavicular dislocation (Tossy stage III) using Balser's hook plate combined with ligament sutures. Injury 19(4):227–232
15. Morrison DS, Lemos MJ (1995) Acromioclavicular separation. Reconstruction using synthetic loop augmentation. Am J Sports Med 23(1):105–110
16. Liu HH, Chou YJ, Chen CH, Chia WT, Wong CY (2010) Surgical treatment of acute acromioclavicular joint injuries using a modified Weaver–Dunn procedure and clavicular hook plate. Orthopedics 33:8
17. Weaver JK, Dunn HK (1972) Treatment of acromioclavicular injuries, especially complete acromioclavicular separation. J Bone Joint Surg Am 54(6):1187–1194
18. Cottom JM, Hyer CF, Philbin TM, Berlet GC (2008) Treatment of syndesmotic disruptions with the Arthrex Tightrope: a report of 25 cases. Foot Ankle Int 29(8):773–780
19. Scheibel M, Ifesanya A, Pauly S, Haas NP (2008) Arthroscopically assisted coracoclavicular ligament reconstruction for chronic acromioclavicular joint instability. Arch Orthop Trauma Surg 128(11):1327–1333
20. Breslow MJ, Jazrawi LM, Bernstein AD, Kummer FJ, Rokito AS (2002) Treatment of acromioclavicular joint separation: suture or suture anchors? J Shoulder Elbow Surg 11(3):225–229
21. Dimakopoulos P, Panagopoulos A, Syggelos SA, Panagiotopoulos E, Lambiris E (2006) Double-loop suture repair for acute acromioclavicular joint disruption. Am J Sports Med 34(7):1112–1119
22. Lafosse L, Baier GP, Leuzinger (2005) Arthroscopic treatment of acute and chronic acromioclavicular joint dislocation. Arthroscopy 21(8):1017
23. Choi SW, Lee TJ, Moon KH, Cho KJ, Lee SY (2008) Minimally invasive coracoclavicular stabilization with suture anchors for acute acromioclavicular dislocation. Am J Sports Med 36(5):961–965
24. Tomlinson DP, Altchek DW, Davila J, Cordasco FA (2008) A modified technique of arthroscopically assisted AC joint reconstruction and preliminary results. Clin Orthop Relat Res 466(3):639–645
25. Baumgarten KM, Altchek DW, Cordasco FA (2006) Arthroscopically assisted acromioclavicular joint reconstruction. Arthroscopy 22(2):228.e1–228.e6
26. Rehbein K, Jung C, Becker U, Bauer G (2008) Treatment of acute AC joint dislocation by transosseal acromioclavicular and coracoclavicular fiberwire cerclage. Z Orthop Unfall 146(3):339–343
27. Wellmann M, Zantop T, Weimann A, Raschke MJ, Petersen W (2007) Biomechanical evaluation of minimally invasive repairs for complete acromioclavicular joint dislocation. Am J Sports Med 35(6):955–961
28. Martetschläger F, Buchholz A, Sandmann G, Siebenlist S, Döbele S, Hapfelmeier A, Stöckle U, Millett PJ, Elser F, Lenich A (2013) Acromioclavicular and coracoclavicular PDS augmentation for complete AC joint dislocation showed insufficient properties in a cadaver model. Knee Surg Sports Traumatol Arthrosc 21(2):438–444
29. Motamedi AR, Blevins FT, Willis MC, McNally TP, Shahinpoor M (2000) Biomechanics of the coracoclavicular ligament complex and augmentations used in its repair and reconstruction. Am J Sports Med 28(3):380–384

34

Functional outcomes of operative fixation of clavicle fractures in patients with floating shoulder girdle injuries

Alex K. Gilde[1,3] · Martin F. Hoffmann[2] · Debra L. Sietsema[3,4] · Clifford B. Jones[3,4]

Abstract

Background Double disruptions of the superior suspensory shoulder complex, commonly referred to as 'floating shoulder' injuries, are ipsilateral midshaft clavicular and scapular neck/body fractures with a loss of bony attachment of the glenoid. The treatment of 'floating shoulder' injuries has been debated controversially for many years. The purpose of this study was to demonstrate the clinical and functional outcomes of patients with 'floating shoulder' injuries who underwent operative fixation of the clavicle fracture only.

Materials and methods Between 2002 and 2010, 32 consecutive floating shoulder injuries were identified in skeletally mature patients at a level I trauma center and followed in a single private practice. Thirteen patients met the inclusion and exclusion criteria for this retrospective study with a minimum 12-month follow-up. Clavicle and scapular fractures were identified by Current Procedural Technology codes and classified based on Orthopaedic Trauma Association/Arbeitsgemeinschaft für Osteosynthesefragen criteria. 'Floating shoulder' injuries were surgically managed with only clavicular reduction and fixation utilizing modern plating techniques. Nonunion, malunion, implant removal, range of motion, need for secondary surgery, pain according to the visual analog scale (VAS), and return to work were measured.

Results All injuries were the result of high-energy mechanisms. Fracture union of the clavicle was seen after initial surgical fixation in the majority of patients (12; 92.3 %). Final pain was reported as minimal (11 cases; 1–3 VAS), moderate (1 case; 4–6 VAS), and high (1 case; 7–10 VAS) at last follow-up. Excellent range of motion (180° forward flexion and abduction) was observed in the majority of patients (8; 61.5 %). The Herscovici score was 12.9 (range 10–15) at 3 months. Unplanned surgeries included two clavicular implant removals and one nonunion revision. None of the patients required reconstruction for scapula malunion after nonoperative management. Twelve patients returned to previous work without restrictions.

Conclusions 'Floating shoulder' injuries with only clavicular fixation return to function despite persistent scapular deformity and some residual pain.

Level of evidence Level IV.

Keywords Clavicle · Floating shoulder · Scapula · Osteosynthesis · Outcome

✉ Martin F. Hoffmann
   martinfhoffmann@gmx.net

   Alex K. Gilde
   Alex.Gilde@grmep.com

   Debra L. Sietsema
   Debra.Sietsema@gmail.com

   Clifford B. Jones
   cbjones230@gmail.com

[1] Grand Rapids Medical Education Partners, Orthopaedic Surgery Residency, Grand Rapids, MI 49503, USA

[2] BG-University Hospital Bergmannsheil, Bochum, Germany

[3] Michigan State University College of Human Medicine, 15 Michigan St NE, Grand Rapids, MI 49503, USA

[4] Orthopaedic Associates of Michigan, 230 Michigan St NE, Suite 300, Grand Rapids, MI 49503, USA

Introduction

Double disruptions of the superior suspensory shoulder complex (SSSC) resulting in ipsilateral midshaft clavicular and scapular body/neck fractures, are commonly referred to as a 'floating shoulder' injury, and result in a loss of bony attachment of the glenoid [1, 2]. Floating shoulder injuries are the result of high-energy mechanisms [3–5] with an incidence of approximately 0.10 % of trauma patients [6]. Although much is known about these fractures when they occur in isolation, evidence is lacking in regard to treatment as concomitant fractures are associated with poor cosmesis, reduced strength, and dyskinesia of the shoulder girdle. Ganz and Noesberger [7] originally suggested that the weight of the arm and the muscles at the humerus would cause caudal and anteromedial displacement of the glenoid. Ada and Miller [3] found high numbers of rotator cuff dysfunction in patients with displaced clavicular and scapular fractures, as the normal lever arm of the rotator cuff is lost with glenoid displacement.

The treatment of 'floating shoulder' injuries has been debated over many years. Several studies recommend that conservative treatment results in acceptable patient outcomes, especially when fractures are minimally displaced [8–13]. Other studies have reported good to excellent outcomes with only clavicular fixation [6, 14–17]. In floating shoulder injuries with significant displacement, some studies have recommended fixation of both clavicular and scapular fractures [11, 13, 18–20]. Despite cited surgical indications for isolated extra-articular and intra-articular scapular fractures [3, 21–25], validated indications for 'floating shoulder' surgical management remain unclear. The purpose of this study was to describe the clinical and functional outcomes of patients with displaced and unstable 'floating shoulder' injury following fixation of only the clavicular fracture.

Materials and methods

This Institutional Review Board-approved retrospective exploratory study reviewed operatively treated midshaft clavicular fractures with associated ipsilateral non-operatively treated scapular fractures. The patients were recruited from a private practice office associated with a level I teaching trauma center. Consecutive patients were identified using Current Procedural Technology coding for operatively fixed clavicle fractures (23515) and a scapular injury database from March 1, 2002 to October 1, 2010.

Operative criteria for clavicular fixation included significant clavicular shortening (>20 mm on either anterior-posterior [AP], cephalad, or caudal radiographs), associated neurological injury, associated unstable scapular injury (glenoid neck, acromion, coracoid, or intra-articular glenoid fractures), double suspensory shoulder instability, open clavicular fractures, published criteria for displacement, impending skin compromise, or polytrauma [26–30]. Inclusion criteria for this study were skeletally mature (age ≥18 years), ipsilateral middle third clavicular fracture and

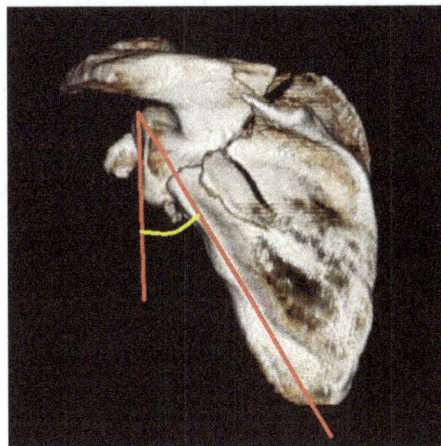

Fig. 1 The glenopolar angle as measured on 3D CT reconstruction. The apex created by *two lines* extending from the superior glenoid pole to the mid-point of the inferior angle and inferior glenoid pole determine the glenopolar angle

scapular fracture meeting the definition of a 'floating shoulder', clavicle fixation utilizing modern plating techniques [27, 31–33], and a minimum 12-month follow-up. A total of 32 patients were identified during this time period. Nineteen patients were excluded due to initial non-operative treatment of the clavicle fracture with subsequent nonunion (1), incarceration (1), insufficient records or imaging (7), and operative treatment of both clavicle and scapular fractures (10). When initially planning surgical management of these patients, the indications for fixation of the scapular fracture were partly based on the preferences of the senior surgeons as well as the patient's clinical condition. All patients in this study, with the exception of two, did not meet currently published indications for fixation of the scapular fracture in 'floating shoulder' injuries [11]. Thirteen 'floating shoulder' injuries in 13 patients formed the basis of this study.

All patients were treated and followed by four fellowship-trained orthopedic trauma surgeons utilizing similar philosophies and techniques. At the time of injury, all patients had computed tomography (CT) scans with three-dimensional (3D) reconstruction of the scapular fracture to assess deformity which included the glenopolar angle [34] (Fig. 1) and medialization/lateralization [35] (Fig. 2) of the scapular fragments [GE LightSpeed VCT 64-slice CT scanner; GE Healthcare, Waukesha, WI, USA (1.25-mm slice thickness); 3D reconstruction with TeraRecon Aquarius iNtuition v.4.4.5.49; TeraRecon, Inc, Foster City, CA, USA].

At 1–2 weeks postoperatively, physical therapy-directed passive range of motion (ROM) was instituted in all patients. At 6 weeks postoperatively, physical therapy-directed active ROM and strengthening was started. Patients were evaluated and imaged at regular intervals of 2, 6, and 12 weeks, and ongoing according to clinical necessity

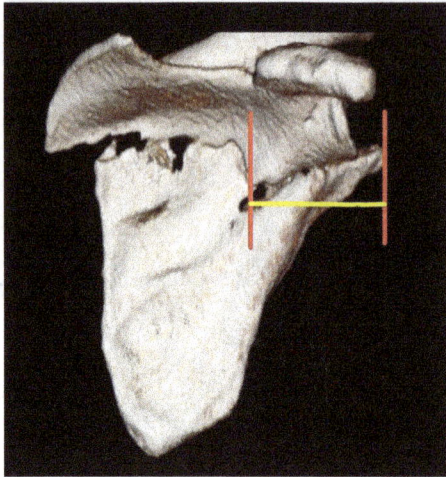

Fig. 2 Medialization/lateralization displacement as measured on 3D CT reconstruction. It is determined by the distance between the *vertical planes* drawn at the lateral-most edge of both scapular fragments

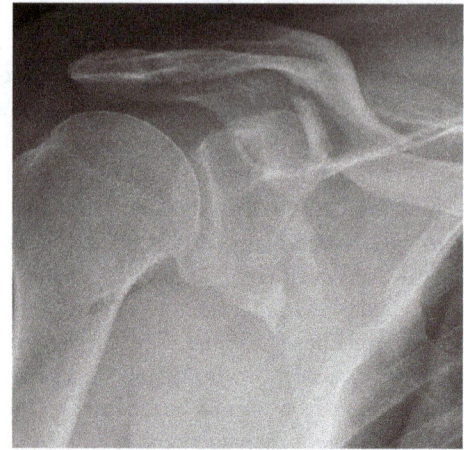

Fig. 3 This patient sustained 15-B2 clavicular and 14-A3.1 scapular fractures in a motorcycle accident

including, but not limited to pain, plate irritation, plate prominence, poor ROM, or not achieving complete clinical healing. Cephalad and caudal views of the clavicle were obtained at each interval to determine healing and alignment [36]. Grashey (true shoulder AP), axillary, and scapular Y views of the shoulder were obtained at each interval to determine scapular healing and morphology. Distances and angles were measured using digital software with a picture archiving and communication system or by manual techniques and protractors. Both clavicle and scapular fracture patterns were classified according to Orthopedic Trauma Association/Arbeitsgemeinschaft für Osteosynthesefragen (OTA/AO) criteria [37].

Pain according to the visual analog scale (VAS) [38] and ROM using basic clinical measurements were recorded. Outcomes were further measured using the Herscovici scoring system which assigns a numerical value (1–4) for pain, lifestyle, ROM, and muscle strength with a value of 16 being the best possible outcome [6]. Return to previous work was assessed. Follow-up was for a minimum of 12 months with radiographic union and return to previous activities and/or employment being established.

Standard statistical analyses were employed. Descriptive statistics, including means, range, standard deviation, and percentages were calculated using SPSS® 18.0 (IBM, Armonk, NY, USA).

Results

The mean follow-up was 16 months (12–45 months). The mean age at time of injury was 46 years (18–60 years) and 10 patients were male. High-energy mechanisms were the cause of all patient injuries including motorcycle accidents (11; 84.6 %) and all-terrain vehicle accidents (2; 15.4 %). None of the fractures were classified as open. Clavicular fracture classification was recorded as type 15-B1 (5; 38.4 %), type 15-B2 (7; 53.9 %), and type 15-B3 (1; 7.7 %). Scapular fracture classification was recorded as type 14-A3.1 (7; 53.9 %), type 14-A3.2 (5; 38.4 %), and type 14-C1.1 (1; 7.7 %) (Fig. 3). All clavicle fractures were unstable with shortening averaging 14 mm (6–30 mm) and translation averaging 10 mm (2–24 mm). Associated injuries were found in 12 of the 13 patients (92.3 %), which included rib fractures (11; 84.6 %), ipsilateral extremity fractures (6; 46 %), pneumothorax (5; 38.4 %), intracranial hemorrhage (2; 15.4 %), and abdominal hemorrhage/laceration (2; 15.4 %). Injury and fracture data are displayed in Table 1.

Eleven of 13 (85 %) patients reported minimal pain (VAS 1–3) upon final examination. One patient (1; 7.7 %) reported moderate levels of pain (VAS 4–6), which was attributed to overlying skin irritation at the surgical site. One patient (1; 7.7 %) reported high levels of pain (VAS 7–10) which was associated with the development of a nonunion. All patients eventually returned to work, 12 of whom had no restrictions. One patient (case 13) returned to function with restrictions secondary to pain despite complete nonunion resolution and full symmetrical strength and ROM.

Eight of 13 patients (62 %) had full symmetrical ROM (180° of forward flexion and abduction) at last follow-up. Three patients without complete restoration of ROM showed adequate ROM and function necessary to perform activities of daily living of the shoulder joint (flexion >121°, abduction >128°) [39]. Two patients exhibited suboptimal ROM at last follow-up. One of these patients (case 7) had a traumatic brain injury that impeded

Table 1 Patient demographic and injury data

Case	Age	Gender	Clavicle fracture classification	Scapula fracture classification	Clavicle translation; shortening (mm) +/−	Glenopolar angle (°)	Scapular medialization/ lateralization (mm)	Associated injuries
1	45	F	15-B1	14-A3.2	8; +17	41	23	1, 3, 4
2	54	M	15-B2	14-A3.1	8; −16	34	0	2, 3
3	45	M	15-B1	14-A3.2	0; +21	34	15	1
4	54	M	15-B2	14-A3.1	2; −8	32	4	1
5	48	M	15-B2	14-C1.1	16; +19	49	0	1
6	41	F	15-B1	14-A3.1	8; −6	44	9	1
7	60	M	15-B2	14-A3.1	17; −12	34	24	1, 2, 3, 4, 5
8	18	M	15-B2	14-A3.2	24; −9	48	6	
9	45	M	15-B3	14-A3.1	4; −8	40	10	1, 2, 3
10	44	M	15-B2	14-A3.1	7; −7	38	42	1, 5
11	40	F	15-B1	14-A3.1	21; −10	34	17	1, 2
12	51	M	15-B1	14-A3.2	10; −15	28	31	1, 2, 3
13	52	M	15-B2	14-A3.2	7; +30	40	28	1, 2

1 rib fracture(s), *2* ipsilateral extremity fractures, *3* pneumothorax, *4* intracranial hemorrhage, *5* abdominal hemorrhage/laceration

formalized therapy and therapy compliance. The mean Herscovici score for all patients was 12.9 at 3-month follow-up (range 10–15). Patient outcome data is categorized in Table 2.

Twelve of 13 (92 %) clavicular fractures initially healed. One infected nonunion successfully healed after debridement, antibiotics, and revision plating. All of the scapular fractures healed with radiographic evidence of malunion without further displacement. None of the scapular fractures required reconstructive surgery to re-align the scapular malunion after initial conservative management.

Discussion

Stable, minimally displaced isolated clavicular and scapular fractures heal quickly and predictably with conservative nonoperative treatment [13, 40–42]. These injuries, however, are different from the unstable, displaced 'floating shoulder' injuries [1, 2]. 'Floating shoulder' injuries are rare with complex fracture patterns. This type of double SSSC injury is usually the result of high-energy trauma and often has associated ipsilateral shoulder and chest trauma.

Previous studies have described clinical outcomes following clavicular fixation of these injuries with varied

Table 2 Patient outcomes

Case number	Final follow-up					3 months
	Forward flexion	Abduction	Pain	Subsequent surgery	Return to work	Herscovici score[a]
1	180	180	Minimal	None	Full return	15
2	180	180	Minimal	None	Full return	10
3	180	180	Minimal	None	Full return	13
4	180	180	Minimal	None	Full return	14
5	150	140	Minimal	None	Full return	15
6	150	150	Minimal	None	Full return	13
7	180	120	Minimal	None	Full return	11
8	160	160	Minimal	None	Full return	15
9	180	180	Minimal	Implant removal	Full return	14
10	140	110	Minimal	None	Full return	11
11	180	180	Moderate	Implant removal	Full return	14
12	180	180	Minimal	None	Full return	13
13	180	180	High	Nonunion revision	Restrictions	10

Minimal, moderate, and high pain levels correspond to VAS of 1–3, 4–6, and 7–10, respectively

[a] Mean Herscovici for all patients at 3 months was 12.9

Table 3 Published results involving only clavicle fixation of floating shoulder injuries

	Number of injuries	Treatment			Patient outcomes
		Conservative	Clavicle fixation	Clavicle and scapular fixation	
Gilde et al. (present study)	13		13		Mean Herscovici score 12.9 at 3 months
Herscovici et al. [6]	9	2	7		1 good, 1 poor: 2 with 'droop' 7 excellent
Yadav et al. [17]	25	13	12		Mean Herscovici score 10.4 at 3 months Mean Herscovici score 13.9 at 3 months
Labler et al. [11]	17	8	6	3	Mean Constant–Murley score 90 (67–100) Mean Constant–Murley score 66 (0–98) Mean Constant–Murley score 93 (86–100)
van Noort et al. [12]	35	28	7		Mean Constant–Murley score 76 (30–100) Mean Constant–Murley score 71 (43–100)
Hashiguchi and Ito [14]	5		5		Mean UCLA score 34.2 (33–35)
Rikli et al. [15]	12		11	1	Mean Constant–Murley—96% match to age- and sex-corrected normal values
Oh et al. [18]	11	3	5	3	Mean Rowe score 77 (55–90) Mean Rowe score 88 (80–90) Mean Rowe score 90 (80–100)
Low and Lam [16]	4		4		Rowe scores—1 (70–84); 3 (85–100)

results (Table 3). Herscovici et al. [6] reported on seven patients who had excellent outcomes with a Herscovici score of 13–16 after surgical fixation of only the clavicle. Two conservatively treated patients had persistent shoulder 'drooping', but could not undergo operative treatment due to severe injuries. An alternative randomized study of 25 patients by Yadav et al. [17] reported a significantly greater mean Herscovici score at 3 and 24 months in patients treated with clavicular fixation only compared to conservative management (13.9 vs 10.4 and 14.9 vs 13.0, respectively). Labler et al. [11] reported on 17 patients treated either conservatively, with clavicular fixation only, or with combined clavicular and scapular fixation. In their operative group, five patients showed good to excellent results (Constant–Murley scores 93–100) and four patients showed bad to fair results (Constant–Murley scores 0–86). The high Constant–Murley scores seen in the nonoperative group correlated with minimally displaced clavicular and scapular fractures suggestive of stable patterns. Van Noort et al. [12] reported that only two of seven patients had a corresponding indirect scapular reduction with only clavicular fixation, and persistent caudal displacement of the glenoid was observed in the other five patients. Fourteen of 28 conservatively treated patients showed persistent 'drooping' of the shoulder. Hashiguchi and Ito [14] found fracture union of all five clavicular and scapular fractures treated with only clavicular plating. Correspondingly high UCLA shoulder scores were noted. Rikli et al. [15] reported healing of 11 clavicular fractures after plating. Nine

of their patients were completely pain free at last follow-up. Four patients changed jobs; however, three of these changes were secondary to concomitant injuries. Oh et al. [18] found improved mean Rowe scores in clavicular fractures treated operatively versus conservative management. Low and Lam [16] reported one good (Rowe score 70–84) and three excellent outcomes (Rowe score 85–100) after only clavicular fixation.

This study also demonstrates that 'good' to 'excellent' outcomes can be observed with only clavicle fixation in patients with floating shoulder injuries. At 3 months after fixation, we observed a mean Herscovici score of 12.9 consistent with near excellent outcomes. Four patients had good outcomes (9–12) and 9 experienced excellent outcomes (13–16) despite the severity of associated injuries and varying levels of shoulder instability. This does not correspond to the outcomes published by Yadav et al.; however, patients with associated neurovascular injuries or rib fractures requiring intervention were included in this study. We agree with previous studies and the recommendations set forth by Labler et al. that the majority of patients with floating shoulder injuries resulting in minimally displaced scapular fractures that are treated with clavicular plating may return to function despite varying levels of pain and scapular deformity [11]. On the basis of our patient outcomes, we recommend only clavicular fracture fixation for minimally displaced 'floating shoulder' injuries.

A weakness of this study is the retrospective design and absence of a standardized functional outcome tool such as the UCLA shoulder score, ASES shoulder scoring scale, Constant–Murley score, and disabilities of arm, shoulder, and hand (DASH) systems. No validated surgical indications for scapular fixation exist in the literature. Without validated surgical indication, surgeon and/or patient preference for nonoperative versus operative management does not exist; therefore, potential patient selection and treatment intervention bias may have occurred. All patterns were complex shoulder girdle injuries with varied stability. The strengths of this study include isolated clavicular fixation of a relatively large number of 'floating shoulder' injuries utilizing modern plating techniques. Patients were followed until complete fracture healing and operative site healing became stable.

Further research efforts are needed to reliably quantify scapular deformities objectively in order to determine surgical indications and the effectiveness of postoperative reduction of the glenoid following clavicular fixation. Three questions still persist regarding the 'floating shoulder'. First, does clavicular fixation actually restore the scapula fracture component to its pre-injury anatomy [43, 44]? Secondly, is residual pain related to the combined shoulder girdle injury, clavicular fixation, and/or the scapular malunion? Lastly, would scapular fracture fixation decrease required formal physical therapy, allow patients to return to work earlier, or improve their overhead strength and endurance.

In conclusion, isolated plate fixation of the clavicular fracture in 'floating shoulder' injuries results in high rates of both clavicular and scapular fracture healing with good to excellent outcomes. Despite varying persistent shoulder girdle pain and scapular malunion, the majority of patients returned to previous work.

Acknowledgments We would like to thank Drs. Terrence Endres, James Ringler, and David Bielema for the contribution of their patients and surgical skill.

Conflict of interest Each author certifies that he or she has no commercial associations (e.g., consultancies, stock ownership, equity interest, patent/licensing arrangements, etc.) that might pose a conflict of interest in connection with the submitted article. No funding was received for this study.

Ethical standards Approval was granted from the Spectrum Health Institutional Review Board. All procedures were in accordance with the ethical standards of the institutional research committee. The need for informed consent was waived by the ethical committee since rights and interests of the patients would not be violated and their privacy and anonymity would be assured by this study design. The authors declare that this study was performed in accordance with the ethical standards of the 1964 Declaration of Helsinki as revised in 2000.

References

1. Owens BD, Goss TP (2006) The floating shoulder. J Bone Joint Surg Br 88B:1419–1424
2. Goss T (1993) Double disruptions of the superior shoulder suspensory complex. J Orthop Trauma 7:99–106
3. Ada JR, Miller ME (1991) Scapular fractures—analysis of 113 cases. Clin Orthop Relat Res (269):174–180
4. Thompson DA, Flynn TC, Miller PW, Fischer RP (1985) The significance of scapular fractures. J Trauma-Injury Infect Crit Care 25:974–977
5. Imatani RJ (1975) Fractures of scapula—review of 53 fractures. J Trauma-Injury Infect Crit Care 15:473–478
6. Herscovici D, Fiennes A, Allgower M, Ruedi TP (1992) The floating shoulder—ipsilateral clavicle and scapular neck fractures. J Bone Joint Surg Br 74:362–364
7. Ganz R, Noesberger B (1975) Treatment of scapular fractures. Hefte Unfallheilkd 126:59–62
8. Edwards SG, Whittle AP, Wood GW (2000) Nonoperative treatment of ipsilateral fractures of the scapula and clavicle. J Bone Joint Surg Am 82A:774–780
9. Ramos L, Mencia R, Alonso A, Ferrandez L (1997) Conservative treatment of ipsilateral fractures of the scapula and clavicle. J Trauma-Injury Infect Crit Care 42:239–242
10. Egol KA, Connor PM, Karunakar MA, Sims SH, Bosse MJ, Kellam JF (2001) The floating shoulder: clinical and functional results. J Bone Joint Surg Am 83A:1188–1194
11. Labler L, Platz A, Weishaupt D, Trentz O (2004) Clinical and functional results after floating shoulder injuries. J Trauma-Injury Infect Crit Care 57:595–602
12. van Noort A, Slaa RLT, Marti RK, van der Werken C (2001) The floating shoulder—a multicentre study. J Bone Joint Surg Br 83B:795–798
13. Cole PA, Gauger EM, Schroder LK (2012) Management of scapular fractures. J Am Acad Orthop Surg 20:130–141
14. Hashiguchi H, Ito H (2003) Clinical outcome of the treatment of floating shoulder by osteosynthesis for clavicular fracture alone. J Shoulder Elbow Surg 12:589–591
15. Rikli D, Regazzoni P, Renner N (1995) The unstable shoulder girdle—early functional treatment utilizing open reduction and internal-fixation. J Orthop Trauma 9:93–97
16. Low CK, Lam AWM (2000) Results of fixation of clavicle alone in managing floating shoulder. Singapore Med J 41:452–453
17. Yadav V, Khare G, Singh S, Kumaraswamy V, Sharma N, Rai A, Ramaswamy A, Sharma H (2013) A prospective study comparing conservative with operative treatment in patients with a 'floating shoulder' including assessment of the prognostic value of the glenopolar angle. Bone Joint J 95-B:815–819
18. Oh CW, Jeon IH, Kyung HS, Park BC, Kim PT, Ihn JC (2002) The treatment of double disruption of the superior shoulder suspensory complex. Int Orthop 26:145–149
19. Leung KS, Lam TP (1993) Open reduction and internal-fixation of ipsilateral fractures of the scapular neck and clavicle. J Bone Joint Surg Am 75A:1015–1018
20. Fleischmann W, Kinzl L (1993) Philosophy of osteosynthesis in shoulder fractures. Orthopedics 16:59–63
21. Khallaf F, Mikami A, Al-Akkad M (2006) The use of surgery in displaced scapular neck fractures. Med Princ Pract 15:443–448

22. Herrera DA, Anavian J, Tarkin IS, Armitage BA, Schroder LK, Cole PA (2009) Delayed operative management of fractures of the scapula. J Bone Joint Surg Br 91B:619–626

23. Jones CB, Cornelius JP, Sietsema DL, Ringler JR, Endres TJ (2009) Modified Judet approach and minifragment fixation of scapular body and glenoid neck fractures. J Orthop Trauma 23:558–564

24. Mayo KA, Benirschke SK, Mast JW (1998) Displaced fractures of the glenoid fossa—results of open reduction and internal fixation. Clin Orthop Relat Res (347):122–130

25. Kavanagh BF, Bradway JK, Cofield RH (1993) Open reduction and internal-fixation of displaced intraarticular fractures of the glenoid fossa. J Bone Joint Surg Am 75A:479–484

26. Lazarides S, Zafiropoulos G (2006) Conservative treatment of fractures at the middle third of the clavicle: the relevance of shortening and clinical outcome. J Shoulder Elbow Surg 15:191–194

27. Zlowodzki M, Zelle BA, Cole PA, Jeray K, McKee MD (2005) Treatment of acute midshaft clavicle fractures: systematic review of 2144 fractures—On behalf of the Evidence-Based Orthopaedic Trauma Working Group. J Orthop Trauma 19:504–507

28. Potter JM, Jones C, Wild LM, Schemitsch EH, McKee MD (2007) Does delay matter? The restoration of objectively measured shoulder strength and patient-oriented outcome after immediate fixation versus delayed reconstruction of displaced midshaft fractures of the clavicle. J Shoulder Elbow Surg 16:514–518

29. Kim W, McKee MD (2008) Management of acute clavicle fractures. Orthop Clin North Am 39:491–505

30. Altamimi SA, McKee MD, Canadian Orthopaedic Trauma S (2008) Nonoperative treatment compared with plate fixation of displaced midshaft clavicular fractures. Surgical technique. J Bone Joint Surg Am 90 Suppl 2 Pt 1:1–8

31. Jones CB, Sietsema DL, Ringler JR, Endres TJ, Hoffmann MF (2013) Results of anterior-inferior 2.7-mm dynamic compression plate fixation of midshaft clavicular fractures. J Orthop Trauma 27:126–129

32. Collinge C, Devinney S, Herscovici D, DiPasquale T, Sanders R (2006) Anterior-inferior plate fixation of middle-third fractures and nonunions of the clavicle. J Orthop Trauma 20:680–686

33. McKee MD, Kreder HJ, Mandel S, McCormack R, Reindl R, Pugh DMW, Sanders D, Buckley R, Canadian Orthopaedic Trauma S (2007) Nonoperative treatment compared with plate fixation of displaced midshaft clavicular fractures—a multicenter, randomized clinical trial. J Bone Joint Surg Am 89A:1–10

34. Bestard E, Schvene H (1986) Glenoplasty in the management of recurrent shoulder dislocation. Contemp Orthop 12:47–55

35. Armitage BM, Wijdicks CA, Tarkin IS, Schroder LK, Marek DJ, Zlowodzki M, Cole PA (2009) Mapping of scapular fractures with three-dimensional computed tomography. J Bone Joint Surg Am 91A:2222–2228

36. Sharr JRP, Mohammed KD (2003) Optimizing the radiographic technique in clavicular fractures. J Shoulder Elbow Surg 12:170–172

37. Marsh JL, Slongo TF, Agel J, Broderick JS, Creevey W, DeCoster TA, Prokuski L, Sirkin MS, Ziran B, Henley B, Audige L (2007) Fracture and dislocation classification compendium-2007—Orthopaedic Trauma Association classification, database and outcomes committee. J Orthop Trauma 21:S1–S133

38. Scott J, Huskisson EC (1976) Graphic representation of pain. Pain 2:175–184

39. Namdari S, Yagnik G, Ebaugh DD, Nagda S, Ramsey ML, Williams GR, Mehta S (2012) Defining functional shoulder range of motion for activities of daily living. J Shoulder Elbow Surg 21:1177–1183

40. Robinson CM, Court-Brown CM, McQueen MM, Wakefield AE (2004) Estimating the risk of nonunion following nonoperative treatment of a clavicular fracture. J Bone Joint Surg Am 86-A:1359–1365

41. Faldini C, Nanni M, Leonetti D, Acri F, Galante C, Luciani D, Giannini S (2010) Nonoperative treatment of closed displaced midshaft clavicle fractures. J Orthop Traumatol: Off J Ital Soc Orthop Traumatol 11:229–236

42. Jones CB, Sietsema DL (2011) Analysis of operative versus nonoperative treatment of displaced scapular fractures. Clin Orthop Relat Res 469:3379–3389

43. Patterson JMM, Galatz L, Streubel PN, Toman J, Tornetta P, Ricci WM (2012) CT evaluation of extra-articular glenoid neck fractures: does the glenoid medialize or does the scapula lateralize? J Orthop Trauma 26:360–363

44. Zuckerman SL, Song YN, Obremskey WT (2012) Understanding the concept of medialization in scapula fractures. J Orthop Trauma 26:350–357

35

Predisposing factors for early infection in patients with open fractures and proposal for a risk score

Marcos Almeida Matos · Lucynara Gomes Lima ·
Luiz Antonio Alcântara de Oliveira

Abstract

Background The primary goals of orthopedic treatment of open fractures are to prevent infection, stabilize bone injury and restore limb function. The objective of the current study was to identify risk factors associated with infection in patients suffering from open fractures, using the strength of association of these factors to propose a score that enables risk stratification in initial care.

Materials and methods A retrospective analysis was performed on 122 patients who underwent open fracture treatment. Clinical and demographic data were collected and the results were divided into two groups: those without infection and those with infection. Both groups were evaluated searching for associated factors that could lead to infection.

Results Thirty-one patients out of 122 were infected (25.4 %). Infection was significantly associated with exposure time up to 24 h (mean 30.3 h; $p = 0.007$). Fractures classified as Gustilo III had a greater chance of infection (74.2 %; $p = 0.042$), especially type IIIB (41.9 %). Fractures classified as Tscherne II and III had a greater chance of infection (48.4 and 25.8 %, respectively; $p = 0.001$).

Conclusions It was possible to show that the exposure time and the types of fracture classified as Gustilo III and Tscherne II and III are associated with the outcome of infection. It was also possible to create a risk score (IRS) for predicting infection in these types of fractures, which can be used in the initial care of the patient, with a sensitivity of 0.840, specificity of 0.544, cut-off of 6.5 and area under the curve of 0.709 ($p = 0.002$).

Level of evidence Level III.

Keywords Fracture · Infection · Treatment · Trauma · Evaluation

Introduction

Orthopedic treatment in open fractures is often performed to prevent infection, to stabilize the bone lesion and to restore limb function. The prevention of infection represents the main measure so that the other objectives may be achieved [1–3].

Post-traumatic bone infection (osteomyelitis) is a devastating event that often compromises the rehabilitation of the patient and their treatment. This infection increases the cost and duration of the treatment, causing physical and social losses, and affecting the quality of life and the functional independence of patients [4].

Early surgical debridement within 6 h and the immediate stabilization of the fracture are the most effective measures for preventing infection in the treatment of open fractures [1–3]. Even though these measures are fundamental, other clinical and environmental factors may contribute to the onset of post-traumatic osteomyelitis. The main risk factors associated with infection include trauma energy, the size of the lesion, devitalization of soft tissues, severity of the bone damage, degree of local contamination, delay in initiating treatment and the immunological status of the patient [5–7].

M. A. Matos (✉) · L. G. Lima
Bahian School of Medicine and Public Health, Rua da Ilha, 378,
Itapuã, Salvador, Bahia 41620-620, Brazil
e-mail: malmeidamatos@ig.com.br

M. A. Matos · L. G. Lima
Roberto Santos General Hospital, Salvador, Bahia, Brazil

L. A. A. de Oliveira
Feira de Santana State University, Feira De Santana, Brazil

The identification of risk factors predictive for infection in the initial clinical evaluation of the patient with an open fracture should therefore be the crucial stage of the orthopedic treatment. The recognition of these indicators could result in more effective therapeutic measures. Thus, in the earliest instance, risk stratification could help the orthopedic surgeon to choose the best treatment for each patient.

Despite recognizing the importance of clinical and environmental risk factors in open fracture prognosis, most studies on this matter are confined to surgical aspects [8–12]. This paper seeks to identify the risk factors for infection in patients with open fractures, using the strength of the association of these factors to propose a score that may enable a risk stratification when a patient is admitted.

Materials and methods

A retrospective study was conducted based on the records of patients who had open fractures and were treated at the Roberto Santos General Hospital (HGRS in Portuguese or RSGH in English), Salvador, Bahia, from March 2009 to December 2009.

All patients over 8 years of age with open fractures admitted through the Emergency Room of the RSGH were included. Patients coming from other units of the Public Health system of the state of Bahia who were referred to the RSGH were also included. Patients with open fractures of the axial skeleton (spine, face, skull, thorax), and those who did not remain at the unit for at least 1 day after the initial procedure, for any reason, were excluded. Patients with incomplete records were also excluded.

The RSGH is the largest public hospital in Northeastern Brazil, and a reference center for trauma surgery. The initial procedure includes filling out a standardized form for the assessment of orthopedic patients, which is attached to the records. This form is updated daily during the patient's admission and records clinical and demographic data, as well as any occurrences related to the patient, including the presence of infection or not. This clinical form rendered this study possible and all the data used in this study was retrieved from it.

The independent variables used in the analysis were: age, sex, marital status (unmarried, married, others), origin (capital or other towns of Bahia), affected bone (upper limb and lower limb), type of accident (traffic: motorcycle, automobile, run over; gunshot wound, fall from height, direct trauma), exposure time of the fracture (time between the trauma and the therapeutic procedure), fracture classification according to Gustilo et al. [13], and classification of soft tissue lesion according to Tscherne and Oestern [14], as well as habits such as drinking and smoking. Primary

treatment methods were considered as follows: cast, external fixation (all types), or internal fixation (either intra- or extra-medullary). The end result "infection" was adopted as a dependent variable.

Early infection (end result variable) was considered to be infections occurring within 2 weeks, as proposed by Willenegger [15]. The criteria to define surgical site infection in patients' evolution followed the rules of the Center for Diseases Control and Prevention [2]. We used clinical signs and symptoms such as purulent drainage, pain, swelling, redness or fever, along with surgeon's confirmation of the diagnosis, and also laboratory findings such as increased white cell count, raised hemosedimentation rate and C-reactive protein (CRP), and fluid cultures [15, 16]. To verify this result, the patients were evaluated at the time of admission and after a 2-week follow-up, regardless of discharge from hospital.

Data on 122 patients who met the inclusion criteria were collected. From these, the end result "infection" (dependent variable) was confirmed in 31 patients, and 91 were free of infection. The patients were thus divided into two groups: patients with and without infection.

Data were presented in tables of frequency distribution for discrete variables, and using the average and standard deviation for continuous variables. The analysis of risk factors associated with infection in both groups (with or without infection) was made using the Student t test for continuous variables and the chi-squared test for discrete variables. The value of $p \leq 0.05$ was adopted as the significance level for all tests.

Considering the statistical significance found in the bivariate analysis, and with the objective of selecting variables predictive of infection, a multivariate analysis was performed. From the final model of logistic regression, the odds ratio was calculated for each variable. Thus, from the identification of variables significantly associated with infection in the bivariate and multivariate analyses, a score was created to predict the risk of infection at the time of admission, even before the initial treatment.

For the construction of the score, which was called the Infection Risk Score (IRS), relevant factors (statistic and clinical) were considered as infection predictors. Thus, three variables were included in the IRS: the Tscherne [14] and Gustilo [13] classifications, as well as the time elapsed since the fracture event. As for the exposure period, it was necessary to categorize this into the following groups: up to 12 h, from 12 to 24 h, and above 24 h. This subdivision was made to transform the time into a categorical variable, and was based on the studies of Patzakis and Wilkins [17].

For the development of the score, the exposure period of the fracture was considered as 1 for a period of up to 12 h, 2 for a period between 12 and 24 h, and 3 for a period over 24 h. For the Gustilo [13] classification, 1 was scored for type I (slight), 2 for type II (moderate), 3 for type IIIA (severe A), 4 for type IIIB (severe B) and 5 for type IIIC (severe C). For the Tscherne [14] classification, 1 was scored for type I, 2 for type II, 3 for type III and 4 for type IV. The variables were thus transformed by means of the sum of the individual scores into the final score designated IRS. These data allow the construction of the IRS, which varies from a score of 3 for the lowest infection risk to a score of 12 for the greatest infection risk.

To identify the association of the IRS with the end result of infection, the Student t test was used to associate the median score in both groups with the infection variable. The IRS was categorized into three levels with the object of identifying the infection risk: level I (low risk), patients with 3, 4 or 5 points in the IRS; level II (intermediate risk) for patients with 6, 7, 8 or 9 points in the IRS; and level III (high risk) for patients with 10, 11 and 12 points. In addition, a receiver operating characteristic (ROC) curve was built to show the accuracy parameters of the IRS.

Results

The demographic characteristics of the 122 patients can be seen in Table 1. The global infection rate was 25.4 % (31 patients) and there was no statistical association between the variables studied. No association was found between infection and the anthropometric measures such as weight, age and body mass index (BMI), despite a significant difference in the height of the patients (Table 2).

For clinical conditions, all the results showed a significant association. The mean time elapsed from the trauma to the surgical treatment was 30.3 h ($\pm$19.5) for the infection group, and 21.4 h ($\pm$12.1) for the group without infection. The earliest treatment was 6 h after the trauma, and the longest length of time until treatment was 76 h after the accident. Infection had a significant association with the exposure time of the fracture. For the Gustilo [13] classification, type III fractures (74.2 %) had a greater probability of infection than other types. For the Tscherne [14] classification, lesions of type III (48.4 %) and type II (25.8 %) presented the greater risk of infection (Table 3).

Internal fixation was the treatment choice in 25 (20.5 %) of the fractures and cast or external fixation was performed in 97 cases (79.5 %). According to the Gustilo classification, internal fixation was the method of choice in 36.45 % ($n = 4$) of type I open fractures, 15.2 % ($n = 7$) of type II, and 23.1 % ($n = 15$) of all type III. There were no statistically significant differences with regard to treatment options and infection (Table 3). There was no association between infection and treatment method when comparing only external versus internal fixation ($p = 0.745$) or cast plus external fixation versus internal fixation ($p = 0.739$).

A multivariate analysis was performed, and odds-ratio values were determined for the variables that were statistically significant in the bivariate analysis (Table 4). However, the bivariate analysis used for the IRS took into account that none of the variables were statistically significant in the multivariate analysis.

The IRS had a mean of 7.12 points. When we compared the means of IRS between the groups, with infection (8.24)

Table 1 Sociodemographic data of patients with open fractures in a public hospital in the state of Bahia, from March to December 2009	Variable	With infection (%)	Without infection (%)	Total (%)	p value
	N (%)	31 (25.4)	91 (74.6)	122	
	Gender	31	91	122	0.96
	Male	26 (83.9)	76 (83.5)	102 (83.6)	
	Female	5 (16.1)	15 (16.5)	20 (16.4)	
	Marital status	26	83	109	0.77
	Unmarried	15 (57.7)	55 (66.3)	70 (64.2)	
	Married	10 (38.5)	25 (30.1)	35 (32.1)	
	Other	1 (3.8)	3 (3.6)	4 (3.7)	
	Origin	31	90	121	0.08
	City of Salvador	12 (38.7)	55 (61.1)	67 (55.4)	
	Other towns	19 (61.3)	35 (38.9)	54 (44.6)	
	Fracture localization	31	91	122	0.34
	Lower limbs	22 (71.0)	56 (61.5)	78 (63.9)	
	Upper limbs	9 (29.0)	35 (38.5)	44 (36.1)	
	Type of trauma	31	91	122	0.14
	Gunshot wound	5 (16.1)	29 (31.9)	34 (27.9)	
	Direct trauma	10 (32.2)	23 (25.3)	33 (27.0)	
	Traffic	16 (51.6)	39 (42.8)	55 (45.1)	

Table 2 Anthropometric profile of patients with open fractures in a public hospital in the state of Bahia, from March to December, 2009

Variable	With infection	Without infection	N total	p value
Age	31.5 (±13.5)	31.7 (±14.3)	118	0.929
Weight	71.9 (±14.2)	67.9 (±14.1)	89	0.269
Height	1.76 (±0.1)	1.71 (±0.1)	84	0.036
Body mass index	23.5 (±3.0)	22.8 (±6.1)	53	0.669

Table 3 Clinical characteristics and treatment options of open fractures in a public hospital in the state of Bahia, from March to December, 2009

Variable	With infection	Without infection	N total	p value
Time of exposure (h)	N = 25	N = 79	94	0.007
	30.3 (±19.5)	21.4 (±12.1)		
Gustilo criteria	N = 31	N = 91	122	0.042
I	1 (3.2 %)	10 (11.0 %)	11	
II	7 (22.6 %)	39 (42.8 %)	46	
IIIA	7 (22.6 %)	20 (22.0 %)	27	
IIIB	13 (41.9 %)	19 (20.9 %)	32	
IIIC	3 (9.7 %)	3 (3.3 %)	6	
Tscherne criteria	N = 31	N = 91	122	0.001
I	6 (19.4 %)	32 (35.2 %)	38	
II	8 (25.8 %)	43 (47.2 %)	51	
III	15 (48.4 %)	15 (16.5 %)	30	
IV	2 (6.4 %)	1 (1.1 %)	3	
Treatment	N = 31	N = 91	122	0.944
Cast	42 (9.8 %)	14 (11.8 %)	56	
External fixation	31 (25.4 %)	10 (8.2 %)	41	
Internal fixation	18 (14.7 %)	7 (5.7 %)	25	

Table 4 Odds ratio for each variable

Variable	Estimate	95 % confidence interval
Gustilo criteria	1.328	0.731–2.411
Tscherne criteria	1.899	0.853–4.225
Exposure time	1.007	1.007–1.076

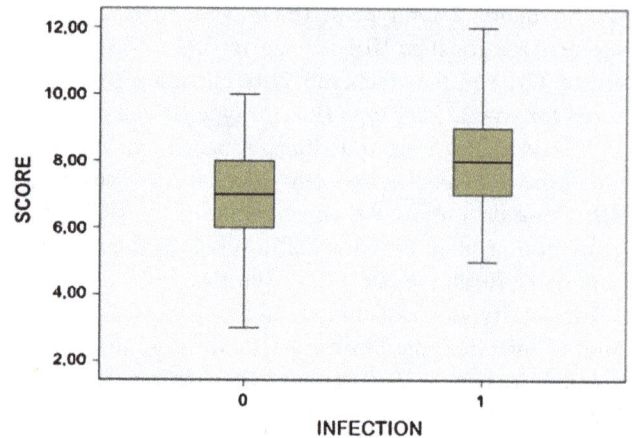

Fig. 1 Boxplot comparing the median scores in the groups with and without infection

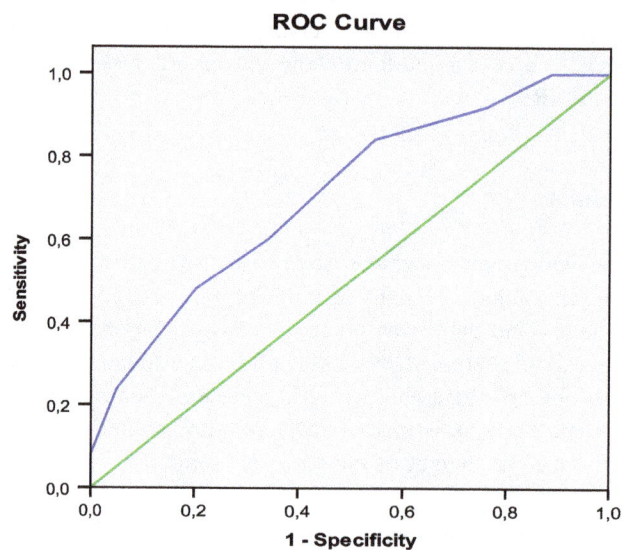

Fig. 2 ROC curve showing the accuracy of the IRS score

and without infection (6.77), a statistically significant difference was observed ($p = 0.001$) (Fig. 1).

The receiver operating characteristic (ROC) curve built from the IRS showed a direct correlation between the IRS and the end result "infection"; the area under the curve had an estimate of 0.709 ($p = 0.002$), a result considered satisfactory for the assessment of the association in clinical studies [18]. The accuracy of the IRS may be assessed from the characteristics of the curve at the cut-off point selected for the end result, which was 6.5. At this point, the curve presents parameters of 0.840 for sensitivity and 0.544 for specificity (Fig. 2).

Discussion

The results of this study reveal that the clinical factors that were significantly associated with the end result "infection" were: time elapsed since the accident, type of open fracture according to Gustilo's criteria [13], and the type of soft tissue damage according to Tscherne's criteria [14]. These three variables were used for the construction of the IRS, resulting in a score that is able to predict the risk of infection of an open fracture at a patient's first evaluation. The IRS had 0.84 sensitivity and 0.55 specificity at the cut-off point of 6.5. The area under the IRS ROC curve was also considered satisfactory for clinical assessment parameters (0.709) [18].

The method of treatment was not associated with the infection outcome. This fact could be explained by considering that treatment is based on infection potential and the severity of the open fracture [1, 5, 7, 8]. Therefore, the methods used were not a predictive variable. As stated in the literature, in the current sample severe open fracture or those at risk of infection were treated by external fixation in order to minimize complications [1, 5, 7, 8].

Though the greater part of the sociodemographic and anthropometric variables did not present a significant association, the assessment of these variables provided important data on the profile of the assisted population. The global infection rate was 25.4 % and in the whole sample there was a high prevalence of males (83.6 %), a mean age of 31.5 years, most were unmarried (64.2 %), lower limbs were the most involved (63.9 %) and traffic accidents represented 45.1 % of all patients in the sample. The high prevalence of alcohol (67.2 %) and tobacco (38.5 %) use should also be noted.

The sociodemographic data of the current study is in accordance with several previous reports on the same subject. Spencer et al. [9] observed a mean age of 45 years, and 40 % was traffic accident. Chua et al. [19] showed a mean age of 36.5 years, with 91.3 % of the sample being male, and traffic accidents accounting for 69 % of the individuals. Müller et al. [3] and Moore et al. [6] also found that most of the patients were male, with average ages of 35.2 and 31 years, respectively. As for the type of trauma, Moore et al. [6] found 52 % of traffic accidents and Müller et al. [3] found a prevalence of 38.4 %. Even though this type of trauma has not been identified as a factor associated with infection, it shows that the frequency of this type of high-energy trauma results in more complex open fractures, with greater chances of infection as the end result.

Bowen and Widmaier [11] show tobacco use and the patient's immunological condition as risk factors for the development of infection. In our study, despite the high number of patients using alcohol and tobacco, this association was not confirmed. In a similar study, Pollak et al. [10] did not find any association between smoking and infection. However, the high prevalence of alcohol use reinforces the study by Arruda et al. [20], who found a strong association between accidents and the use of alcohol and illicit drugs prior to the trauma.

The overall infection rate in the current study is higher than the rates reported in previous studies. Kamat et al. [21] found an infection rate of 11.6 %, Singh et al. [22] found 14.9 %, and Spencer et al. [9] showed 14.6 % cases of infection. These reports slightly differ from the present paper. In the study by Kamat et al. [21] there were only

21.3 % of Gustilo type III fractures and all the cases were operated within a period of less than 17 h, 93 % of the Gustilo type III patients (49.5 %) in the study by Spencer et al. [9] were treated within 12 h of the injury, and 69 % of the type III fractures were treated within 6 h in the report by Singh et al. [22].

In contrast, the report by Pollak et al. [10] showed 27 % of infected fractures, which is very similar to our rate of 25.4 %. All the fractures in that study were Gustilo type III and produced by high-energy trauma, and 41.7 % of the patients were treated more than 10 h after the trauma. Our study comprised 53.3 % of Gustilo type III fractures and debridement occurred in an average of 30.3 h for the infection group, and 21.4 h for the group without infection. We believe that this higher infection rate can be explained by both severity of the wounds and a long delay in the time to treatment. Individuals coming from other towns showed greater chances of developing infection compared with those from the city of Salvador. Therefore, it is possible that some individuals, often in the most severe cases, have been referred to the RSGH because of a lack of hospital units or adequate therapeutic means.

The classifications by Gustilo [13] and Tscherne [14] have been shown in this study to be important predictive factors for infection. This agrees with most papers using Gustilo's classification, but there are also a few studies that evaluate infection predictors using Tscherne's classification. Gustilo et al. [23] showed in their paper a 0 % infection rate for type I fractures, 2.5 % for type II, 13.7 % for type IIIA, 5 % for type IIIB and 44.4 % for type IIIC. In comparison, Müller et al. [3] demonstrated an infection rate of 68.8 % for Gustilo type III for an exposure time greater than 6 h. Recently, Chua et al. [19] have shown a rate of 8.5 % of infection in type I, 9.4 % in type II, 21.8 % in type IIIA and 44.6 % in types IIIB and IIIC. The lesions more strongly associated with infection found in our study, according to Tscherne's soft tissue lesion classification, were type II and III. These findings also agree with Müller et al. [3], who found a high rate of infection in Tscherne type III and IV lesions.

Although there is no consensus in the orthopedic literature regarding the correlation between time and infection, there is evidence of its strength. Spencer et al. [9], Kamat et al. [21] and Singh et al. [22] did not find an association between infection and time to first debridement. Conversely, in our study, this variable was statistically significant, and thus an important predictive factor for infection in open fractures. Kindsfater and Jonassen [24] made a comparative study of tibial fractures grades II and III in which there were different statistical results in relation to osteomyelitis in the groups operated earlier and later than 5 h after the trauma (7 and 38 %, respectively). In the study by Pollak et al. [10], infection was not associated with the time delay from injury to debridement, but time from injury to admission was a predictor of infection, considering time as a continuous variable. In the same study, considering time as a categorical variable, there was a significant chance of infection when time to admission was longer than 2 h (5.4 times more likely to have development of infection) and the risk of infection was significantly higher when patients were transferred to the trauma center after 11 h.

All these previous studies presented time as a categorical variable divided into multiples of 5 or 6 h. However, only a few fractures were treated after 12 h: for instance, just eight (7 %) in the study by Spencer et al. [9]. In our study, time was also used as a categorical variable. Thus, we used intervals of 12 h, similar to the model adopted by Patzakis and Wilkins [17]. This division was used because only nine fractures (7.3 %) were treated in less than 6 h after the time of exposure; the majority were treated after 12 h. Therefore, we believe that time from injury to admission (or debridement) as a categorical variable is a significant predictor when the delay is more than 12 h, and that may conform with and elucidate some of the previous findings in the orthopedic literature.

Though orthopedists agree that prevention of infection is a crucial matter in the treatment of open fractures, few studies have been dedicated to the assessment of predictive factors in these cases. Our study analyzed factors associated with infection and those factors with a stronger association were combined to build a score designated IRS. This score has been shown to be satisfactory in its objectives and especially adequate regarding its sensitivity for infection (84 %). No similar scores have been found in the literature, though much emphasis has been given to individual variables associated with infection, especially the time elapsed between the accident and actual treatment, and the severity of the lesion according to Gustilo [13].

The basic utility of the IRS is to create a useful tool for predicting the risk of infection in open fractures at the moment of the patient's admission to the Emergency Room, keeping in mind that all variables used for the IRS are collected at the initial clinical assessment, and thus post-operative or laboratory results are not necessary for this tool. The IRS could, therefore, guide an orthopedic surgeon in the first surgical approach, which would be as cautious as the infection risk requires. Factors such as debridement extension, primary closure of the lesion, type and time of antibiotics, and type of fracture fixation could be decided based on the IRS. Post-operative therapeutics, nursing care and patient rehabilitation could also be provided according to the IRS score.

This paper was developed using data from patient's records which were not always complete, thus preventing a complete analysis that could have complemented the study.

In addition, some statistical sub-analyses could have suffered distortions as the sample size was calculated specifically for the infection end result. Time was also a limitation factor in constructing the score, because exposure time was categorized in a subjective way, trying to categorize time as homogeneously as possible.

This paper furnishes the literature with several original contributions on the theme. Our data has reinforced the association between infection and time of exposure and lesion severity variables in open fractures. Gustilo's classification has already been related to infection several times in the literature, but our study represents one of the few in which Tscherne's classification has been used, thus supporting its strongest association among all factors. Creating a risk score (IRS) to predict infection with 0.840 sensitivity and 0.544 specificity which may be used at the initial presentation of the patient may also constitute an important contribution which could be used in future studies bearing in mind its validation.

Conflict of interest None.

Ethical standards The study was authorized by Ethics and Research Committee of the Bahian School of Medicine and Public Health and was performed in accordance with the ethical standards of the 1964 Declaration of Helsinki as revised in 2000. All procedures were in accordance with the ethical standards of the institutional and national research committee, and the informed consent of the patients was waived by the committee.

References

1. Ashford RU, Mehta JA, Cripps R (2004) Delayed presentation is no barrier to satisfactory outcome in the management of open tibial fractures. Injury 35:411–416
2. Harley BJ, Beaupre LA, Jones CA et al (2002) The effect of time to definitive treatment on the rate of nonunion and infection in open fractures. J Orthop Traum 16:484–490
3. Müller SS, Sadenberg T, Pereira GJC et al (2003) Epidemiological, clinical and micorbiological prospective study of patients with open fractures assisted at a university hospital. Acta Ortop Bras 11:158–169
4. Silva AGP, Silva FBA, Santos ALG et al (2008) Infection after intramedullary stabilization of diaphyseal fractures of the lower limbs: treatment protocol. Acta Ortop Bras 16:266–269
5. Cleveland KB (2006) Infection: general principles. In: Canale ST (ed) Orthopedic surgery Campbell (Translation of Maurice Kfuri Junior). 10th edn. Editora Manole, São Paulo, pp 643–659
6. Moore TJ, Mauney C, Barron J (1989) The uses of quantitative bacterial counts in open fractures. Clin Orthop Relat Res 248:227–230
7. Khatod M, Botte MJ, Hoyt DB et al (2003) Outcomes in open tibia fractures: relationship between delay in treatment and infection. J Trauma 55:949–954

8. Skaggs DL, Friend L, Alman B et al (2005) The effect of surgical delay on acute infection following 554 open fractures in children. J Bone Joint Surg Am 87:8–12

9. Spencer J, Smith A, Woods D (2004) The effect of time delay on infection in open long-bone fractures: a 5-year prospective audit from a district general hospital. Ann R Coll Surg Eng 86:108–112

10. Pollak AN, Jones AL, Castillo RC et al (2012) The relationship between time to surgical debridement and incidence of infection after open high-energy lower extremity trauma. J Bone Joint Surg Am 92:7–15

11. Bowen TR, Widmaier JC (2005) Hast classification predicts infection after open fracture. Clin Orthop Relat Res 433:205–211

12. Lima ALLM, Zumiotti AV, Uip DE et al (2004) Predictors of infection in patients with fractures of the lower limbs. Acta Ortop Bras 12:32–39

13. Gustilo R, Mendonza R, Williams D (1984) Problems in the management of type III (severe) open fractures: a new classification of type III open fractures. J Trauma 24:742–746

14. Oestern HJ, Tscherne H (1984) Pathophysiology and classification of soft tissue injuries associated with fractures. In: Tscherne H, Gotzen L (eds) Fractures with soft tissue injuries. Springer, Berlin, pp 1–8

15. Willenegger H, Roth B (1986) Treatment tactics and late results in early infection following osteosynthesis. Unfallchirurgier 12:241–246

16. Garner JS (1985) CDC guideline for prevention of surgical wound infection. Infect Control 7:190–200

17. Patzakis MJ, Wilkins J (1989) Factors influencing infection rate in open fracture wounds. Clin Orthop 243:36–40

18. Ludbrook J (2002) Statistical techniques for comparing measurers and methods of measurement: a critical review. Clin Exp Pharmacol Physiol 29:527–536

19. Chua W, Murphy D, Siow W et al (2012) Epidemiological analysis of outcomes in 323 open tibial diaphyseal fractures: a nine-year experience. Singap Med J 53(6):385

20. Arruda LRP, Silva MAC, Malerba FG et al (2009) Fractures: epidemiological and descriptive. Acta Ortop Bras 17:326–330

21. Kamat AS (2011) Infection rates in open fractures of the tibia: is the 6-hour rule fact or fiction? Orthop Adv 2011:1–4

22. Singh J, Rambani R, Hashim Z et al (2012) The relationship between time to surgical debridement and incidence of infection in grade III open fractures. Strategies Trauma Limb Reconstr 7:33–37

23. Gustilo RD (1989) Management of open fractures in orthopeadic infection. Diagnoses and treatment. Saunders, Philadelphia, pp 87–117

24. Kindsfater K, Jonassen EA (1995) Osteomyelitis in grade II and III open tibia fractures with late debridement. J Orthop Trauma 9:121–127

36

Does the position of shoulder immobilization after reduced anterior glenohumeral dislocation affect coaptation of a Bankart lesion? An arthrographic comparison

Omid Reza Momenzadeh[1] · Masoome Pourmokhtari[2] · Sepideh Sefidbakht[3] ·
Amir Reza Vosoughi[1]

Abstract

Background The position of immobilization after anterior shoulder dislocation has been a controversial topic over the past decade. We compared the effect of post-reduction immobilization, whether external rotation or internal rotation, on coaptation of the torn labrum.

Materials and methods Twenty patients aged <40 years with primary anterior shoulder dislocation without associated fractures were randomized to post-reduction external rotation immobilization (nine patients) or internal rotation (11 patients). After 3 weeks, magnetic resonance arthrography was performed. Displacement, separation, and opening angle parameters were assessed and analyzed.

Results Separation (1.16 ± 1.11 vs 2.43 ± 1.17 mm), displacement (1.73 ± 1.64 vs 2.28 ± 1.36 mm), and opening angle (15.00 ± 15.84 vs 27.86 ± 14.74 °) in the externally rotated group were decreased in comparison to the internally rotated group. A statistically significant difference between groups was seen only for separation ($p = 0.028$); p values of displacement and opening angle were 0.354 and 0.099, respectively.

Conclusion External rotation immobilization after reduction of primary anterior shoulder dislocation could result in a decrease in anterior capsule detachment and labral reduction.

Level of evidence Level 2.

Keywords Shoulder · Dislocation · Bankart lesion · External rotation

Introduction

The most commonly dislocated joint in the human body is the glenohumeral joint [1]. Trauma is the main cause of primary anterior shoulder dislocation [2]. Recurrent dislocations and instabilities are the most common sequelae of primary anterior shoulder dislocation and are seen especially in young and active persons [3, 4]. A Bankart lesion or traumatic anterior detachment of the capsulolabrum complex is the principle pathology of further instabilities [5]. Treatment of anterior shoulder dislocation includes immobilization, immediate surgery or delayed surgery [4, 6].

Traditionally, to prevent recurrence of shoulder dislocation, the initial management of first-time anterior shoulder dislocation was immobilization in internal rotation after reduction followed by strengthening exercises of muscles around the shoulder joint. In recent years, multiple published articles reported better results after immobilizing the shoulder in external rotation [1, 7–12]. This prospective clinical trial was carried out to compare the effect of post-reduction shoulder immobilization positions, whether internal rotation or external rotation, on coaptation of the torn labrum.

✉ Amir Reza Vosoughi
vosoughiar@hotmail.com

[1] Bone and Joint Diseases Research Center, Department of Orthopedic Surgery, Chamran Hospital, Shiraz University of Medical Sciences, Shiraz, Iran

[2] Department of Orthopedic Surgery, Jahrom University of Medical Sciences, Jahrom, Iran

[3] Medical Imaging Research Center, Department of Radiology, Namazi Hospital, Shiraz University of Medical Sciences, Shiraz, Iran

Materials and methods

Of the 60 patients with traumatic anterior shoulder dislocation from March 2012 to July 2012, only 35 cases were eligible to participate in this study. Exclusion criteria included associated fracture of the glenoid or the greater tuberosity approved by X-rays and computed tomography (CT), nerve damage, non-primary anterior dislocation, open reduction, and patients >40 years of age. Finally, 25 cases provided written informed consent before enrollment. After successful reduction, patients were randomized to either externally or internally rotated immobilization. All patients in the internal rotation group used a sling and swathe. Because of the high cost of a special external rotation brace, the arm was immobilized in a light comfortable shoulder spica cast with 10° external rotation (Fig. 1). Immobilization was continued for 3 weeks as performed in previous research [8, 11, 18]. Radiographic evaluation was then performed by an experienced radiologist blinded to the groups.

Before injection, routine magnetic resonance imaging (MRI) sequences including T1 tse, T2 tse, and PD tse images in the oblique coronal plane and T2 tse and PD tse axial images as well as PD fat-saturated images in the oblique sagittal plane were obtained on a 1.5T GE scanner. A needle was then introduced into the glenohumeral joint through the rotator cuff interval [13]. A mixture of 10 cc omnipaque, 0.1 cc omniscan, 0.1 cc epinephrine, and 10 cc distilled water was injected under CT guidance. The patient was immediately taken to the MR scanner where T1 fat-saturated images in all three planes were obtained after immobilization of the arm using sandbags on the neutral/supinated hand. The slice thickness was 4 mm with a gap of 0.8 mm (Fig. 2).

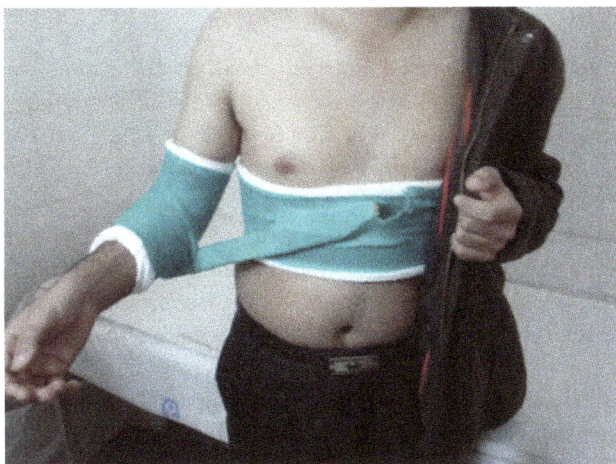

Fig. 2 MRA of a 24-year-old male in the internal rotation group shows a Bankart lesion

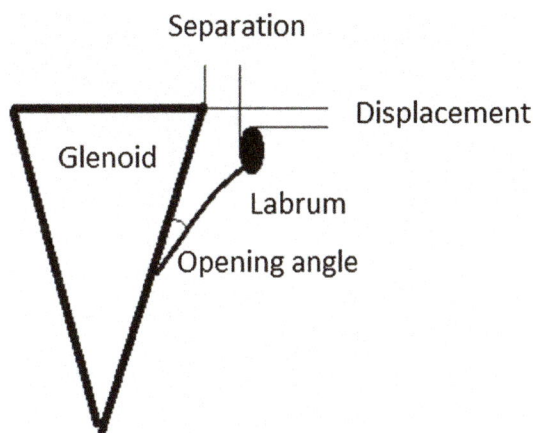

Fig. 3 Schematic picture depicts radiographic parameters, i.e., displacement, separation, and opening angle

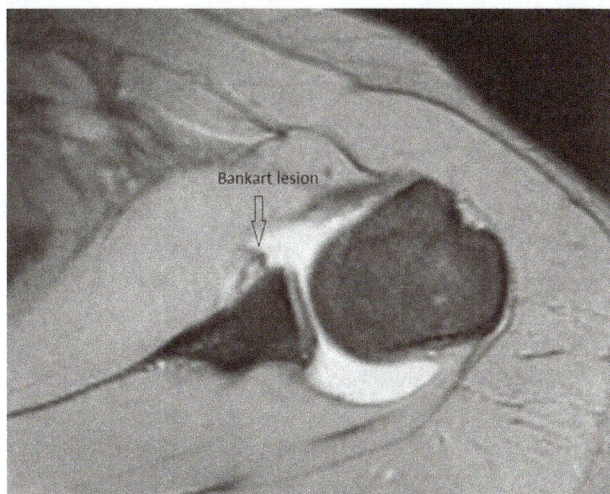

Fig. 1 Shoulder spica cast to fix the arm in external rotation

Parameters defined by Itoi et al. [7] were assessed in magnetic resonance arthrography (MRA). Separation is the distance in millimeters between the inner margin of the labrum and the anterior part of the glenoid neck. Displacement is defined as the distance in millimeters between the tip of the labrum and the tip of the glenoid rim. The opening angle is the angle between the articular aspect of the glenoid neck and a line tangential to the capsule at its glenoid insertion (Fig. 3). It is necessary to mention that separation and opening angle are not directly correlated because separation shows labrum translation at the level of the most lateral part of the glenoid but opening angle reveals the extent of capsular detachment from the glenoid.

SPSS version 18.0 for Windows was used for statistical analyses (SPSS Inc. Chicago, IL, USA). A Mann–Whitney test was performed.

Table 1 Demographic features and MRI parameters of all cases

Case number	Age (years)	Gender	Immobilization	Shoulder	Separation (mm)	Displacement (mm)	Angle (°)
1	31	M	External	Right	2.0	3.0	30
2	21	M	External	Right	2.5	5.0	43
3	19	M	External	Right	0	2.0	20
4	35	M	External	Left	0	0	0
5	32	M	External	Left	0	0	0
6	30	M	External	Right	2.0	2.0	22
7	18	M	External	Right	0	1.5	20
8	25	M	External	Left	2.0	2.1	0
9	34	M	External	Right	2.0	0	0
10	20	M	Internal	Right	3.1	2.0	57.5
11	40	M	Internal	Right	1.0	2.0	25
12	35	M	Internal	Right	0	0	17
13	22	M	Internal	Right	1.8	3.6	37
14	21	F	Internal	Right	3.4	4.0	30
15	25	M	Internal	Right	4.0	3.2	21
16	33	M	Internal	Right	3.2	1.8	0
17	28	M	Internal	Left	2.0	2.0	18
18	18	M	Internal	Right	2.2	0	30
19	19	M	Internal	Right	3.0	3.5	31
20	22	M	Internal	Right	3.1	3.0	40

mm millimeters, *M* male, *F* female

Table 2 Description of age, radiographic parameters, and *p* values

	Mean age (years)	Separation (mean ± SD)	Displacement (mean ± SD)	Open angle (mean ± SD)
Externally rotated immobilization group	27.2	1.16 ± 1.11 mm	1.73 ± 1.64 mm	15.00 ± 15.84°
Internally rotated immobilization group	25.7	2.43 ± 1.17 mm	2.28 ± 1.35 mm	27.86 ± 14.74°
p value		0.028	0.354	0.099

SD standard deviation, *mm* millimeters

Results

Five patients were lost to follow-up. Hence, the externally rotated immobilization group consisted of nine patients and the internally rotated immobilization group consisted of eleven patients; all patients were male except one in the internally rotated group (Table 1).

Comparison of the imaging parameters of the two groups, as shown in Table 2, shows all variables decreased in the externally rotated immobilization group; therefore, the labrum coaptated in a near anatomical position when the arm immobilized in external rotation. The labrum of two patients in the externally rotated group (20 % of cases) had been perfectly located in its original position with a zero measurement for displacement, separation, and open angle.

Discussion

Traditionally, reduced anterior shoulder dislocation was immobilized in adduction and internal rotation and reduced posterior dislocation was immobilized in abduction and external rotation [14]. Approximately 15 years ago, Itoi et al. [15] defined the coaptation zone of a Bankart lesion to the glenoid in a cadaveric study. Itoi et al. [7] then evaluated coaptation of the torn labrum in internal rotation and external rotation using MRI. They concluded that external rotation immobilization approximates the Bankart lesion more than internal rotation. Moreover, another study by Itoi et al. [1] reported a decrease in recurrence rate of anterior shoulder dislocation at a mean follow-up of 15.5 months in patients with the arm immobilized in external rotation after glenohumeral reduction. Other studies in cadavers [16] and in humans using MRI [9, 12] and arthroscopy [10] showed coaptation of the labrum and increase of the labrum—glenoid contact force after immobilization in external rotation. This position improves approximation of the Bankart lesion by placing greater tension on the subscapularis, anterior capsule, and ligaments, closing the anterior joint cavity, and bringing the labrum back to the glenoid rim [1, 7].

Clinically, satisfactory results with regard to instabilities and recurrence rates of dislocation (0.0–19.0 %) have been reported [1, 8, 11, 17, 18]. Although patients with primary anterior shoulder dislocation immobilization in external rotation may have more benefits than in internal rotation, some reported contradictions and controversies should be mentioned.

1. The optimum position of immobilization in external rotation and its duration has not been clearly determined [4, 12, 19].
2. Multiple studies reported conflicting results on acceptance of external rotation braces by patients [1, 20].
3. External rotation immobilization after first-time anterior shoulder dislocation has not been well accepted by orthopedic surgeons, e.g., approximately 93 % of orthopedic surgeon in England preferred internal rotation immobilization after reduction of anterior shoulder dislocation [21].
4. Recent multiple clinical trials have not supported the effectiveness of immobilization in external rotation compared with internal rotation to prevent further instabilities [22–26].

In our study, separation decreased to a larger extent in the externally rotated immobilization group than in the internally rotated group (1.16 ± 1.11 vs 2.43 ± 1.17 mm; $p = 0.028$); the p value of displacement and opening angle showed no statistically significant difference. Our results are the same as those reported by Liavaag et al. [9].

The main limitation of this study is the small number of cases in each group. Moreover, the review of MRA by only one radiologist, the lack of clinical confirmation of stability of the joint especially in the long-term follow-up period, and the absence of questioning patient satisfaction are other limitations.

We would suggest external rotation immobilization after reduction of primary anterior shoulder dislocation for decreasing anterior capsule detachment and labral reduction. Long-term clinical trials may be required to confirm its clinical usage.

Acknowledgments This article has been obtained from a thesis submitted to the Shiraz University of Medical Sciences in partial fulfillment of the requirement for the degree of specialty in orthopedic surgery. The project is sponsored by the Bone and Joint Diseases Research Center, Shiraz University of Medical Sciences.

Conflict of interest The authors declare that they have no conflict of interest related to the publication of this manuscript.

Ethical standards All patients gave informed consent prior to being included in the study. All procedures performed in this study involving human participants were approved by the Ethical Committee of Shiraz University of Medical Sciences and conform to the 1964 Helsinki declaration and its later amendments.

1. Itoi E, Hatakeyama Y, Kido T, Sato T, Minagawa H, Wakabayashi I, Kobayashi M (2003) A new method of immobilization after traumatic anterior dislocation of the shoulder: a preliminary study. J Shoulder Elb Surg 12:413–415
2. Hayes K, Callanan M, Walton J, Paxinos A, Murrell GA (2002) Shoulder instability: management and rehabilitation. J Orthop Sports Phys Ther 32:497–509
3. Owens BD, DeBerardino TM, Nelson BJ, Thurman J, Cameron KL, Taylor DC, Uhorchak JM, Arciero RA (2009) Long-term follow-up of acute arthroscopic Bankart repair for initial anterior shoulder dislocations in young athletes. Am J Sports Med 37:669–673
4. Arliani GG, Astur DD, Cohen C, Ejnisman B, Andreoli CV, Pochini AC, Cohen M (2011) Surgical versus nonsurgical treatment in first traumatic anterior dislocation of the shoulder in athletes. Open Access J Sports Med 2:19–24
5. Hintermann B, Gächter A (1995) Arthroscopic findings after shoulder dislocation. Am J Sports Med 23:545–551
6. Emami MJ, Solooki S, Meshksari Z, Vosoughi AR (2011) The effect of open Bristow-Latarjet procedure for anterior shoulder instability: a 10-year study. Musculoskelet Surg 95:231–235
7. Itoi E, Sashi R, Minagawa H, Shimizu T, Wakabayashi I, Sato K (2001) Position of immobilization after dislocation of the glenohumeral joint. A study with use of magnetic resonance imaging. J Bone Jt Surg Am 83-A:661–667
8. Itoi E, Hatakeyama Y, Sato T, Kido T, Minagawa H, Yamamoto N, Wakabayashi I, Nozaka K (2007) Immobilization in external rotation after shoulder dislocation reduces the risk of recurrence. A randomized controlled trial. J Bone Jt Surg Am 89:2124–2131
9. Liavaag S, Stiris MG, Lindland ES, Enger M, Svenningsen S, Brox JI (2009) Do Bankart lesions heal better in shoulders immobilized in external rotation? Acta Orthop 80:579–584
10. Hart WJ, Kelly CP (2005) Arthroscopic observation of capsulolabral reduction after shoulder dislocation. J Shoulder Elb Surg 14:134–137
11. Seybold D, Gekle C, Fehmer T, Pennekamp W, Muhr G, Kälicke T (2006) Immobilization in external rotation after primary shoulder dislocation. Chirurg 77:821–826
12. Scheibel M, Kuke A, Nikulka C, Magosch P, Ziesler O, Schroeder RJ (2009) How long should acute anterior dislocations of the shoulder be immobilized in external rotation? Am J Sports Med 37:1309–1316
13. Mulligan ME (2008) CT-guided shoulder arthrography at the rotator cuff interval. Am J Roentgenol 191:W58–W61
14. Rezazadeh S, Vosoughi AR (2011) Closed reduction of bilateral posterior shoulder dislocation with medium impression defect of

the humeral head: a case report and review of its treatment. Case Rep Med 2011:124581

15. Itoi E, Hatakeyama Y, Urayama M, Pradhan RL, Kido T, Sato K (1999) Position of immobilization after dislocation of the shoulder. A cadaveric study. J Bone Jt Surg Am 81:385–390

16. Miller BS, Sonnabend DH, Hatrick C, O'leary S, Goldberg J, Harper W, Walsh WR (2004) Should acute anterior dislocations of the shoulder be immobilized in external rotation? A cadaveric study. J Shoulder Elb Surg 13:589–592

17. Königshausen M, Schliemann B, Schildhauer TA, Seybold D (2014) Evaluation of immobilization in external rotation after primary traumatic anterior shoulder dislocation: 5-year results. Musculoskelet Surg 98(2):143–151

18. Taşkoparan H, Kılınçoğlu V, Tunay S, Bilgiç S, Yurttaş Y, Kömürcü M (2010) Immobilization of the shoulder in external rotation for prevention of recurrence in acute anterior dislocation. Acta Orthop Traumatol Turc 44:278–284

19. De Baere T, Delloye C (2005) First-time traumatic anterior dislocation of the shoulder in young adults: the position of the arm during immobilisation revisited. Acta Orthop Belg 71:516–520

20. Schliemann B, Seybold D, Muhr G, Gekle C (2009) Immobilisation of the shoulder in external rotation after traumatic first-time dislocation—what is reasonable? A retrospective survey. Sportverletz Sportschaden 23:100–105

21. Chong M, Karataglis D, Learmonth D (2006) Survey of the management of acute traumatic first-time anterior shoulder dislocation among trauma clinicians in the UK. Ann R Coll Surg Engl 88:454–458

22. Finestone A, Milgrom C, Radeva-Petrova DR, Rath E, Barchilon V, Beyth S, Jaber S, Safran O (2009) Bracing in external rotation for traumatic anterior dislocation of the shoulder. J Bone Jt Surg Br 91:918–921

23. Handoll HH, Hanchard NC, Goodchild L, Feary J (2006) Conservative management following closed reduction of traumatic anterior dislocation of the shoulder. Cochrane Database Syst Rev 1:CD004962

24. Whelan DB, Litchfield R, Wambolt E, Dainty KN (2014) External rotation immobilization for primary shoulder dislocation: a randomized controlled trial. Clin Orthop Relat Res 472:2380–2386 [In conjunction with the Joint Orthopaedic Initiative for National Trials of the Shoulder (JOINTS)]

25. Vavken P, Sadoghi P, Quidde J, Lucas R, Delaney R, Mueller AM, Rosso C, Valderrabano V (2014) Immobilization in internal or external rotation does not change recurrence rates after traumatic anterior shoulder dislocation. J Shoulder Elb Surg 23:13–19

26. Tanaka Y, Okamura K, Imai T (2010) Effectiveness of external rotation immobilization in highly active young men with traumatic primary anterior shoulder dislocation or subluxation. Orthopedics 33:670

37

Is acromioplasty necessary in the setting of full-thickness rotator cuff tears? A systematic review

Filippo Familiari[1,2] · Alan Gonzalez-Zapata[1] · Bruno Iannò[2] · Olimpio Galasso[2] · Giorgio Gasparini[2] · Edward G. McFarland[1]

Abstract

Background The benefits of acromioplasty in treating rotator cuff disease have been debated. We systematically reviewed the literature regarding whether acromioplasty with concomitant coracoacromial (CA) release is necessary for the successful treatment of full-thickness rotator cuff tears.

Materials and methods We identified randomized controlled trials that reported on patients who underwent rotator cuff repair with or without acromioplasty and used descriptive statistics to summarize the findings.

Results Four studies fulfilled the inclusion criteria. They reported on 354 patients (mean age, 59 years; range 3–81 years) with a mean follow-up of 22 months (range 12–24 months). There were two level-I and two level-II studies. Two studies compared rotator cuff repair with versus without acromioplasty, and two studies compared rotator cuff repair with versus without subacromial decompression (acromioplasty, CA ligament resection, and bursectomy). The procedures were performed arthroscopically, and the CA ligament was released in all four studies. There were no statistically significant differences in clinical outcomes between patients treated with acromioplasty compared with those treated without acromioplasty.

Conclusions This systematic review of the literature does not support the routine use of partial acromioplasty or CA ligament release in the surgical treatment of rotator cuff disease. In some instances, partial acromioplasty and release of the CA ligament can result in anterior escape and worsening symptoms. Further research is needed to determine the optimum method for the operative treatment of full-thickness rotator cuff tears.

Level of evidence Level I, systematic review of level I and II studies.

Keywords Acromioplasty · Surgery · Rotator cuff tear · Subacromial decompression · Coracoacromial ligament · Systematic review

✉ Edward G. McFarland
editorialservices@jhmi.edu

[1] Division of Shoulder Surgery, Department of Orthopaedic Surgery, The Johns Hopkins University, 10753 Falls Road, Pavilion II, Suite 215, Lutherville, MD 21093, USA

[2] Department of Orthopaedic and Trauma Surgery, Magna Græcia University, Catanzaro, Italy

Introduction

Shoulder pain has been described as the second-most common musculoskeletal disorder after low back pain [1–4]. Disorders of the rotator cuff, commonly called "impingement," have been reported to be the leading cause of pain in the shoulder [5, 6]. In 1949, Armstrong [7] first suggested that compression of the bursa and rotator cuff tendons under the acromion causes supraspinatus syndrome. Subsequently, Neer [8] stated that 95 % of rotator cuff tears were caused by mechanical impingement and reported successful treatment with partial anterior acromioplasty. Later, the same author described three stages in the development of impingement: stage I, involving edema and hemorrhage; stage II, an irreversible stage involving tendinitis and fibrosis; and stage III, involving severe tendon degeneration and tearing [9]. A subsequent study using conventional radiographs reported a relationship between the shape of the acromion [flat (type I), curved (type II), or hooked (type III)] and the presence of rotator cuff disease [10]. Although these studies confirmed an association between rotator cuff disease and acromial shape, a causal relationship between the shape of the acromion and rotator cuff disease was not established [11, 12].

The procedure of reshaping the acromion with a partial acromioplasty to relieve mechanical pressure on the rotator cuff was widely adopted in open rotator cuff repair. The ability to perform an arthroscopic partial acromioplasty was first described by Ellman [13] in 1987. The risks and benefits of open acromioplasty compared with the arthroscopic approach have been identified in a series of studies, as summarized by Spangehl et al. [14]. The major advantage of the open procedure was that it was technically easier to perform and required less surgeon expertise [14]. The advantages of the arthroscopic approach theoretically included improved cosmetic appearance of the surgical scar, preservation of the deltoid muscle, and faster recovery [14].

Subsequent studies questioned the role of the acromion in the production of rotator cuff disease [15, 16]. Tibone et al. [17] found that partial acromioplasty did not result in improvement of pain in athletic individuals with "impingement." Published reviews of the efficacy of partial acromioplasty for rotator cuff symptoms found that the results were not as good as expected, with failure rates of 15–20 % [18, 19].

In 2001, Goldberg et al. [20] reported the first clinical study to suggest that acromioplasty for full-thickness rotator cuff tears was not necessary for a successful surgical result; this was subsequently confirmed by McAllister et al. [21]. Both studies reported on full-thickness rotator cuff repairs performed without acromioplasty, thus preserving the integrity of the coracoacromial (CA) arch and the deltoid insertion. They found statistically significant improvements in all clinical outcomes evaluated and advocated abandonment of partial acromioplasty and CA ligament release for the treatment of rotator cuff disease [20, 21].

These studies led to a reassessment not only of the role of the acromion in the development of rotator cuff disease but also of the concept of "impingement" itself [22, 23]. Most of these studies suggest that rotator cuff disease is a multifactorial process of both intrinsic causes (rotator cuff degeneration with age) and extrinsic causes (contact with other structures, high tensile load) [24, 25]. However, subsequent clinical studies have indicated that the role of partial acromioplasty and CA ligament release in the surgical treatment of rotator cuff disease should be reassessed. It has been shown that acromioplasty with CA ligament release may lead to increases in anterosuperior and superior glenohumeral instability [26–28].

The purpose of this review was to systematically evaluate published clinical studies as they relate to the need for partial acromioplasty with concomitant release of the CA ligament in the treatment of full-thickness rotator cuff tears.

Materials and methods

Three independent reviewers (F.F., A.G.Z., and E.G.M.) performed a review of the literature using the MEDLINE/PubMed, Excerpta Medica/EMBASE, and Cochrane Register of Controlled Trials databases. Our purpose was to identify and include all English-language randomized controlled trials (level I or II) on the role of acromioplasty with concomitant release of the CA ligament in the treatment of full-thickness rotator cuff tears. We searched using the keywords "acromioplasty," "arthroscopic acromioplasty," "open acromioplasty," "subacromial decompression," and "coracoacromial ligament" ("Appendix"). Only prospective, randomized studies that reported on patients who underwent rotator cuff repair with or without acromioplasty were included.

Our search identified 96 pertinent abstracts or full-text articles. Reference sections of all accessed papers were searched for any undetected studies. These articles were reviewed and cross-referenced to exclude repeated references. Nineteen of these were considered relevant, and the full text of each was reviewed to determine eligibility. Seventy-seven articles were excluded on the basis of titles or abstracts, and 15 were excluded on the basis of full-text review. Biomechanical reports, animal and cadaver studies, in vitro studies, case reports, literature reviews, technical notes, letters to the editor, instructional courses, studies comparing different techniques, study protocols with no results, and studies of nonsurgical interventions were excluded. The remaining four articles [29–32] met the inclusion criteria and were analyzed in this systematic review (Fig. 1).

This review includes only articles that meet accepted quality standards for design and reporting as described by Wright et al. [33] and Spindler et al. [34] and according to the CONSORT statement [35].

For studies that used similar outcome measures, we pooled the results to generate a summary outcome—the frequency-weighted mean (calculated by weighting the mean value for each study by the number of patients in that study). If both preoperative and postoperative values for the outcome were available, we used the frequency-weighted means to calculate a P value for the change; a value of $P < 0.05$ was considered statistically significant.

We extracted the following data: study year, country, study design, and presence of control group; primary and secondary hypotheses; primary and secondary outcomes; basic study characteristics, including number of enrolled

Fig. 1 Flowchart for the
literature search

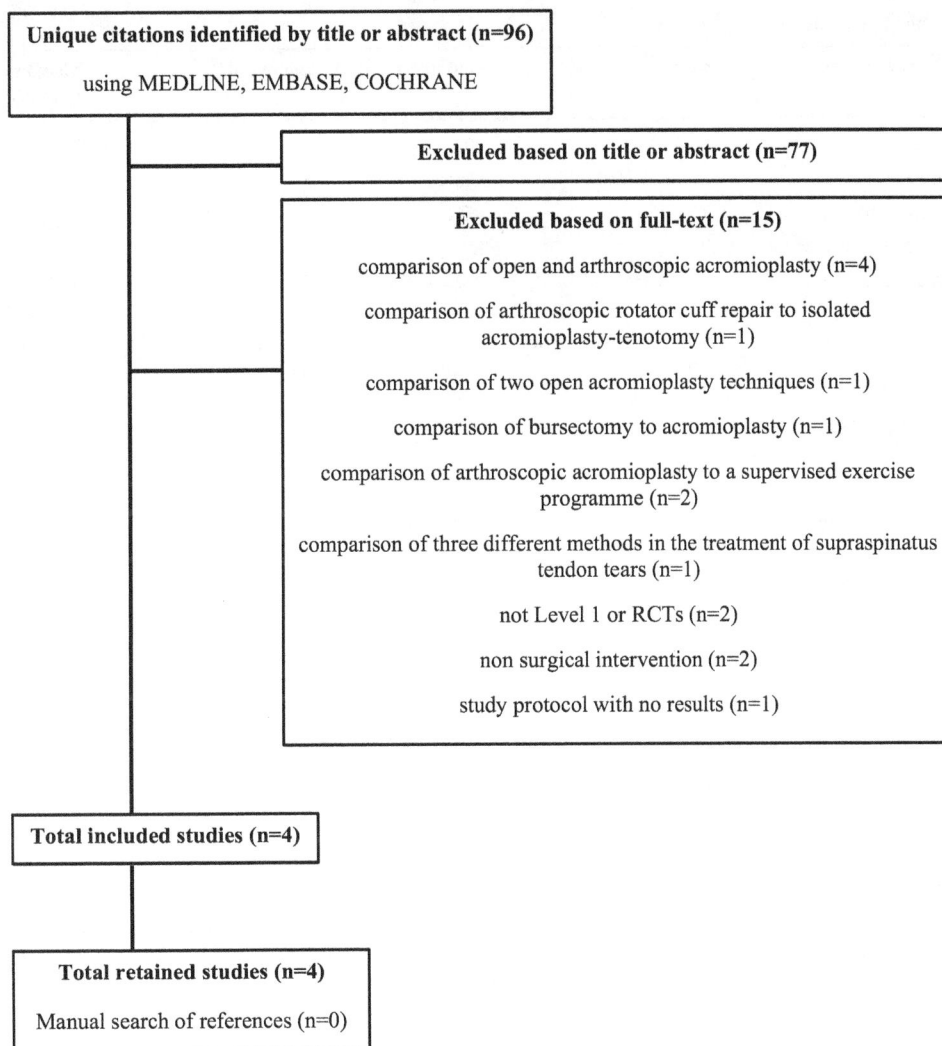

Fig. 1 Flowchart for the literature search

patients, patient age, patient sex, length of follow-up, and study group comparability at baseline; potential sources of bias; use of validated questionnaires; statistical methods and consultation with a biostatistician; presence of independent examiners; differences in rehabilitation protocols between groups; and results (Table 1). Data were extracted from each of the selected papers independently by two evaluators (F.F. and A.G.Z.). There was agreement regarding inclusion or exclusion in all cases. Specific data extracted included the degree of rotator cuff abnormality, the outcome measures (where available), preoperative versus postoperative range of motion, and patient satisfaction and pain relief.

Results

There were two level-I [31, 32] and two level-II studies [29, 30] that met the inclusion criteria. These four studies reported on a total of 354 patients (range 80–95 per study)

[29–32]. The mean patient age was 59 years (range 3–81). Three studies indicated patients' sex, with 159 (63 %) males and 93 (37 %) females [29, 31, 32]. Two studies compared rotator cuff repair with and without acromioplasty [29, 31], and two studies compared rotator cuff repair with and without subacromial decompression (acromioplasty, CA ligament resection, and bursectomy) [30, 32]. The procedures were performed arthroscopically, and the CA ligament was released in all four studies [29–32]. Patients were followed for a mean of 22 months (range 12–24 months).

The outcomes included pain relief [29–31], range of motion [29, 31], and patient- and disease-specific outcome measures (disease-specific quality of life, shoulder-specific outcome measures) [29–32] at final follow-up (Table 2). None of the studies evaluated postoperative patient satisfaction or rotator cuff integrity. There were no statistically significant differences in clinical results between patients treated with acromioplasty versus those treated without

Table 1 Details of included studies

Characteristics	Abrams et al. [29]	Gartsman and O'Connor [30]	MacDonald et al. [31]	Milano et al. [32]
Year	2014	2004	2011	2007
Country	United States	United States	Canada	Italy
Study design	RCT	RCT	RCT	RCT
Level of evidence	II	II	I	I
Procedures	ACR versus ACR-A	ACR versus ACR-SD	ACR versus ACR-A	ACR versus ACR-SD
Inclusion criteria	Full-thickness superior rotator cuff tear	Isolated, repairable full-thickness supraspinatus tendon tear and type 2 acromion	Full-thickness rotator cuff tear	Full-thickness rotator cuff tear and type 2 or 3 acromion
No. of patients	95	93	86	80
Mean age in years	58.8 (SD ±8.1)	59.7 (range 37–81)	56.8 (range 33–77)	60.3 (SD ±8.3)
Mean follow-up in months	24	15.6 (SD ±3.3)	24	24
Study outcome measures	ASES, SST, UCLA, VAS, Constant–Murley	ASES	ASES, ROM, WORC	Constant–Murley, DASH, Work-DASH
Study characteristics comparable at baseline	Yes	Yes	Yes	Yes
Use of validated questionnaires	Yes	Yes	Yes	Yes
Presence of independent examiners	Yes	No	Not reported	Yes
Difference in rehabilitation protocols in groups	No	No	Yes	No

ACR Arthroscopic cuff repair, *ACR-A* arthroscopic cuff repair with acromioplasty, *ACR-SD* arthroscopic cuff repair with subacromial decompression, *ASES* American Shoulder and Elbow Surgeons score, *DASH* Disabilities of the Arm, Shoulder, and Hand questionnaire, *RCT* randomized controlled trial, *ROM* range of motion, *SD* standard deviation, *SST* Simple Shoulder Test, *UCLA* University of California–Los Angeles score, *VAS* Visual Analog Scale for pain, *WORC* Western Ontario Rotator Cuff Index, *Work-DASH* Work-Disabilities of the Arm, Shoulder, and Hand questionnaire

Table 2 Postoperative results of validated questionnaires

Study	Procedure	ASES	WORC	UCLA	CM	VAS	SST	DASH	Work-DASH
MacDonald et al. [31]	ACR	85.6	80.7						
	ACR-A	90.5	87.5						
Gartsman and O'Connor [30]	ACR-SD	91.5							
	ACR	89.2							
Milano et al. [32]	ACR-SD				103.6			18.2	23.7
	ACR				96.1			23.1	26.2
Abrams et al. [29]	ACR	89.0		17.4	78.7	1.0	10.5		
	ACR-A	91.5		17.2	75.0	0.7	10.5		

There were no significant differences between the scores by procedure type. *ACR* Arthroscopic cuff repair, *ACR-A* arthroscopic cuff repair with acromioplasty, *ACR-SD* arthroscopic cuff repair with subacromial decompression, *ASES* American Shoulder and Elbow Surgeons score, *CM* Constant–Murley score, *DASH* Disabilities of the Arm, Shoulder, and Hand questionnaire, *SST* Simple Shoulder Test, *UCLA* University of California, Los Angeles score, *VAS* visual analog scale for pain, *WORC* Western Ontario Rotator Cuff Index, *Work-DASH* Work-Disabilities of the Arm, Shoulder, and Hand questionnaire

acromioplasty in all studies [29–32]. The variability in functional outcome measures reported across trials made a pooled analysis possible for only American Shoulder and Elbow Surgeons scores [29–31] and Constant–Murley scores [29, 32], and no statistically significant differences were found ($P = 0.938$ and $P = 0.673$, respectively)

Table 3 Pooled analysis of ASES and Constant–Murley scores (frequency-weighted means)

Study	Scoring system	Mean (SD) score with acromioplasty	Mean (SD) score no acromioplasty	P value
Abrams et al. [29]; Gartsman and O'Connor [30]; MacDonald et al. [31]	ASES	30.0 (±7.0)	29.6 (±5.2)	0.938
Abrams et al. [29]; Milano et al. [32]	CM	44.5 (±2.0)	46.7 (±6.1)	0.673

ASES American Shoulder and Elbow Surgeons score, *CM* Constant-Murley score, *SD* standard deviation

(Table 3). None of the studies measured patient satisfaction or outcomes in a nonparametric manner such as poor, fair, good, or excellent.

Discussion

Our systematic review of the literature showed no difference in short-term clinical results between patients with full-thickness rotator cuff tears who are treated with versus without acromioplasty and CA ligament release. Our results support the findings of the American Academy of Orthopaedic Surgeons [36], which gave acromioplasty a "moderate" recommendation for the treatment of rotator cuff disease. On the basis of two studies [30, 32] they suggested that "routine acromioplasty is not required at the time of rotator cuff repair," and that despite theoretic benefits of acromioplasty in the setting of rotator cuff repair, it has little or no effect on postoperative clinical outcomes. Furthermore, one published systematic review and meta-analysis of three studies of patients undergoing arthroscopic rotator cuff repair treated with subacromial decompression found no difference from those treated without subacromial decompression [18].

There are several challenges when performing studies and interpreting the results of studies about rotator cuff disease. The first is the wide range of abnormalities that can be included under the umbrella of rotator cuff disease. The patient with "impingement" pain without any rotator cuff abnormality at the time of arthroscopy may be an entirely different entity from the patient who has a partial-thickness or full-thickness rotator cuff tear. Similarly, the degree of partial tear (in terms of percentage of depth of the tendon involved) may be a critical factor in determining the treatment [37]. The size of full-thickness rotator cuff tears has been shown to be a major factor in the success or failure of their treatment, and it is nearly impossible to have a study of the effect of treatment in patients with only one size of tear. Other abnormalities may also contribute to pain in this group of patients, such as biceps tendon abnormality or stiffness of the shoulder; these factors are rarely addressed in studies of the treatment of rotator cuff disease. Lastly, the origin of the pain in rotator cuff disease has not yet been established, making surgical treatment empirical.

There are other limitations of our study. There is wide variability in the reporting of results of surgery for rotator cuff disease. The results of any clinical study should include subjective patient measures (e.g., satisfaction, pain relief), patient- or disease-specific outcomes, preoperative versus postoperative range of motion, strength testing, and integrity of the rotator cuff repair at least 1–2 years after surgery. None of the studies reported here included all of these elements (Table 4). This variability makes it difficult to compare the results of all of the factors important to the surgeon and the patient. For example, in our systematic review, the variability in functional outcome measures reported across studies made a pooled analysis possible for only American Shoulder and Elbow Surgeons and Constant–Murley scores. Moreover, although this review included all RCTs reporting on outcomes after arthroscopic treatment of rotator cuff tears and/or "impingement syndrome," the surgical techniques in the studies may have varied, creating the potential for performance bias. Lastly, the follow-up periods in the included studies ranged from 1 to 2 years. Larger studies with longer follow-up will be required to corroborate the reported findings regarding the need for partial acromioplasty with CA ligament release.

Although Neer [8, 9] remarked that acromioplasty should be reserved for "carefully selected patients with mechanical impingement" and proposed that this procedure should be performed only for patients with reasonable life expectancy and persistent disability despite at least 1 year of nonoperative treatment, Vitale et al. [38] showed that the incidence of acromioplasty has increased dramatically in recent decades. They analyzed the New York Statewide Planning and Research Cooperative System ambulatory surgery database from 1996 to 2006 and the American Board of Orthopaedic Surgery database from 1999 to 2008 to identify patients who had undergone acromioplasty. They reported a 254 % increase in the Statewide Planning and Research Cooperative System group versus a 142 % increase in the American Board of Orthopaedic Surgery group for the number of acromioplasties over their respective time periods. Yu et al. [39] also evaluated the rising incidence of anterior acromioplasty using medical records of residents in Olmsted County, Minnesota, who underwent isolated acromioplasty between 1980 and 2005. They found a 576 % increase over this time period, further showing the widespread popularity of this procedure. It is likely that because acromioplasty is no

Table 4 Parameters evaluated in the included studies

Study	Pain relief	Patient satisfaction	Rotator cuff tear integrity	Shoulder strength testing	Patient- or disease-specific outcome measures
Abrams et al. [29]	Yes	No	No	Yes	Yes
Gartsman and O'Connor [30]	Yes	No	No	No	Yes
MacDonald et al. [31]	Yes	No	No	No	Yes
Milano et al. [32]	No	No	No	No	Yes

longer reimbursed by some insurers in the United States, the incidence of acromioplasty will begin to decrease.

Another issue that we were not able to address in this systematic review was the role of CA ligament release alone in the treatment of rotator cuff disease. Moorman et al. [40] performed a biomechanical study of the CA ligament and found that it was an important restraint to superior subluxation of the humeral head. They concluded that the CA ligament was not vestigial and served an important function in shoulder stability [40]. As a result, standard performance of the procedure has some theoretical disadvantages, including superior subluxation of the humeral head in some patients [40]. Unfortunately, there is no strong evidence for or against CA ligament release alone or in combination with other procedures for the treatment of the different stages and abnormalities of rotator cuff disease.

There is an increasing number of published reports examining the role of acromioplasty with concomitant CA ligament release in the treatment of rotator cuff disease. The current literature suggests that patients have similar outcomes at short-term and intermediate follow-up independent of whether acromioplasty was performed, regardless of acromion morphology. These findings do not support the routine use of acromioplasty as an adjunct to arthroscopic rotator cuff repair. However, current knowledge is limited by the unknown pathophysiology of rotator cuff disease and the inability to know exactly what produces a satisfactory result with rotator cuff surgery. Further study is needed to evaluate the role of acromioplasty and bursectomy alone in the treatment of rotator cuff disease.

Conflict of interest The authors declare that they have no conflict of interest.

Compliance with ethical standards The paper involves no human or animal research.

Appendix: Search strategy

MEDLINE/PubMed

1. Acromioplasty/
2. Acromioplasty*.mp.
3. Exp acromioplasty/
4. Exp arthroscopic acromioplasty/
5. Exp open acromioplasty/
6. Exp subacromial decompression/
7. Exp coracoacromial ligament/
8. Arthroscopic acromiop*.mp.
9. Open acromiop*.mp.
10. Subacromial decomp*.mp.
11. Coracoacromial lig*.mp.
12. 1 or 2 or 3
13. 4 or 5 or 6 or 7 or 8 or 9 or 10 or 11
14. 12 and 13

Excerpta Medica/EMBASE

1. Acromioplasty/
2. Acromioplasty*.mp.
3. Exp acromioplasty/
4. Exp arthroscopic acromioplasty/
5. Exp open acromioplasty/
6. Exp subacromial decompression/
7. Exp coracoacromial ligament/
8. Arthroscopic acromiop*.mp.
9. Open acromiop*.mp.
10. Subacromial decomp*.mp.
11. Coracoacromial lig*.mp.
12. 1 or 2 or 3
13. 4 or 5 or 6 or 7 or 8 or 9 or 10 or 11
14. 12 and 13

Cochrane Register of Controlled Trials

A text-search strategy was performed using the terms "acromioplasty AND (arthroscopic* OR open* OR subacromial decompression* OR coracoacromial ligament*)".

References

1. Makela M, Heliovaara M, Sainio P, Knekt P, Impivaara O, Aromaa A (1999) Shoulder joint impairment among Finns aged 30 years or over: prevalence, risk factors and co-morbidity. Rheumatology (Oxford, UK) 38(7):656–662

2. Picavet HS, Schouten JS (2003) Musculoskeletal pain in the Netherlands: prevalences, consequences and risk groups, the DMC(3)-study. Pain 102(1–2):167–178

3. Pope DP, Croft PR, Pritchard CM, Silman AJ (1997) Prevalence of shoulder pain in the community: the influence of case definition. Ann Rheum Dis 56(5):308–312

4. Urwin M, Symmons D, Allison T, Brammah T, Busby H, Roxby M, Simmons A, Williams G (1998) Estimating the burden of musculoskeletal disorders in the community: the comparative prevalence of symptoms at different anatomical sites, and the relation to social deprivation. Ann Rheum Dis 57(11):649–655

5. Khan Y, Nagy MT, Malal J, Waseem M (2013) The painful shoulder: shoulder impingement syndrome. Open Orthop J 7:347–351. doi:10.2174/1874325001307010347

6. van der Windt DAWM, Koes BW, de Jong BA, Bouter LM (1995) Shoulder disorders in general practice: incidence, patient characteristics, and management. Ann Rheum Dis 54(12):959–964

7. Armstrong JR (1949) Excision of the acromion in treatment of the supraspinatus syndrome; report of ninety-five excisions. J Bone Jt Surg Br 31(3):436–442

8. Neer CS II (1972) Anterior acromioplasty for the chronic impingement syndrome in the shoulder: a preliminary report. J Bone Jt Surg Am 54(1):41–50. doi:10.2106/JBJS.8706.cl

9. Neer CS II (1983) Impingement lesions. Clin Orthop 173:70–77. doi:10.1097/00003086-198303000-00010

10. Bigliani LU, Morrison DS, April EW (1986) The morphology of the acromion and its relationship to rotator cuff tears (abstr). Orthop Trans 10:216

11. Bigliani LU, Ticker JB, Flatow EL, Soslowsky LJ, Mow VC (1991) The relationship of acromial architecture to rotator cuff disease. Clin Sports Med 10(4):823–838

12. Morrison DS, Bigliani LU (1987) Roentgenographic analysis of acromial morphology and its relationship to rotator cuff tears. Orthop Trans 11:439

13. Ellman H (1987) Arthroscopic subacromial decompression: analysis of one- to three-year results. Arthrosc J Arthrosc Relat Surg Off Publ Arthrosc Assoc North Am Int Arthrosc Assoc 33:173–181

14. Spangehl MJ, Hawkins RH, McCormack RG, Loomer RL (2002) Arthroscopic versus open acromioplasty: a prospective, randomized, blinded study. J Shoulder Elb Surg 11(2):101–107. doi:10.1067/mse.2002.120915

15. Gill TJ, McIrvin E, Kocher MS, Homa K, Mair SD, Hawkins RJ (2002) The relative importance of acromial morphology and age with respect to rotator cuff pathology. J Shoulder Elb Surg 11(4):327–330

16. Shin SJ, Oh JH, Chung SW, Song MH (2012) The efficacy of acromioplasty in the arthroscopic repair of small- to medium-sized rotator cuff tears without acromial spur: prospective

comparative study. Arthroscopy 28(5):628–635. doi:10.1016/j.arthro.2011.10.016

17. Tibone JE, Jobe FW, Kerlan RK, Carter VS, Shields CL, Lombardo SJ, Yocum LA (1985) Shoulder impingement syndrome in athletes treated by an anterior acromioplasty. Clin Orthop 198:134–140

18. Chahal J, Mall N, MacDonald PB, Van Thiel G, Cole BJ, Romeo AA, Verma NN (2012) The role of subacromial decompression in patients undergoing arthroscopic repair of full-thickness tears of the rotator cuff: a systematic review and meta-analysis. Arthroscopy 28(5):720–727. doi:10.1016/j.arthro.2011.11.022

19. Shi LL, Edwards TB (2012) The role of acromioplasty for management of rotator cuff problems: where is the evidence? Adv Orthop 2012:467571. doi:10.1155/2012/467571

20. Goldberg BA, Lippitt SB, Matsen FA III (2001) Improvement in comfort and function after cuff repair without acromioplasty. Clin Orthop 390:142–150

21. McCallister WV, Parsons IM, Titelman RM, Matsen FA III (2005) Open rotator cuff repair without acromioplasty. J Bone Jt Surg Am 87(6):1278–1283

22. McFarland EG, Maffulli N, Del Buono A, Murrell GAC, Garzon-Muvdi J, Petersen SA (2013) Impingement is not impingement: the case for calling it "rotator cuff disease". Muscles Ligaments Tendons J 3(3):196–200

23. Papadonikolakis A, McKenna M, Warme W, Martin BI, Matsen FA III (2011) Published evidence relevant to the diagnosis of impingement syndrome of the shoulder. J Bone Jt Surg Am 93(19):1827–1832. doi:10.2106/jbjs.j.01748

24. Mehta S, Gimbel JA, Soslowsky LJ (2003) Etiologic and pathogenetic factors for rotator cuff tendinopathy. Clin Sports Med 22(4):791–812

25. Ozaki J, Fujimoto S, Nakagawa Y, Masuhara K, Tamai S (1988) Tears of the rotator cuff of the shoulder associated with pathological changes in the acromion. A study in cadavera. J Bone Jt Surg Am 70(8):1224–1230

26. Lee TQ, Black AD, Tibone JE, McMahon PJ (2001) Release of the coracoacromial ligament can lead to glenohumeral laxity: a biomechanical study. J Shoulder Elb Surg 10(1):68–72

27. Scheibel M, Lichtenberg S, Habermeyer P (2004) Reversed arthroscopic subacromial decompression for massive rotator cuff tears. J Shoulder Elb Surg 13(3):272–278. doi:10.1016/s1058274604000242

28. Su WR, Budoff JE, Luo ZP (2009) The effect of coracoacromial ligament excision and acromioplasty on superior and anterosuperior glenohumeral stability. Arthrosc J Arthrosc Relat Surg Off publ Arthrosc Assoc North Am Int Arthrosc Assoc 25(1):13–18. doi:10.1016/j.arthro.2008.10.004

29. Abrams GD, Gupta AK, Hussey KE, Tetteh ES, Karas V, Bach BR Jr, Cole BJ, Romeo AA, Verma NN (2014) Arthroscopic repair of full-thickness rotator cuff tears with and without acromioplasty: randomized prospective trial with 2-year follow-up. Am J Sports Med 42(6):1296–1303. doi:10.1177/0363546514529091

30. Gartsman GM, O'Connor DP (2004) Arthroscopic rotator cuff repair with and without arthroscopic subacromial decompression: a prospective, randomized study of one-year outcomes. J Shoulder Elb Surg 13(4):424–426. doi:10.1016/s1058274604000527

31. MacDonald P, McRae S, Leiter J, Mascarenhas R, Lapner P (2011) Arthroscopic rotator cuff repair with and without acromioplasty in the treatment of full-thickness rotator cuff tears: a multicenter, randomized controlled trial. J Bone Jt Surg Am 93(21):1953–1960. doi:10.2106/jbjs.k.00488

32. Milano G, Grasso A, Salvatore M, Zarelli D, Deriu L, Fabbriciani C (2007) Arthroscopic rotator cuff repair with and without subacromial decompression: a prospective randomized study. Arthroscopy 23(1):81–88

33. Wright RW, Brand RA, Dunn W, Spindler KP (2007) How to write a systematic review. Clin Orthop 455:23–29. doi:10.1097/BLO.0b013e31802c9098

34. Spindler KP, Kuhn JE, Dunn W, Matthews CE, Harrell FE Jr, Dittus RS (2005) Reading and reviewing the orthopaedic literature: a systematic, evidence-based medicine approach. J Am Acad Orthop Surg 13(4):220–229

35. Moher D, Schulz KF, Altman DG (2001) The CONSORT statement: revised recommendations for improving the quality of reports of parallel-group randomised trials. Lancet 357(9263):1191–1194

36. Pedowitz RA, Yamaguchi K, Ahmad CS, Burks RT, Flatow EL, Green A, Iannotti JP, Miller BS, Tashjian RZ, Watters WC 3rd, Weber K, Turkelson CM, Wies JL, Anderson S, St Andre J, Boyer K, Raymond L, Sluka P, McGowan R (2011) Optimizing the management of rotator cuff problems. J Am Acad Orthop Surg 19(6):368–379

37. McConville OR, Iannotti JP (1999) Partial-thickness tears of the rotator cuff: evaluation and management. J Am Acad Orthop Surg 7(1):32–43

38. Vitale MA, Arons RR, Hurwitz S, Ahmad CS, Levine WN (2010) The rising incidence of acromioplasty. J Bone Jt Surg Am 92(9):1842–1850. doi:10.2106/jbjs.i.01003

39. Yu E, Cil A, Harmsen WS, Schleck C, Sperling JW, Cofield RH (2010) Arthroscopy and the dramatic increase in frequency of anterior acromioplasty from 1980 to 2005: an epidemiologic study. Arthroscopy 26(9 Suppl):S142–S147. doi:10.1016/j.arthro.2010.02.029

40. Moorman CT, Warren RF, Deng XH, Wickiewicz TL, Torzilli PA (2012) Role of coracoacromial ligament and related structures in glenohumeral stability: a cadaveric study. J Surg Orthop Adv 21(4):210–217

38

Nitric oxide-associated chondrocyte apoptosis in trauma patients after high-energy lower extremity intra-articular fractures

Daniel E. Prince[1] · Justin K. Greisberg[2]

Abstract

Background The primary goal of this study was to identify nitric oxide (NO)-induced apoptosis in traumatized chondrocytes in intra-articular lower extremity fractures and the secondary goal was to identify the timeline of NO-induced apoptosis after injury.

Materials and methods This is a prospective collection of samples of human cartilage harvested at the time of surgery to measure apoptotic cell death and the presence of NO by immunohistochemistry. Three patients met the criteria for control subjects and eight patients sustained high-energy intra-articular fractures and were included in the study. Subjects who sustained intra-articular acetabular, tibial, calcaneal and talus fracture had articular cartilage harvested at the time of surgical intervention. All 8 patients underwent open reduction and internal fixation of the displaced intra-articular fractures. The main outcome measures were rate of apoptosis, degree of NO-induced apoptosis in chondrocytes, and the timeline of NO-induced apoptosis after high-energy trauma.

Results The percentage of apoptotic chondrocytes was higher in impacted samples than in normal cartilage (56 vs 4 %), confirming the presence of apoptosis after intra-articular fracture. The percentage of cells with NO was greater in apoptotic cells than in normal cells (59 vs 20 %), implicating NO-induction of apoptosis. The correlation between chondrocyte apoptosis and increasing time from injury was found to be -0.615, indicating a decreasing rate of apoptosis post injury.

Conclusions The data showed the involvement of NO-induced apoptosis of chondrocytes after high-energy trauma, which decreased with time from injury.

Keywords Apoptosis · Chondrocyte · Nitric oxide · Intra-articular fractures · Post-traumatic osteoarthritis

Introduction

Post-traumatic arthritis remains a problem after intra-articular fractures. Anatomic reduction of displaced articular fragments is the gold standard to restore articular congruency. However, anatomic reduction does not guarantee viable chondrocytes and functional articular cartilage in the zone of injury. Post-traumatic arthritis develops in many patients with pilon, calcaneus, or acetabular fractures despite a good reduction [1–3]. Earlier studies of blunt trauma in canine articular cartilage found biochemical aberrations in addition to structural full-thickness damage to the cartilaginous matrix of chondrocytes when subjected to intra-articular fractures without obvious displacement of the subchondral bone [4–6]. In recent years, attention has been directed to the chondrocyte and to finding alterations in chondrocyte viability in human and animal cartilage after blunt trauma [7–9]. Chondrocytes may die by necrosis (physical disruption of the cell) or by apoptosis (programed cell death). Apoptosis was first identified in thymocytes 30 years ago [10] as a logical means of eliminating unwanted cells. Chondrocyte apoptosis is a normal physiological event in the physis, which allows osteoblasts to lay down osteoid; however, chondrocyte apoptosis has also been identified as a pathologic process in osteoarthritic

✉ Daniel E. Prince
princed@mskcc.org

[1] Memorial Sloan Kettering Cancer Center, 1275 York Avenue, Howard 1013, New York, NY 10065, USA

[2] New York Presbyterian Hospital, Columbia University, New York, NY, USA

articular cartilage [11–16]. It is speculated that loss of chondrocytes may be an essential step in arthritis [12], i.e., without chondrocytes to maintain the matrix, the joint inevitably progresses to end-stage arthritis. Nitric oxide (NO) can induce chondrocyte apoptosis in vitro [14, 17–20] and has been found in both rheumatoid and osteoarthritic cartilage [12]. Researchers have suggested that NO may be a signaling molecule for chondrocyte apoptosis in vivo [21].

Therefore, we hypothesized that (1) the percentage of cells with NO is greater in apoptotic chondrocytes than in non-apoptotic cells, (2) the percentage of chondrocytes with NO-induced apoptosis is greater in cartilage specimens from intra-articular fractures than in control specimens, and (3) the duration of cell death secondary to apoptosis will be determined over time.

Materials and methods

The study design was a prospectively collected series of cartilage specimens from both high-energy intra-articular trauma patients and a control group of specimens from patients undergoing elective first tarsometatarsal fusions. The specimens were stained for viability, presence of NO, and apoptosis and the percentage of stained cells for each variable was calculated for each specimen.

The study included adult patients presenting at our institution who had sustained intra-articular (OTA type B and C) high-energy lower extremity trauma requiring open reduction and internal fixation. The cartilage specimens were from the injured area and were sufficiently small so that reconstruction of the fragment was not possible at the time of definitive surgical repair. Exclusion criteria for both control and cohort groups were age >65 years, history of prior pain, surgery or arthritis in the affected joint, diabetes or a history of systemic inflammatory disease. All control specimens were obtained from healthy young adults who met the same exclusion criteria undergoing first tarsometatarsal arthrodesis for distal hallux deformity via Lapidus fusion. One trauma patient had single medication-controlled hypertension and had previously undergone an uneventful cholecystectomy many years before. Another patient had medication-controlled gastro-esophageal reflux disease, and another patient had an anxiety disorder, while the remaining trauma and control patients had no prior preoperative medical or surgical conditions.

Eight specimens were harvested from eight patients. Four patients sustained tibial plateau fractures after being struck by a car; one patient had a talus fracture, one had a calcaneus fracture, and one had tibial pilon injury (all resulting from a fall from a height); and another had an acetabular fracture after a car accident. Specimens were immediately fixed in formalin, embedded in paraffin, and then cut into 5-μm sections in a direction that captured all levels (surface to subchondral bone). A power analysis was performed after refining the staining technique utilizing three control and three fracture specimens. The analysis determined that a total of 8 fracture specimens would be necessary for a power of 0.91. This study was approved by the Institutional Review Board and was performed in accordance with the ethical standards of the 1964 Declaration of Helsinki as revised in 2000.

Paraffin-embedded tissues were rehydrated and then permeabilized in 0.1 % triton X-100 in 0.1 % sodium citrate solution. Slides were incubated with 0.5 % sheep testicular hyaluronidase (Sigma-Aldrich, St Louis, MO, USA). Staining was performed with a dUTP terminal transferase-mediated nick-end labeling (TUNEL) assay (In Situ Cell Death Detection kit; Roche Molecular Biochemicals, Indianapolis, IN, USA). The TUNEL assay labels the characteristic DNA strand breaks of apoptosis with fluorescent nucleotides. Because normal cells have few strand breaks, little or no fluorescence is incorporated into normal cells. Nucleotides were labeled with fluorescein, which fluoresces green. Negative controls were performed with the TUNEL In Situ Cell Death Detection kit without applying the terminal transferase enzyme. Positive controls were performed using the TUNEL enzyme DNase I (30,000 U/mL) prior to the labeling procedure.

NO reacts with the tyrosine residues of intracellular proteins to form nitrotyrosine [15, 22]. Antibodies to nitrotyrosine can be used to mark sites of NO production [14, 23]. After staining for apoptosis with the TUNEL kit, the same tissue sections were blocked with 5 % normal goat serum and were then exposed to 1:200 anti-nitrotyrosine rabbit antibody (Sigma-Aldrich). We counterstained the sections with a 1:100 goat anti-rabbit antibody labeled with Rhodamine Red-X (Jackson ImmunoResearch, West Grove, PA, USA), which fluoresces red. Slides were then mounted in media containing 1.5 ug/mL 4′,6-diamidino-2-phenylindole (Vector Shield with DAPI; Vector Laboratories, Burlingame, CA, USA), a fluorescent blue non-specific nuclear stain. Following the protocol, all cells with intact nuclei fluoresce blue, apoptotic cells fluoresce green, and cells containing NO fluoresce red under fluorescent microscopy (Figs. 1, 2).

We prepared three nonconsecutive slides from each cartilage sample. One image from each slide was photographed with a fluorescent microscope (Axiovert 200; Carl Zeiss Light Microscopy, Oberkochen, Germany) at 200× magnification under blue, green, and red fluorescence. The image was taken from the interior of the cartilage (to avoid the edge necrosis effect) in a nonrandom manner to capture a large number of cells in the frame. We only included cells with intact nuclei in the analysis. This

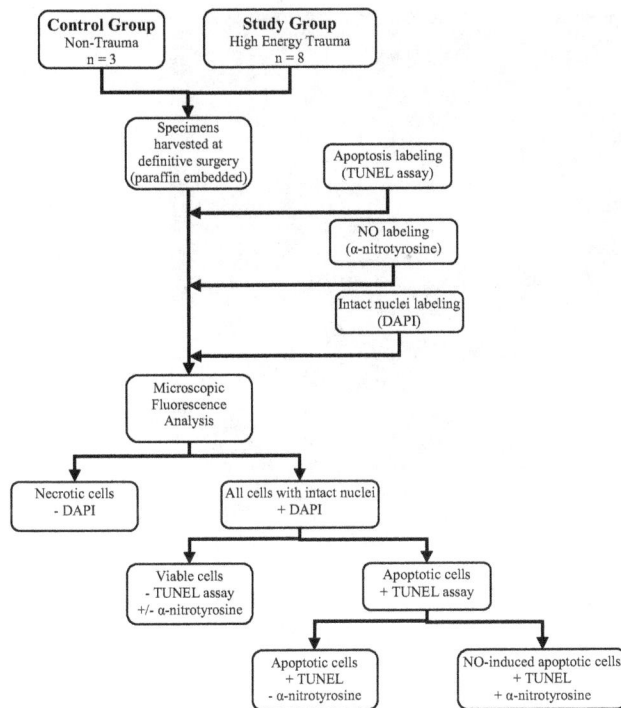

Fig. 1 Study Design. Specimens from both groups were stained for all three assays and analyzed under fluorescence microscopy. Cells with intact nuclei were then determined to be apoptotic based on the TUNEL assay. Apoptotic cells were then sub-classified based on the presence of NO

resulted in a mean of 19 cells analyzed per section (range 7–45). The section was then photographed with blue, green, and red fluorescence, and the number of cells positive for each was counted (Fig. 2).

A total of 24 slides from the eight test specimens and 9 slides from the three control patients were analyzed. One of the authors (DEP) was blinded to the origin of the samples and reviewed each of the 33 slides. The observed variability by the reviewer between the 3 slides of each specimen was found to be 0.684. The percentage of cells staining positive for apoptosis and NO in each section was calculated based on the number of viable cells on each section. The three slides were then averaged to determine the value per specimen. In this manner, each specimen was weighted equally and cell density was thus normalized for each specimen. The percentage of cells positive for apoptosis and/or NO was calculated for the test and control specimens.

The percentage of cells that stained positive for both apoptosis and NO were compared with the percentage of cells staining positive only for apoptosis in the test specimens using Student's t test, as the cells were all exposed to the same staining procedure and the means and variance for both populations were assumed to be equal. For each specimen, the percentage of cells with apoptosis and NO was plotted against time from injury and correlation

coefficients were calculated (SPSS 15.0 for Windows; IBM, Somers, NY, USA).

Results

There was no difference ($p = 0.127$) between the mean age of the trauma patients (47.8 years; range 23–56) and the control group (36 years; range 31–39). There was no difference in gender or comorbidities between the groups— there were 6 males in the trauma group and 1 male in the control group ($p = 0.219$) and 3 comorbidities in the trauma group and none in the control group ($p = 0.148$). The comorbidities of the trauma patients were hypertension, gastroesophageal reflux disease and anxiety, which the authors do not believe influenced the control specimens. The specimens were harvested at a mean time of 211 h (range 72–456) after injury and ranged in size from 4–16 mm in maximum dimension.

No difference in the percentage of intact cells, NO-positive cells, or apoptotic cells was found amongst the different anatomic locations—tibial plateau, tibial pilon, acetabulum, and calcaneus ($p > 0.05$). No difference was found in all outcomes between specimens harvested from the most frequent location, the tibial plateau and all other locations ($p > 0.05$). Additionally, no trend was found in the percentage of NO-positive cells or apoptotic cells based on the number of viable cells in each specimen ($p > 0.05$).

The percentage of cells with apoptosis was greater ($p < 0.001$) in the fracture group than in the control group—55.8 versus 4.3 %, respectively (Table 1). Similarly, the percentage of cells with NO was greater ($p < 0.02$) in the fracture group than in the control group— 39.2 versus 10.9 %, respectively (Table 1).

For chondrocytes staining positive for apoptosis, the percentage of cells co-staining for NO was greater ($p < 0.001$) in the fracture group than in the control group—58.7 versus 19.6 % (Table 2). There was no difference in percentage of cells co-staining for NO and apoptosis in the control subjects. Given the small sample size, a sensitivity analysis for outliers was performed and found no individual samples had a significant skew effect on the data to be considered an outlier.

There was a negative correlation of −0.615 ($p = 0.01$) between the percentage of chondrocytes positively co-staining for apoptosis and NO and increasing time from injury (Fig. 3); the coefficient of determination for this correlation was 38 %. There was no correlation between the percentage of cells staining positive independently for NO, apoptosis, or the total number of intact cells with time from injury. There were insufficient data points to calculate a best-fit trend line to determine if the rate of apoptosis was logarithmic, linear, or variable.

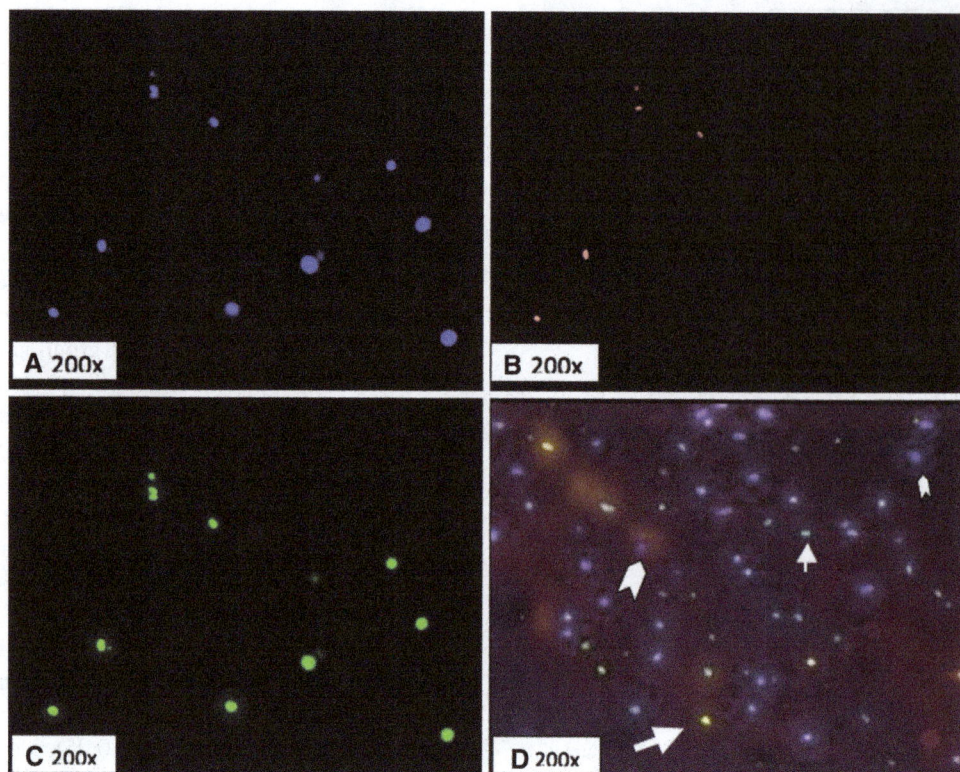

Fig. 2 Fluorescence staining of cartilage slides. **a** Cells with intact nuclei (DAPI, ×200). **b** NO-containing cells (Rhodamine-X, ×200). **c** Apoptotic cells (TUNEL, ×200). **d** Computer-generated combined overlay image (×200). *Large arrow* indicates a cell staining positive for both NO and apoptosis. *Small arrow* indicates a cell staining positive for apoptosis and negative for NO. *Large arrowhead* indicates a cell positive for NO and negative for apoptosis. *Small arrowhead* indicates a cell negative for both NO and apoptosis

Table 1 Percentage of NO and apoptosis in fracture and control cartilage samples

Percentage of chondrocyte staining positive	Fracture cartilage		Control cartilage		p
	$n = 24$ (range)	SD (%)	$n = 9$ (range)	SD (%)	
Apoptosis (TUNEL)	55.8 % (6–100)	30.9	4.3 % (0–15)	5.7	<0.001
NO (α-nitrotyrosine)	39.2 % (6–100)	31.7	10.9 % (0–31)	12.2	<0.02

n is the number of microscopic slides reviewed; percentage was calculated per section of cartilage

Table 2 Prevalence of nitric oxide in apoptotic chondrocytes in fracture

Positive for nitric oxide	Positive for apoptosis	SD	Negative for apoptosis	SD	P
Fracture group $n = 24$	58.7 % (0–100)	36.3 %	19.6 % (0–93)	28.7 %	<0.001
Control group $n = 9$	11.1 % (0–100)	33.3 %	9.9 % (0–27)	10.4 %	0.919

Percentage was calculated per section of cartilage; n is the number of chondrocytes evaluated in each group

Discussion

Chondrocyte apoptosis has been identified in osteoarthritic cartilage in animal models and in human samples taken at the time of implant arthroplasty [12, 14]; however, more recently it has also been implicated in post-traumatic osteoarthritis [39–41]. Cyclic loading [24], matrix lacerations [25], and blunt impact [8, 26–28] all decrease chondrocyte viability in cartilage explants. It is speculated that loss of chondrocytes is a key step in the development of arthritis; without cells to maintain the cartilage matrix, the joint inevitably progresses to osteoarthritis. Studies have also identified NO in arthritic cartilage [12, 14], while others found NO could induce apoptosis in cultured chondrocytes [12]. NO synthase inhibitors seemed to reduce the progression of arthritis in animal models [29, 30], suggesting

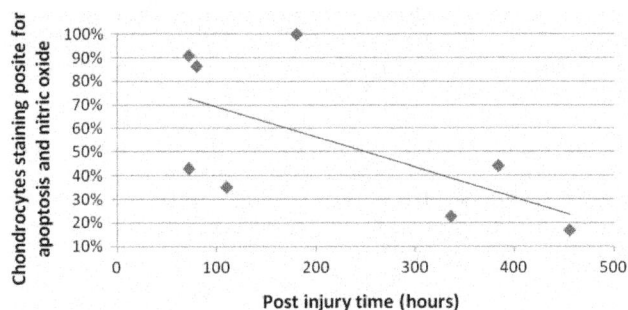

Fig. 3 Timing of chondrocyte apoptosis. The rate of chondrocyte apoptosis has a moderate correlation of 0.62 with a coefficient of demonstration (r^2) of 0.38 ($p = 0.01$) indicating that 38 % of the decreasing rate of chondrocyte apoptosis is the result of increasing time from injury

NO may be a signal for human chondrocyte apoptosis in vivo [18]. Chondrocytes subjected to high-energy trauma undergo apoptosis [16]. This first aim of this study was to identify the presence of NO-induced apoptosis in traumatized human chondrocytes after injury. The second aim of this study was to attempt to demonstrate a greater degree of NO-induced apoptosis in chondrocytes subjected to high-energy trauma compared to non-traumatized chondrocytes, indicating that the apoptosis in these chondrocytes is due to the presence of NO. The study also attempted to identify the timeline of chondrocyte NO-induced apoptosis after high-energy injury.

We acknowledge limitations to our study. First, we had a small number of specimens from various joints, with varying forces and orientations across each cartilaginous surface. It is unclear how these differences influence the rate, induction, or timing of chondrocyte apoptosis; however, no significant differences were found in all outcomes between the specimens harvested from the various locations, implying that NO-induced apoptosis is not influenced by the location or force of the fracture, but may be a unified down-stream result of intra-articular damage. Despite, the small size, a power analysis using the eight study subjects and three control subjects yielded a power of 0.91 to determine differences in the percentage of cells staining positive for NO and apoptosis between the control and fracture groups. This was based on a determined standard deviation of 30.3 % and a 0.05 two-tailed significance level [31]. Second, co-localization of NO and apoptosis does not imply causality, merely correlation; however, other studies have elucidated the role of NO in apoptosis [17, 22, 32–34]. The study design did not allow for determination of the intra- and inter-observer variability of the methods; however, the variability between the three specimens from each specimen was determined to be good ($R = 0.684$). Third, the specimens used were small pieces that would otherwise be discarded at the time of surgery. It is likely that these samples are the most traumatized

sections of the cartilage, resulting in a sampling error that biases the results toward the null hypothesis and may not be representative of the remainder of the articular cartilage; however, these fragments may be more subject to mechanical cell death rather than apoptotic cell death subsequently, which would bias the results against the hypothesis of this study. Fourth, the controls were not normal cartilage because they was harvested from midfoot joints with deformity and pain and the properties of the cartilage of this joint may be different from traumatized joints. This bias would favor the null hypothesis showing no difference with traumatized cartilage regardless of the underlying cause. It is possible that using arthritic cartilage as a control would only lead to a bias towards rejecting the hypotheses of this study, because the control cartilage is more likely to have higher rates of cell death than completely normal cartilage. Fifth, the TUNEL assay was the primary test for apoptosis in this study, but the TUNEL assay has been criticized for accurately detecting apoptosis [35]. Other studies have compared the TUNEL assay to other methods of detection such as enzyme-linked immunosorbent assay (ELISA), flow cytometry, and caspase-3 assays, finding good correlation among the various methods [32–34]. Although the TUNEL assay and nitrotyrosine stains were titrated carefully in control and fracture samples so as not to give false-negatives or false-positives, these techniques are inherently subject to both positive and negative error. The data should be interpreted more qualitatively than quantitatively.

This study found a higher percentage of chondrocytes staining independently for apoptosis in fracture specimens than in the control specimens. This concurs with Murray et al. [16] who found a high percentage of apoptotic cells in cartilage samples from patients with intra-articular fractures. Sena et al. [41] found similar results in cultured chondrocytes from calcaneal fractures that had sustained high-energy trauma.

Second, our study found a greater percentage of traumatized chondrocytes showed co-staining for NO and apoptosis compared to chondrocytes from control specimens. This supports the role of NO-induced apoptosis after high-energy trauma in human chondrocytes. Blanco et al. [17] hypothesized, based on the study of cultured chondrocytes, that NO is the primary inducer of apoptosis. Although NO is not the sole catalyst of post-traumatic chondrocyte death, it plays a central role [15, 35, 36]. Several studies suggest several factors inhibit the NO-induced apoptotic pathway, including hyaluronic acid, cilostazol, and other agents [15, 17, 30, 33–38]. A better understanding of the chondrocyte apoptotic pathway could lead to intervention and prevention of chondrocyte death. Administration of NO-inhibiting agents at the time of initial presentation or surgery may be a novel treatment in the future [15].

Finally, our study found persistent co-staining of NO and apoptosis with increasing time from injury as a negative correlation, which is supported by the literature. Lima et al. [26] found chondrocyte death increased until 7 days after a single impact injury, and the percentage of dead cells was decreased by apoptosis inhibitors. In a bovine cartilage explants model, Loening et al. [32] showed via TUNEL staining that apoptosis peaked 24 h after the simulated loading event and persisted for 2 days and other signs of cartilage injury increased for 6 days. Tew et al. [9] also found in bovine cartilage explants damaged by cutting that apoptotic cells detected by TUNEL staining remained in the tissue for 20 days following injury. This study, with few time points cannot determine the rate or the pattern of NO-induced apoptosis to be parabolic, logarithm, linear or variable. Additional time points would aide in affirming the theory that apoptosis increases initially and diminishes with increasing time to injury. More detailed studies analyzing the timing of the NO cascade in vivo are necessary to delineate this pathway.

In conclusion, we found the percentage of cells with apoptosis is increased in cartilage from trauma patients, and that those cells are more likely to contain NO, implicating NO-induced apoptosis after intra-articular fracture. Our study found a decreasing number of NO-induced apoptotic chondrocytes with increasing time from injury without being able to show the specific time course of apoptosis after trauma. Future studies should focus on animal models to assess the rate of chondrocyte cell death due to NO-induced apoptosis compared to other causes of both immediate and delayed cell death as well as determining the viability of remaining chondrocytes to survive. The degree to which NO-induced apoptosis is the ultimate cause of post-traumatic arthritis will have to be further elucidated with models both inducing and blocking NO-apoptosis in animal models. This should be performed in both normal and traumatized cartilage to account for the presence and contribution of post-traumatic fibrocartilage after injury. Additional time points will be necessary to elucidate the rate and pattern of NO-induced apoptosis. We believe it is important to focus on NO-induced apoptosis because of existing therapies to block NO that may be applicable to patients undergoing intra-articular fractures.

Acknowledgments We thank Dr. Seong Sil Chang for her assistance in optimizing the TUNEL assay and Mr. Thomas Gardner for his guidance with the fluorescence microscope. No funding was received from any of the following organizations—National Institutes of Health (NIH), Wellcome Trust, and the Howard Hughes Medical Institute (HHMI). This work was performed at Columbia University, Department of Orthopaedic Surgery, Center for Orthopaedic Research, New York, NY, USA.

Conflict of interest The authors declare that they have no conflict of interest related to the publication of this manuscript. Each author certifies that he or she has no commercial associations (e.g., consultancies, stock ownership, equity interest, patent/licensing arrangements, etc.) that might pose a conflict of interest in connection with the submitted article.

Ethical standards This study was approved by the Institutional Review Board and was performed in accordance with the ethical standards of the 1964 Declaration of Helsinki as revised in 2000. All patients signed informed consent for participation in the study via IRB approved documentation.

References

1. Letournel E (1978) Surgical repair of acetabular fractures more than 3 weeks after injury, apart from total hip replacement. Int Orthop 2:305–313
2. Thermann H, Hufner T, Schratt HE et al (1999) Subtalar fusion after conservative or surgical treatment of calcaneus fracture. A comparison of long term results. Unfallchirurg 102:13–22
3. Dupont WD, Plummer WD (1990) Power and sample size calculations: a review and computer program. Control Clin Trials 11:116–128
4. Thompson RC, Oegema TR, Lewis JL et al (1991) Osteoarthritic changes after acute transarticular load. An animal model. J Bone Joint Surg Am 73:990–1001
5. Thompson RC, Vener MJ, Griffiths HJ et al (1993) Scanning electron-microscopic and magnetic resonance-imaging studies of injuries to the patellofemoral joint after acute transarticular loading. J Bone Joint Surg Am 75:704–771
6. Borrelli J, Tinsley K, Ricci WM et al (2003) Induction of chondrocyte apoptosis following impact load. J Orthop Trauma 17:635–641
7. Kerr JF, Wyllie AH, Currie AR (1972) Apoptosis: a basic biological phenomenon with wide-ranging implications in tissue kinetics. Br J Cancer 26:239–257
8. Radin EL, Paul IL, Lowy M (1970) A comparison of the dynamic force transmitting properties of subchondral bone and articular cartilage. J Bone Joint Surg Am 52:444–456
9. Kühn K, Shikhman AR, Lotz M (2003) Role of nitric oxide, reactive oxygen species, and p38 MAP kinase in the regulation of human chondrocyte apoptosis. J Cell Physiol 197:379–387
10. Bendele AM, White SL (1987) Early histopathologic and ultrastructural alterations in femorotibial joints of partial medial meniscectomized guinea pigs. Vet Path 24:436–443
11. Blanco FJ, Guitian R, Vazquez-Martul E et al (2004) Osteoarthritis chondrocytes die by apoptosis: a possible pathway for osteoarthritis pathology. Arthritis Rheum 41:284–289
12. Jang D, Murrell GAC (1998) Nitric oxide in arthritis. Free Radic Biol Med 24:1511–1519
13. Jang D, Szabo C, Murrell GAC (1996) S-substituted isothioureas are potent inhibitors of nitric oxide biosynthesis in cartilage. Eur J Pharmacol 312:341–347
14. Kurz B, Lemke AK, Fay J et al (2005) Pathomechanisms of cartilage destruction by mechanical injury. Ann Anat 187(5–6): 473–485

15. Murray MM, Zurakowski D, Vrahas MS (2004) The death of articular chondrocytes after intra-articular fracture in humans. J Trauma 56:128–131

16. Blanco FJ, Ochs RL, Schwarz H et al (1995) Chondrocyte apoptosis induced by nitric oxide. Am J Pathol 146:75–85

17. Haddad IY, Pataki G, Hu P et al (1994) Quantitation of nitrotyrosine levels in lung sections of patients and animals with acute lung injury. J Clin Invest 94:2407–2413

18. Jarvinen TAH, Moilanen T, Jarvinen TLN et al (1995) Nitric oxide mediates interleukin-1 induced inhibition of glycosaminoglycan synthesis in rat articular cartilage. Mediators Inflamm 4:107–111

19. Jeffrey JE, Gregory DW, Aspden RW (1995) Matrix damage and chondrocyte viability following a single impact load on articular cartilage. Arch Biochem Biophys Acta 322:87–96

20. Kim HT, Lo MY, Pillarisetty R (2002) Chondrocyte apoptosis following intraarticular fracture in humans. Osteoarthritis Cartilage 10:747–749

21. Van der Vliet A, Eiserich JP, Kaur H et al (1996) Nitrotyrosine as biomarker for reactive nitrogen species. Methods Enzymol 269:175–184

22. Hashimoto S, Takahashi K, Amiel D et al (1998) Chondrocyte apoptosis and nitric oxide production during experimentally induced osteoarthritis. Arthritis Rheum 41:1266–1274

23. Chen CT, Burton-Wurster N, Borden C et al (2001) Chondrocyte necrosis and apoptosis in impact damaged articular cartilage. J Orthop Res 19:703–711

24. Tew SR, Kwan APL, Hann A et al (2000) The reactions of articular cartilage to experimental wounding. Arthritis Rheum 1:215–225

25. Duda GN, Eilers M, Loh L et al (2001) Chondrocyte death precedes structural damage in blunt impact trauma. Clin Orthop Relat Res 393:302–309

26. Greisberg J, Bliss M, Terek R (2002) The prevalence of nitric oxide in apoptotic chondrocytes of osteoarthritis. Osteoarthritis Cartilage 10:207–211

27. Rundell SA, Baars DC, Phillips DM et al (2005) The limitation of acute necrosis in retro-patellar cartilage after a severe blunt impact to the in vivo rabbit patello-femoral joint. J Orthop Res 23:1363–1369

28. Kaur H, Halliwell B (1994) Evidence for nitric oxide-mediated oxidative damage in chronic inflammation. FEBS Lett 350:9–12

29. Peng H, Zhou JL, Liu SQ et al (2010) Hyaluronic acid inhibits nitric oxide-induced apoptosis and dedifferentiation of articular chondrocytes in vitro. Inflamm Res 59:519–530

30. Grogan SP, Aklin B, Frenz M et al (2002) In vitro model for the study of necrosis and apoptosis in native cartilage. J Pathol 198:5–13

31. Loening AM, James IE, Levenston ME, Badger AM et al (2000) Injurious mechanical compression of bovine articular cartilage induces chondrocyte apoptosis. Arch Biochem Biophys 381(2):205–212

32. Lee SW, Song YS, Shin SH, Kim KT et al (2008) Cilostazol protects rat chondrocytes against nitric oxide-induced apoptosis in vitro and prevents cartilage destruction in a rat model of osteoarthritis. Arthritis Rheum 58:790–800

33. Wu GJ, Chen TG, Chang HC et al (2007) Nitric oxide from both exogenous and endogenous sources activates mitochondria-dependent events and induces insults to human chondrocytes. J Cell Biochem 101:1520–1531

34. Cherng YG, Chang HC, Lin YL et al (2008) Apoptotic insults to human chondrocytes induced by sodium nitroprusside are involved in sequential events, including cytoskeletal remodeling, phosphorylation of mitogen-activated protein kinase kinase kinase-1/c-Jun N-terminal kinase, and Bax-mitochondria-mediated caspase activation. J Orthop Res 26(7):1018–1026

35. Yang JH, Lee HG (2010) 2,3,7,8-Tetrachlorodibenzo-p-dioxin induces apoptosis of articular chondrocytes in culture. Chemosphere 79:278–284

36. Stefanovic-Racic M, Meyers K, Meschter C et al (1995) Comparison of the nitric oxide synthase inhibitors methylarginine and aminoguanidine as prophylactic and therapeutic agents in rat adjuvant arthritis. J Rheumatol 22:1922–1928

37. Hashimoto S, Ochs RL, Komiya S et al (2004) Linkage of chondrocyte apoptosis and cartilage degradation in human osteoarthritis. Arthritis Rheum 41:1632–1638

38. Houard X, Godlring MB, Berenbaum F (2013) Homeostatic mechanisms in articular cartilage and role of inflammation in osteoarthritis. Curr Rheumatol Rep 15:375

39. Byun S, Sinskey YL, Lu YC et al (2013) Transport of anti-IL-6 antigen binding fragments into cartilage and the effects of injury. Arch Biochem Biophys 532:15–22

40. Li Y, Frank EH, Wang Y et al (2013) Moderate dynamic compression inhibits pro-catabolic response of cartilage to mechanical injury, tumor necrosis factor-a and interleukin-6, but accentuates degradation above a strain threshold. Osteoarthritis Cartilage 21:1933–1941

41. Sena P, Manfredini G, Benincasa M et al (2014) Up-regulation of the chemo-attractive receptor ChemR23 and occurrence of apoptosis in human chondrocytes isolated from fractured calcaneal osteochondral fragments. J Anat 224:659–668

39

Surgical site infection in high-energy peri-articular tibia fractures with intra-wound vancomycin powder: a retrospective pilot study

Keerat Singh[1] · Jennifer M. Bauer[1] · Gregory Y. LaChaud[1] · Jesse E. Bible[1] ·
Hassan R. Mir[1]

Abstract

Background Surgical site infections (SSI) continue to be a significant source of morbidity despite the introduction of perioperative intravenous antibiotics. Our objective was to assess the efficacy of local vancomycin powder on lowering deep SSI rates in high-energy tibial plateau and pilon fractures.

Materials and methods A retrospective review of all tibial plateau and pilon fractures treated in 2012 at our level I trauma center identified 222 patients. Of these, 107 patients sustained high-energy injuries that required staged fixation, and 93 had minimum 6 month follow-up. Ten patients received 1 gram vancomycin powder directly into the surgical wound at the time of definitive fixation, and the remaining 83 patients served as controls. SSI was defined according to criteria from the Centers for Disease Control. Demographic data, patient comorbidities, injury and treatment details, and infection details were recorded. Descriptive and comparative statistics were performed.

Results Amongst the vancomycin powder group, 1 patient (10 %) developed a deep SSI; in the control group, 14 (16.7 %) developed deep SSI. The rate of deep SSI between the groups was not statistically significantly different ($P = 1.0$). The groups were statistically similar with regard to injuries, treatment, comorbidities, and infectious outcomes (P values range = 0.06–1.0).

Conclusions The application of local vancomycin powder into surgical wounds of high-energy tibial plateau and pilon fractures did not reduce the rate of deep SSI in this retrospective review. There is a need to find effective, cheap, and widely available methods for prevention of SSI. Basic science and larger prospective clinical studies are needed to further delineate the role of local vancomycin powder as a modality to reduce deep SSI in extremity trauma.

Level of evidence Level III, therapeutic.

Keywords Tibial plateau · Tibial plafond · Pilon · Vancomycin powder · Infection

Introduction

Infection is a well-known complication of operative fixation of extremity fractures. Such infections have a significant effect on patients and often require repeat surgery, prolonged systemic antibiotic use and lead to delay in fracture healing and rehabilitation. The risk of mortality doubles in a patient with a surgical site infection (SSI) and the cost of care increases significantly [1]. Risk factors for post-traumatic infection include open fractures, smoking, alcoholism, sustained intensive care unit stay, inadequate debridement at the fracture site and malnutrition [2, 3]. In a patient sustaining high-energy trauma, immune system dysfunction results, as evidenced by decreased ability of polymorphonuclear leukocytes (PMNs) in chemotaxis, decreased superoxide formation and decreased microbial elimination [4]. In the setting of fractures, bone that is devoid of periosteum and other surrounding devitalized tissue serve as an ideal medium for bacterial colonization and replication. Introduction of hardware to appropriately manage a fracture becomes yet another suitable medium for bacterial proliferation given that most metals are electrochemically active and promote molecular adhesion [5].

✉ Hassan R. Mir
hassan.mir@vanderbilt.edu

[1] Division of Orthopaedic Trauma, Vanderbilt Orthopaedic Institute, Suite 4200 MCE, South Tower, Nashville, TN 37232, USA

Some authors have reported infection rates of 14–60 % in high-energy lower extremity fractures [6–11]. Systemic antibiotics reduce surgical site infections, but they are limited by the risk of toxicity. Additionally, traumatic tissues have a compromised blood supply, further limiting the effectiveness of systemic antibiotics. Local antibiotics avert this by sterilizing the wound and preventing the development of a biofilm. The development of a complex glycocalyx biofilm around bacterial colonies greatly impedes the delivery of systemic antibacterial agents and allows bacteria to become more virulent than in their non-adherent state [12, 13].

Administration of perioperative, intravenous antibiotics prior to making a surgical incision has become standard of care and has been effective at reducing surgical infections [14, 15]. Vancomycin is a glycopeptide that inhibits bacterial cell wall synthesis and is used mostly in the prophylaxis and treatment of Gram-positive bacteria. Topical vancomycin offers advantages over systemic administration because higher local concentrations can be achieved and directed to the site of need. Additionally, organisms that may be otherwise resistant to a given systemic therapeutic concentration may be sensitive to the local concentrations [16]. Local antibiotics are commonly delivered via cement beads and spacers. However, these are not always practical, as they require space for placement and necessitate late removal.

Topical vancomycin powder has become popular over the last decade as its efficacy in spine surgery has been demonstrated. A meta-analysis pooling 5888 spine patients that evaluated the effectiveness of topical vancomycin powder at preventing SSI and deep incisional infections showed a significant protective effect of vancomycin powder [17]. Despite extensive research into vancomycin powder efficacy in the spine literature and some work in the field of vascular surgery, no literature exists on vancomycin powder use in prevention of surgical wound infection in extremity injuries.

The objective of our retrospective review was to assess the efficacy of intraoperative vancomycin powder administration on preventing deep SSI in high-energy lower extremity trauma of the tibial plateau and pilon. We hypothesized that the use of intrawound vancomycin powder would reduce the incidence of deep SSI in the treatment group as compared to well-matched controls.

Materials and methods

Inclusion/exclusion criteria, treatment, and data collection

The study protocol was approved by the institutional review board at the participating level I trauma center.

Inclusion criteria consisted of patients older than 18 years of age who had undergone staged operative fixation of their high-energy tibial plateau or pilon injury. Staged treatment (external fixation, limited internal fixation, or splinting) was defined as definitive internal fixation at a minimum of 5 days post-injury after swelling had resolved. Exclusion criteria consisted of patients with follow-up less than 6 months.

A total of 222 adult patients were found in the institutional database to have sustained tibial plateau and pilon fractures between 1 January 2012 and 31 December 2012. Of these injuries, 50 were treated non-operatively, and 65 did not require staged fixation. The remainder of these injuries ($n = 107$) were treated by the six board-certified orthopaedic trauma surgeons at our institution. Of the 107 patients, 14 had a follow-up time of less than 6 months, leaving 93 patients in the final analysis group. Charts and operative reports of all injuries were reviewed, and ten patients (10.8 %) were documented to have received 1 gram vancomycin powder (Hospira, Lake Forest, IL) directly into the surgical wound at time of definitive fixation at the discretion of the treating surgeon. The remaining 83 patients served as the control group.

All patients received standard systemic antibiotic prophylaxis consisting of 1 g IV cefazolin within 1 h of surgical incision, followed by 1 g IV cefazolin every 8 h for 24 h postoperatively. If the patient was allergic to penicillin, 900 mg IV clindamycin was used instead. Patient demographics (age and gender), injury type (location, open versus closed), smoking status, presence of diabetes, staged treatment with external fixation, presence of single or dual incision, presence of concomitant compartment syndrome and time (in days) from presentation to definitive surgery were all recorded. All patients records were evaluated for signs of SSI for a minimum of 6 months post-operatively. A deep SSI was defined as one requiring operative irrigation and debridement. Wound site erythema without the presence of fluctuance, drainage or purulence was defined as a superficial SSI. Amongst the deep SSI patients, intraoperative microbiological data was also collected.

Statistics

Using SPSS 22.0 software, dichotomous data was compared using Fisher's exact tests, while independent t tests and Mann–Whitney U tests were used for comparisons of parametric and non-parametric data, respectively. Statistical significance was set at $P < 0.05$.

Outcome measure

The primary outcome measure was the occurrence of deep SSI.

Results

Demographic parameters did not differ statistically between the two groups. The average age of the vancomycin-treated group was 55 years (range 38–73 years), and the control age was 46 years (range 17–82 years), $P = 0.064$. Of the 10 vancomycin-treated patients, 6 were male (60 %) and 4 were female (40 %), and of the 83 control patients, 55 (54 %) were male and 38 (46 %) were female ($P = 1.0$). Thirty-six (43 %) out of the 83 control subjects were smokers and 2 (20 %) of the vancomycin-treated were smokers ($P = 0.191$). Six (7 %) of the 83 control patients were diabetic whereas no patient in the vancomycin-treated group had diabetes ($p = 1.0$). Of the ten vancomycin-treated patients, five (50 %) sustained a tibial plateau injury and five (50 %) sustained a tibial plafond (pilon) injury. Forty-six injuries in the control group were pilon injuries and 37 were plateau injuries. Comparison of injury type amongst the two groups was not statistically significant ($P = 0.751$). A total of 3 injuries (30 %), all pilon, were open injuries in the vancomycin-treated group, and 23 (28 %) injuries were open in the control group ($P = 1.0$). Patient characteristics and outcomes for the treatment and control groups are presented in Table 1.

Amongst the vancomycin-treated group, one patient (10 %) developed a deep SSI. In the control group of 83 patients, 14 patients (16.8 %) developed deep SSI. The rate of deep SSI was not statistically different between the two groups ($P = 1.0$). Seven (50 %) of the 14 patients in the control group that developed a deep SSI initially had an open injury. The one patient with a deep infection in the vancomycin-treated group had an injury that was initially open. There were no cases of superficial SSI in the vancomycin-treated group and 7 cases (8 %) of superficial SSI in the control group of 83 patients. The rate of superficial SSI was not statistically different between the two groups ($P = 1.0$). Seven (8 %) of the 83 control patients and one (10 %) of the ten vancomycin-treated patients had concomitant compartment syndrome requiring surgical release. The incidence of compartment syndrome was not statistically significant amongst the two groups ($P = 1.0$).

There was no significant difference in average time (in days) to definitive surgical treatment amongst the two groups (15.6 vs 19.8) for the control and vancomycin-treated groups, respectively ($P = 0.149$). The groups were statistically similar in terms of pre-operative temporizing management with 74/83 (89 %) of control group and 9/10 (90 %) of the vancomycin-treated patients being externally fixed prior to definitive management ($P = 1.0$). Thirty-four (41 %) of the 83 control patients underwent dual-incision operations at time of definitive fixation of their plateau and pilons, and 59 % (49/83) had a single incision. In the vancomycin-treated group, four out of ten (40 %) had single incisions and 60 % had dual incisions. The number of incisions did not differ statistically among the two groups ($P = 1.0$).

In the vancomycin-treated group, the surgical site cultures obtained from the one clinically infected patient at time of surgical irrigation and debridement showed no growth of pathogen at 6 months. Of the 14 infections in the control group, 6 yielded Methicillin-sensitive *Staphylococcus aureus* (MSSA), 4 resulted in Methicillin-resistant *Staphylococcus aureus* (MRSA), 1 grew *Staphylococcus epidermidis*, and 3 had no microbiology data available.

Table 1 Patient demographics, injury, treatment characteristics and rate of infection

	Control	Treatment	P value
Total (n)	83	10	
Average age (years)	46	55	0.06
Gender			
M	45	6	1.00
F	38	4	1.00
Smoker n (%)	36 (43 %)	2 (20 %)	0.19
Diabetic n (%)	6 (7 %)	0 (0 %)	1.00
Pilon injuries n (%)	46 (55 %)	5 (50 %)	0.75
Plateau injuries n (%)	37 (45 %)	5 (50 %)	0.75
Open injuries n (%)	23 (28 %)	3 (30 %)	1.00
Staged treatment with external-fixation n (%)	74 (89 %)	9 (90 %)	1.00
Time to definitive fixation (days)	15.6	19.8	0.15
Single incision n (%)	34 (41 %)	4 (40 %)	1.00
Dual incision n (%)	49 (59 %)	6 (60 %)	1.00
Presence of compartment syndrome n (%)	7 (8 %)	1 (10 %)	1.00
Superficial infection n (%)	7 (8 %)	0 (0 %)	1.00
Deep infection n (%)	14 (16.8 %)	1 (10 %)	1.00

One of the patients that grew MRSA concomitantly grew *Escherichia coli*, and one patient with MSSA cultures also grew *Enterobacter aerogenes*.

Discussion

Even with timely preoperative IV antibiotic prophylaxis, meticulous attention to sterile technique, and less invasive surgical procedures, postoperative infections continue to occur in high-energy lower extremity fractures. Wound infections can dramatically increase health care resource utilization and further increase morbidity, especially in patients with extremity trauma. The post-operative infection rates in the lower extremity are reported to be as high as 60 % [6–11]. The objective of the present study was to investigate the efficacy of vancomycin powder in the prevention of deep SSI in high-energy lower extremity fractures—something previously not studied.

We found no significant difference in the rate of deep or superficial SSI high-energy tibia fractures when intra-wound vancomycin powder was administered. There are several possible unanswered questions with the use of local vancomycin powder that necessitate more refined study. The amount of local vancomycin necessary is unknown, and it is possible that 1 g intra-wound vancomycin does not achieve a therapeutic concentration, or does not do so for a sufficient period of time. Perhaps in such a challenging environment an antibiotic-eluting vehicle would be beneficial such that prolonged local concentrations can be maintained.

Pathogen resistance or targeting of inappropriate pathogens may be another reason for antibiotic failure. No cases of vancomycin resistance were seen in the infected patients of the control group ($n = 14$), illustrating that vancomycin resistance is not a significant issue in our region. Only one of the patients in the treatment group had an infection, and cultures from the surgical site did not grow any pathogens. It is difficult to surmise a connection between vancomycin administration and culture-negative infection given the $n = 1$.

Our results are consistent with the work of Martin et al. [19], who demonstrated no change in deep SSI in spinal deformity cases ($n = 305$), and Mohammed et al. [20] who showed no difference in SSI in the inguinal region after vascular procedures ($n = 424$) with the administration of intraoperative vancomycin. Martin et al. [19] mentions that spinal deformity patients are at higher risk for infection due to very large incisions, greater time of surgery, greater blood loss, greater exposure to instruments and increased amount of instrumentation. With regards to inefficacy of vancomycin in inguinal wounds, the authors postulated that the wound bed was not vascular enough for systemic absorption of vancomycin, which could have helped combat deep infections.

Several limitations of this study should be noted. The small sample size limits the statistical power of our study and the results must be interpreted with caution. The lack of patient randomization could have led to surgeon bias and treatment of the worst-appearing wounds with vancomycin, falsely giving the impression of vancomycin inefficacy. The incorporation of data from multiple surgeons also introduces bias. Operative time, a factor known to contribute to postoperative infections was not recorded. Additional factors, such as limited mobility, malnutrition, and various medical comorbidities, contribute to infection and were not controlled for in this study as we were unable to reliably obtain complete information due to the study's retrospective nature.

With the high cost of managing the sequelae of SSI and the growing emphasis of the health care system on reduction of readmissions, it is important to investigate methods of reducing such complications. There is a need to find effective, cheap, and widely available methods for prevention of SSI. At a cost of approximately US $7 for 1 g vancomycin powder, it is a low-cost measure that has shown efficacy in lowering SSI rates for some surgeries, and should be investigated further [18]. Our study provides an initial look at vancomycin use in orthopaedic extremity trauma and recommends the need for further study. Basic science and larger prospective clinical studies are needed to further delineate the role of local vancomycin powder as a modality to reduce deep SSI in extremity trauma.

Conflict of interest H.R.M. is a paid consultant for Smith and Nephew and Acumed. The remaining authors have no disclosures.

Ethical standards All procedures were in accordance with the declaration of Helsinki and the ethical standards of our institutional IRB. Informed consent for participants was waived by the IRB for this retrospective study.

References

1. Kirkland KB, Briggs JP, Trivette SL, Wilkinson WE, Sexton DJ (1999) The impact of surgical-site infections in the 1990s: attributable mortality, excess length of hospitalization, and extra costs. Infect Control Hosp Epidemiol Off J Soc Hosp Epidemiol Am 20(11):725–730. doi:10.1086/501572
2. Evans RP, Nelson CL, Harrison BH (1993) The effect of wound environment on the incidence of acute osteomyelitis. Clin Orthop Relat Res 286:289–297

3. Toh CL, Jupiter JB (1995) The infected nonunion of the tibia. Clin Orthop Relat Res 315:176–191

4. Hoch RC, Rodriguez R, Manning T, Bishop M, Mead P, Shoemaker WC, Abraham E (1993) Effects of accidental trauma on cytokine and endotoxin production. Crit Care Med 21(6):839–845

5. Gristina AG (1987) Biomaterial-centered infection: microbial adhesion versus tissue integration. Science 237(4822):1588–1595

6. Bosse MJ, MacKenzie EJ, Kellam JF, Burgess AR, Webb LX, Swiontkowski MF, Sanders RW, Jones AL, McAndrew MP, Patterson BM, McCarthy ML, Travison TG, Castillo RC (2002) An analysis of outcomes of reconstruction or amputation after leg-threatening injuries. New Engl J Med 347(24):1924–1931. doi:10.1056/NEJMoa012604

7. Barei DP, Nork SE, Mills WJ, Henley MB, Benirschke SK (2004) Complications associated with internal fixation of high-energy bicondylar tibial plateau fractures utilizing a two-incision technique. J Orthop Trauma 18(10):649–657

8. Harris AM, Althausen PL, Kellam J, Bosse MJ, Castillo R (2009) Complications following limb-threatening lower extremity trauma. J Orthop Trauma 23(1):1–6. doi:10.1097/BOT.0b013e31818e43dd

9. Patterson MJ, Cole JD (1999) Two-staged delayed open reduction and internal fixation of severe pilon fractures. J Orthop Trauma 13(2):85–91

10. Owens BD, Kragh JF Jr, Wenke JC, Macaitis J, Wade CE, Holcomb JB (2008) Combat wounds in operation Iraqi Freedom and operation Enduring Freedom. J Trauma 64(2):295–299. doi:10.1097/TA.0b013e318163b875

11. Starr AJ (2008) Fracture repair: successful advances, persistent problems, and the psychological burden of trauma. J Bone Joint Surg Am 90(Suppl 1):132–137. doi:10.2106/JBJS.G.01217

12. Tompkins LS (1992) The use of molecular methods in infectious diseases. New Engl J Med 327(18):1290–1297. doi:10.1056/NEJM199210293271808

13. Webb LX, Holman J, de Araujo B, Zaccaro DJ, Gordon ES (1994) Antibiotic resistance in staphylococci adherent to cortical bone. J Orthop Trauma 8(1):28–33

14. Gillespie WJ, Walenkamp GH (2010) Antibiotic prophylaxis for surgery for proximal femoral and other closed long bone fractures. Cochrane Database Syst Rev 3:CD000244. doi:10.1002/14651858.CD000244.pub2

15. Page CP, Bohnen JM, Fletcher JR, McManus AT, Solomkin JS, Wittmann DH (1993) Antimicrobial prophylaxis for surgical wounds. Guidelines for clinical care. Arch Surg 128(1):79–88

16. Burdon DW (1982) Principles of antimicrobial prophylaxis. World J Surg 6(3):262–267

17. Chiang HY, Herwaldt LA, Blevins AE, Cho E, Schweizer ML (2013) Effectiveness of local vancomycin powder to decrease surgical site infections: a meta-analysis. Spine J 14:397–407 doi:10.1016/j.spinee.2013.10.012

18. DrugBank (2014) Vancomycin. Drugbank. http://www.drugbank.ca/drugs/DB00512. Accessed 23 July 2014

19. Martin JR, Adogwa O, Brown CR et al (2014) Spine (Phila Pa 1976) 39:177–184

20. Mohammed S, Pisimisis GT, Daram SP et al (2013)Impact of intraoperative administration of local vancomycin on inguinal wound complications.J Vasc Surg 57:1079–1083

40

Short uncemented stems allow greater femoral flexibility and may reduce peri-prosthetic fracture risk: a dry bone and cadaveric study

Christopher Jones · Adeel Aqil · Susannah Clarke ·
Justin P. Cobb

Abstract

Background Short femoral stems for uncemented total hip arthroplasty have been introduced as a safe alternative to traditional longer stem designs. However, there has been little biomechanical examination of the effects of stem length on complications of surgery. This study aims to examine the effect of femoral stem length on torsional resistance to peri-prosthetic fracture.

Materials and methods We tested 16 synthetic and two paired cadaveric femora. Specimens were implanted and then rapidly rotated until fracture to simulate internal rotation on a planted foot, as might occur during stumbling. 3D planning software and custom-printed 3D cutting guides were used to enhance the accuracy and consistency of our stem insertion technique.

Results Synthetic femora implanted with short stems fractured at a significantly higher torque (27.1 vs. 24.2 Nm, $p = 0.03$) and angle (30.3° vs. 22.3°, $p = 0.002$) than those implanted with long stems. Fracture patterns of the two groups were different, but showed remarkable consistency within each group. These characteristic fracture patterns were closely replicated in the pair of cadaveric femora.

Conclusions This new short-stemmed press-fit femoral component allows more femoral flexibility and confers a higher resistance to peri-prosthetic fracture from torsional forces than long stems.

Keywords Short stem · Total hip arthroplasty · Mechanical testing · Fracture

Introduction

Short femoral stems for uncemented total hip arthroplasty (THA) have been introduced widely, with the suggestion that they may facilitate easier revision [1], distribute stress anatomically [2] and cause fewer intra-operative complications than longer stem designs [3]. With some series reporting 10–16-year survival rates of 99–100 % [4, 5], short stems may be considered a safe alternative to traditional longer stem designs. However, there has been little biomechanical examination of the effects of stem length on complications of surgery.

Peri-prosthetic fracture following primary THA is estimated to occur in approximately 1 % of cases, rising to 4 % within 5 years for revision cases where longer stems are used [6, 7]. Fracture is associated with increased morbidity and dysfunction [8, 9]. Previous studies in cemented stems have found that short stems do not confer a higher risk of peri-prosthetic fracture [10]. The majority of stems inserted worldwide are uncemented and little has been published about the effect of stem length on peri-prosthetic fracture pattern in these press-fit stems. The fracture pattern is also relevant, as it determines treatment and may affect subsequent morbidity [11, 12].

The aim of this study was to examine the impact of femoral stem length on (1) the resistance to fracture of implanted stems subjected to torsional forces, and (2) the peri-prosthetic fracture patterns in a synthetic bone model. Finally, we wished to assess the clinical relevance of this model by comparing tested synthetic femurs to results obtained by testing a single pair of cadaveric bones.

C. Jones · A. Aqil (✉) · S. Clarke · J. P. Cobb
MSK Lab, 7th Floor, Lab Block, Department of Surgery and Cancer, Imperial College London, Charing Cross Hospital, Fulham Palace Road, London W6 8RF, UK
e-mail: a.aqil@imperial.ac.uk

Materials and methods

In order to compare the two femoral prostheses, we implanted them into synthetic (and later paired cadaveric) femurs. These femurs were then subjected to torsional mechanical testing.

This study compared a successful uncemented long-stem design with a shorter one. From shoulder to tip, the longer stems measured 152 mm, while the shorter ones were 100 mm. Besides the apparent difference in length, the shorter stem had a wider proximal section, and was reduced laterally to make insertion easier and minimise the risk of fracture of the greater trochanter. Both stems were fully hydroxyapatite-coated with 12/14 neck tapers and collars to prevent implantation past the required depth (Fig. 1). These stems also required different femoral preparations. The short-stem rasps were designed to be more bone-sparing by impacting loose bone, while the longer stem rasp was designed for more bone extraction.

Left-sided "medium"-sized synthetic composite femoral bones (Sawbone Model Number 1121; Sawbones Europe AB, Sweden) were used for their consistency of geometry and to aid a repeatable and controllable methodology (Fig. 2). These bones were dual density, with a foam polyurethane cortical shell. Bones from the same batch were used to avoid any inter-batch variation in mechanical properties. One synthetic bone was scanned by computed tomography (CT) to generate a digital three-dimensional (3D) model, which was later used for planning and validation of correct implant positioning.

A 3D surgical plan was made by one of the authors (S.C.) using the CT scan data from the synthetic bone, and

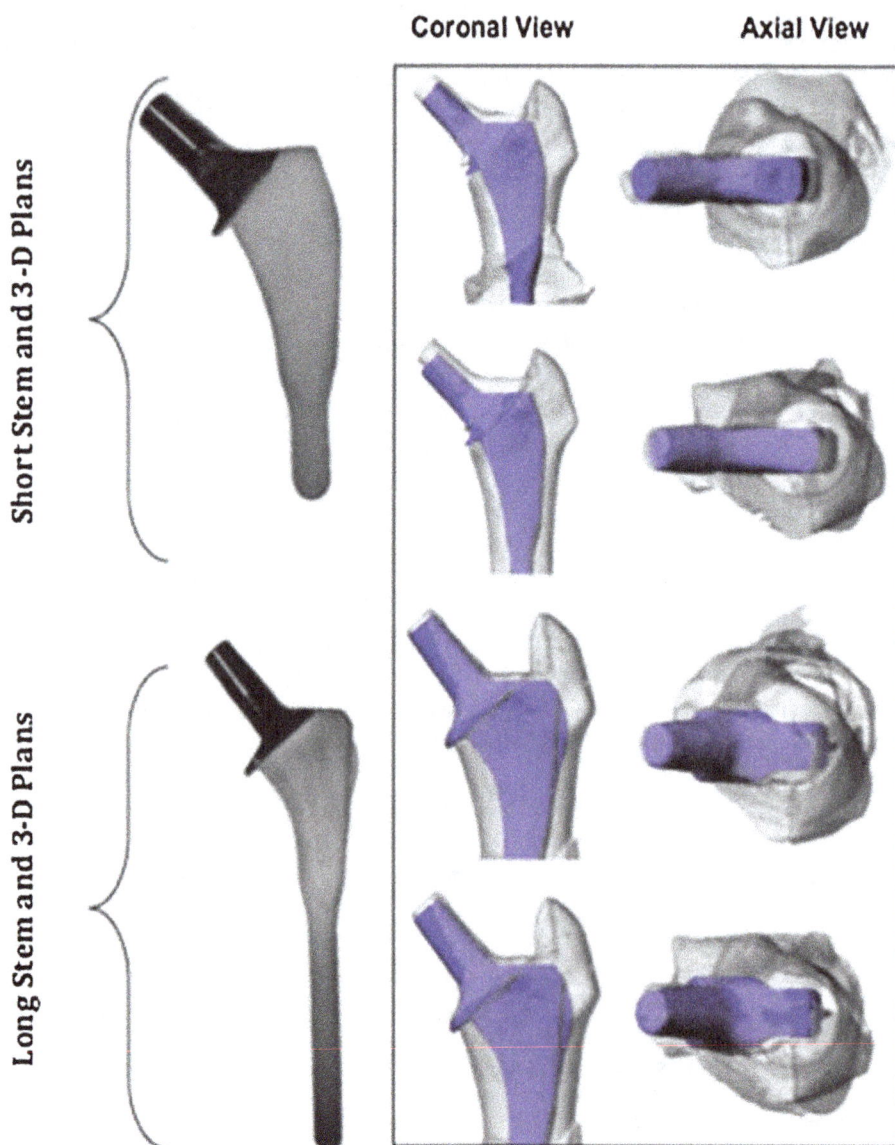

Fig. 1 Photograph of the short- and long-stemmed prostheses with three-dimensional rendered images of implanted femurs (shown in *grey*) and the planned positioning of the implant (shown in *blue*) (colour figure online)

Fig. 2 Photograph of a synthetic femur in antero-posterior and lateral plane, following osteotomy of femoral neck using the three-dimensional cutting guide (Embody, UK)

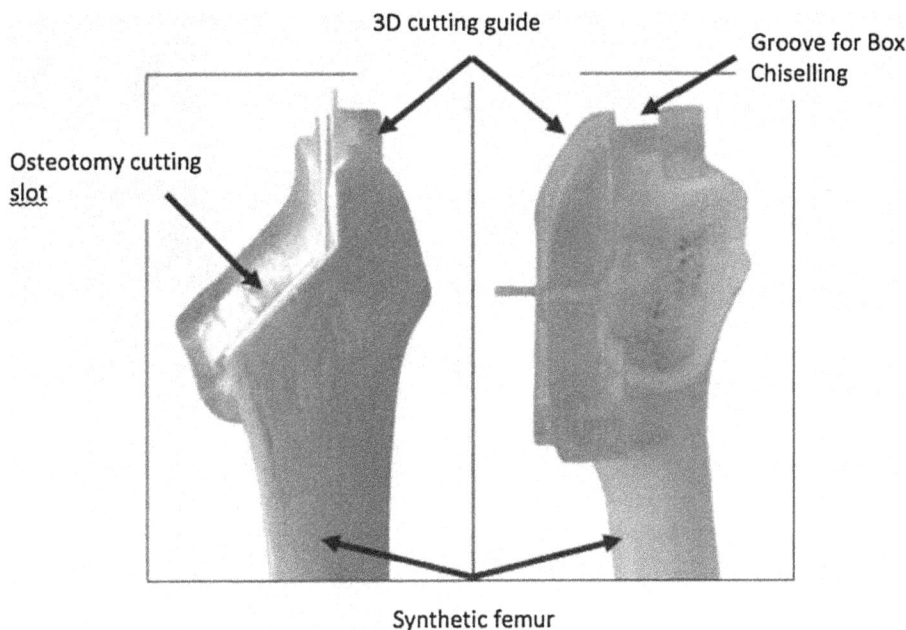

3D data files of the implants. Ideal positioning for each implant was determined based on alignment of the implant neck and head within the original bone (Fig. 1). From this data, the optimal position for the neck osteotomy and box chiselling entry point could be determined and planned.

Two 3D cutting guides (Embody, UK)—one for each femoral stem—were produced to ensure accuracy and repeatability of our osteotomy cuts and our box chiselling. These guides are designed to precisely match the surface anatomy of the bone (Fig. 2).

Use of these guides ensured that cutting and box chiselling of bone was restricted to areas pre-defined by the 3D planning. Subsequent reaming and rasping thus began in the correct location and planes.

We began by pinning the cutting guide to the specimen. The specimen-matched guide then directed the neck osteotomy and box chiselling of the femoral shaft (Fig. 2). Each bone was sequentially reamed and rasped according to the manufacturer's instructions.

An experienced surgeon (J.P.C.) used standard intra-operative techniques to determine the appropriate implant size. A size 11 was used for the long, and a size 12 for the short stem. The prostheses were then inserted until seated.

The distal 18 cm of each femur were sawn off, and the implanted proximal femurs were potted in poly-methylmethacrylate (PMMA) bone cement (within a metal cylinder). The cement was fixed to the cylinder with three screws to prevent rotation and left for 30 min to cure.

The metal cylinder was mounted to the base of a ser-vohydraulic testing machine (Instron 8874 Biaxial Testing System; Instron Corporation, MA, USA) using a bespoke adjustable vice. The potted bone was aligned such that the plane of the femoral stem was vertical, and directly un-derneath the centre of the servohydraulic crosshead. A 6-mm hex key was attached to the crosshead and lowered into the 6-mm hex hole in the implant (this hole is aligned with the centre of the distal femoral stem). This allowed the stem to be rotated about its central axis (Fig. 3).

Throughout the testing a small constant vertical load of 10 N was applied, to counteract any vertical loosening, and to ensure engagement of the hex key in the implant hex hole. Before each test, the Instron crosshead was manually positioned in a neutral position, fully engaged with the implant but with no vertical or rotational force.

To test resistance to femoral fracture, the implant was rotated clockwise through 90° in 1 s. This testing protocol has been described previously [13], and is designed to simulate peri-prosthetic fracture due to internal rotation on a planted foot, as might occur during stumbling.

Torque, rotation, vertical load and vertical position data were sampled 50 times per second throughout the testing protocols, and were exported to a data spreadsheet file (Microsoft Excel; Microsoft Corporation, WA, USA).

Following ethical approval, a single pair of cadaveric femurs were extracted from an embalmed cadaver donated to the Human Anatomy Unit (Charing Cross Hospital, London, UK). The cadaver had been embalmed with a mixture of formaldehyde, phenol, polyethylene glycol and alcohol, which has been shown not to significantly affect the stiffness of bone [14].

An experienced surgeon used a posterior approach and standard intra-operative techniques to implant and size the short and long femoral stems. The femurs were then care-fully dissected from the cadavers and stripped of soft tissues.

Fig. 3 Image showing
standardised set-up of
equipment

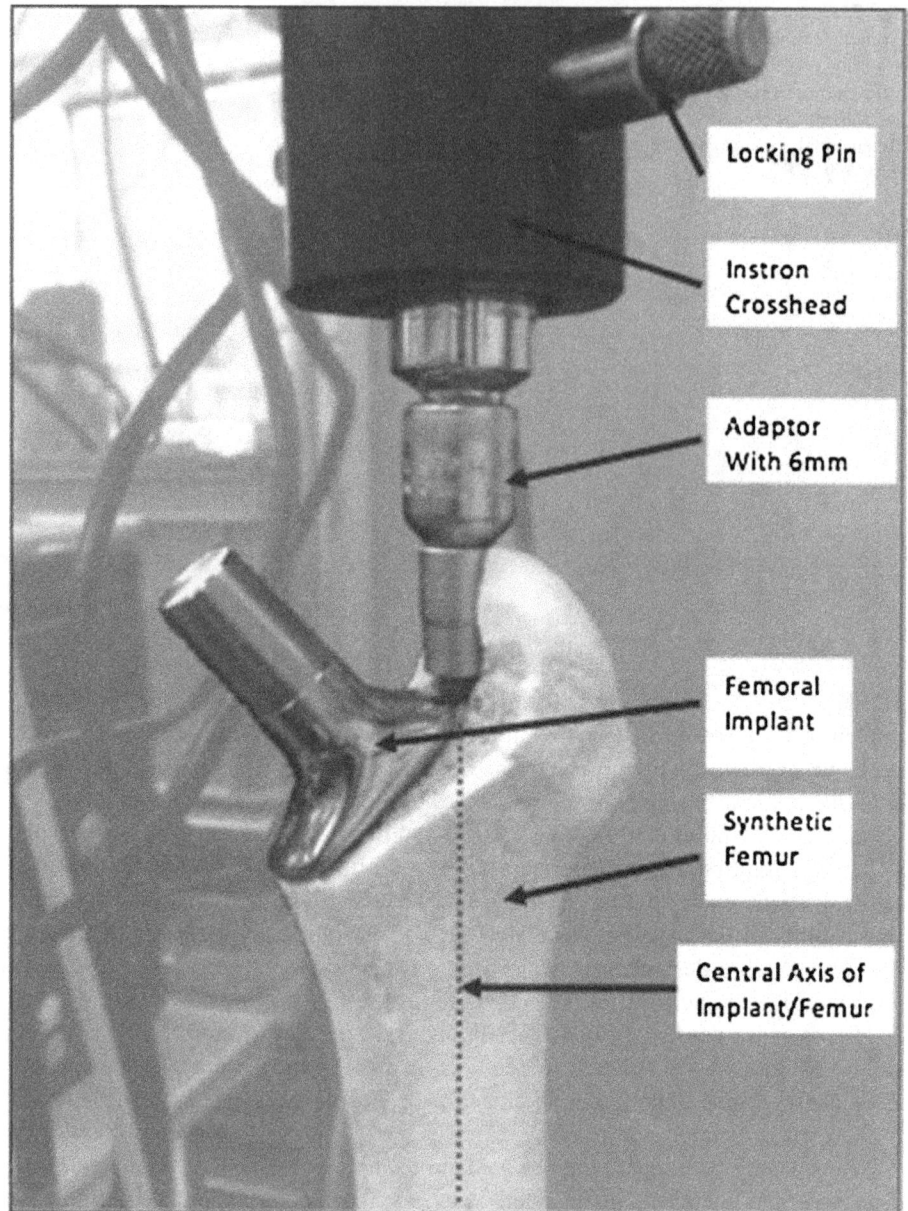

The implanted femurs underwent the same experimental setup as the synthetic bones. Testing was in a clockwise direction on the left, and anticlockwise on the right femur to ensure both hips were torqued in internal rotation. The data was analysed using SPSS (IBM SPSS Statistics, version 20) using a Mann–Whitney U test as data was not found to be parametric.

Results

The torsional force required to fracture the short-stem implanted femurs [mean 27.1 Nm, range 24.4–30.3, standard deviation (SD) 2.1] was significantly greater than that of the long stems (mean 24.2 Nm, range 21.1–30.1, SD 2.8) (Fig. 1; $p = 0.03$). The ranges of fracture torque for the short (24.4–30.3 Nm) and long (21.1–25.7 Nm) stems show only partial overlap, with the exception of a single outlier (30.1 Nm) in the long-stemmed group (excluding this value, the range was 21.05–25.70 Nm). The torsional force required to fracture the short-stem implanted cadaveric femur (27.8 Nm) was higher than that for the long stem (14.7 Nm).

The angular deformation at fracture for the short stems (mean 30°, range 24°–36°, SD 5.2) was significantly greater than that of the long stems (mean 22°, range 19°–25°, SD 3.2, $p = 0.002$), (Fig. 1). The ranges of fracture angle for the short (24.3°–35.9°) and long (18.6°–27.7°) stems show only partial overlap. Fracture torque and angle

Fig. 4 Box plots of the fracture angles and torque of long and short implanted stems

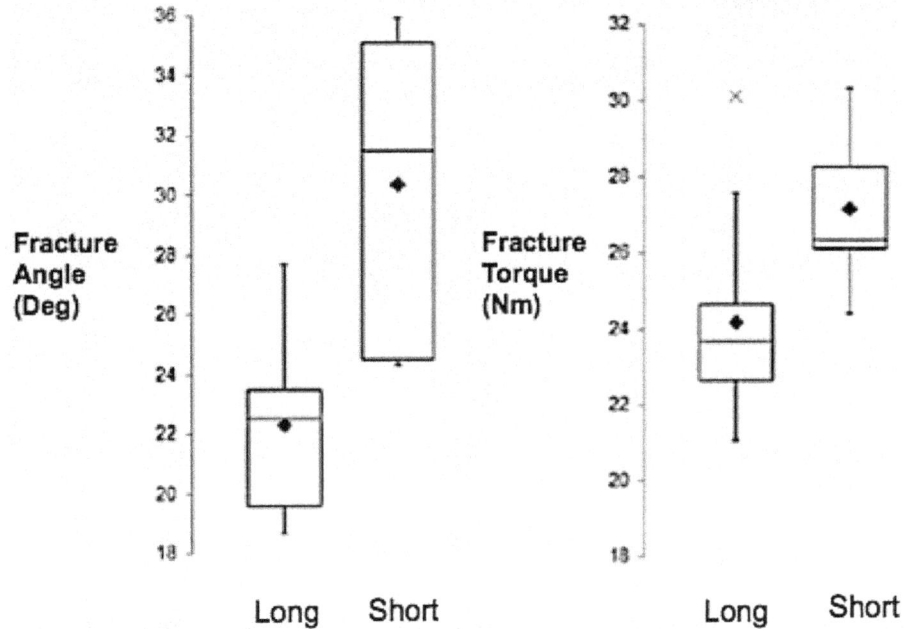

Mean fracture angles for each group are shown as filled diamonds (◆)

data are presented in Fig. 4. The cadaveric bone fracture angle was 14.5° for the short stem, but was not clearly determinable for the longer stem.

The fracture patterns for the two implants were consistent but different. Both stems displayed a spiral fracture pattern with the apex of fracture 3 cm below the lesser trochanter. However, the long-stem group had a butterfly segment of the anterior part of the greater trochanter but the short-stem group's involved the entire greater trochanter (Fig. 5). The single outlier from the long-stem group (which fractured at 30.1 Nm) had a similar fracture pattern to the short stems.

Discussion

In this study, we sought to compare the pattern and force required to induce a peri-prosthetic fracture of femurs implanted with uncemented short- and long-stem hip replacements. We found that bones implanted with the short-stemmed implants required a significantly higher force before fracture. Implanted femurs were also found to be more flexible and deformed more prior to fracture in the short-stem group. Although limited, testing in paired cadaveric femurs demonstrated a similar fracture torque and pattern to the results seen with synthetic bones. Our findings are consistent with a similar study [13] where the torsional fracture strength of *cemented* femoral components (in a synthetic bone model) demonstrated fracture torques of 25–40 Nm and fracture angles of 20°–35°.

Jakubowitz et al. [10] compared the grit-blasted short uncemented Mayo® hip (Zimmer, Warsaw, IN, USA) to an equivalent uncemented long-stem design. Whilst these implants differed from those in our study in many ways, the authors similarly found that the short-stem implants compared favourably to the long-stemmed equivalent with respect to the risk of a peri-prosthetic fracture.

As the short stem in our study is a relatively new addition to the implant market, we are not able to evaluate the fracture patterns we observed against clinical reports of peri-prosthetic fracture. However, given the clear and consistent difference between the fracture patterns of the two groups in synthetic and paired cadaveric femurs (Fig. 5), we can be confident that this difference is significant. Furthermore, Van Eynde et al. [15] have reported a typical fracture pattern in an uncemented long-stem series that was very similar to the fracture pattern we described for our long-stemmed implants.

The peri-prosthetic fracture pattern can have implications for recovery and treatment; however, as both fractures created an unstable femoral stem, revision of the stem would be necessary if they occurred in the early post-operative period [16].

Previous work by Cristofolini et al. [17] has demonstrated that the mechanical strength variability of cadaveric femurs may be up to 200 times that of composite synthetic femurs. These results help rationalise our choice in using mainly synthetic bones, which benefit from consistent geometries and mechanical properties. Their use also enabled accurate and reproducible implant positioning. In

Fig. 5 Photograph showing fracture patterns of the long- and short-stem groups

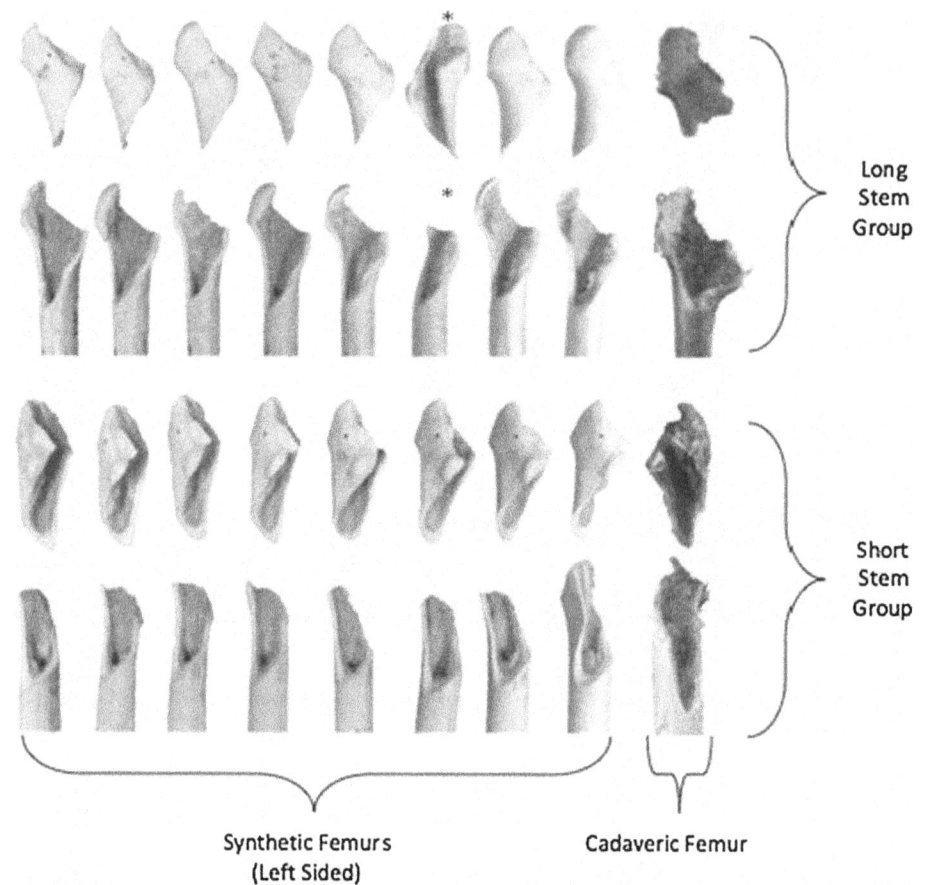

Long Stem Group

Short Stem Group

Synthetic Femurs
(Left Sided)

Cadaveric Femur

addition, previous studies have shown they do behave similarly to human femurs in mechanical testing protocols [13, 18–20]. Synthetic femurs may thus be a reasonable surrogate for human bone and our cadaveric testing results further support this conclusion.

A limitation of this in vitro study is that we are only able to simulate initial implant behaviour. The on-growth of bone onto the implanted femoral stems, promoted by the hydroxyapatite (HA) coating, only occurs in living bone. HA in living subjects would therefore increase the strength of implant fixation [21]. The present study is therefore most relevant in the context of implant behaviour in the early post-operative period, before full bony on-growth occurs.

We are also limited in our interpretation of the data by the fact that we only tested one size of each implant in a "medium"-sized synthetic femur. We cannot therefore comment on how implant sizing might affect biomechanical behaviour. Further work could investigate the effects of implant sizing on peri-prosthetic fracture risk.

In conclusion, we found that the peri-prosthetic fracture pattern of the two stems were different. In spite of this, both patterns would require stem revision and hence present a similar revision dilemma. However, the new short-stemmed press-fit femoral component allows more femoral flexibility and confers a higher resistance to peri-prosthetic

fracture from torsional forces than the long stem. This higher resistance to fracture is an important consideration when selecting implants for elderly female patients who are both more likely to fall and to have osteoporotic bone.

Acknowledgments   We wish to thank the Human Anatomy Unit at Charing Cross Hospital (Imperial College London, London, UK), for their assistance in this study and Joint Replacement Instruments (JRI Ltd.), for providing the femoral components. We would also like to thank Embody for designing and manufacturing the specimen-matched guides.

Conflict of interest   The authors declare that they have no conflict of interest related to the publication of this manuscript. No benefits in any form have been received or will be received from a commercial party related directly or indirectly to the subject of this article. Tested implants were from Joint Replacement Instruments (JRI Ltd.).

Ethical standards   "This article does not contain any studies with human participants or animals performed by any of the authors". Ethical approval was sought and gained prior to commencement of the trial. All investigations were conducted in conformity with ethical principles of research. This work was performed at Imperial College London, Charing Cross Campus, London, UK.

References

1. Lombardi AV Jr, Berend KR, Ng VY (2011) Stubby stems: good things come in small packages. Orthopedics 34:e464–e466

2. McElroy MJ, Johnson AJ, Mont MA, Bonutti PM (2011) Short and standard stem prostheses are both viable options for minimally invasive total hip arthroplasty. Bull NYU Hosp Jt Dis 69(Suppl 1):S68–S76

3. Molli RG, Lombardi AV Jr, Berend KR, Adams JB, Sneller MA (2012) A short tapered stem reduces intraoperative complications in primary total hip arthroplasty. Clin Orthop Relat Res 470:450–461

4. McLaughlin JR, Lee KR (2010) Cementless total hip replacement using second-generation components: a 12- to 16-year follow-up. J Bone Joint Surg Br 92:1636–1641

5. Sariali E, Mouttet A, Mordasini P, Catonne Y (2012) High 10-year survival rate with an anatomic cementless stem (SPS). Clin Orthop Relat Res 470:1941–1949

6. Berry DJ (1999) Epidemiology: hip and knee. Orthop Clin North Am 30:183–190

7. Meek RM, Norwood T, Smith R, Brenkel IJ, Howie CR (2011) The risk of peri-prosthetic fracture after primary and revision total hip and knee replacement. J Bone Joint Surg Br 93:96–101

8. Lindahl H, Oden A, Garellick G, Malchau H (2007) The excess mortality due to periprosthetic femur fracture. A study from the Swedish national hip arthroplasty register. Bone 40:1294–1298

9. Schmidt AH, Kyle RF (2002) Periprosthetic fractures of the femur. Orthop Clin North Am 33:143–152 ix

10. Jakubowitz E, Seeger JB, Lee C, Heisel C, Kretzer JP, Thomsen MN (2009) Do short-stemmed-prostheses induce periprosthetic fractures earlier than standard hip stems? A biomechanical ex vivo study of two different stem designs. Arch Orthop Trauma Surg 129:849–855

11. Learmonth ID (2004) The management of periprosthetic fractures around the femoral stem. J Bone Joint Surg Br 86:13–19

12. Corten K, Vanrykel F, Bellemans J, Frederix PR, Simon JP, Broos PL (2009) An algorithm for the surgical treatment of periprosthetic fractures of the femur around a well-fixed femoral component. J Bone Joint Surg Br 91:1424–1430

13. Harris B, Owen JR, Wayne JS, Jiranek WA (2010) Does femoral component loosening predispose to femoral fracture?: an in vitro comparison of cemented hips. Clin Orthop Relat Res 468:497–503

14. van Haaren EH, van der Zwaard BC, van der Veen AJ, Heyligers IC, Wuisman PI, Smit TH (2008) Effect of long-term preservation on the mechanical properties of cortical bone in goats. Acta Orthop 79:708–716

15. Van Eynde E, Hendrickx M, Scheerlinck T (2010) Uncemented femoral stem design influences the occurrence rate of postoperative fractures after primary hip arthroplasty: a comparison of the image and profile stems. Acta Orthop Belg 76:189–198

16. Sledge JB 3rd, Abiri A (2002) An algorithm for the treatment of vancouver type B2 periprosthetic proximal femoral fractures. J Arthroplasty 17:887–892

17. Cristofolini L, Viceconti M, Cappello A, Toni A (1996) Mechanical validation of whole bone composite femur models. J Biomech 29:525–535

18. Zdero R, Olsen M, Bougherara H, Schemitsch EH (2008) Cancellous bone screw purchase: a comparison of synthetic femurs, human femurs, and finite element analysis. Proc Inst Mech Eng H 222:1175–1183

19. Gardner MP, Chong AC, Pollock AG, Wooley PH (2010) Mechanical evaluation of large-size fourth-generation composite femur and tibia models. Ann Biomed Eng 38:613–620

20. Heiner AD, Brown TD (2001) Structural properties of a new design of composite replicate femurs and tibias. J Biomech 34:773–781

21. Cook SD, Thomas KA, Dalton JE, Kay JF (1991) Enhanced bone ingrowth and fixation strength with hydroxyapatite-coated porous implants. Semin Arthroplasty 2:268–279

Permissions

All chapters in this book were first published in JOT, by Springer; hereby published with permission under the Creative Commons Attribution License or equivalent. Every chapter published in this book has been scrutinized by our experts. Their significance has been extensively debated. The topics covered herein carry significant findings which will fuel the growth of the discipline. They may even be implemented as practical applications or may be referred to as a beginning point for another development.

The contributors of this book come from diverse backgrounds, making this book a truly international effort. This book will bring forth new frontiers with its revolutionizing research information and detailed analysis of the nascent developments around the world.

We would like to thank all the contributing authors for lending their expertise to make the book truly unique. They have played a crucial role in the development of this book. Without their invaluable contributions this book wouldn't have been possible. They have made vital efforts to compile up to date information on the varied aspects of this subject to make this book a valuable addition to the collection of many professionals and students.

This book was conceptualized with the vision of imparting up-to-date information and advanced data in this field. To ensure the same, a matchless editorial board was set up. Every individual on the board went through rigorous rounds of assessment to prove their worth. After which they invested a large part of their time researching and compiling the most relevant data for our readers.

The editorial board has been involved in producing this book since its inception. They have spent rigorous hours researching and exploring the diverse topics which have resulted in the successful publishing of this book. They have passed on their knowledge of decades through this book. To expedite this challenging task, the publisher supported the team at every step. A small team of assistant editors was also appointed to further simplify the editing procedure and attain best results for the readers.

Apart from the editorial board, the designing team has also invested a significant amount of their time in understanding the subject and creating the most relevant covers. They scrutinized every image to scout for the most suitable representation of the subject and create an appropriate cover for the book.

The publishing team has been an ardent support to the editorial, designing and production team. Their endless efforts to recruit the best for this project, has resulted in the accomplishment of this book. They are a veteran in the field of academics and their pool of knowledge is as vast as their experience in printing. Their expertise and guidance has proved useful at every step. Their uncompromising quality standards have made this book an exceptional effort. Their encouragement from time to time has been an inspiration for everyone.

The publisher and the editorial board hope that this book will prove to be a valuable piece of knowledge for researchers, students, practitioners and scholars across the globe.

List of Contributors

Malhar N. Kumar, M. R. Ravishankar and Ravikiran Manur
HOSMAT Hospital, 45, McGrath Road, Bangalore 560025, India

Frank A. Liporace and Richard S. Yoon
Division of Orthopaedic Trauma, Department of Orthopaedic Surgery, NYU Hospital for Joint Diseases, 301 E 17th Street, Suite 1402, New York, NY 10003, USA

Eric A. Breitbart, Erin Doyle, David N. Paglia and Sheldon Lin
Division of Orthopaedic Trauma, Department of Orthopaedic Trauma, UMDNJ, New Jersey Medical School, Newark, NJ 07101, USA

M. Cappuccio, F. De Iure, L. Amendola and A. Martucci
Department of Orthopedics and Traumatology - Spine Surgery, Maggiore Hospital, Largo Nigrisoli, 2, 40100 Bologna, Italy

Babak Shadgan
Trauma Orthopaedic Division, Department of Orthopaedics, University of British Columbia, #110-828W 10th Ave, Vancouver, BC V5Z 1L8, Canada
5440-ICORD, Blusson Spinal Cord Centre, 818 West 10th Avenue, Vancouver, BC V5Z-1M9, Canada

Gavin Pereira
University Hospital Coventry and Warwickshire, Clifford Bridge Road, Coventry CV2 2DX, UK

Matthew Menon
Division of Orthopaedic Surgery, University of Alberta, 10150-121 Street, Edmonton, AB T5N 1K4, Canada

Siavash Jafari
School of Population and Public Health, Faculty of Medicine, University of British Columbia, 2206 East Mall, Vancouver, BC V6T 1Z3, Canada

W. Darlene Reid
Department of Physical Therapy, University of Toronto, 160-500 University Avenue, Toronto, ON M5G 1V7, Canada

Peter J. O'Brien
Trauma Orthopaedic Division, Department of Orthopaedics, University of British Columbia, #110-828W 10th Ave, Vancouver, BC V5Z 1L8, Canada

John T. Capo
Division of Hand Surgery, Department of Orthopaedic Surgery, NYU Hospital for Joint Diseases, New York, NY 10009, USA

Ben Shamian, Ramces Francisco, Virak Tan, Jared S. Preston and Linda Uko
Division of Hand and Microvascular Surgery, Department of Orthopaedic Surgery, Rutgers New Jersey Medical School, Newark, NJ, USA

Richard S. Yoon and Frank A. Liporace
Division of Orthopaedic Trauma, Department of Orthopaedic Surgery, NYU Hospital for Joint Diseases, 301 E 17th Street Suite 1402, New York, NY 10003, USA

Riazuddin Mohammed
Wrightington Hospital, Appley Bridge, Wigan WN6 9EP, UK

Keith Hayward, Sanjay Mulay, Frank Bindi and Murray Wallace
Queens Hospital, Burton Hospitals NHS Foundation Trust, Burton on Trent DE13 0RB, UK

Amin Bigham-Sadegh
Department of Veterinary Surgery and Radiology, Faculty of Veterinary Medicine, School of Veterinary Medicine, Shahrekord University, Shahrekord, Iran

Iraj Karimi
Veterinary Pathology, School of Veterinary Medicine, Shahrekord University, Shahrekord, Iran

Mohamad Shadkhast
Veterinary Histology, School of Veterinary Medicine, Shahrekord University, Shahrekord, Iran

Mohamad-Hosein Mahdavi
School of Veterinary Medicine, Shahrekord University, Shahrekord, Iran

Thomais Goula, Alexandros Kouskoukis, Georgios Drosos, Alexandros-Savvas Tselepis, Athanasios Ververidis, Christos Valkanis, Athanasios Zisimopoulos and Konstantinos Kazakos
Department of Orthopaedics, Democritus University of Thrace, University General Hospital of lexandroupolis, Dragana, Alexandroupolis 68100, Greece

Zhe Yu, Haoran Gao and Xinwen Zhao
Department of Orthopedic Surgery, Tangdu Hospital, Fourth Military Medical University, Xi'an 710038, Shaanxi, People's Republic of China

Jie Geng
Medical Department of Tangdu Hospital, Fourth Military Medical University, Xi'an 710038, Shaanxi, People's Republic of China

Jingyuan Chen
Faculty of Military Preventive Medicine, Fourth Military Medical University, 169 Changle West Road, Xi'an 710032, Shaanxi, People's Republic of China

M. van Heumen, B. A. Swierstra, G. G. Van Hellemondt and J. H. M. Goosen
Department of Orthopaedic Surgery, Sint Maartenskliniek, PO Box 9011, 6500 GM Nijmegen, The Netherlands

P. J. C. Heesterbeek
Department of Research, Sint Maartenskliniek, Nijmegen, The Netherlands

Giovanni Merolla
Unit of Shoulder and Elbow Surgery, D. Cervesi Hospital, Cattolica, AUSL della Romagna Ambito Territoriale di Rimini, Rimini, Italy

Mahendar G. Bhat, Paolo Paladini and Giuseppe Porcellini
Unit of Shoulder and Elbow Surgery, D. Cervesi Hospital, Cattolica, AUSL della Romagna Ambito Territoriale di Rimini, Rimini, Italy
Biomechanics Laboratory "Marco Simoncelli", D. Cervesi Hospital, Cattolica, AUSL della Romagna Ambito Territoriale di Rimini, Rimini, Italy

Bruno Battiston
III Orthopaedic Division, Department of Orthopaedics and Traumatology, Orthopaedic and Trauma Center, Turin, Italy

Stefano Artiaco
IV Orthopaedic Division, Department of Orthopaedics and Traumatology, Orthopaedic and Trauma Center, Via Zuretti 29, 10126 Turin, Italy

Raimondo Piana and Elena Boux
Oncologic Orthopaedic Division, Department of Orthopaedics and Traumatology, Orthopaedic and Trauma Center, Turin, Italy

Pierluigi Tos
Microsurgery Unit, Department of Orthopaedics and Traumatology, Orthopaedic and Trauma Center, Turin, Italy

Haroon Majeed
University Hospital of North Staffordshire, Stoke-on-Trent ST4 6QG, UK

SaravanaVail Karuppiah and Kohila Vani Sigamoney
Trauma and Orthopaedics, Royal Derby Hospital, Derby, UK

Guido Geutjens and Robert G. Straw
Royal Derby Hospital, Derby, UK

K. B. Ferguson, O. Bailey, I. Anthony, I. G. Stother and M. J. G. Blyth
Department of Orthopaedics and Trauma, Glasgow Royal Infirmary, 84 Castle Street, Glasgow G4 0SF, Scotland, UK

P. J. James
Department of Orthopaedics and Trauma, Nottingham City Hospital, Nottingham, UK

Daniel J. Johnson, Sarah E. Greenberg, Vasanth Sathiyakumar, Rachel Thakore, Jesse M. Ehrenfeld, William T. Obremskey and Manish K. Sethi
The Vanderbilt Orthopaedic Institute Center for Health Policy, Vanderbilt University, Suite 4200, South Tower, MCE, Nashville, TN 37221, USA

Volker Brinkmann, Florian Radetzki, Karl Stefan Delank, David Wohlrab and Alexander Zeh
Department of Orthopaedics and Traumatology, Faculty of Medicine, Martin-Luther-University of Halle-Wittenberg, Ernst-Grube-Strasse 40, 06120 Halle/Saale, Germany

Ahmed Shawkat Rizk
Orthopaedics and Traumatology Department, Faculty of Medicine, Benha University, Benha, Egypt
Shebeen el-kanater, Qualiobia, Egypt

A. Clemente and F. Bergamin
Department of Hand, Plastic and Reconstructive Surgery, Maria Vittoria Hospital, Turin, Italy

C. Surace
Laboratory of Bio-inspired Nanomechanics "Giuseppe Maria Pugno", Department of Structural, Building and Geotechnical Engineering, Politecnico di Torino, Turin, Italy

E. Lepore
Laboratory of Bio-inspired and Graphene Nanomechanics, Department of Civil, Environmental and Mechanical Engineering, University of Trento, Via Mesiano 77, 38123 Trento, Italy

N. Pugno
Laboratory of Bio-inspired and Graphene Nanomechanics, Department of Civil, Environmental and Mechanical Engineering, University of Trento, Via Mesiano 77, 38123 Trento, Italy
Centre of Materials and Microsystems, Bruno Kessler Foundation, Via Santa Croce 77, 38122 Trento, Italy
School of Engineering and Materials Science, Queen Mary University, Mile End Rd, London E1 4NS, UK

Ramesh Chand Meena, Umesh Kumar, Meena Sahil Gaba and Gopal Lal Gupta
Department of Orthopaedics, SMS Medical College and Hospital, Jaipur 302004, India

Nitesh Gahlot
Department of Orthopaedics, Postgraduate Institute of Medical Education and Research, Chandigarh, India

Sattar Alshryda and T. Lou
Departments of Trauma and Orthopaedics, Central Manchester University Hospitals, Oxford Road, Manchester M13 9WL, Lancashire, UK

James M. Mason
School of Medicine and Health, Wolfson Research Centre, Queen Campus, Durham University, Stockton on Tees TS17 6BH, UK

Praveen Sarda
Departments of Trauma and Orthopaedics, Medway Maritime Hospital, Windmill Road, Gillingham, Kent ME7 5NY, UK

Martin Stanley, Junjie Wu and Anthony Unsworth
Centre for Biomedical Engineering School of Engineering and Computing Sciences, Durham University, Durham DH1 3LE, UK

Takashi Kanamoto and Shinji Hirabayashi
Department of Rehabilitation, Osaka Rosai Hospital, 1179-3 Nagasone-cho, Kita-ku, Sakai, Osaka 597-8025, Japan

Yoshinari Tanaka, Yasukazu Yonetani, Keisuke Kita, Hiroshi Amano, Masashi Kusano and Shuji Horibe
Department of Orthopaedic Surgery, Osaka Rosai Hospital, 1179-3 Nagasone-cho, Kita-ku, Sakai, Osaka 597-8025, Japan

Mie Fukamatsu
Department of Clinical Laboratory, Osaka Rosai Hospital, 1179-3 Nagasone-cho, Kita-ku, Sakai, Osaka 597-8025, Japan

Pier Paolo Mariani
Università Roma 4-Foro Italico, Piazza L. de Bosis 5, 00136 Rome, Italy

Germano Iannella, Guglielmo Cerullo and Marco Giacobbe
Clinic "Villa Stuart", via Trionfale 5952, 00136 Rome, Italy

Ill Ho Park, Su Chan Lee, Il Seok Park, Chang Hyun Nam, Hye Sun Ahn, Ha Young Park, Viral kumar Harilal Gondalia and Kwang Am Jung
Joint and Arthritis Research, Department of Orthopaedic Surgery, Himchan Hospital, 20-8, Songpa-dong, Songpa-gu, Seoul, Korea

Giovanni Merolla
Unit of Shoulder and Elbow Surgery, "D. Cervesi" Hospital, AUSL della Romagna, Ambito Territoriale di Rimini, L.V Beethowen 5, 47841 Cattolica, RN, Italy

Arpit C. Dave, Paolo Paladini, Fabrizio Campi and Giuseppe Porcellini
Unit of Shoulder and Elbow Surgery, "D. Cervesi" Hospital, AUSL della Romagna, Ambito Territoriale di Rimini, L.V Beethowen 5, 47841 Cattolica, RN, Italy

Biomechanics Laboratory "Marco Simoncelli", D. Cervesi Hospital, Cattolica, AUSL della Romagna, Ambito Territoriale di Rimini, Cattolica, Italy

Luigi Tarallo, Raffaele Mugnai, Francesco Fiacchi, Francesco Zambianchi and Fabio Catani
Department of Orthopaedic Surgery, University of Modena and Reggio Emilia, Modena, Italy

Roberto Adani
Department of Hand Surgery, University Hospital of Verona, Verona, Italy

Luca Pierannunzii, Andrea Fossali, Orazio De Lucia and Arturo Guarino
Gaetano Pini Orthopaedic Institute, P.zza Cardinal Ferrari, 1, 20122 Milan, Italy

Luis Natera
Hospital de la Santa Creu i Sant Pau, Universitat Auto`noma de Barcelona, C/Sant Antoni Maria Claret 167, 08025 Barcelona, Spain

Pablo E. Gelber
Hospital de la Santa Creu i Sant Pau, Universitat Auto`noma de Barcelona, C/Sant Antoni Maria Claret 167, 08025 Barcelona, Spain
Hospital Universitari Quiro´n Dexeus, Universitat Auto`noma de Barcelona, C/Sabino Arana, 5-19, 08028 Barcelona, Spain

Juan Carlos Monllau
Hospital de la Santa Creu i Sant Pau, Universitat Auto`noma de Barcelona, C/Sant Antoni Maria Claret 167, 08025 Barcelona, Spain
Hospital Universitari Quiro´n Dexeus, Universitat Auto`noma de Barcelona, C/Sabino Arana, 5-19, 08028 Barcelona, Spain

Juan I. Erquicia
Hospital Universitari Quiro´n Dexeus, Universitat Auto`noma de Barcelona, C/Sabino Arana, 5-19, 08028 Barcelona, Spain

Michele Vasso and Alfredo Schiavone Panni
Department of Medicine and Science for Health, University of Molise, Via Francesco De Sanctis, Campobasso, Italy

Muhammad Naeem, Muhammad Kazim Rahimnajjad, Nasir Ali Rahimnajjad, Zaki Idrees, Ghazanfar Ali Shah and Ghulam Abbas
B-8, Akbar Apartments, Bleak House Road, Civil Lines, Cantt. Karachi, Karachi 74200, Pakistan

Ozkan Kose and Ferhat Guler
Department of Orthopaedics and Traumatology, Antalya Education and Research Hospital, Kultur mah. 3025 sk. Durukent Sit. F Blok Daire 22, Kepez, Antalya, Turkey

Mert Keskinbora
Faculty of Medicine, Department of Orthoapedics and Traumatology, Medipol University, Istanbul, Turkey

C. E. Uzoigwe, M. Venkatesan, N. Johnson, K. Lee, S. Magaji and L. Cutler
Department of Trauma and Orthopaedics, University Hospitals of Leicester, Infirmary Square, Leicester LE1 5WW, UK

Andrea Piccioli
Oncologic Center, "Palazzo Baleani", Teaching Hospital Policlinico Umberto I, Rome, Italy

Giulio Maccauro and Maria Silvia Spinelli
Department of Geriatrics, Orthopedics and Neurosciences, Agostino Gemelli University Hospital, School of Medicine, Catholic University of the Sacred Heart, Rome, Italy

Roberto Biagini and Barbara Rossi
Unit of Oncological Orthopaedics, Regina Elena National Cancer Institute, Rome, Italy

Ferran Abat
Department of Sports Orthopaedics, ReSport Clinic, Barcelona, Spain
Department of Traumatology and Orthopaedic Surgery, Hospital de la Santa Creu i Sant Pau, Universitat Autónoma de Barcelona, Sant Quintı´, 89, Barcelona 08026, Spain

Juan Sarasquete and Luis Gerardo Natera
Department of Traumatology and Orthopaedic Surgery, Hospital de la Santa Creu i Sant Pau, Universitat Autónoma de Barcelona, Sant Quintı´, 89, Barcelona 08026, Spain

Ángel Calvo and Néstor Zurita
Hospital IMED Elche, Alicante, Spain

Juan Carlos del Real and Eva Paz-Jimenez
Engineering School (ICAI), University of Comillas, Madrid, Spain

Francisco Forriol
Universidad San Pablo CEU, Madrid, Spain

Manuel Pérez-España and Jesús Ferrer
Shoulder and Elbow Pathology Unit Shoulder of Madrid, Madrid, Spain

Alex K. Gilde
Grand Rapids Medical Education Partners, Orthopaedic Surgery Residency, Grand Rapids, MI 49503, USA

Martin F. Hoffmann
BG-University Hospital Bergmannsheil, Bochum, Germany

Debra L. Sietsema and Clifford B. Jones
Michigan State University College of Human Medicine, 15 Michigan St NE, Grand Rapids, MI 49503, USA
Orthopaedic Associates of Michigan, 230 Michigan St NE, Suite 300, Grand Rapids, MI 49503, USA

Marcos Almeida Matos and Lucynara Gomes Lima
Bahian School of Medicine and Public Health, Rua da Ilha, 378, Itapuã, Salvador, Bahia 41620-620, Brazil
Roberto Santos General Hospital, Salvador, Bahia, Brazil

Luiz Antonio Alcântara de Oliveira
Feira de Santana State University, Feira De Santana, Brazil

Omid Reza Momenzadeh and Amir Reza Vosoughi
Bone and Joint Diseases Research Center, Department of Orthopedic Surgery, Chamran Hospital, Shiraz University of Medical Sciences, Shiraz, Iran

Masoome Pourmokhtari
Department of Orthopedic Surgery, Jahrom University of Medical Sciences, Jahrom, Iran

Sepideh Sefidbakht
Medical Imaging Research Center, Department of Radiology, Namazi Hospital, Shiraz University of Medical Sciences, Shiraz, Iran

Filippo Familiari
Division of Shoulder Surgery, Department of Orthopaedic Surgery, The Johns Hopkins University, 10753 Falls Road, Pavilion II, Suite 215, Lutherville, MD 21093, USA
Department of Orthopaedic and Trauma Surgery, Magna Græcia University, Catanzaro, Italy

Alan Gonzalez-Zapata and Edward G. McFarland
Division of Shoulder Surgery, Department of Orthopaedic Surgery, The Johns Hopkins University, 10753 Falls Road, Pavilion II, Suite 215, Lutherville, MD 21093, USA

Bruno Iannó, Olimpio Galasso and Giorgio Gasparini
Department of Orthopaedic and Trauma Surgery, Magna Græcia University, Catanzaro, Italy

Daniel E. Prince
Memorial Sloan Kettering Cancer Center, 1275 York Avenue, Howard 1013, New York, NY 10065, USA

Justin K. Greisberg
New York Presbyterian Hospital, Columbia University, New York, NY, USA

Keerat Singh, Jennifer M. Bauer, Gregory Y. LaChaud, Jesse E. Bible and Hassan R. Mir
Division of Orthopaedic Trauma, Vanderbilt Orthopaedic Institute, Suite 4200 MCE, South Tower, Nashville, TN 37232, USA

Christopher Jones, Adeel Aqil, Susannah Clarke and Justin P. Cobb
MSK Lab, 7th Floor, Lab Block, Department of Surgery and Cancer, Imperial College London, Charing Cross Hospital, Fulham Palace Road, London W6 8RF, UK